Disabled Village Children

A guide for community health workers, rehabilitation workers, and families

By David Werner
with the help of many friends

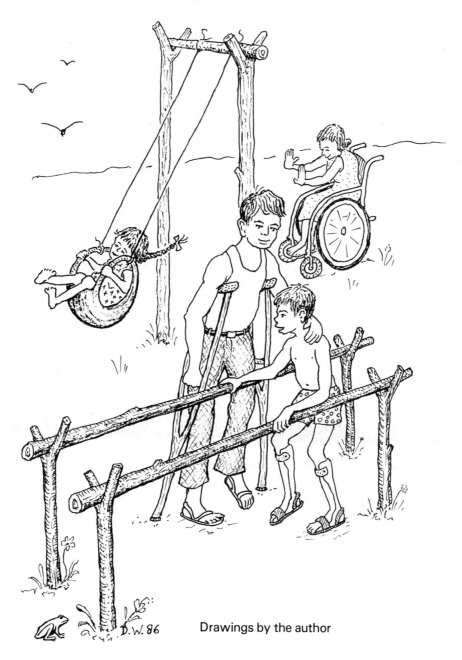

D.W. 86

Drawings by the author

Library of Congress Cataloging-in-publicaton data

Includes Index

1. Medicine, Popular—Handbooks, manuals, etc.
2. Rehabilitation—Handbooks, manuals, etc.
3. Community Health Aids—Handbooks, manuals, etc.

Catalog Card No.: 86-81738

Werner, David, 1943 —
Disabled Village Children
Palo Alto, CA: Hesperian Foundation
672 p.
ISBN: 0-942364-06-6

PUBLISHED BY:

The Hesperian Foundation
1919 Addison St., #304
Berkeley, California 94704
United States of America

2nd edition, 7th printing, June 2006

This book is dedicated to disabled children everywhere,
with the hope that they and their families
will help lead the world
to be more loving, understanding,
and just for everyone.

REQUEST FOR YOUR SUGGESTIONS, CRITICISMS, AND IDEAS

This book is an attempt to pull together basic information to help you meet the needs of village children with a wide range of disabilities.

We have done the best we can, given our limitations. We know the book is not perfect and that it has weaknesses and perhaps some mistakes.

We urge anyone reviewing or using the book, whether a disabled person, parent, health worker, or professional, to send us all your criticism and suggestions. Help us to make improvements for a later edition. Thank you.

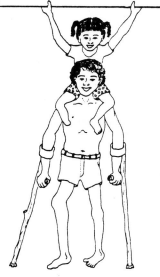

WE WOULD APPRECIATE ANY SUGGESTIONS YOU MAY HAVE FOR WAYS THAT THIS BOOK MIGHT BE IMPROVED TO SERVE YOUR RURAL AREA BETTER.

CONTENTS

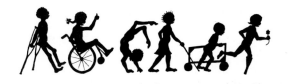

THANKS

This book has been a cooperative effort. Many persons have contributed in different ways. Some have helped to write or rewrite different sections; some have criticized early drafts; some have used it in their programs and sent us feedback; some have sent original ideas or technologies that we have tested and then included. In all, persons or programs from 27 countries on 6 continents (North and South America, Africa, Asia, Europe, Australia) have contributed.

The entire book has been carefully reviewed by specialists in related fields: physical therapists (PTs), occupational therapists (OTs), orthotists, prosthetists, wheelchair designers, rehabilitation engineers, and leaders from among the disabled. We cannot include the names of all those who have helped in so many ways, but the help of the following has been outstanding:

Sophie Levitt, PT; Ann Hallum, PT; Terry Nordstrom,PT; Anne Affleck, OT; Mike Miles, rehab planner and critic; Christine Miles, special educator; Farhat Rashid, PT; Bruce Curtis, peer disabled group counselor; Ralf Hotchkiss, wheelchair rider/engineer; Alice Hadley, PT; Jan Postma, PT; Jean-Baptiste Richardier, prosthetist, Claude Simonnot, MD/prosthetist; Wayne Hampton, MD/prosthetist; Jim Breakey, prosthetist; Wally Motlock, orthotist; Valery Taylor, PT; Dr. P. K. Sethi, orthopedic surgeon/prosthetist; Pam Zinkin, pediatrician/CBR expert; Paul SilvWa, wheelchair builder; David Morley, pediatrician; Elia Landeros, PT; Teresa Paez, social worker; Rafiq Jaffer, rehab specialist; Kris Buckner, parent of many adopted disabled children; Barbara Anderson, PT; Don Caston, rehab engineer; Greg Dixon, Director, Partners' Appropriate Technology In Health; Susan Hammerman, Director, Rehabilitation International; Carole Coleman, specialist in sign language; Suzanne Reier, recreation therapist; Sarah Grossman, PT; Donal Laub, plastic surgeon; Jean Kohn, MD in rehabilitation; Bob Friedricks, orthotist; Katherine Myers, spinal cord injury nurse; Grace Warren, PT in leprosy; Jean M. Watson, PT in leprosy; David Sanders, pediatrician; Jane Neville, leprosy expert; Stanley Browne, MD, leprosy; Alexandra Enders, OT; John McGill, prosthetist; Victoria Sheffield, Rita Leavell, MD, Jeff Watson, J. Kirk Horton, Lawrence Campbell, Helen Keller International; Owen Wrigley, IHAP; Roswitha and Kenneth Klee, Winfried Lichtemberger, Jeanne R. Kenmore, Christoffel Blindenmission; Judy Deutsch, PT; Jane Thiboutot, PT; R.L. Huckstep, MD; Linda Goode, PT; Susan Johnson, PT; David Hall, child health consultant; Ann Goerdt, PT for WHO; Mira Shiva, MD; Nigel Shapcott, seating specialist; Ann Yeadon, educator; Charles Reilly, sign language consultant; Eli Savanack, Gallaudet College; John Gray, MD; Molly Thorburn, MD; Lonny Shavelson, MD; Margaret Mackenzie, medical anthropologist; Rainer Arnhold, MD, Gulbadan Habibi, Caroline Arnold, Philip Kgosa a, Garren Lumpkin, UNICEF.

Above all, we would like to thank the team of disabled village rehabilitation workers in Project PROJIMO, Ajoya, Sinaloa, Mexico, along with the hundreds of disabled children and their families. Their involvement and interaction in exploring, testing, inventing, and discovering simplified alternatives has led to the formation of this book. Key among the PROJIMO team are: Marcelo Acevedo, Miguel Álvarez, Adelina Bastidas, Roberto Fajardo, Teresa Gárate, Bruce Hobson, Concepción Lara, Inés León, Ramon León, Polo Leyva, Armando Nevárez, María Picos, Adelina Pliego, Elijio Reyes, Cecilia Rodríguez, Josefa Rodríguez, Concepción Rubio, Moisés Salas, Rosa Salcido, Asunción Soto, Javier Valverde, Florentino Velázquez, Efrain Zamora, Miguel Zamora.

For this book we have borrowed information, ideas, illustrations, methods, and designs from many sources, published and unpublished. Often credit has been given, but not always. If you notice we have 'borrowed' from your material and neglected to give you credit, please accept our unspoken thanks and apologies.

For their excellent and dedicated work in preparing the manuscript for publication, special thanks go to: Jane Maxwell, editing, page design, and art production; Irene Yen, editing and paste-up; Kathy Alberts, Elizabeth de Avila, Martín Bustos, Mary Klein, Carlos Romero and Marjorie Wang, paste-up; Martin Bustos and Anna Muñoz-Briggs, Spanish translation; Myra Polinger, typing; Lynn Gordon, Bill Bower, Phil Pasmanick and Dan Perlman, general review; Alison Davis, reference section research; Elizabeth de Ávila, Don Baker, Agnes Batteiger, Jane Bavelas, Leda Bosworth, Renee Burgard, Michael Lang, Betty Page, Pearl Snyder, Tinker Spar, Paula Tanous and Roger Wilson, proofreading; Lino Montebon, Joan Thompson and David Werner, drawings; Richard Parker, John Fago, Carolyn Watson, Tom Wells and David Werner, photography; Dyanne Ladine, art production; Martin Bustos and Richard Parker, photo production; Hal Lockwood and Helen Epperson of Bookman Productions, Tim Anderson and Linda Inman of Reprographex, typesetting and layout; and Trude Bock for giving so wholeheartedly of herself and her home for the preparation of this book.

We want to give an extra word of thanks to Carol Thuman for coordination, typing, and correspondence and Janet Elliott for graphics, artwork, and paste-up, and to both for sharing the responsibility for the preparation and quality of this book.

The main costs of preparing this book were met with grants from the Public Welfare Foundation, whose continued friendship and support of the Hesperian Foundation's publications is deeply appreciated. Additional funding was generously provided by the Gary Wang Memorial Fund, UNICEF, OXFAM UK, the Swedish International Development Agency, MISEREOR, and May and Stanley Smith Charitable Trust. We would also like to thank the Thrasher Research Fund, and Mulago Foundation for helping meet the costs of Project PROJIMO, from which this book evolved.

For updating this book, we thank Manisha Aryal, Martín Bustos, Darlena David, Iñaki Fernández de Retana, Todd Jailer, Jane Maxwell, Susan McCallister, Gail McSweeney, Elena Metcalf, Christine Sienkiewicz, and Sarah Wallis.

Finally, we would like to thank David Werner for his careful and hard work in preparing this book. His vision and advocacy for disabled people around the world is reflected throughout the book.

The Hesperian Foundation

ABOUT THIS BOOK

A TRUE STORY: CRUTCHES FOR PEPE

A teacher of village health workers was helping as a volunteer in the mountains of western Mexico. One day he arrived on muleback at a small village. A father came up to him and asked if he could cure his son. The health worker went with the father to his hut.

The boy, whose name was Pepe, was sitting on the floor. His legs had been paralyzed by polio, from when he was a baby. Now he was 13 years old. Pepe smiled and reached up a friendly hand.

The health worker, who also had a physical disability, examined Pepe. "Have you ever tried to walk with crutches?" he asked. Pepe shook his head.

"We live so far away from the city," his father explained.

"Let's try to make some crutches," said the health worker.

The next morning the health worker got up at dawn. He borrowed a long curved knife and went into the forest. He looked and looked until he found 2 forked branches the right size.

He took the branches back to Pepe's home and began to make them into crutches, like this.

The father came and seeing the crutches, he said, "They won't work!"

The health worker frowned. "Wait and see!" he said.

When both crutches were finished, they showed them to Pepe, who was eager to try them. His father lifted Pepe to a standing position and the health worker placed the crutches under the boy's arms.

But as soon as Pepe put his weight on the crutches, they bent and broke.

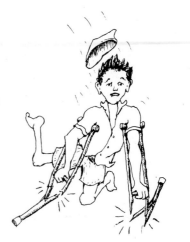

"I tried to tell you they wouldn't work," said the father. "It's the wrong kind of tree. Wood's weak as water! But now I see your idea. I'll go cut some branches of 'jútamo'. Wood's tough as iron, but light! Don't want the crutches too heavy."

He took the knife and went into the forest. Fifteen minutes later he was back with 2 forked branches of 'jútamo'. He began making the crutches, his strong hands working rapidly. The health worker and Pepe helped him.

When these crutches were finished, Pepe's father tested them by putting his own weight on them. They supported him easily, yet were lightweight. Then Pepe tried them. At first, he had trouble balancing, but soon he could hold himself up. By afternoon, he was walking with the crutches! But they rubbed under his arms.

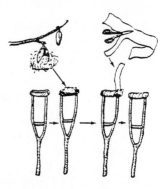

"I have an idea," said Pepe's father. He ran to a wild kapok tree, and picked several of the large ripe fruits. He gathered the soft cotton from the pods and put a cushion of kapok on the top crosspiece of each crutch. He wrapped the kapok in place with strips of cloth. Pepe tried the crutches again. They were comfortable.

"Thanks, Papa, you fixed them great!" he said, smiling at his father with pride. "Look how well I can walk now!" He moved about quickly in front of them.

"I'm proud of you, son!" said his father, smiling too.

As the health worker prepared to leave, the whole family came to say good-bye.

"I can't thank you enough," said Pepe's father. "It's so wonderful to see my son walking. I don't know why I never thought of making crutches before. . . ."

"I should be thanking you," said the health worker. "You have taught me a lot."

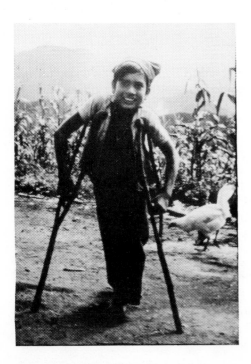

After leaving, the health worker smiled to himself. He thought, "How foolish of me not to have asked the father's advice in the beginning. He knows the trees better than I do. And he is a better craftsperson.

"But it was good that the crutches I made broke. Making them was my idea, and the father felt bad for not thinking of it himself. But when my crutches broke, he made much better ones. That made us equal again!"

So the health worker learned many things from Pepe's father—things that he had never learned in school. He learned what kind of wood is best for making crutches. He also learned how important it is to use the skills and knowledge of the local people—because a better job can be done, and because it helps maintain people's dignity. People feel equal when they learn from each other.

HOW THIS BOOK WAS WRITTEN

The story of Pepe's crutches is an example of the lessons we have learned that helped to create this book. We are a group of village health and rehabilitation workers who have worked with people in farming communities of western Mexico to form a 'villager-run' rehabilitation program. Most of us on the rehabilitation 'team' are disabled ourselves.

From our experience of trying to help disabled children and their families to meet their needs, we have developed many of the methods, aids, and ideas in this book. We have also gathered ideas from books, persons, and other programs, and have adapted them to fit the limitations and possibilities of our village area. We hope this book will be useful to village people in many parts of the world. So we have asked for cooperation and included suggestions from community program leaders in more than 20 countries.

This book was *not* written by experts,

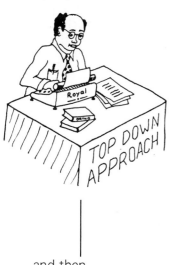

and then 'field tested' with community workers.

Unlike most handbooks for village workers and families, this book was not written by 'professionals' and then 'field tested'. Instead, it grew out of the practical experience of a team of disabled village health workers as we looked for information to help meet the most common problems we face.

However, a large number of professionals have helped in important ways. Many are well-known leaders in their fields. They include physical and occupational therapists, special educators, nurses, doctors, brace and limb makers, and rehabilitation engineers. They have carefully reviewed and even helped to rewrite sections of this book. Some have also helped to teach and advise our village team.

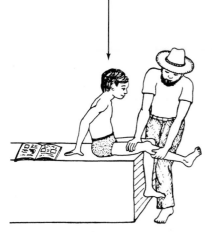

Instead, it was written by and with community workers,

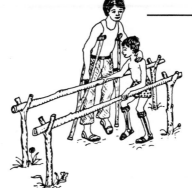

and then reviewed and corrected by experts.

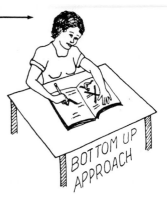

HOW THIS BOOK DIFFERS FROM OTHER 'REHABILITATION MANUALS'

This book was written from the 'bottom up', working closely with disabled persons and their families. We believe that those with the most personal experience of disability can and should become leaders in resolving the needs of the disabled. In fact, the main author of this book (David Werner) and many of its contributors happen to be disabled. We are neither proud nor ashamed of this. But we do realize that in some ways our disabilities contribute to our abilities and strengths.

In many rehabilitation manuals, disabled persons are treated as objects to be worked upon, to be 'normalized' or made as normal as possible. As disabled persons, we object to attempts by the experts to fit us into the mold of normal. Too often 'normal' behavior in our society is selfish, greedy, narrow-minded, prejudiced—and cruel to those who are weaker or different from others. We live in a world where too often it is 'normal' and acceptable for the rich to live at the expense of the poor, and for health professionals to earn many times the wages of those who produce their food but cannot afford their services. We live on a wealthy planet where most children do not get enough to eat, where half the people have never seen a trained health worker, and where poverty is a major cause of disability and early death. And yet the world's leaders spend 50 billion dollars every 3 weeks on the instruments of war—an amount that could provide primary health care to everyone on earth for an entire year!

Instead of being 'normalized' into such an unkind, unfair, and unreasonable social structure, we disabled persons would do better to join together with all who are treated unfairly, in order to work for a new social order that is kinder, more just, and more sane.

This large book, then, is a small tool in the struggle not only for the liberation of the disabled, but for their solidarity in the larger effort to create a world where more value is placed on being human than on being 'normal'—a world where war and poverty and despair no longer disable the children of today, who are the leaders of tomorrow.

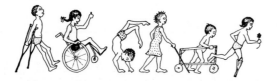

Top-down rehabilitation manuals too often only give orders telling the 'local trainer', family member, and disabled person exactly what they 'must do'. We feel that this is a limiting rather than liberating approach. It encourages people to obediently fit the child into a standard 'rehabilitation plan', instead of creating a plan that fits and frees the child. Again and again we see exercises, lessons, braces, and aids incorrectly, painfully, and often harmfully applied. This is done both by community rehabilitation workers and by professionals, because they have been taught to follow standard instructions or pre-packaged solutions rather than to respond in a flexible and creative way to the needs of the whole child.

In this book we try *not* to tell anyone what they *must* do. Instead we provide information, explanations, suggestions, examples, and ideas. We encourage an imaginative, adventurous, thoughtful, and even playful approach. After all, each disabled child is different and will be helped most by approaches and activities that are lovingly adapted to her specific abilities and needs.

As much as we can, we try to **explain basic principles** and **give reasons for doing things.** After village rehabilitation workers and parents understand the basic principles behind different rehabilitation activities, exercises, or aids, they can begin to make adaptations. They can make better use of local resources and of the unique opportunities that exist in their own rural area. In this way many rehabilitation aids, exercises, and activities can be made or done in ways that **integrate rather than separate** the child from the day-to-day life in the community.

This is not the first handbook of 'simplified rehabilitation'. We have drawn on ideas from many other sources. We would like to give special credit to the world Health Organization's manual, *Training the Disabled in the Community,* and to UNICEF and Rehabilitation International's *Childhood Disability: Prevention and Rehabilitation at the Community Level,* a shortened and improved version of the WHO manual. The WHO manual has recently been rewritten in a friendlier style that invites users to take more of a problem-solving approach instead of simply following instructions.

This handbook is not intended to replace these earlier manuals. It provides additional information. It is for families, village health workers, and community rehabilitation workers who want to do a more complete job of meeting the needs of physically disabled children.

HOW WE DECIDED WHICH DISABILITIES TO INCLUDE

Because this book is written for village use in many countries, it was not easy to decide what to include. People in different parts of the world give importance to different disabilities. This is partly because some disabilities are much more common in one area than another. For example,

- **polio** in some countries is the most common disability. In others, it is rare because of effective vaccination programs.

- **deafness** and **mental retardation** are much more common in certain mountain regions because of lack of iodine in the diet (or in salt).

- **blindness** due to lack of vitamin A is common in some poor, crowded communities, and depends a lot on local food habits.

- **rickets** is still common in regions where children are wrapped up or kept in dark places so much that they do not get enough sunlight.

- **burn deformities** are frequent where people cook and sleep on the ground near open fires and in war zones.

- **amputations** are a big problem in war zones, refugee camps, and 'shanty towns' along railway tracks.

- disability from **tuberculosis, leprosy, measles, malnutrition,** and **poor sanitation** are especially common where lack of social justice lets some people live in great wealth while most live in extreme poverty.

As more communities around the world are affected by the HIV/AIDS epidemic, more children are being born to HIV infected mothers. Many more children are surviving and living with the long-term effects of HIV disease. This book does not separately address illness and disability related to HIV/AIDS, but many of the sections will be useful for children with HIV/AIDS (care for pressure sores, assistive walking devices, etc.). For more information, see a general health book like *Where There is No Doctor* or a book specific to care for people with HIV like *HIV, Health and Your Community* (to order, see page 642).

Local beliefs also affect how people see different disabilities. In an area where people believe that **fits** are the work of the devil, a child with fits may be feared, teased, or kept hidden. But in places where everyone accepts fits as 'just something that happens to certain persons' a child who sometimes has fits may participate fully in the day-to-day life of the community, without being seen as 'handicapped'. Both of these children need medicine. But probably only the mistreated one needs 'rehabilitation'.

It is important to consider how local people see a child who is in some way 'different'. How do they accept or treat the child who learns slowly, limps a little, or occasionally has fits?

Many reports say that in both rich and poor countries, 1 in 10 children are disabled. However, this number can be misleading. Although 1 child in 10 may show some defect if examined carefully, most of these defects are so minor that they do not affect the child's ability to lead a full, active life. In rural areas, children who are physically strong but are slow learners often fit into the life and work of the village without special notice. In India, a study found that only 1 in 7 of those recorded as mentally retarded by screening tests were seen as retarded by the community.

Studies in several countries show that, on the average, only 2 or 3 children in 100 are considered disabled by the community. These are the children most likely to benefit from 'rehabilitation'.

CAUTION: If the community does not consider a child 'disabled', and the child manages well, it may be wiser *not* to bring attention to her condition. To do so might actually 'disable' the child more in the eyes of the community, and make life harder for her. Think carefully before deciding to do a 'complete survey' on disability.

When we started to write this book, we planned to include only physical disabilities. This is because **concerned villagers and health workers in rural Mexico considered physical handicaps to be the area of greatest need.**

This is understandable. In poor farming communities, where many day-to-day activities depend on physical strength, and where schooling for most children is brief, the physically disabled child can have an especially difficult time fitting in. By contrast, in a middle-class city neighborhood, where children are judged mainly by their ability in school, it is the mentally slow child who often has the hardest time.

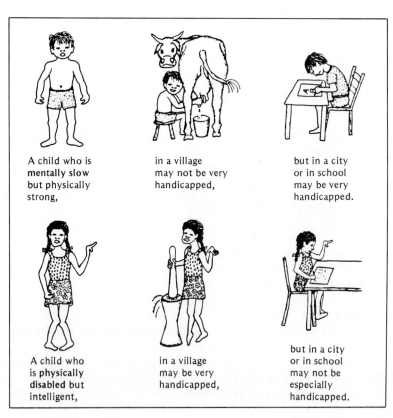

A child who is **mentally slow but physically strong,**

in a village may not be very handicapped,

but in a city or in school may be very handicapped.

A child who is **physically disabled but intelligent,**

in a village may be very handicapped,

but in a city or in school may not be especially handicapped.

The team of disabled village workers in Mexico was at first concerned mostly with physical disabilities. But they soon realized that they also had to learn about other disabilities. Even children whose main problem was physical, like polio, were often held back by other (secondary) emotional, social or behavioral disabilities. And many children with brain damage not only had difficulties with movement, but also were slow learners, had fits, or could not see or hear.

As the PROJIMO team's need for information on different disabilities has grown, so has this book. **The main focus is still on physical disabilities** which are covered in more detail. However, the book now includes a fairly complete (but less detailed) coverage of **mental retardation and developmental delay** (slow learning). **Fits** (epilepsy) are also covered.

Blindness and deafness are included, but only in a very brief, beginner's way. This is partly because we at PROJIMO still do not have much experience in these areas. And partly it is because seeing and hearing disabilities require so much special information that they need to be covered in separate books. Some fairly good instructional material is available on these disabilities, especially on blindness. We list some of the best materials that we know on p. 639 and 640.

Note: This book does *not* include disabilities which are mainly in the area of internal medicine, such as asthma, chronic lung problems, severe allergies, heart defects, diabetes, bleeding problems, cancers or HIV/AIDS. And except for brief mention, it does *not* include very local disabilities such as lathyrism (parts of India). In local areas where such disabilities are common, rehabilitation workers should obtain information separately.

To decide which disabilities to put in this book and how much importance to give to each, we used information from several sources, including the records of Project PROJIMO in Mexico. We found that the numbers of children with different disabilities who came to PROJIMO were fairly similar to those in studies done by WHO, UNICEF, and others in different areas of the world.

On the next page is a chart showing how many children with each disability might be seen in a typical village area. (Of course, there is no such thing as a 'typical' village. The patterns of disability in some areas will be quite different from those shown on the chart.) The chart is based mainly on our records from PROJIMO over a 3-year period.

Notice that in the chart, the number of children with each disability corresponds more or less to the relative importance that we give to each disability in this book. In certain cases we have made exceptions. For example, few persons with leprosy have come to PROJIMO. But we have included a long chapter on leprosy because we realize it is a big problem in some places.

IMPORTANT: The disabilities discussed in this book are those that are most common in rural areas in many countries. But not all disabilities are included. Also, certain disabilities may be difficult to identify, or require special tests or analyses. **When in doubt, try to get advice from persons with more training and experience.**

Clearly you cannot solve every problem. But **there is much you can do.** By asking questions, carefully examining the child, and using whatever information and resources you can find, you may be able to learn much about what these children need and to figure out ways to help them manage better.

HOW COMMON ARE DIFFERENT DISABILITIES

The little 'stick people' in this chart show how many children might have each disability in an average group of 100 significantly disabled village children. These figures are based on records of 700 children seen at PROJIMO, Mexico (1982–1985), and other studies. The numbers in your area may be similar or very different from these, depending on local factors.

TYPICAL FREQUENCY OF DISABILITIES
PER 100 SIGNIFICANTLY DISABLED CHILDREN
(based on records of 700 children seen at PROJIMO, Mexico)

Primary or main disabilities

Movement disabilities

Polio

Brain damage and cerebral palsy

Birth defects (includes club feet)

Injury, burns, amputations

Spina bifida

Spinal cord injury

Muscular dystrophy and atrophy

Juvenile arthritis and other joint pain

Bone infections (includes tuberculosis of the spine)

Hip problems

Leprosy

Arthrogryposis

Other

Seeing disabilities

Hearing and speech disabilities

Fits

Developmental delay (slow learners)

Secondary or additional disabilities

Contractures (mostly with polio and cerebral palsy)

Spinal curve

Developmental delay (mostly with cerebral palsy)

Fits (mostly with cerebral palsy)

Seeing (mostly with cerebral palsy)

Hearing and speech (mostly with cerebral palsy)

Behavioral problems

(plus those occurring with cerebral palsy = 8 per 100)

(plus those occurring with cerebral palsy = 10 per 100)

(plus those occurring with cerebral palsy = 14 per 100)

(plus those occurring with cerebral palsy = 16 per 100)

Note: Seeing and hearing disabilities, fits, and developmental delay are listed in 2 places, depending on whether they are the main disability or occur in addition to some other disability.

HOW THIS BOOK IS ORGANIZED

This book is divided into 3 parts: 1, "Working with the Child and Family," 2, "Working with the Community," and 3, "Working in the Shop."

The disabilities that villagers usually consider most important are discussed in early chapters, beginning with Chapter 7. In many countries, more than half of the disabled children have either polio or cerebral palsy. For this reason, we start with them. Other disabilities are arranged partly in order of their relative importance, and partly to place near to each other those disabilities that are similar, related, or easily confused.

Notice that in the chart on p. A8, certain 'secondary disabilities' occur very often. ('Secondary disabilities' are problems that result after the main disability.) For example, contractures (joints that no longer straighten) can develop with many disabilities. In many villages, there will be more children who have contractures than who have any single primary disability. For this reason we include some of the important secondary problems in separate chapters.

Common disabilities that are often 'secondary' to other disabilities include:

Contractures, Chapter 8

Dislocated Hips (either a primary or secondary disability), Chapter 18

Spinal Curve (either primary or secondary), Chapter 20

Pressure Sores (often occurs with spinal cord injury, spina bifida, or leprosy), Chapter 24

Urine and Bowel Management (with spinal cord injury and spina bifida), Chapter 25

Behavior Disturbances, Chapter 40

Other disabilities that are often the primary problem but commonly occur with other disability—usually with cerebral palsy—include fits (Chapter 29), blindness (Chapter 30), and deafness and speech problems (Chapter 31).

IMPORTANT: Some important information in this book applies to many disabilities. In order not to make the book longer than it is now, we have not repeated all of this information in each chapter on specific disabilities. Instead we have put it in separate chapters.

This means that **to meet the needs of a specific child, you will often have to look in several different chapters.** We have tried to make this as easy for you as possible (see "How To Use This Book," inside the back cover).

 FOR MANY DISABILITIES IT IS VERY IMPORTANT THAT YOU READ INFORMATION FROM SEVERAL CHAPTERS.

Note to

REHABILITATION PROFESSIONALS, PROGRAM PLANNERS, AND THERAPISTS

You may think that this book is 'too complex' or 'too long' for community health workers or rehabilitation workers, or family members. At first, for many, it may be. This is a book to grow into—a simplified but detailed work book and reference book.

But remember, **almost all the ideas and information in this book are right now being put into practice by village workers with little schooling, together with disabled children and their families.** The book was developed for and with a team of village workers who have an average of 3 years primary school education.

Some health workers and parents will be able to make fairly good use of the book, or parts of it, without special training. Others will not.

This book is not intended to be a substitute for 'learning through guided practice'. People learn best when someone with more experience shows and explains things to them in a real situation (working with disabled children and their families). Skills for making aids and teaching exercises are also learned best by working with an experienced rehabilitation worker or craftsperson.

In some places, or when a village program is just beginning, this book may at first be used mainly by program leaders, therapists, and instructors to help you learn to teach in ways that communicate clearly and that encourage a problem-solving approach. The book can also be a resource to help you answer questions that village workers will have after they start working with disabled children.

We have observed that when making decisions about what a child needs, some rehabilitation professionals, therapists, aid makers, and surgeons do not think enough about the whole child, the situation where she lives, the money problems, or the resources within the family and community. As a result, much too often the professionals make decisions that are not practical or that sometimes do more harm than good (see Chapter 56). Often their recommendations fail because they have tried to fit the child into their textbook, instead of adapting the textbook to fit the child and her situation. This comes partly from many years of conventional schooling, which encourages 'following instructions' more than 'thinking things through' and 'being creative'.

There will never be enough highly-trained rehabilitation professionals to attend to the needs of more than a small part of the world's millions of disabled persons. Most rehabilitation and therapy can and should take place in the home and community with loving support of family, neighbors, and friends.

You rehabilitation professionals and therapists can play an extremely important role in 'community-directed rehabilitation'. By simplifying and sharing your knowledge and skills, you can reach many more children. But to do this you will need to go out of the large city rehabilitation centers and into neighborhoods and villages. You will need to meet and work with the people on their terms, as learners, teachers, and information providers. You can help disabled persons, parents, and other concerned individuals to organize small, community-directed centers or programs. You can teach those who have the most interest to become teachers. You can help local craftspersons to figure out or improve low-cost designs for rehabilitation aids (and they can help you). You can encourage village leaders to improve paths and entrances to schools and public places. You can help local people to understand basic principles and to avoid common mistakes, so that they can be more effective leaders and participants in home and community rehabilitation.

IMPORTANT: RESPECT THE KNOWLEDGE AND SKILLS OF THE PEOPLE

Villagers are often much better than city persons at figuring out how to do things, at using whatever happens to be available, and at making and fixing things with their hands. In short, they are more 'resourceful'. They have to be to survive! **This 'resourcefulness' of village people can be one of the most valuable 'resources' for rehabilitation in rural areas.**

But for this to happen, **we need to help people understand basic principles and 'concepts'—not just tell them what to do.** Above all, we need to respect their intelligence, their knowledge of the local situation, and **their ability to improve on our suggestions.**

Whenever possible, arrange for village workers to learn to use this book with guidance from experienced rehabilitation workers. Those rehabilitation workers should be able to listen to the people, respect their ideas, and relate to them as equals.

For best learning, the teacher, or 'guide' should stay as much in the background as possible, offering friendly advice when asked, and always asking the learners what they think before giving instructions and answers.

It is our hope that this book may help disabled persons, their families, village workers, and rehabilitation professionals to **learn more from each other,** and to help each other to become more capable, more caring, human beings.

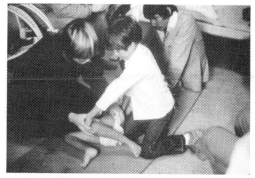

A visiting therapist at PROJIMO teaches the older brother of a disabled girl how to do stretching exercises of her hip to correct a contracture.

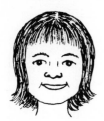
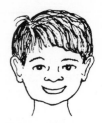

NOTE ON LANGUAGE
USED IN THIS BOOK
Speaking of the Disabled Child—
'SHE' or 'HE'

Many studies have shown that more boys are disabled than girls. It is sometimes argued that this is because boys are more exposed to physical stress and danger, or because of sex-linked 'genetic' factors.

But there may also be other, more disturbing reasons why reports show so many more disabled boys than girls:

- Of those who are disabled, more of the boys than the girls are taken to medical centers where their disabilities are recorded.

- Disabled girls often are not cared for as well as disabled boys; therefore more of the girls die when they are babies or small children.

In short, **disabled boys often receive better attention than do disabled girls.** This, of course, is not surprising: in most countries, non-disabled boys also get better treatment, more food, and more opportunities than do non-disabled girls.

Most literature on disabled children speaks of the disabled child as 'he'. This is partly because male dominance is built into our language. However, we feel this can only add to the continued neglect of the so-called 'weaker sex'.

In this book, therefore, we have made an effort to be fair. But rather than to always speak of the child as 'he-or-she' or 'they', which is awkward, we sometimes refer to her as 'she' and sometimes as 'he'.

If at times this is confusing, please pardon us. And if we sometimes slip and give more prominence to 'he' than 'she', either in words or pictures, please criticize but forgive us. We too are products of our language and culture. But we are trying to change.

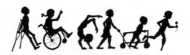

Speaking of the Author(s):
'WE' or 'I'

Although one person has done most of the writing of this book, many persons have shared in its making (see the 'Thanks' page at the beginning of this book.) Therefore, when speaking from our authors-advisers' viewpoint, we usually use 'we'. This book is a group effort.

PART 1

WORKING WITH THE CHILD AND FAMILY

Information on Different Disabilities

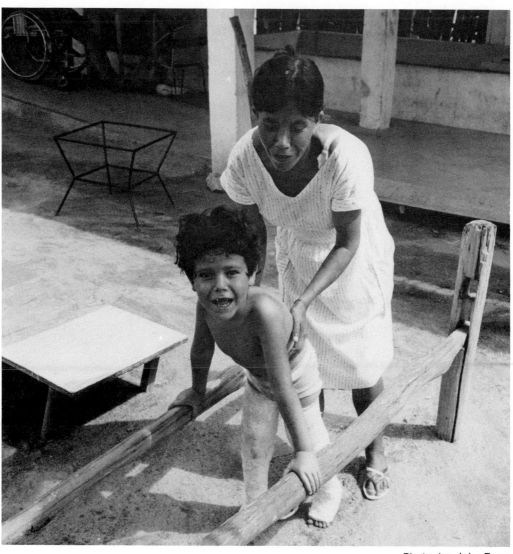

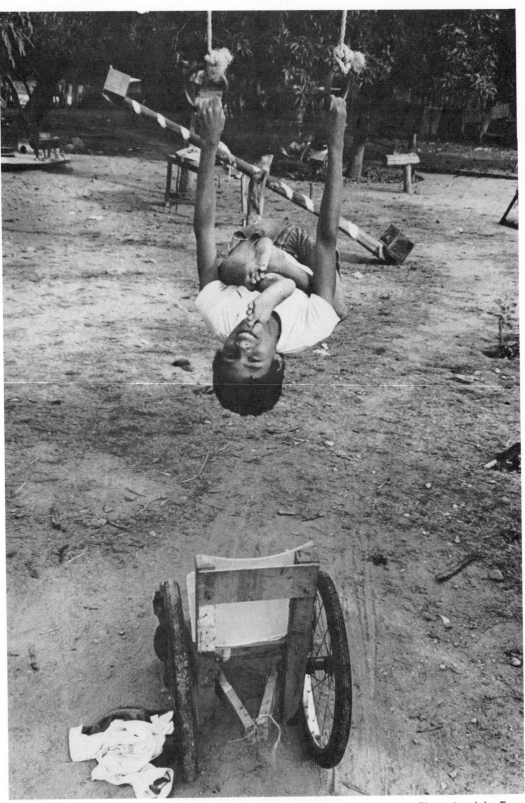

Photo by John Fago

INTRODUCTION TO PART 1

Making Therapy Functional and Fun

Most disabled people in the world live in villages and poor communities where they never see a 'rehabilitation expert' or 'physical therapist'. But this does not always mean that they have no 'rehabilitation' or 'therapy'. In many villages and homes, family members, local craftspersons, traditional healers, and disabled people themselves have figured out ways for persons with disabilities to do things better and move about more easily.

We have seen examples where local carpenters, tinsmiths, leatherworkers or blacksmiths have put together simple crutches, carts, wooden legs and other aids. We know parents who have figured out ways of adapting daily activities so that their children can help do farm work or housework—and at the same time get much of the exercise (therapy) they need.

Sometimes the 'rehabilitation' that families and communities figure out by themselves works better in their situation than do methods or aids introduced by outside professionals. Here are 2 examples:

1. In India, I met a villager who had lost a leg in a house-building accident. Using his imagination, he had made himself an artificial leg with a flexible foot out of strong wire with strips of an old cotton blanket for padding. After several months, he had the chance to go to a city where a professional 'leg maker' (prosthetist) made him a costly modern fiberglass leg. The man tried using the new limb for a couple of months, but it was heavy and hot. It did not let his stump breathe like his 'wire cage' leg. And he could not squat to eat or do his toilet, as he could with his homemade leg. Finally, he stopped using the costly new leg and went back to the one he had made. For the climate and customs where he lived, it was more appropriate.

Two words often used by people who work with disabled persons are *'rehabilitation'* and *'therapy'*.

Rehabilitation means **returning of ability,** or helping a disabled person to manage better at home and in the community.

Therapy basically means treatment. *Physical therapy*—or physiotherapy—is the art of improving position, movement, strength, balance, and control of the body. *Occupational therapy* is the art of helping a disabled person learn to do useful or enjoyable activities.

We speak of 'therapy' as an **art** rather than a science because there are many different beliefs and approaches, and because the human feeling that goes into therapy is as important as the methods.

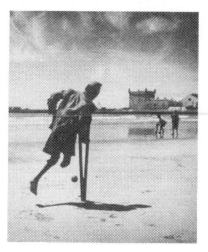

All children, as much as possible, should get the exercise they need through daily work and play. (Morocco. Photo by Charles Trieschmann)

2. In a small village in Mexico, over the years, the community together with its deaf citizens has developed a simple but expressive 'sign language' using their hands, faces, mouths, and whole bodies to communicate. As a result, children who are born deaf quickly and gracefully learn to express themselves. They are well accepted in the community, and some have grown up to become creative and respected craftspersons. This village method of 'total communication' allows the deaf children to learn a useful language more quickly, easily, and effectively than does the 'lip reading and speech' method now taught in the cities. For children who are born deaf, attempts to teach only lip-reading-and-spoken-language often end in cruel disappointment (see p. 264). **The 'special educators' in the cities could learn a lot from these villagers.**

Disabled children—if allowed—often show great imagination and energy in figuring out ways to move about, communicate, or get what they need. Much of what they do is, in effect, 'therapy', artfully adapted for and by each child.

With a little help, encouragement, and freedom, the disabled child can often become her own best therapist. One thing is certain: she will make sure her therapy is 'functional' (useful), always changing it to meet her immediate needs. A disabled child, like other children, instinctively knows that life is to be lived NOW and that her body and her world are there to be explored, used, and challenged. **The best therapy is built into everyday activities: play, work, relationship, rest, and adventure.**

The challenge, then, for health workers and parents (as well as for therapists), is to look for ways that children can get the 'therapy' they need in ways that are easy, interesting, and functional.

This takes imagination and flexibility on the part of all those working with disabled children. But mostly, it takes understanding. When family members clearly understand the reasons for a particular therapy and the basic principles involved, they can find many imaginative ways to do and adapt that therapy.

'Physical therapy' to improve control of the head, strength of the back, and use of both arms and hands together:

(a) in a city clinic

(b) in a village home

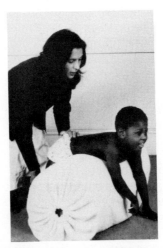

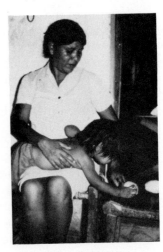

Photo: Cheyne Walk
Spastic's Centre

Photo: PROJIMO,
Ajoya, Mexico

Appropriate therapy helps the child to enjoy himself, be useful, and take part with others, while mastering the skills for daily living.

Physical therapy and rehabilitation techniques have been developed mostly in cities. Yet most of the world's disabled children live in villages and farms. Their parents are usually very busy growing the food and doing the chores to keep the family fed and alive from day to day. In some ways, this makes home therapy more difficult. But in other ways **it provides a wide range of possibilities for exciting therapy in which the child and his family can meet life's needs together.**

Here is a story that tells how therapy can be adapted to village life.

Maricela lives in a small village on a river. She has cerebral palsy. When she was 4 years old, she was just beginning to walk.

But her knees bumped together when she tried to take steps. So she did not try often. Also, her arms and hands were weak and did not work very well.

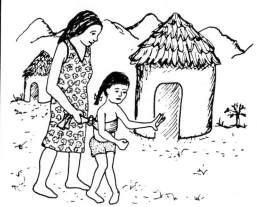

Her family saved money and took Maricela to a rehabilitation center in the city. After a long wait, a therapist examined her. He explained that Maricela needed to stretch the muscles on the inner side of her thighs, so her knees would not press together as much.

He recommended that her parents do special exercises with her, and that they buy a special plastic seat to hold her knees wide apart.

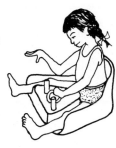

He said she also needed exercises to strengthen and increase the control of her hands and arms.

He suggested buying her some special toys, game boards, and aids to practice handling and gripping things.

Maricela's family could not afford these costly things. So back in her village her father used whatever he could find to make similar aids at low cost. First he made a special seat of sticks.

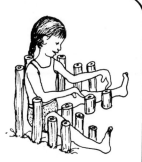

Later he made a better seat with pieces of wood, and an old bucket to hold her legs apart.

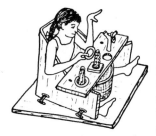

Then, using a board, corn cobs and rings cut from bamboo, he added a small table so that she could play games to develop hand control.

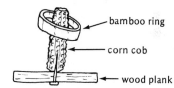

← bamboo ring

← corn cob

← wood plank

He also made a hand exerciser out of bamboo.

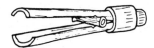

At first, while they were strange and new, Maricela used her special seat and played with her special toys. But soon, she got bored and stopped using them. She wanted to do the things that other children did. She wanted to go with her father and brother to the cornfield. She wanted to help her mother prepare food and wash the clothes. She wanted to be helpful and grown up.

(story continued on next page)

So she broke her special toys and refused to sit in her special seat. Her parents were furious with her—and she loved it! She would sit for hours with her knees together and her legs bent back. Walking began to get more difficult for her, so she did not walk much.

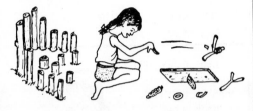

Her parents then visited a small rehabilitation center in a neighboring village. The village team suggested that they look for new ways to help Maricela keep her knees apart and improve control of her arms and hands—ways that would be exciting and help her to develop and practice useful skills together with the rest of her family. Here are some of the ideas that Maricela and her parents came up with:

When she was good (and sometimes even if she was not) her father would let her help shell corn with him and the other children. Because she had trouble holding the corn and snapping off the grain with her fingers, her father made a special holder and scraper.

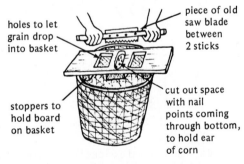

holes to let grain drop into basket

piece of old saw blade between 2 sticks

stoppers to hold board on basket

cut out space with nail points coming through bottom, to hold ear of corn

The basket between her legs held her knees apart, and the shelling of the corn strengthened her arms, gave her practice gripping, and improved her coordination and control.

shelling corn (taking the dried grain off the cobs)

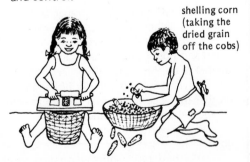

It was hard, important work that Maricela found she could do. And she loved it!

Maricela's mother sometimes invited her to help wash the clothes at the river. Maricela would sit at the river's edge with a big 'washing rock' between her legs. She would wash the clothes by squeezing and beating them against the rock—just like her mother.

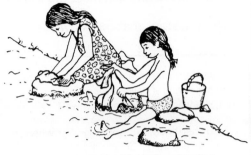

The rock kept her knees apart and the squeezing and banging strengthened her hands and improved her control. But what mattered was getting the clothes clean. It was hard work. But she found it easy—and fun!

Coming back from the river, Maricela just had to walk. It was too far to crawl. And besides, she had to help her mother carry back the washed clothes. This was hard, but she tried hard, and could do it!

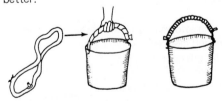

Carrying the pails of clothes helped her learn to walk without bending and jerking her arms so much.

To help Maricela grip the handle of the pail easier, her father wrapped a long strip of old bicycle inner tube very tightly around the handle. But when Maricela's hand sweated, the smooth rubber got slippery. So her father wound a thin rope around the rubber. This way, Maricela could hold it better.

As time passed she learned how to carry a bucket of clothes on her head—then a bucket of water. To do this took a lot of practice with balance and control of movement. She just had to keep her legs farther apart to keep her balance.

Her mother was almost afraid to let her try carrying the water. But Maricela was stubborn—and she did it! Maricela also discovered that if she floated a gourd dipper (or a big leaf) on top of the water, it helped keep the water from splashing out.

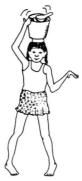

So, by trying different things, Maricela's family, and Maricela herself, learned ways to create therapy and aids that were effective, useful, and enjoyable.

Maricela did learn to walk better, and to use her hands and arms to do many things. But this took a long time. Sometimes she would try something that was too hard, and almost give up. But when her little brother would say she could not do it, she would keep trying until she succeeded.

Even when Maricela liked doing something, because she was a child she would get bored and not keep doing it for long. Her parents always had to look for new ways for her to get her therapy. It became a challenge and a game for them, too.

Of course, Maricela loved horses. So her father made her a rocking horse out of old logs, branches of trees, and a piece of rope for a tail.

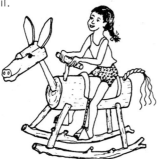

Her father noticed that she was beginning to walk on tiptoe, so he made special stirrups for the rocking horse. With these, when she rocked, her feet stretched up in a more normal position.

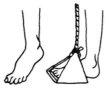

The rocking horse kept her knees apart, strengthened her hands, and helped her improve her balance. Maricela loved her horse and sometimes rocked for an hour or more. When she got off, it seemed she could walk better.

After Maricela had learned to ride the rocking horse, she wanted to ride the real thing. She begged and begged. So one day her father let her ride with him to the cornfield on his donkey. He suggested she ride in front of him where he could hold her. But she insisted on riding behind, like other children do.

So he fixed some stirrups and let her ride behind. Her legs were spread wide and she hung on tightly. It was excellent therapy— but nobody called it that.

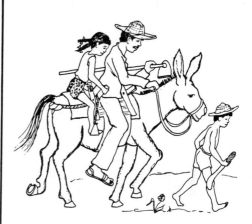

In the cornfield she helped her father and brother clean the weeds out from among the young corn plants. That was good for the young plants—and for her, too! But after several trips to the cornfield on the donkey with her father, Maricela begged him to let her ride alone. He was nervous, but he let her try.

She could do it—and what confidence it gave her! Soon Maricela was preparing lunch for her father and brother and taking it to them in the cornfield—all by herself. Now she found she could do many other things she never thought she could. Although she was still awkward, and at times had to look for special ways to do things, she found she could do most anything she wanted or needed to.

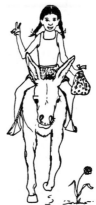

The example of Maricela's 'therapy' cannot and should not be copied—but instead, learned from. In fact, the story suggests that **no approach to rehabilitation should be copied exactly.** Our challenge is to understand each child's needs, and then to look for ways to **adapt her rehabilitation to both the limitations and possibilities within her family and community.** We must always look for ways to make therapy functional and fun.

Recently, some 'appropriate technology' groups have tried to adapt standard 'rehabilitation aids' to poor rural communities. However, many of their designs are modeled fairly closely after the same old city originals, using bamboo and string instead of plastic and aluminum. Some of these low-cost designs are excellent. But more effort is needed to make use of the unique possibilities for rehabilitation and therapy that exist in the village, farm, or fishing camp.

Maricela's family did just this. The basket of corn, the washing rock, the rocking horse, and the donkey all became 'therapy aids' to help Maricela spread her spastic legs, and at the same time, to take part in the life of her family and community.

But not every family shells corn in baskets, washes clothes on rocks, or has a donkey. And not every disabled child has Maricela's needs and strengths. So we repeat:

> We should encourage each family to observe the specific needs and possibilities of their disabled child, to understand the basic principles of the therapy needed, and then to look for ways to adapt the therapy to the child's and family's daily life.

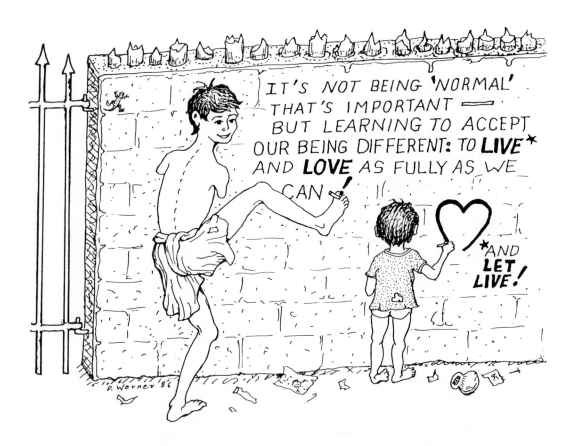

Ideas for Sharing Information from This Book

Most of the information in this book will be useful to health workers and village rehabilitation workers who see many disabled children. *Some* of the information will also be useful for the family of a disabled child. However, a family with one disabled child will usually not need, or be able to afford this whole book. It has information about so many different disabilities, that parents may have difficulty finding the information that applies to their child.

Also, learning from a book is often not the best way to learn something. A lot of methods, aids, and exercises can be learned more easily from other persons, through watching and through guided practice. But after a village worker has taught parents how to do certain exercises, or shown them an example of a homemade aid, **printed instruction sheets with clear drawings can be a big help.** Sometimes they can make the difference between whether the recommendations are followed at home, or not.

There are certain pages or parts of this book that you may want to give to families after you explain and teach to them selected exercises or activities. For example, to the family of a girl with arthritis, you may want to give some of the "Exercise Instruction Sheets" at the end of Chapter 42, and the "Information Sheet on Aspirin" on p. 134. You may also want to give them pages from Chapter 16 on arthritis, and to mark the exercises and activities that are important to their child.

To the family of a young child who is slow to develop, you may want to give pages from the chapters on child development and early stimulation activities (Chapters 34 and 35). For a more advanced child you could give the family material from the chapters on self-care (Chapters 36 to 39).

Depending on the interest and reading ability of the family, you may want to give them a whole chapter (or chapters) about their child's disability. For example, the chapters on cerebral palsy (Chapter 9) or deafness (Chapter 31). An older child who is paralyzed from a broken back might appreciate having a copy of the chapter on spinal cord injury. Letting him and his family take home the chapters on pressure sores and urine and bowel control could even save his life! His family may also want to take home plans for making a low-cost wheelchair, to see if the carpenter and blacksmith in their village could make one.

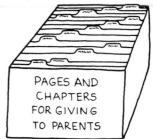

PAGES AND CHAPTERS FOR GIVING TO PARENTS

In Project PROJIMO in Mexico, the village rehabilitation team keeps a big file box with copies of the different pages and chapters that they have found most useful for giving to families. (In fact, the exercise sheets at the end of Chapter 42 were originally prepared separately to give to families. Later, we decided to include them in this book.)

Suggestion: Keep a file of pages, chapters, and information sheets to give to families.

Marking the information that applies to the child

On any page or chapter that you give to parents, some of the information or suggestions will apply more than others to their child.

We suggest that you **circle the activities or suggestions that would be most helpful to the child in his present condition or level of development.** You could also put an "X" through anything that should not be done or might be harmful for that child.

Here is an example. If the child is spastic and beginning to sit, the first 3 activities on p. 307 can help her to improve balance and to develop controlled body movement. So circle these. The next 3 activities will still be too difficult and could increase *spasticity.* Put an "X" through these so the family does not do them.

DEVELOPMENT ACTIVITIES   **307**

To help your child gain balance sitting, first sit her on your knees facing you.

Hold her **loosely** so her body can adapt to leaning.

Slowly lift one knee to lean her gently to one side. Then the other, so that she learns to bend her body to stay seated.

Later, you can sit her facing out so that she can see what is going on around her.

You can do the same thing with the child sitting on a log.

As he gets better balance, move your hands down to his hips and then thighs, so that he depends less on your support.

Give him something to hold so that he learns to use his body and not his arms to keep his balance.

With an older child who has difficulty with balance, you can do the same thing on a 'tilt board'.

At first let her catch herself with her arms.

Later, see how long she can do it holding her hands together. Make it a game.

Or you can do the same on a large ball.

Tilt it to **one side and the other** and also **forward** and **back.**

Note: You can also do these exercises by sitting the child on a table and gently pushing him backward, sideways, and forward. But **it is better to tip what he is sitting on.**

Pushing him causes him to 'catch himself' from falling with his arms.

Tilting him causes him to use his body to keep his balance, which is a more advanced skill.

Making copies of pages can be costly. Or you may have to go a long way for them. Also, there will be times when you want to give a family written suggestions or drawings that you have not copied in advance.

Perhaps some of the children or young people who are at the village center, either for rehabilitation or as learners-and-workers, can help trace drawings from the book. If they have some artistic skill, they can make the drawings larger, or make the child in the drawing look like the child that they are to be used with.*

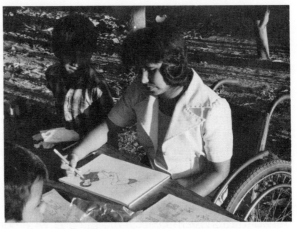

Minerva, a girl with polio who is working and learning at PROJIMO, helps adapt drawings from this book to the needs of specific children.

---

*Ideas for drawing and for copying drawings at larger size are in *Helping Health Workers Learn,* p. 12–1 to 12–21. (See p. 637.)

If someone prepares a set of large drawings in advance, perhaps a disabled child who visits the village center can trace the drawings of exercises he needs to do at home. Giving the child this responsibility from the start makes it more likely that he will do the exercises at home.

If you make your own 'hand out' sheets (instead of just copying pages of this book) you can use the local language and villagers' way of saying things. You can also adapt the drawings to the hair style and dress that people feel 'at home' with.

Whatever you do, try to keep both your language and drawings **simple** and **clear.** Avoid unfamiliar words.

———————•———————

Also, try to **think of ways of adapting exercises or activities to the local situation.**

For example, **suppose you live in a fishing village,** and want to make copies of a drawing showing an aid for strengthening the wrist. Instead of just copying a method like this from a book,

you might add a drawing like this one. This will encourage parents to think of ways to do exercises that involve their child in the life and action of their community.

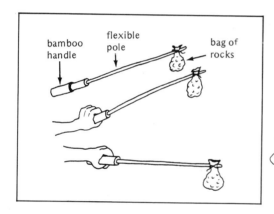

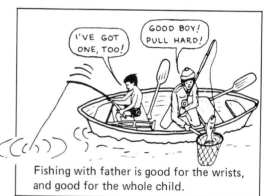

Fishing with father is good for the wrists, and good for the whole child.

Remember: Written pages and drawings can be a big help, but they should not be a substitute for teaching and showing. To help a family understand activities or exercises that are needed:

1. First show and explain.

2. Guide them in doing it until they do it right and understand why.

3. Then, give them the instruction sheet and explain the main points.

These steps are explained with examples and drawings on p. 382.

As much as you can, try *not* to use this book for giving exact instructions on how to do things. Instead, encourage everyone to use it as a source of ideas, in order to figure out better ways to help **their children** lead fuller lives and manage better **in their communities.**

REMEMBER . . .

One of the best ways to share information from this book is to:

1. **SHOW** other people how to do things.

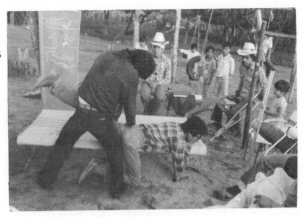

Village rehabilitation
workers and family members
learn in an outdoor class.
Here they practice a hip-
stretching exercise.
Behind them, drawings on
the blackboard show which
muscles are stretched.

2. Then help them **LEARN BY DOING** it themselves—under your guidance.

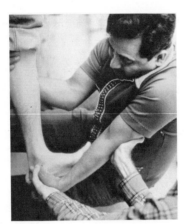

Teaching a village health
worker how to stretch a
tight heel cord (see p. 83.)

3. And to help them remember, give them a **DRAWING** or **INSTRUCTION SHEET**.

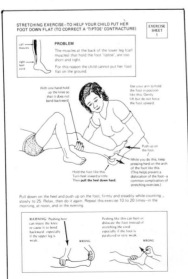

IMPORTANT: Try to help people
to understand not only **what** to
do, but also **why.** Perhaps you
can hold classes using information
from this book. Try to combine
hands-on practice with discussion
of **principles and reasons.**

CHAPTER 3

Prevention of Disabilities

Because this is a book on *'rehabilitation'*, it is mostly about children who are already disabled. However, preventing *disabilities* is also very important. For this reason, in most chapters on specific disabilities, we include suggestions for preventing them.

Notice that **we place the discussion of prevention at the end of each chapter,** not at the beginning. This is because people are usually not concerned about disability until someone they love becomes disabled. Then their first concern is to help that person. *After* we have helped a family to do something for their disabled child, we can interest them in ways to prevent disability in other members of the family and community.

We mention this because when health professionals design community programs, often they try to put prevention first—and find that people do not show much interest. However, when a group of parents comes together to help their disabled children, after their immediate needs are being met, they may work hard for disability prevention.

> **For a community program to be successful, start with what the people feel is important, and work from there.**

To prevent disabilities, we must understand the causes. In most parts of the world, **many causes of disability relate to poverty.** For example:

- **When mothers do not get enough to eat** during pregnancy, often their babies are born early or underweight. These babies are much more likely to have cerebral palsy, which is one of the most common severe disabilities. Also, some birth defects are related to poor nutrition during the first months of pregnancy.

- **When babies and young children do not get enough to eat,** they get infections more easily and more seriously. Diarrhea in a fat baby is usually a mild illness. But in a very thin, malnourished baby, diarrhea often leads to serious dehydration, high fever, and sometimes brain damage with fits or cerebral palsy.

- **Poor sanitation and crowded living conditions,** together with poor food, make diseases such as tuberculosis—and the severe disabilities it causes—much more common.

- **Lack of basic health and rehabilitation services** in poor communities makes disabilities more common and more severe. Often secondary disabilities develop that could be prevented with early care.

To prevent the disabilities that result from poverty, big changes are needed in our social order. There needs to be fairer distribution of land, resources, information, and power. Such changes will happen only when the poor find the courage to organize, to work together, and to demand their rights. **Disabled persons and their families can become leaders in this process.** Only through a more just society can we hope for a long-term, far-reaching answer to the prevention of disabilities caused by poverty.

Although the most complete prevention of disabilities related to poverty depends on social change, this will take time. However, more immediate actions at family, community, and national levels can help prevent some disabilities. For example,

- **Polio,** in certain situations, can be prevented through *vaccination.* (However, effective vaccination depends on much more than good vaccine. See the box.) ——————→

In places where vaccination is not available or not fully effective, families and communities can help to lower the chance of *paralysis* from polio by breast feeding their children as long as possible (see p. 74).

Why, since a good vaccine exists, is there still so much polio in so many countries?

EFFECTIVE VACCINATION DEPENDS ON MANY FACTORS:

TECHNICAL Production and supply of safe, effective, vaccine.

ECONOMIC (Cost of vaccine and of getting it to the children.) Leaders in poorer countries must decide that stopping polio is worth the expense.

MANAGEMENT Knowledge of needs, planning, transportation, and distribution of the vaccine.

KEEPING POLIO VACCINE FROZEN (In many countries, 1/3 of vaccines are spoiled by the time they reach the children.)

EDUCATION People must understand the value of vaccination and want to cooperate. Health workers must know how important it is to keep polio vaccine frozen.

POLITICAL Vaccination programs are most successful where the government fairly represents the people and has their full participation in country-wide vaccination campaigns.

ETHICAL (Honesty and good will) Doctors, health workers, and citizens must try to see that vaccine reaches *all* children. (In some countries, some doctors throw vaccines away and fill out false reports, and health inspectors do not care enough to try to stop what is happening.)

- **Brain damage** and **fits** can become less frequent if mothers and midwives take added **precautions during pregnancy** and childbirth, and if they vaccinate children against measles. (See p. 107.)

- Some **birth defects** and **mental retardation** can be prevented if mothers **avoid most medicines** during pregnancy, and spend the money they save on **food.**

- **Spinal cord injury** could be greatly reduced if fathers would spend on **education and community safety** what they now spend on **alcohol and guns.**

- **Leprosy** could mostly be prevented if people would **stop fearing and rejecting persons with leprosy.** By being more supportive and encouraging early home treatment, the community could help prevent the spread of leprosy, since persons being treated no longer spread it. (See p. 215.)

- **Blindness** in young children in some countries is caused by not eating enough foods with **vitamin A.** Again this relates to poverty. However, many people do not know that they can prevent this blindness by feeding their children dark green leafy vegetables, yellow fruits, or even certain weeds and wild fruit. Also, some kinds of **deafness** and **mental retardation** can be prevented by using **iodized salt** during pregnancy (see p. 276 and 282).

- **Disability caused by poisons in food, water, air, or workplace.** The recent, common, worldwide use of chemicals to kill insects and weeds has become a major health problem. Often villagers use these pesticides without any knowledge of their risks, or of the precautions they should take. As a result, many become paralyzed, blind, or disabled in other ways.

  To prevent these problems, people need to learn about the dangers, not only to themselves and their children but to animals, birds, land, and to the whole 'balance of nature'. Less dangerous ways to control pests give better results over time. Laws are also needed to prohibit the most dangerous products and to provide clear warnings.

- **Poisonous foods** in some areas are a major cause of disability. In parts of India, thousands of farm workers who are paid with a poisonous variety of lentils suffer paralysis from **'lathyrism'**. The poor know the danger but have nothing else to eat. Fair wages and less corruption are needed to correct this situation.

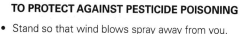

TO PROTECT AGAINST PESTICIDE POISONING

- Stand so that wind blows spray away from you.
- Wear protective clothing, covering the whole body.

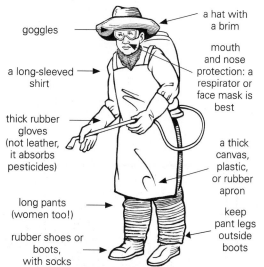

goggles

a hat with a brim

mouth and nose protection: a respirator or face mask is best

a long-sleeved shirt

thick rubber gloves (not leather, it absorbs pesticides)

a thick canvas, plastic, or rubber apron

long pants (women too!)

keep pant legs outside boots

rubber shoes or boots, with socks

- Wash whole body and change clothes immediately after spraying.
- Wash clothes after spraying.
- Do not let wash water get into drinking supply.
- Do not use spray containers for food or water.
- Do not let children play with spray containers.

CAUTION: Make sure that children, and women who are pregnant or breast feeding, stay away from all pesticides.

- **Fluoride poisoning** (fluorosis), mainly from drinking water, is a common cause of bone deformities (knock-knees) in parts of India and other places. Public health measures are needed to provide safe water. *

> The 4 biggest causes of 'crippling' in India, affecting over 2 million people, are reported to be polio, iodine deficiency, fluorosis, and lathyrism. **Given the political will, all could be completely prevented!**

- **Dangerous work conditions,** poisons in the air, and lack of basic safety measures result in many disabilities. These include burns, amputations, blindness, and back and head injuries. In some countries, the use of asbestos for roofs or walls in schools, work places, and homes causes disabling lung diseases. Strict public health measures and an informed, organized people are needed to bring improvements.

- **Certain dangerous medicines,** known to sometimes cause disabilities, are now prohibited in the countries that make them, but are still sold in other countries. For example, diarrhea medicines containing clioquinol caused thousands of cases of blindness and paralysis in Japan. (A good book discussing dangerous medicines in poor countries is *Bitter Pills* by Dianna Melrose. See p. 641.)

  The high cost, overuse, and misuse of medicines in general adds greatly to the amount of poverty and disability in the world today. Better education of both doctors and people, and more effective international laws are needed to bring about more sensible supply and use of medicines.

Note: Although too much fluoride is harmful, some is necessary for healthy bones and teeth. In some areas fluoride needs to be removed from drinking water; in other areas it needs to be added.

WHO SHOULD BE RESPONSIBLE FOR DISABILITY PREVENTION

Notice that many of the specific preventive measures we have discussed, just like the more general social measures, depend on increased awareness, community participation, and new ways of looking at things. These changes do not just happen. They require a process of education, organization, and struggle led by those who are most deeply concerned.

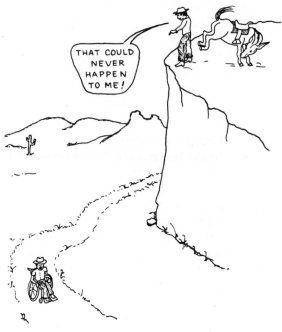

Most able-bodied persons are not very concerned about disability or trying to prevent it. Often people think, "Oh, that could never happen to me!"—until it does.

Those who are most concerned about disability are usually disabled persons themselves and their families. Based on this concern, they can become leaders and community educators for disability prevention.

Disability can affect everybody, and sometime in our lives it usually does.

They can do this in an informal, person-to-person way. For example,

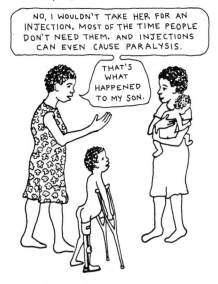

Or disabled children and families can join together to form prevention campaigns. In one village, mothers put on short plays to inform the whole community about the importance of breast feeding and vaccination. (See p. 74.) In Project PROJIMO, Mexico, disabled rehabilitation workers have helped to vaccinate children in remote mountain villages.

In PART 1 of this book, where we discuss different disabilities, we also include basic information on prevention. **We hope that those of you who use this book for children who are already disabled, will also work actively towards disability prevention.**

PREVENTING SECONDARY DISABILITIES

So far we have talked mainly about preventing original or 'primary' disabilities, such as polio or spinal cord injury. But the prevention of 'secondary' disabilities is also very important, and is one of the main concerns of rehabilitation.

By 'secondary' disabilities we mean further disabilities or complications that can appear after, and because of, the original disability.

For example, consider a child with polio or cerebral palsy who at first is unable to walk. She gradually loses the normal range-of-motion of joints in her legs. Shortened muscles, called *'contractures'*, keep her legs from straightening. This secondary disability may limit the child's ability to function or to walk even more than the original paralysis:

This child, after polio, gradually developed contractures in her

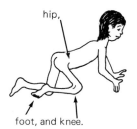

hip,

foot, and knee.

The contractures (not the original paralysis) kept her from being able to stand or walk.

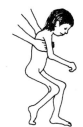

If the contractures had been prevented through early and continued range-of-motion exercises, the child would have been able to stand and walk.

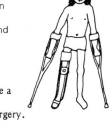

Most contractures can be corrected. But it may take a long time and a lot of expense—perhaps even surgery. It is far better to:
PREVENT CONTRACTURES BEFORE THEY START.

Because contractures develop as a common complication in many disabilities, we discuss them in a separate chapter (Chapter 8). Range-of-motion exercises to help prevent and correct contractures are described in Chapter 42. Use of plaster casts to correct contractures is described in Chapter 59.

Many other secondary disabilities will also develop unless preventive measures are taken. Some examples are **pressure sores** in children with spinal cord injury (see Chapter 24), **spinal curve** in a child with a weak back or with one leg shorter than the other (see Chapter 20), **head injuries** due to fits (see p. 235). Preventive measures for many other secondary disabilities are discussed in the chapters on the specific disabilities.

In several places we discuss problems or **disabilities that are commonly caused by medical treatment or orthopedic aids.** For example,

- The **medicine for fits,** phenytoin, produces serious swelling of the gums in some children. This can partly be prevented by brushing the teeth regularly. (See p. 238.)

- **Crutches** that press hard under the armpit can damage nerves and gradually paralyze the hands. Shorter crutches, or lower-arm crutches (like those shown above) prevent this problem. (See p. 393.)

- **Surgery** is sometimes done to remove contractures that actually help a child to move or function better. So worse difficulties result. The benefits or possible harm of surgery should be carefully evaluated **before** it is done. (See p. 530.)

- Some braces or aids that help a child at first, may later actually hold her back. (See p. 526 to 529.)

To prevent these mistakes, it is essential to **evaluate the needs of each child carefully, and repeat evaluations periodically.** We must take great care to prevent further disability caused by treatment.

> **The first responsibility of a rehabilitation worker or parent, like the healer, should be to:**
> **DO NO HARM**

In addition to secondary disabilities that are physical, others may be psychological or social (affecting the child's mind, behavior, or place in the community).

Some disabled children develop serious **behavior problems.** This is often because they find their bad behavior brings them more attention and 'rewards' than their good behavior. Chapter 40 discusses ways that parents can help prevent tantrums and bad behavior in disabled children.

The biggest secondary handicap for many disabled children (and adults) usually comes from the lack of understanding and acceptance by other people. PART 2 of this book talks about how the community can be involved in taking a more active, supportive role in relating to the disabled and helping them to meet their needs. In PART 2 we also discuss what disabled persons and their families can do, in the community, to promote better understanding and prevent disability from becoming a serious handicap.

Prevention of secondary disability is a basic part of rehabilitation.

THE NEED FOR MORE SENSIBLE AND LIMITED USE OF INJECTIONS

DANGER!

The overuse and misuse of medicines in the world today has become a major cause of health problems and disabilities. This is partly because medicines are so often prescribed or given wrongly (for example, certain medicines taken in pregnancy can cause birth defects, see p. 119). And it is partly because both poor families and poor nations spend a great deal of money on overpriced, unnecessary, or dangerous medicines. The money could be better spent on things that protect their health—such as food, vaccinations, better water, and more appropriate education. Some medicines, of course, when correctly used are of great importance to health. But most are not. **Of the 30,000 medicinal products sold in most countries, the World Health Organization says that only about 250 are needed.**

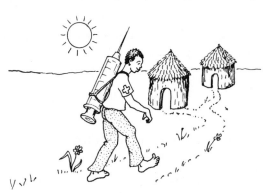
In most of the world, doctors, health workers, and the people make giving and getting injections too big a part of health care.

In many countries, **injections have become the 'modern magic'.** People demand them because doctors and health workers often prescribe them, and doctors and health workers prescribe them too often because people demand them.

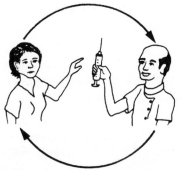
I HAVE FAITH IN INJECTIONS BECAUSE MY DOCTOR PRESCRIBES THEM.

I PRESCRIBE SO MANY INJECTIONS BECAUSE MY PATIENTS HAVE FAITH IN THEM.

HOW INJECTIONS DISABLE CHILDREN

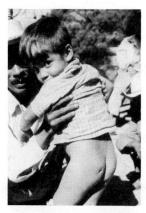
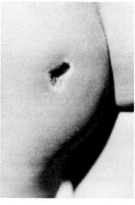

This child was injected with a needle that was not sterile (clean). The dirty needle caused an infected abscess (pocket of pus) that burst. The child had been injected for a cold. It would have been better to give him no medicine at all.

When used correctly, certain injected medicines, like some vaccinations, are important to protect a child's health and prevent disability. However, giving injections with an unclean needle or syringe is a common cause of infection and can pass the germs that cause **HIV/ AIDS** and other serious diseases like **hepatitis** (see *Where There Is No Doctor*, pages 399 to 401, and 172).

Dirty needles and syringes can also cause infections that lead to **paralysis** or **spinal cord injury** (see the story on p. 192), or death. **A needle or syringe must never be used to inject more than one person without first disinfecting it again.**

Also, some injected medicines can cause **dangerous allergic reactions, poisoning, and deafness.** And the overuse of **injectable hormones** to speed up childbirth and 'give force' to the mother is a major cause of babies born with **brain damage.**

How to clean and disinfect injection needles and syringes

Most syringes and needles are disposable (are used only once) and come in sterile packages. Some of them can be taken apart, boiled, and reused several times before they fall apart. We do not recommend this, but if you must reuse them, follow these instructions first:

1. Put on a pair of heavy gloves to protect your hands.

2. Draw clean water (or even better, mix 1 part bleach with 7 parts water) up through the needle into the syringe barrel. **If you use bleach, make a fresh solution each day or it will not be strong enough to kill germs anymore.**

3. Squirt out the water or bleach. Do this several times.

4. If you have used bleach, rinse everything several times with clean water.

5. Take apart the syringe and needle and boil them in water for 20 minutes (as long as it takes to cook rice), or steam them for 20 minutes.

   Note: **For both boiling and steaming, start counting the 20 minutes after the water is fully boiling.**

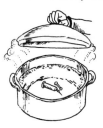

To boil them, make sure water covers everything in the pot the entire time. If possible, put a lid on the pot.

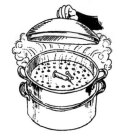

To steam them, you need a steamer pot with a lid (a pot with holes in it that fits inside another pot). Use enough water to keep steam coming out the side of the lid for 20 minutes.

Storing your needles and syringes

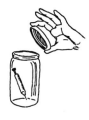

When the needle and syringe have dried, store them carefully in a dry container, like a glass jar with a screw-on lid. Make sure these have also first been cleaned and disinfected. If you are not able to store them this way, boil or steam the needle and syringe again before use.

The **worldwide epidemic of unnecessary injections** each year sickens, kills, or disables millions of persons, especially children. An international campaign is needed to re-educate doctors, nurses, health workers, traditional healers (many of whom also now overuse injections), and the people themselves.

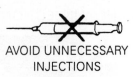

AVOID UNNECESSARY
INJECTIONS

Combatting misuse and overuse of medicines is as important to health as vaccination, clean water, or the correct use of latrines. Health workers, school teachers, and community organizers should all work to help people **weigh the possible risks and benefits** of using any medication. For ideas on teaching about the danger of unnecessary injections, see *Helping Health Workers Learn*, Chapters 18, 19, and 27.

WAR AS A CAUSE OF CHILD DISABILITY

Armed violence is increasing and has become more deadly. In today's wars, most of the people killed or injured are women and children—not soldiers. And the weapons used in wars, like landmines, cluster bombs, and chemical agents, have become even more dangerous and threatening to everyone.

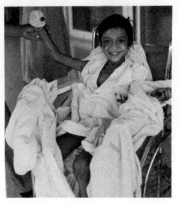

In the past decade, millions of children have died in wars, and at least 6 million have been injured or disabled. Children, especially boys, are sometimes forced to fight as soldiers, and many are either killed or injured and disabled. Girls are sometimes also forced to be "sex-slaves" for soldiers. Not only are these children disabled physically, but their mental health is also badly affected.

Nicaraguan child disabled by a 'Contra' bomb. The Contras were rebel troops supported by the US Government to overthrow the popular government in Nicaragua. (Photo by Marc Krizack, *Links*.)

The increased poverty and 'hard times' caused by war also lead to many disabilities. There are more than 20 million refugees around the world, many living under dangerous and unhealthy conditions. 170 million children in poor countries are underweight, mainly from lack of food. Millions are homeless. Yet world leaders continue to spend billions of dollars on war and arms.

> Terrorism is too often fought with terrorism.
>
> **"AN EYE FOR AN EYE WILL MAKE THE WHOLE WORLD BLIND."** –Mahatma Gandhi

War, terrorism, and torture have become tools of the powerful for economic, political and social control. When the peoples of poor countries dare to get rid of their dictators and form popular governments that work toward fairer distribution, the rich, powerful countries often try to destroy those new governments. They pay for terrorism, long wars, and the destruction of schools, health centers, and production. The result is still more poverty, disease, and disability.

To help change this situation, we disabled persons of the world must join with all who are disadvantaged or treated unfairly, to struggle for a new, more truly human, world order.

Land-mines and cluster bombs cause more disabilities in the world today than anything else does, especially among children. Thousands of children are killed or severely injured by them each year—while they are carrying out their daily work activities or simply playing. Often after an explosion, the child's leg has to be amputated. But only about 1 of every 4 children injured gets a new leg, because they are usually expensive or difficult to get. A group in India has found a way to make a good quality, low-cost, artificial leg called the Mukti Limb (see page 642).

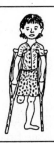

Examining and Evaluating the Disabled Child

To decide what kind of special help, if any, a disabled child may need, first we need to learn as much as we can about the child. Although we may be concerned about her difficulties, we must always try to **look at the whole child.** Remember that:

> **A child's** *abilities* **are more important than her** *disabilities.*

The aim of *rehabilitation* is to help the child to *function* better at home and in the community. So when you examine a child, try to **relate all your observations to what the child can do, cannot do, and might be able to do.**

What a child is and does depends partly on other persons. So we must also look at the child's abilities and difficulties in relation to her home, her family, and her village or neighborhood.

LOOK FIRST AT MY STRENGTHS, NOT AT MY WEAKNESSES

To evaluate a child's needs, try to answer these questions:

- **What can the child do and not do?** How does this compare with other children the same age in your community?

- What **problems** does the child have? How and when did they begin? Are they getting better, worse, or are they the same?

- In what ways are the child's **body, mind, senses, or behavior** affected? **How does each specific problem affect what she does?**

- What **secondary problems** are developing? (Problems that result after and because of the original problem.)

- What is the **home situation** like? What are the **resources and limitations within the family and community** that may increase or hold back the child's possibilities?

- In what way has the child **adjusted to her disability,** or learned to manage?

To find the answers to these questions, a health or rehabilitation worker needs to do 3 things:

1. **Observe the child** carefully—including her interaction with the family and with other persons.

2. **Take a 'history'.** Ask the parents and child (if old enough) for all information they can provide. Obtain medical records if possible.

3. **Examine the child** to find out how well and in what way different parts of her body and mind work, how developed they are, and how much they affect her strengths, weaknesses or problems.

BE SURE TO LOOK AT THE WHOLE CHILD—NOT JUST THE DISABILITY

Observation of the child can begin from the first moment the health worker or rehabilitation worker sees the child and her family. It can begin in the waiting area of a village center, the home, or the street, and should continue through the history-taking, examination, and follow-up visits. Therefore, we do not discuss 'observation' separately, but include it with these other areas.

It is usually best to **ask questions BEFORE beginning to examine the child**—so that we have a better idea what to look for. Therefore, we will discuss history-taking and then examination. But first a word about keeping records.

RECORD KEEPING

For a village rehabilitation worker who helps many children, writing notes or records can be important for following their progress. Also, parents of a disabled child may find that keeping simple records gives them a better sense of how their child is doing.

Six sample RECORD SHEETS are on pages 37 to 41, 50, 292, and 293. You can use these as a guide for getting and recording basic information. But you will want to follow with more detailed questions and examination, depending on what you find.

Sample RECORD SHEETS included in this book	RECORD SHEET number	page
Child history	1	37 and 38
Physical examination	2	39
Tests of nervous system	3	40
Factors affecting child development	4	41
Evaluation of progress	5	50
Child development chart	6	292 and 293

Sheets 1 and 2 will be useful for most disabled children. Sheets 3, 4, and 6 are for children who may have brain damage or seem slow for their age. Sheet 5 is a simple form for evaluating the progress of children 5 years old or older.

HISTORY TAKING

On pages 37 and 38 you will find a record sheet for taking a child's history. You can use it as a guide for the kinds of questions it is important to ask. (Of course, some of the questions will apply more to some children than others, so ask only where the information might be helpful.)

When asking questions, we rehabilitation workers must always remember that **parents and family are the only real 'experts' on their child.** They know what she can and cannot do, what she likes and does not like, in what ways she manages well, and where she has difficulties.

However, sometimes part of the parents' knowledge is hidden. They may not have put all the pieces of knowledge together to form a clear picture of the child's needs and possibilities. The suggestions in this chapter, and the questions on the RECORD SHEETS, may help both rehabilitation workers and parents to form a clearer picture of their child's needs and possibilities.

> **Rehabilitation workers and parents can work together to figure out the child's needs.**

EXAMINING THE DISABLED CHILD

After finding out what we can by asking questions, our next step is to examine the child. In as friendly a way as possible, we carefully observe or test what parts of the child work well, what parts work poorly, and how this affects the child's ability to do things and respond to the world around him.

CAUTION: Although we sometimes examine separately different aspects of the child's body and mind, our main purpose is **to find out how well the child's body and mind work together as a whole: what can the child do and not do, and why?** This information helps us decide how to help the child to do things better.

In examination of a disabled child, we may check on many things:

- **The senses:** How well does the child see? hear? feel?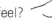

- **Movement:** How well does the child move or control her movements?

- **Form and structure:** How well formed, deformed, or damaged are different parts of the body: the joints, 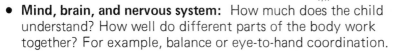 the backbone, and skin?

- **Mind, brain, and nervous system:** How much does the child understand? How well do different parts of the body work together? For example, balance or eye-to-hand coordination.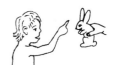

- **Developmental level:** How well does the child do things, compared to other local children her age?

In addition, a ***complete*** physical examination would include checking the health of **systems inside the body.** Although this part of the examination, if needed, is usually done by health workers, rehabilitation workers need to know that with certain disabilities inner body systems may also be affected. Depending on the disability, these may include:

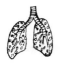 the breathing system (respiratory system)

 the body's cleaning system (urinary tract)

 the heart and blood system (circulation system)

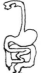 the food processing system (digestive system)

Rehabilitation workers need to work in close cooperation with health workers.

A detailed examination of *all* a child's parts and functions could take hours or days. Fortunately, in most children this is not necessary. Instead, **start by observing the child in a general way.** Based on the questions you have already asked and your general observations, try to **find anything that seems unusual or not quite right.** Then **examine in detail any body parts or functions that might relate to the disability.**

Part of the art of examining a child is KNOWING WHEN TO STOP. It is important to check everything that might help us understand the child's needs. But it is equally important to win the child's confidence and friendship. Too much examining and testing can push any child to the point of fear and anger. Some children reach their limit long before others. So we must learn how much each child can take—and try to examine the child in ways that she accepts.

Some children require a much more complete examination than others. For example:

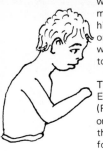

Juan lost one hand in an accident 2 years ago, but otherwise seems normal. Probably he will need little or no physical examination other than to see how he uses his arms, stump, and hand. You will also want to check how much he can do with his other hand, with only his stump, and when using both together.

The Physical Examination Form (RECORD SHEET 2 on p. 39) is probably the only examination form you need to fill out.

However, it would be wise to learn about how Juan's family and others treat him now, and how he feels about himself and his ability to do things. Does he keep his stump hidden when he is with strangers? With family members? What are his hopes and fears? You can write this information on the back of the form.

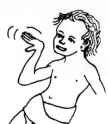

Ana is 2 years old and still does not sit by herself. She has strange uncontrolled movements. She does not play with toys or respond much to her parents.

Ana seems to have many problems.

We will need to check:

- how well she sees and hears.
- how strong, weak, or stiff different parts of her body are.
- in what ways her development is slow (what she can do and not do).
- how much she understands.
- signs of brain damage, and how severe.
- her sense of balance and position.
- what positioning or support gives her better control and function.

It may take weeks or months of repeated examining and testing to figure out all of Ana's difficulties, and how to best help her to function better. It could be a mistake to try to do all the needed examining at one time.

To record all the useful information on a child like Ana, you will find RECORD SHEETS 1, 2, 3, 4, and 6 helpful.

Examining techniques: Winning the child's confidence

Depending on how you go about it, the physical examination can help you become a child's friend or turn you into his enemy. Here are a few suggestions:

- **Dress as one of the people,** not as a professional. White uniforms often scare a child—especially if at some time he was injected by a nurse or doctor.

- Before starting the examination, **take an interest in the child as a person.** Speak to him in a gentle, friendly way. Help him relax. Touch him in ways that show you are a friend.

- Approach the child from the same height, not from above. (Try to have your head at the same level as his.)

- Start the examination with the child sitting or lying **on mother's lap, on the floor, or wherever he feels most safe and comfortable.**

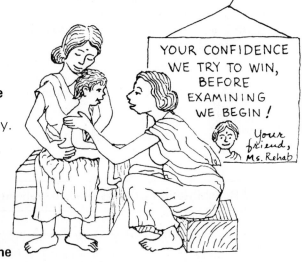

YOUR CONFIDENCE WE TRY TO WIN, BEFORE EXAMINING WE BEGIN!

Your friend, Ms. Rehab

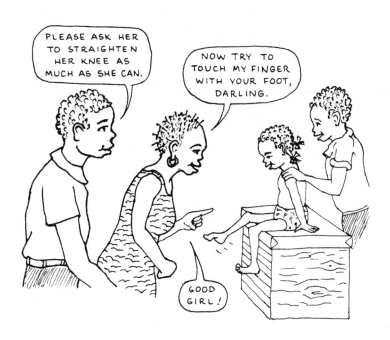

- If the child seems nervous about a stranger touching or examining her, **have the parent do as much of it for you as possible.** This will let the mother know that you respect and want to include her. And she may learn more.

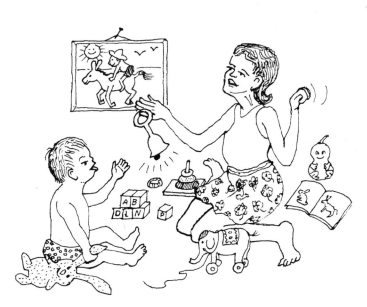

- Make the waiting area and place where you do the examining as **pleasant and as much like home** as you can. Have lots of toys, from very simple to complex, where the children can choose and play with them. By watching **if, how, for how long, with what, and with whom** a child plays, you can learn a lot about what a child can and cannot do, his level of physical and mental development, the types of problems he has, and the ways he has (or has not yet) adapted to them.

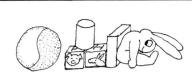 Watching how a child plays— by herself, with people, and with toys—is an essential part of evaluating the child.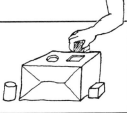

- Try to **make the examination interesting and fun** for the child. Turn it into a game whenever possible. For example:

  When you want to test a child's 'eye-to-hand coordination' (for possible balance problems or brain damage) you might make a game out of having the child touch the nose of a doll. Or have her turn on a flashlight (torch) by pushing its button

  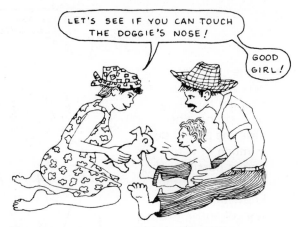

  Also, when he begins to get restless, stop examining for a while and play with him, or let him rest.

 It is best to examine a child when he is *well-rested, well-fed,* **and in a** *'good mood'*—**and when you are, too.** (We know this will not always be possible.)

- When a child is weaker or has less control on one side than the other, **first test the stronger side,**   **and then the weaker side.**

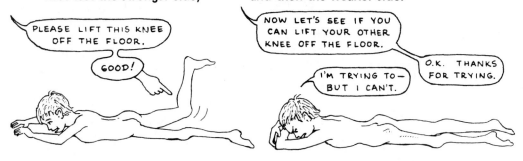

By testing the good side first, you start by giving the child encouragement with what he can do well. Also, if the child does not move the weaker side, you will know it is because he cannot, and not because he does not understand or is not trying.

- As you examine the child, **give her lots of praise and encouragement.** When she tries to do something for you and cannot, praise her warmly for trying.

  Ask her to **do things she can do well and not just the things she finds difficult,** so that she gains a stronger sense of success.

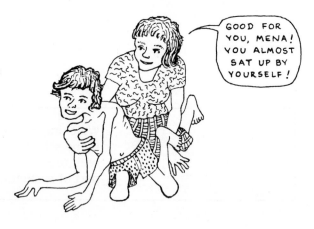

TESTING RANGE OF MOTION OF JOINTS AND STRENGTH OF MUSCLES

Children who have disabilities that affect how they move often have **some muscles that are weak or** *'paralyzed'*. As a result, they often do not move parts of their bodies as much as is normal.

Loss of strength and active movement may in time lead to a stiffening of joints or shortening of muscles (*contractures,* **see Chapter 8**). As a result, **the affected part can no longer be moved through its complete, normal range of motion.**

ACTIVE MOVEMENT | PASSIVE MOVEMENT

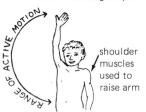

Normally the shoulder muscles can raise the arm until it is straight up.

shoulder muscles used to raise arm

Lifting the arm like this with the arm's own muscles is called **ACTIVE MOTION.**

When the shoulder muscles are paralyzed, the child can no longer actively lift his arm.

shoulder muscles small and weak

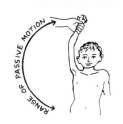

REDUCED RANGE OF ACTIVE MOTION

At first the paralyzed arm can be lifted straight up with help. This is called **PASSIVE MOTION.**

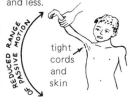

Unless the normal range of motion is kept through daily exercises, the passive range of motion will steadily become less and less.

tight cords and skin

Now the arm cannot be raised straight up, even with help.

In the physical examination of a child with any weakness or paralysis of muscles, or joint pain, or scarring from injuries or burns, it is a good idea to **test and record both RANGE OF MOTION and MUSCLE STRENGTH of all parts of the body that might have contractures or be affected.** There are 2 reasons for this:

- Knowing which parts of the body have contractures or are weak, and how much, can help us to understand why a child moves or limps as she does. This **helps us to decide what activities, exercises, braces, or other measures may be useful.**

- Keeping accurate records of changes in muscle strength and range of motion can help tell us if certain problems are getting better or worse. Regular testing therefore **helps us evaluate how well exercises, braces, casts, or other measures are working,** and whether the child's condition is improving, and how quickly.

For testing range of motion and muscle strength, it helps to first know what is normal. You can practice testing non-disabled, active persons. They should be of the *same ages* as the disabled children you will test. Age matters because babies are usually weaker and have much more flexible joints than older children. For example:

A baby's back and hips bend so much he can lie across his straight legs.

A young child bends less but can usually touch his toes with his legs straight.

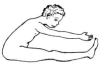

Around 11 to 14 it is harder to touch toes. His legs grow faster and become longer than his upper body.

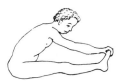

Later, upper body growth catches up with legs. He can again touch toes more easily.

In different children (and sometimes in the same child) you may need to check range of motion and strength in the hips, knees, ankles, feet, toes, shoulders, elbows, wrists, hands, fingers, back, shoulder blades, neck, and jaw. Some joints have 6 or more movements to test: bending, straightening, opening, closing, twisting in, and twisting out. See, for example, the different hip movements (range-of-motion exercises) on p. 380 in Chapter 42.

To test both 'range of motion' and 'strength', first check 'range of motion'. Then you will know that when a child cannot straighten a joint, it is not just because of weakness.

Range-of-motion testing: **Example:**

Knee

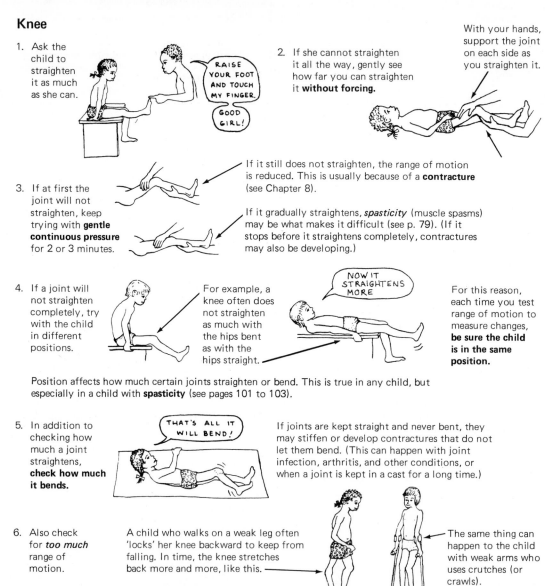

1. Ask the child to straighten it as much as she can.

RAISE YOUR FOOT AND TOUCH MY FINGER. GOOD GIRL!

2. If she cannot straighten it all the way, gently see how far you can straighten it **without forcing.**

With your hands, support the joint on each side as you straighten it.

3. If at first the joint will not straighten, keep trying with **gentle continuous pressure** for 2 or 3 minutes.

If it still does not straighten, the range of motion is reduced. This is usually because of a **contracture** (see Chapter 8).

If it gradually straightens, *spasticity* (muscle spasms) may be what makes it difficult (see p. 79). (If it stops before it straightens completely, contractures may also be developing.)

4. If a joint will not straighten completely, try with the child in different positions.

For example, a knee often does not straighten as much with the hips bent as with the hips straight.

NOW IT STRAIGHTENS MORE

For this reason, each time you test range of motion to measure changes, **be sure the child is in the same position.**

Position affects how much certain joints straighten or bend. This is true in any child, but especially in a child with **spasticity** (see pages 101 to 103).

5. In addition to checking how much a joint straightens, **check how much it bends.**

THAT'S ALL IT WILL BEND!

If joints are kept straight and never bent, they may stiffen or develop contractures that do not let them bend. (This can happen with joint infection, arthritis, and other conditions, or when a joint is kept in a cast for a long time.)

6. Also check for *too much* range of motion.

A child who walks on a weak leg often 'locks' her knee backward to keep from falling. In time, the knee stretches back more and more, like this.

The same thing can happen to the child with weak arms who uses crutches (or crawls).

Usually the best positions for checking range of motion are the same as those for doing range-of-motion and stretching exercises. These are shown in Chapter 42.

For methods of measuring and recording range of motion, see Chapter 5.

Precautions when testing for contractures

Testing range of motion of the **ankles, knees,** and **hips** is important for evaluating many disabled children. We have already discussed knees. Here are a few precautions when testing for contractures of ankles and hips.

Ankle

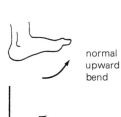

normal
upward
bend

Test the range of motion with the knee as straight as it will go.

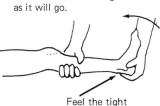

Feel the tight heel *cord* here.

With the knee bent, the foot will usually bend up more. But for walking, we need to know how far it bends with the knee straight.

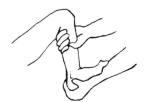

Note: To check ankle range of motion in a child with spasticity:

With his body and knee straight, it may be hard to bend the ankle.

So first bend his neck, body, and knees and then slowly bend up the ankle.

Then slowly straighten his knee while keeping the ankle bent.

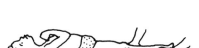
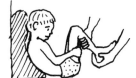
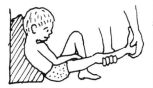

Other precautions for testing ankle range of motion are on p. 383.

(CP)

Hip

To check how far the hip joint straightens, have the child hold his other knee to his chest, like this, so that his lower back is flat against the table. If his thigh will not lower to the table without the back lifting, he has a bent-hip contracture. (See p. 79.)

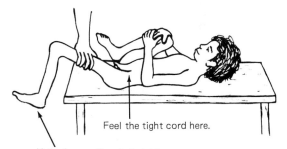

Feel the tight cord here.

If the knee will not straighten, test him with his leg over the edge of a table.

CAUTION The hips will often straighten more at an angle to the body. So be sure to lower the leg in a straight line with the body, or you can miss contractures that need to be corrected before the child can walk.

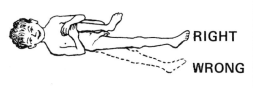

RIGHT

WRONG

Muscle testing

Muscle strength can be anywhere between *normal* and *zero.* Test it like this:

If the child can lift the weight of leg all the way, press down on it, to check if she can hold up as much weight as is normal for a girl her age. If she can, her strength is NORMAL.

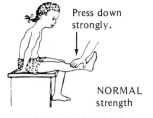 Press down strongly.

NORMAL strength

If she can hold **some extra weight,** but not as much as is normal, she rates GOOD.

Press down lightly.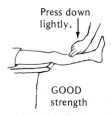

GOOD strength

If she can just hold up the weight of her leg, but no added weight, she rates FAIR.

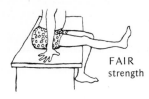

FAIR strength

If she cannot hold up the weight of her leg, have her lie on her side and try to straighten it. If she can, she rates POOR.

POOR strength

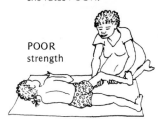

If she cannot straighten her knee at all, put your hand over the muscles as she tries to straighten it. If you can feel her muscles tighten, rate her TRACE.

Muscles move, but not leg:

TRY AS HARD AS YOU CAN TO STRAIGHTEN YOUR LEG.

TRACE strength

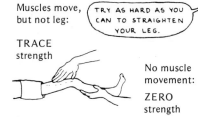

No muscle movement:
ZERO strength

Test the strength of all muscles that might be affected. Here are some of the **muscle tests that are most useful** for figuring out the difficulties and needs of different children.

> *Note:* These tests are simple and mostly test the strength of groups of muscles. *Physical therapists* know ways to test for strength of individual muscles.

Ankle and Foot

If the child can walk, see if she can stand and walk on her heels and her toes.

DOWN 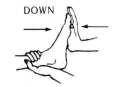 UP   BEND IN  BEND OUT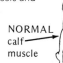

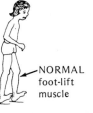

NORMAL calf muscle — NORMAL foot-lift muscle

Note: Sometimes when the muscles that normally lift the feet are weak, the child uses his toe-lifting muscles to lift his foot.

If he lifts his foot with his toes bent up, like this,

see if he can lift it with his toes bent down, like this.

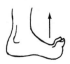 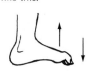

Also notice if the foot tips or pulls more to one side. This may show 'muscle imbalance'. (See p. 78.)

EXAMPLES OF REASONS FOR TESTING

1. If strength to lift up the foot is WEAK and strength to push down is STRONG, tiptoe contractures may develop—unless steps are taken to prevent them. (See p. 383.)

2. An ankle with POOR or very uneven strength may be helped by an ankle brace. But if strength is FAIR, exercise may strengthen it— and a brace may weaken it more!

3. Lifting the foot with only the toe muscles may lead to a high-arch deformity.

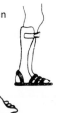

To learn about which muscles move body parts in different ways, as you test muscle strength, feel which muscles and cords tighten.

Knee

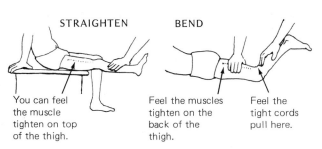

STRAIGHTEN   BEND

You can feel the muscle tighten on top of the thigh.

Feel the muscles tighten on the back of the thigh.

Feel the tight cords pull here.

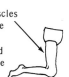

EXAMPLES OF REASONS FOR TESTING

1. POOR or NO strength for straightening knee may mean an above-knee brace is needed.

2. Stronger muscles in back of the thigh than in front can lead to a bent-knee contracture.

Hips

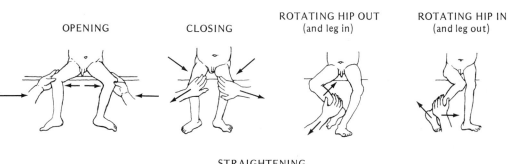

OPENING   CLOSING   ROTATING HIP OUT (and leg in)   ROTATING HIP IN (and leg out)

STRAIGHTENING

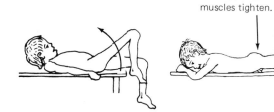

BENDING

Feel the butt muscles tighten.

If the hip has contractures, test with legs off end of table.

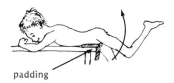

padding

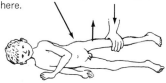

SIDEWAYS LIFT

Feel the side-of-hip muscles tighten here.

Note: Weak hip muscles sometimes lead to **dislocation** of the hip. Be sure to check for this, too. (See p. 155.)

Testing side-of-hip muscles is important for evaluating why a child limps or whether a hip-band may be needed on a long-leg brace.

TEST FOR WEAK SIDE-OF-HIP MUSCLES IN THE CHILD WHO CAN STAND

Have the child *stand on the weaker leg.*

NORMAL

The child stands straight. The hip tilts up on the lifted leg.

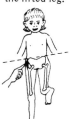

NOT NORMAL

The hip tilts down on the lifted side.

Or the child shifts his whole weight so it balances over the weak hip.

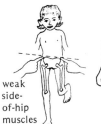

weak side-of-hip muscles

This child dips to the side on each step of the weak leg.

(This is often seen with polio.)

Note: Dipping to one side when walking is caused more by weak side-of-hip muscles than by a shorter leg. But a shorter leg can make dipping worse.

Stomach and Back

To find out how strong the stomach muscles are, see if the child can do 'sit ups' (or at least raise his head and chest).

To test the back muscles, see if he can bend backward like this.

Sitting up with knees bent uses (and tests) mainly the stomach muscles. Feel stomach muscles tighten.

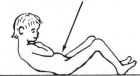

Sitting up with knees straight uses the hip-bending muscles and stomach muscles.

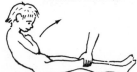

Feel the muscles tighten on either side of the backbone. Notice if they look and feel the same or if one side seems stronger.

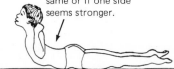

You can check a child's **trunk control** and **strength of stomach, back, and side muscles** like this. Have him hold his body upright over his hips, then lean forward and back, and side to side, and twist his body.

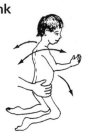

If a child's stomach and back muscles are weak, he may need braces with a body support—or a wheelchair.

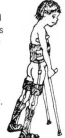

IMPORTANT: Be sure to check for **curvature of the spine**—especially in children with muscle imbalance or weakness of the *trunk*.

Shoulders, Arms, and Hands

When a child's legs are severely paralyzed but she has FAIR or better trunk strength, she may be able to walk with crutches *if* her shoulders, arms, and hands are strong enough.

Therefore, an important test is this.

Can she lift her butt off the seat like this?

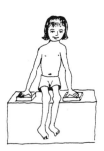

If she can, she has a good chance for walking with crutches.

If she cannot lift herself, check the strength in her shoulders and arms:

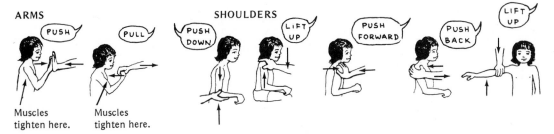

ARMS
PUSH
PULL
Muscles tighten here. Muscles tighten here.

SHOULDERS
PUSH DOWN
LIFT UP
PUSH FORWARD
PUSH BACK
LIFT UP

If the shoulder pushes down strongly but her elbow-straightening muscles are weak, she may be able to use a crutch with an elbow support.

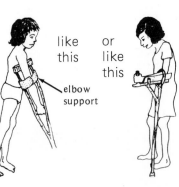

like this

or like this

elbow support

Or, if her elbow range of motion is normal, she may learn to 'lock' her elbow back like this. However, this can lead to elbow problems.

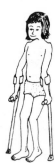

You may want to make a chart something like this and hang it in your examining area, as a reminder.

In muscle testing, it is especially important to note the difference between FAIR and POOR.

This is because FAIR is often strong enough to be fairly useful (for standing, walking, or lifting arm to eat). POOR is usually too weak to be of much use.

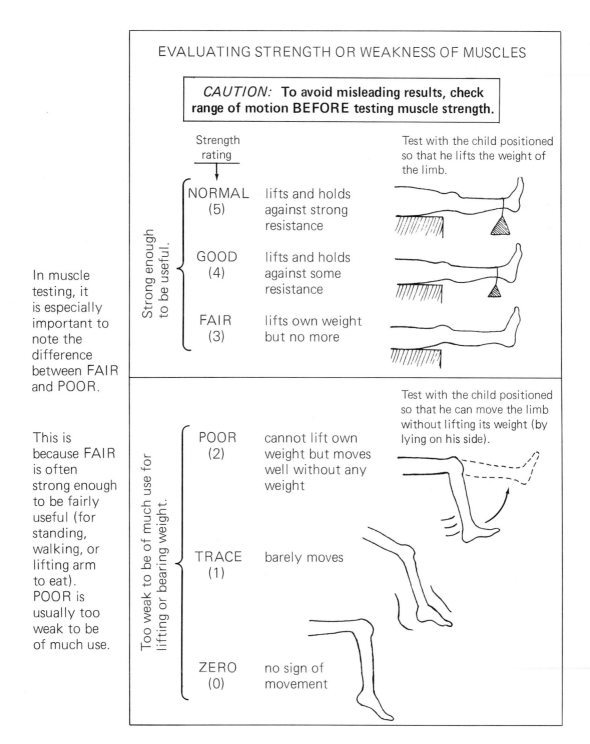

EVALUATING STRENGTH OR WEAKNESS OF MUSCLES

CAUTION: **To avoid misleading results, check range of motion BEFORE testing muscle strength.**

Strength rating

Strong enough to be useful.

Test with the child positioned so that he lifts the weight of the limb.

NORMAL (5) — lifts and holds against strong resistance

GOOD (4) — lifts and holds against some resistance

FAIR (3) — lifts own weight but no more

Too weak to be of much use for lifting or bearing weight.

Test with the child positioned so that he can move the limb without lifting its weight (by lying on his side).

POOR (2) — cannot lift own weight but moves well without any weight

TRACE (1) — barely moves

ZERO (0) — no sign of movement

Sometimes with exercise POOR muscles can be strengthened to FAIR; this can greatly increase their usefulness. It is much less common for a TRACE muscle to increase to a useful strength (FAIR), no matter how much it is exercised. (However, if muscle weakness is due to lack of use, as in severe arthritis, rather than to paralysis, a POOR muscle can sometimes be strengthened with exercise to GOOD or even NORMAL. Also, in very early stages of recovery from polio or other causes of weakness, POOR or TRACE strength sometimes returns to FAIR or better.)

Other things to check in a physical examination

Difference in leg length. When one leg is weaker, it usually grows slower, and becomes shorter than the other leg. An extra thick sole on the sandal might help the child stand straighter, limp less, and avoid curving of the spine. A short leg may also be a sign of a dislocated hip. So it helps to check for, and to measure, difference in leg length. (For tests, see p. 155 and 156.)

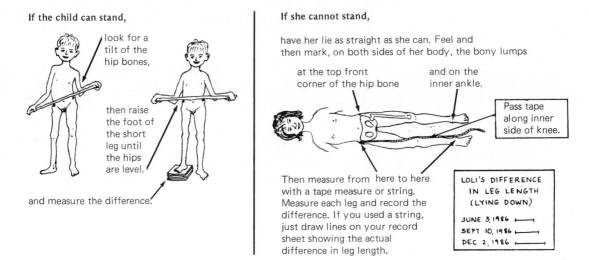

If the child can stand,

look for a tilt of the hip bones,

then raise the foot of the short leg until the hips are level.

and measure the difference.

If she cannot stand,

have her lie as straight as she can. Feel and then mark, on both sides of her body, the bony lumps

at the top front corner of the hip bone

and on the inner ankle.

Pass tape along inner side of knee.

Then measure from here to here with a tape measure or string. Measure each leg and record the difference. If you used a string, just draw lines on your record sheet showing the actual difference in leg length.

LOLI'S DIFFERENCE IN LEG LENGTH (LYING DOWN)

JUNE 3, 1986
SEPT 10, 1986
DEC 2, 1986

Curve of the spine

Especially when one leg is shorter or there are signs of muscle imbalance in the stomach or back, be sure to check for abnormal curve of the spine (back bone). The 3 main types of spinal curve (which may occur separately or in combination) are:

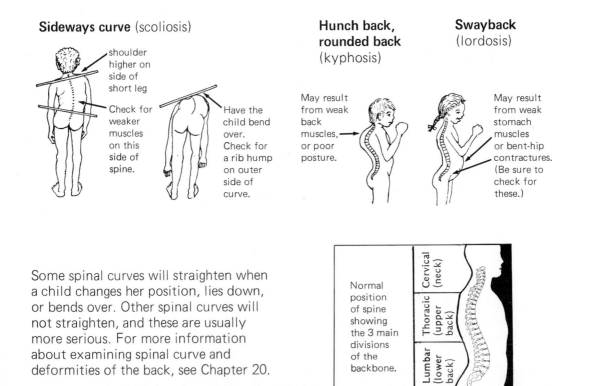

Sideways curve (scoliosis)

shoulder higher on side of short leg

Check for weaker muscles on this side of spine.

Have the child bend over. Check for a rib hump on outer side of curve.

Hunch back, rounded back (kyphosis)

May result from weak back muscles, or poor posture.

Swayback (lordosis)

May result from weak stomach muscles or bent-hip contractures. (Be sure to check for these.)

Some spinal curves will straighten when a child changes her position, lies down, or bends over. Other spinal curves will not straighten, and these are usually more serious. For more information about examining spinal curve and deformities of the back, see Chapter 20.

Normal position of spine showing the 3 main divisions of the backbone.

Cervical (neck)

Thoracic (upper back)

Lumbar (lower back)

EXAMINING THE NERVOUS SYSTEM

Sometimes physical disability results from problems in the muscles, bones, or joints themselves. But often it comes from a problem in, or damage to, the nervous system.

Depending on what part of the nervous system is affected, the disability will have different patterns.

For example, **polio** affects only certain **action nerves** at points in the spinal cord (or brain stem). It therefore affects movement. It never affects sensory *nerves,* so sight, hearing, and feeling stay normal. (See Chapter 7.)

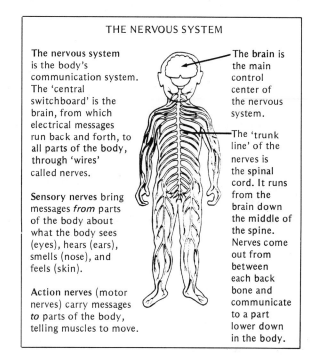

THE NERVOUS SYSTEM

The nervous system is the body's communication system. The 'central switchboard' is the brain, from which electrical messages run back and forth, to all parts of the body, through 'wires' called nerves.

Sensory nerves bring messages *from* parts of the body about what the body sees (eyes), hears (ears), smells (nose), and feels (skin).

Action nerves (motor nerves) carry messages *to* parts of the body, telling muscles to move.

The **brain** is the main control center of the nervous system.

The 'trunk line' of the nerves is the spinal cord. It runs from the brain down the middle of the spine. Nerves come out from between each back bone and communicate to a part lower down in the body.

A **spinal-cord injury,** however, can damage or cut both the sensory and action nerves, so that both movement and feeling are lost. (See Chapter 23.)

Unlike polio and spinal-cord injury, which come from damage to nerves in the spine, **cerebral palsy** comes from damage to the brain itself. Because any part or parts of the brain may be damaged, any or all parts of the body may be affected: **movement, sense of balance, seeing, hearing, speech,** and **mental ability.** (See Chapter 9.)

Therefore, how completely you examine the workings of the nervous system will depend partly on what disability the child appears to have. If it is fairly clear the disability comes from polio, little examination of the nervous system is needed. But sometimes polio and cerebral palsy can be confused. If you have any suspicion that the disability might be caused by brain damage, you will want to do a fairly complete exam of nervous system function. **Damage to the brain or nervous system can cause problems in any of these areas:**

- seeing (See Chapter 30.)

- eye movement or position (See pages 40 and 301.)

- fits or seizures (epilepsy) (See Chapter 29.)

- balance, coordination, and sense of position (See pages 90 and 105.)

- hearing (See Chapter 31.)

- use of mouth and tongue, and speech (See pages 313 to 315.)

- mental ability; level of development (See pages 278 and 288.)

- feeling (pain and touch) (See pages 39 and 216.)

- unusual or strange behaviors; signs of self-damage (See page 364.)

- muscle tone (patterns of unusual floppiness, tightness, spasms, or movements). (See Chapter 9.)

- reflexes; muscle jerks (See pages 40 and 88.)

- urine and bowel control (See Chapter 25.)

Methods for testing some of these things are included on the next few pages and on the RECORD SHEETS 2, 3, and 4. Other tests that you will need less often, we include with specific disabilities. Refer to the page numbers listed above.

EVALUATION OF A CHILD WHOSE DEVELOPMENT IS SLOW

For the child who cannot do as much as other children do at the same age, a special developmental evaluation may be helpful. Additional information about the child's mother during pregnancy, or any difficulties during or after birth may explain possible causes. Measurement of the distance around the head may show possible causes of problems or other important factors. Repeated head-size measurements (once a month at first) may tell us even more.

 For example, a child who has had meningitis (brain infection) at age 1, and whose head almost stops growing from that age on, will probably remain quite retarded. We should not expect a lot. However, if the child's head continues to grow normally, the child may have better possibilities for learning and doing more (although we cannot be sure).

A child who is born with a 'sack on the back' (spina bifida, see p. 167) may have a head that is bigger than average. If the head continues to grow rapidly, this is a danger sign (see p. 41 and 169). Unless the child has surgery, she may become severely retarded or die. If, however, the monthly measurements show that the head has stopped growing too fast, the problem may have corrected itself. She may not need surgery.

RECORD SHEET 4, on page 41, covers additional questions relating to child development, and includes a chart for recording and evaluating head size.

To help the child who is developmentally delayed, you will first want to evaluate her level of physical and mental development. Chapter 34, pages 287 to 300, explains ways to do this.

You can use the Child Development Chart on pages 292 and 293 to find a child's developmental level, to plan her step-by-step activities, and to evaluate and record her progress. We have marked this 2-page chart, RECORD SHEET 6.

RECORD SHEETS

On the next 5 pages are the sample RECORD SHEETS that we discussed on p. 22. You are welcome to copy and use them. However, they are not perfect. They were developed for use by the village rehabilitation team in Mexico, and we are still trying to improve them. Before you make copies, we suggest that you adapt them to meet the needs of your area.

> **Be sure you have copies made of the RECORD SHEETS you will need *before* you need to use them.**

In addition to the 4 RECORD SHEETS here, you may also want copies of RECORD SHEET 5 "Evaluation of Progress," page 50, and RECORD SHEET 6, "Child Development Chart," pages 292 and 293.

Note on RECORD SHEET 1 (CHILD HISTORY):

The box at the top of RECORD SHEET 1 is to be filled out *after* you examine the child. It gives brief, essential information. This will make it easier to find out which disabilities you have seen most often, and to check on what you still need to do for different children.

The last few questions on page 2 of RECORD SHEET 1 are for a study PROJIMO is doing on medical causes of disability. Adapt them to study special concerns in your area.

File Number	TYPE OF DISABILITY	Movement _____	Future action:	Date:	Done:	RECORD SHEET 1 (page 1)

Movement _____

Deformity _____

Retarded _____

Blindness _____

Deafness _____

Speech _____

Fits _____

Behavior _____

Other _____

Future action: Date: Done:

_____ come back again   _____ _____

_____ refer to specialist   _____ _____

_____ visit at home   _____ _____

_____ other _____   _____ _____

File Number

Code

TYPE OF DISABILITY

Specific disability if known: _____

CHILD'S HISTORY (First visit)

Name: _____ Sex:

Date of birth: _____ Address: _____

Age: _____ Weight: _____ Height: _____ _____

Mother: _____ _____

Father: _____ Telephone: _____

How did you learn about the program?_____

WHAT IS THE CHILD'S MAIN PROBLEM? _____

_____

_____

When did it begin? _____ How? (Cause?) _____

Other problems? _____

Is the disability improving?_____Getting worse?_____About the same? _____

Explain: _____

How do you hope your child will benefit from coming here? _____

Do other family members or relatives have a similar problem? _____ Who?_____

Has the child received medical attention? _____ What? _____

_____ Where? _____

Use any braces or other aids? _____ What? _____

Has he used any in the past?_____ Explain: _____

_____

How is the child's general health? _____

Is he fat? _____ Very thin? _____Other? _____

Hears and sees well? _____ Explain: _____

Comment on the child's developmental abilities or difficulties: normal for age?

head control _____ _____

use of hands _____ _____

creeping or crawling _____ _____

standing, walking _____ _____

play_____ _____

feeding or drinking_____ _____

toileting _____ _____

personal hygiene _____ _____

dressing _____ _____

Does the child speak? _____ How much or well? _____ Began when? _____

What other things can the child do? _____

_____

What things can the child not do? _____

_____

What new skills or abilities would you like to see your child gain? _____

_____

Is the child mentally normal? _____

Retarded? _____ How severely? _____

Why do you think so? _____

Does the child have fits? _____ How often? _____

Describe: _____

Takes medicine? _____ What? _____

For what? _____ Results (good or bad): _____

Behavior normal for age? _____

Behavioral or emotional problems? _____ Explain: _____

_____

_____

Goes to school? _____ What year? _____

With whom does the child live? _____

Number of brothers and sisters: _____ Ages: _____ | AVERAGE EARNINGS

Father works? _____ At what? _____ | _____

Mother works? _____ At what? _____

The child seems: well-cared for? _____ spoiled or overprotected? _____

neglected? _____ happy? _____ self-confident? _____ withdrawn? _____

other? _____

Important details of family situation: _____

_____

_____

What has the family done, made, or obtained to help the child function better? _____

_____

Other observations, information or drawings:
(Use an additional sheet if necessary.)

_____

_____

_____

_____

_____

_____

History of illness	Date
measles	_____
chicken pox	_____
whooping cough	_____
other _____	_____
_____	_____

Vaccinations:	How many	Dates	Allergies
BCG (TB)	_____		
polio	_____		
D.P.T	_____		
Hep B (Hepatitis B)	_____		
measles	_____		
tetanus	_____		
other	_____		

How much have you spent for your child's disability? _____ For what? _____

_____

Were disability or complications caused by improper medical treatment or therapy? _____
Explain: _____

FOR CHILDREN WITH PARALYSIS:

Was your child injected before becoming paralyzed? _____

SAMPLE RECORD SHEET FOR PHYSICAL EXAM

RECORD SHEET 2

Child's name _____

File number _____

Mark on the drawings where you find the problems. Use lines and circles together with abbreviations shown on this page. For example: → OW-J++ 2 CTR 4

Where necessary, make new drawings on another sheet.

Parts of body affected

L or R _____ other _____ (indicate)

OW: Pain
OW-J pain in joints
OW-M pain in muscles

0 none
+little
++a lot
+++so much that she does not move it

CTR: contractures
___ tight muscles do not yield with pressure

SP: spasticity
___ *tight muscles yield slowly with pressure

Spine

hunchback (kyphosis) sideways curve (scoliosis) swayback (lordosis) hard bump (TB?)

curve fixed___ curve can straighten___ (See p. 161.)

Strength or weakness of muscles: Use this code

NORMAL 5 lifts and holds against strong resistance
GOOD 4 moves against some resistance
FAIR 3 lifts own weight but no more
POOR 2 moves some but cannot lift own weight
TRACE 1 barely moves
ZERO 0 no sign of movement

T: ability to feel, touch, pain, etc.

R or L	normal	*reduced	*absent
other			

Problems with
___ *Eyes or sight. What: _____
___ *Ears or hearing. What: _____

Deep tendon reflexes:

	*nothing 0	*little +	normal ++	*brisk +++	*extreme ++++
Right knee					
Left knee					
Other ___					

HT: hips tilt
R leg shorter ___
L leg shorter ___ by ___ cm

DL: dislocations:

	R	L	from birth	old	new
hip					
knee					
elbow					
other ___					

*Spina bifida
soft sac
*large head (hydrocephalus)

back already operated___ date___
head already operated___ date___
extent of paralysis _____
_____
extent of feeling lost _____
_____

*Spinal cord injury
what level _____

	Good	Poor	None
Bowel control			
Bladder control			

Other problems
___ *pressure sores
___ *unusual movements
___ *tremors
___ *fits
___ *poor balance
___ *developmental delay

IMPORTANT: This form does *not* cover all the tests and information you will want to record when examining a child. Put other information on the back of this sheet. Or use separate sheets or forms.

*If you check any problem area marked with a star (*), a more complete check of the nervous system is needed. You can use the RECORD SHEETS 3, 4, and 6.

RECORD SHEET: ADDITIONAL TESTS AND OBSERVATIONS OF THE
NERVOUS SYSTEM

These tests are *often not needed* but may sometimes be useful when you are not
sure if a child has *brain damage*. For other signs of brain damage, see Chapter 9
on Cerebral Palsy. For tests of seeing and hearing, see p. 447 to 454.

RECORD
SHEET
3

Eye movement

___ eyes jerk, flutter, or roll up unexpectedly and
repeatedly (brain damage, possible epilepsy—
p. 233)

___ one eye looks in a different direction or moves
differently from the other (possible brain damage)

Move finger or toy
in front of eyes
from side to side
and up and down.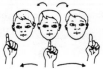

___ eyes follow smoothly (normal)

___ eyes follow in jumps or jerks (possible brain
damage)

Eye to hand coordination

___ moves finger from nose to
object and back again
almost without error—
with eyes open, and also
closed (normal)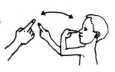

___ misses or has difficulty
with eyes open (poor
coordination, poor balance,
or loss of position sense)

___ has much more
difficulty with
eyes closed
(loss of position
sense)

Body movements

___ awkwardness or difficulty in controlling
movements

___ sudden or rhythmic uncontrolled movements

___ parts of body twist or move strangely when child
tries to move, reach, walk, speak, or do certain
things

(All these may be signs of brain damage;
see Chapter 9.)

Details of any of the above: _____
_____
_____

Fits of different kinds (See Chapter 29.)

___ sudden loss of consciousness with strange
movements,

___ brief periods of strange movements or positions,

___ blank stares, ___ eye fluttering, ___ twitching.

Developmental delay: Is the child unable to do
many different things that others her age can do?
Which? (See Chapter 34.)

___ head control   ___ sucking

___ use of hands   ___ eating

___ rolling   ___ playing

___ creeping and crawling   ___ communication or
                                speech
___ sitting
                            ___ behavior
___ standing and walking
                            ___ self-care activities

Balance

With the child in a sitting or standing position,
gently rock or push him off balance.

___CHILD DOES NOT TRY TO KEEP FROM FALLING
(poor balance—sign of brain damage in child over 1
year)

___ CHILD TRIES NOT TO FALL by putting out his
hands (fair balance)

___ CHILD KEEPS FROM FALLING by correcting
body position (good balance)

GOOD   POOR   GOOD   POOR

Balance test for the older, more stable child

Have child stand with feet together.

___ balance difficulty with eyes open—
may be brain damage (or muscle-joint
problem)

___ balance difficulty much greater
with eyes closed (probably nervous
system damage)

'Knee jerks' and other 'muscle jump' reflexes

With the leg relaxed and partly bent, tap the
cord just below the knee cap.

NORMAL	REDUCED	OVER ACTIVE	KEEPS JUMPING
The knee jumps a little.	The leg moves *very little* or not at all. Typical of polio, muscular dystrophy, and other floppy paralyses.	A slight tap causes a *big jump*. Typical of spasticity from cerebral palsy, spinal cord injury, and other brain or spinal cord damage.	One tap causes the limb to jerk many times. Happens with spinal cord injury and some cerebral palsy.

You can also
tap the heel
cord and
other cords
near joint.

Great toe reflex

Stroke the foot toward the toe with a
somewhat pointed object (like a pen).

NORMAL   NOT NORMAL
                (in a child over 2)
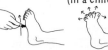
toes bend down   toes bend up
                  and spread

This is a sign of
brain or spinal
cord damage
(Babinski's sign)
May occur in a
normal child
under 2 years.

RECORDS OF FACTORS POSSIBLY AFFECTING CHILD DEVELOPMENT
(mainly for children with possible brain damage or developmental delay)

RECORD
SHEET
4

Added history

Was the child born before 9 months? _____ at how many months? _____

Was the child born smaller or thinner than normal? _____ weight at birth? _____

Was the birth of the child normal? _____ slow or difficult? _____

    Explain: _____

Did the child seem normal at birth? _____ If not, describe problems: delayed breathing? _____

    very floppy? _____ other? _____

Did the mother have problems in pregnancy? _____ German measles _____ at _____ months.

    Other? _____. Medicines or drugs during pregnancy: _____ What? _____

    Age of mother _____ and father _____ at time of child's birth.

Physical exam

Does the child show signs of brain damage? (Use RECORD SHEETS 3 and 4.)

    What? _____

Does the child show signs of Down syndrome (mongolism)? _____

    What? (wide, slanted eyes _____, crease in hand _____, other _____. See p. 279.)

Other physical signs, possibly related to retardation _____

Does the child's head seem smaller _____ or larger _____ than normal?

Distance around head? _____ cm. Difference from normal _____ cm.

Average at her age (from chart) _____ cm. Difference from average _____ cm.

Record of the child's head size

On the chart put a dot where the up-and-down line of the child's age crosses the sideways line of her head size:

Measure around the widest part of the head.

If the dot is *below* the shaded area the head is smaller than normal. The child may be **microcephalic** (small-brained, see p. 278).

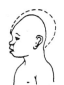

If the dot falls *above* the shaded area, the head is bigger than normal. The child may have **hydrocephalus** (see p. 169).

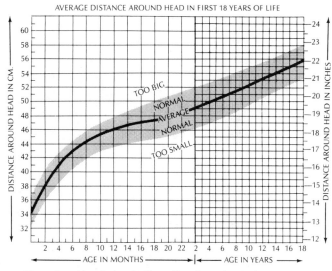

AVERAGE DISTANCE AROUND HEAD IN FIRST 18 YEARS OF LIFE

Note: Boys' heads average from ½ to 1 cm. larger than girls' heads. Also head size may vary somewhat with different races. If possible get local charts.

Use the chart for a continuing record. Every month put a new dot on the chart.* If the difference from normal increases, the problem is more likely to be serious. For example,

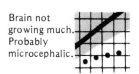

Brain not growing much. Probably microcephalic.

Brain growing well. Probably not serious.

Head too big; growing fast. Hydrocephalus or tumor. Getting worse.

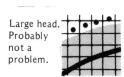

Large head. Probably not a problem.

*Filling out this chart every month is especially important for children with spina bifida or suspected hydrocephalus (see p. 169). If you do not know how to use the chart, ask a local schoolteacher.

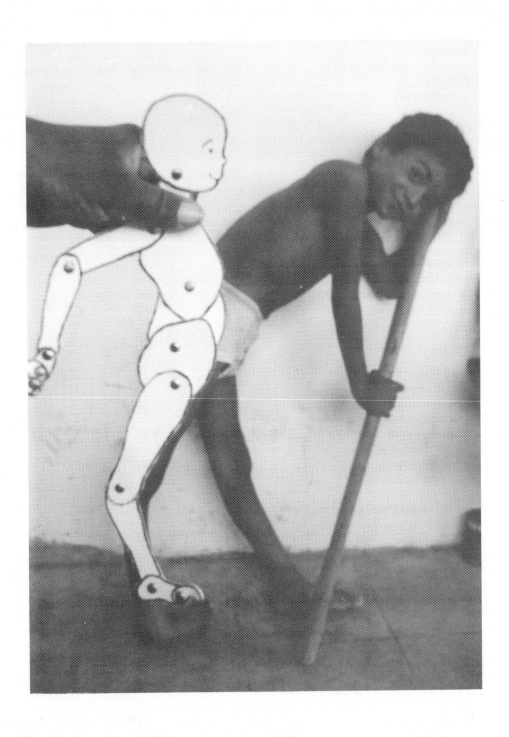

Simple Ways to Measure and Record a Child's Progress

It is important to keep records of each child's progress. Careful records help workers and parents to **follow the change in the individual child, and to evaluate the effectiveness of advice, therapy, and aids.**

We need a clear view of the progress of the **whole child in all areas**—physical, mental, and social. The Child Development Chart on p. 292 and 293 will help us to do this for younger children. For children over 5, at the end of this chapter there is a simple chart (RECORD SHEET 5) for evaluating a child's increasing ability to do things.

When the parents and child themselves regularly measure and record a child's progress, they become more aware of gradual improvements. But let them know that **the child's progress may be very slow and it may take several weeks, or even months, before they notice any real improvement**. Encourage them to be patient and to continue with the important exercises, aids, and activities.

Unfortunately, the standard way of recording physical deformities and *contractures* requires knowledge of angles, degrees, and symbols that many people do not understand. **For evaluation to become a family tool, we need a way to measure, record, and interpret information that is as simple, clear, and enjoyable as possible.** Here are some ideas.

MEASURING JOINT POSITIONS AND CONTRACTURES

You can make a simple measuring tool using 2 flat pieces of wood, plastic, or cardboard. (Tongue depressors work well.)

Other simple methods for recording joint positions are on p. 79.

1. Rivet the pieces together on one end.

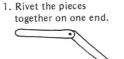

2. Line them up exactly with the joint.

3. Trace the angle on paper.

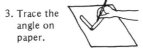

4. Do this again every 1 or 2 weeks to see if the joint is straightening with exercise.

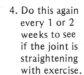

March	∨
April	∨
May	∨
June	∨

The 'flexikin'—an aid to measure and encourage progress

Flexikins are cardboard dolls with joints. Disabled and non-disabled children can make and play with them. They are **so easy to use that even parents who cannot read can measure and record their children's contractures.** Because the periodic measurements are recorded as a line of pictures, anyone can see the child's progress at a glance.

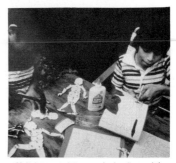

Children making and playing with flexikins. In the PROJIMO village rehabilitation center, all the flexikins used are made by disabled children and the local school children.

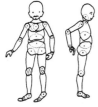

Flexikins—front and side view models

We have found that when families follow their child's progress using flexikins, both the child and parents are more likely to keep doing stretching exercises. As a result, many contractures can be partly or completely straightened in the home, and there is less need for casting and surgery.

Examples of how flexikins are used

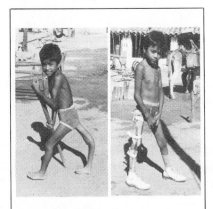

Village rehabilitation workers have just made a brace for a child with polio whose leg bends back severely. They want to know if the leg will gradually get better (bend back less). So they ask the mother to measure it every month.

The mother places the flexikin's leg in the same position as her son's leg, bent back as far as it goes. She then traces it onto a large sheet of paper.

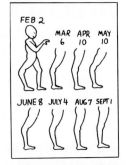

Each month she does the same and records the date. (In April her son did not use the brace for 2 weeks and she saw the knee was getting worse. This convinced both mother and boy of the importance of using the brace.)

The flexikins can be used to record a wide variety of positions, deformities, contractures, and limitations in range of motion, mainly of the arms and legs but also of the neck, back, hips, and body:

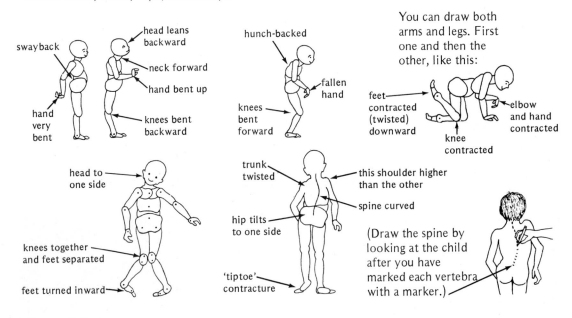

In addition to using the small flexikins for record keeping, you can make large flexikins for group teaching. Or use them to keep body proportions correct when making drawings for instruction sheets.

Note: For recording contractures, we have found the side-view flexikin more useful than the front-view one. The side-view flexikin is also easier to make. It is probably the only one you will need for evaluating a child's progress.

How to make the flexikins

1. Trace the patterns of different pieces (p. 47 and 48) onto very thick paper or thin, firm cardboard. Or use old X-ray film.

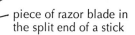

   You can do this using *carbon paper*. (Make your own carbon paper by completely blackening a sheet of paper with a soft-leaded pencil.)

   cardboard
   carbon paper
   pattern sheet

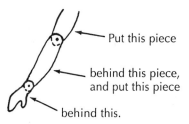

   Or you can glue a copy of the pattern sheet directly to the cardboard.

   (If your program plans to make many flexikins, or have children make them, we suggest you have the patterns printed or mimeographed directly on sheets of thin, firm cardboard.)

2. Cut out the pieces with strong scissors, shears, or a piece of razor blade.

   piece of razor blade in the split end of a stick

3. Place the pieces together as shown in the drawings.

   Make sure the pieces that overlap with dotted lines go behind those with complete lines.

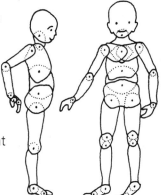

   Put this piece

   behind this piece, and put this piece

   behind this.

4. Fasten the pieces together at the black dots with metal or plastic rivets, sewing thread or yarn, or sewing pins.

Metal or plastic rivets usually work best.

For metal rivets: Use the smallest metal rivets you can find. First punch a hole through each black dot. Put the rivets through and **hammer them just enough so that the cardboard joints are tight enough to hold their position but can be moved without tearing.**

For plastic rivets: Use small pieces of plastic cut from a plastic drinking straw, or a plastic knitting needle or crochet hook. A drinking straw will be easier to use, but make sure it is made from plastic and not paper. Put small pieces of the plastic into each hole you have punched. Then use a lighted candle to heat a knife or metal blade to press and melt the plastic so it will get soft, spread, and hold the cardboard pieces together. Do not melt it too much or the 2 pieces of cardboard will stick together and you will not be able to move the flexikin 'joint'.

Or use **sewing pins**

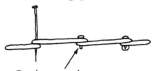

Cut here and put a drop of very strong glue (like epoxy) here.

Or use **thin wire or string** and tie knots.

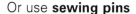

Or string the joints together with **thread or yarn** (this does not work as well).

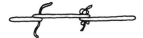

You can copy this sheet, or one like it, and give it to parents together with a flexikin. Be sure that you also **show them** how to use it and then **watch them use it.**

INSTRUCTIONS FOR USING THE FLEXIKIN

We have given you a 'flexikin' so that you can measure and see the progress that your child is making with his exercises or aids.

We suggest you take a new measurement every_____ .
Do it like this:

1. Have your child take the position you want to measure (for example, straighten his knee as much as he can).

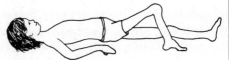

2. Put the flexikin in exactly the position the child is in. To do this **hold the flexikin at a distance between your eye and the child so that it appears the same size as the child.** This will let you line it up exactly.

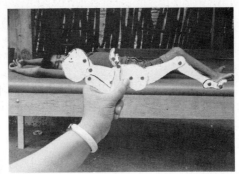

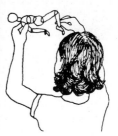

3. Without moving the position of the flexikin, trace it onto a large piece of paper. The first time trace the whole body. Each time measure the child in the same posture.

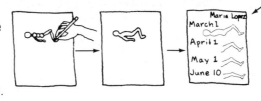

This example shows how exercises have helped straighten a contracted knee.

> María Lopez
> March 1
> April 1
> May 1
> June 10

For later recordings, you only need to trace the part or parts you are measuring. Each time you record a measurement, write the date.

In certain cases you may want to measure how far the child can straighten an arm or leg by herself, and how far you are able to straighten it for her (little by little without forcing).

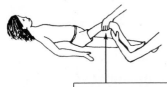

CAUTION: When you straighten the limb, support it close to the joint. This prevents injury.

Make 2 columns. In one, record how far the child can move it by herself. In the other column record how far she can move it with help.

Here you see the progress of a leg until it became straight and a brace could be made for it.

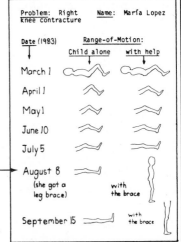

Problem: Right Knee contracture		Name: María Lopez
Date (1983)	**Range-of-Motion:** Child alone	with help
March 1		
April 1		
May 1		
June 10		
July 5		
August 8 (she got a leg brace)		with the brace
September 15		with the brace

SIDE-VIEW FLEXIKIN

*Patterns of pieces
for making it*

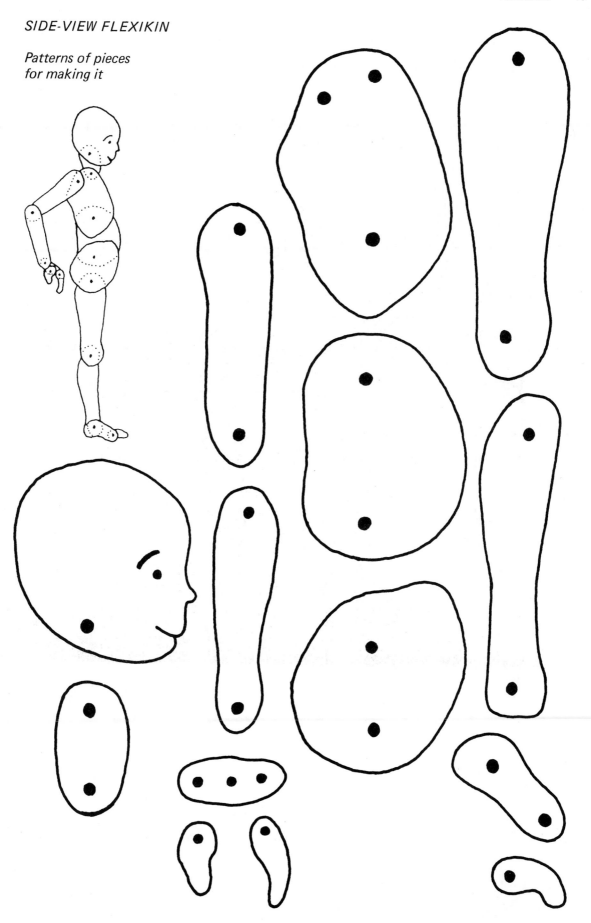

FRONT-VIEW FLEXIKIN

*Patterns of pieces
for making it*

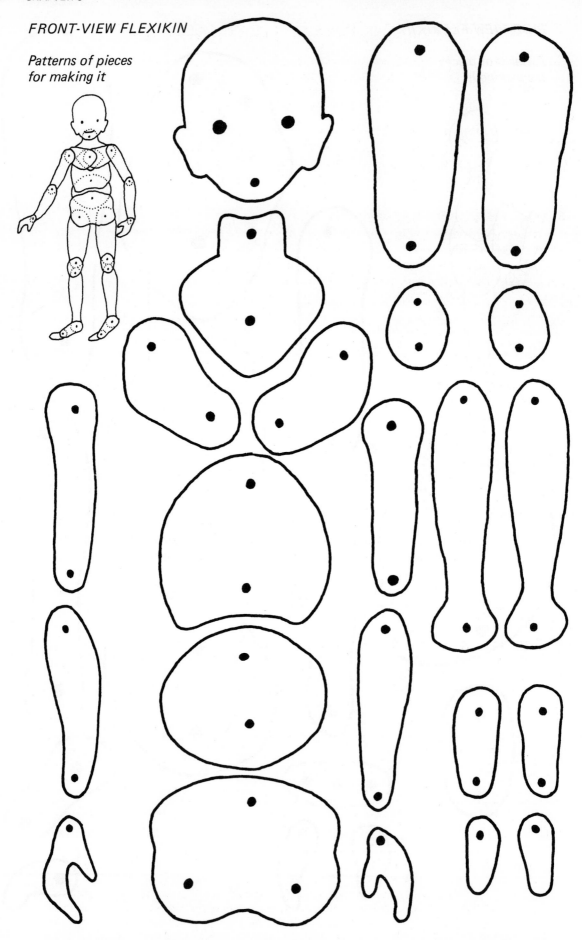

EVALUATING THE PROGRESS OF THE WHOLE CHILD

A simple way for rehabilitation workers and parents to evaluate how a child is progressing as a whole is to keep a record of her ability to do different things. Each month, or during each visit to the community rehabilitation center, the child's different abilities are reviewed, tested, or observed. Any changes are recorded.

For children under 5 years old, one way of evaluating a child's development is to use the RECORD SHEET 6 (p. 292). This chart shows the developmental levels ('milestones') for different skills and activities. The first time the child is evaluated, circle the drawing that shows what the child can do in each area.

Each time the child is evaluated, on the same sheet, again circle the appropriate drawing, **but use a different color** (or a dotted, dashed, or zigzag line). This way, you can see where the child is moving ahead well and where he is behind.

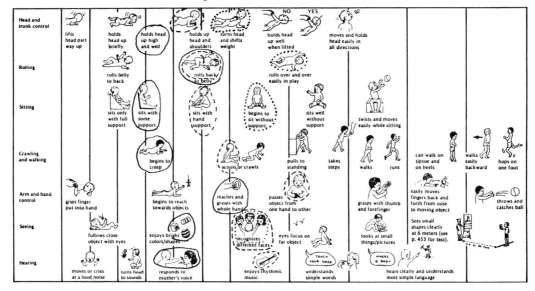

For evaluating the progress of children over age 5, the charts on the next page may help. Two different approaches are used. Chart A is more **objective** (requires less personal judgment or opinion) but does not allow for small improvements. Chart B is more **subjective** (is based more on personal judgments). It considers **quality** of improvement, not just quantity. You can try both and see which you think gives truer, more useful results.

To use Chart A: For each skill, circle whether the child can do it "without help," "with a little help," or "with lots of help." Add all the numbers you circle. Compare the scores of the first and second visits. For example:

	First visit			Second visit		
	without help	little help	lots of help	without help	little help	lots of help
How does the child eat?	4	②	0	④	2	0
How does the child drink?	4	②	0	4	②	0

Here we see the child has improved his eating skills but not his drinking skills.

To use Chart B: In each area, on the second visit, circle whether the child is doing a lot better, a little better, or the same. Add it all up. The higher the score, the more the child has improved.

> *NOTE:* We question whether the use of numbers may not be misleading. But we think the questions themselves may be a useful guideline. None of these evaluation forms will show all areas of change or improvement. They are not substitutes for **detailed notes, drawings, and a good memory!**

EVALUATION OF PROGRESS — CHILD OVER AGE 5

Name_____ Age_____ Disability _____

CHART A Daily activities	First visit (date____)			Second visit (date _____)		
	without help	little help	lots of help	without help	little help	lots of help
Feeding						
1. How does the child eat?	4	2	0	4	2	0
2. How does the child drink?	4	2	0	4	2	0
Dressing and washing						
3. Does child wash face and body?	4	2	0	4	2	0
4. Does child dress?	4	2	0	4	2	0
5. Does child put on orthopedic equipment?	4	2	0	4	2	0
Bowel and bladder care and control						
6. Does child stay clean (bowel control)?	4	2	0	4	2	0
7. Does child clean herself after shitting?	4	2	0	4	2	0
8. Does child stay dry during the day?	4	2	0	4	2	0
9. Does child stay dry at night?	4	2	0	4	2	0
Mobility/transfers						
10. Does child move from chair to bed and back? . .	4	2	0	4	2	0
11. Does child move from floor to bed and back? . .	4	2	0	4	2	0
Movement						
12. Walks on flat surface?	4	2	0	4	2	0
13. Walks on uneven surface?	4	2	0	4	2	0
14. Climbs up and down stairs?	4	2	0	4	2	0
15. Uses a wheelboard or wheelchair?	4	2	0	4	2	0
16. Does child crawl?	4	2	0	4	2	0
Social activities/communication						
17. Does child help with housework or farm work? . .	4	2	0	4	2	0
18. Does child play with other children?	4	2	0	4	2	0
19. Does child go to school?	4	2	0	4	2	0
20. Does child speak?	4	2	0	4	2	0
21. Does child communicate with signs or gestures? . .	4	2	0	4	2	0
		Total _____			Total _____	

CHART B Quality of activities	First visit	Second visit			
	make notes for comparison here	much better	a little better	same	worse
Does child move about better?		4	2	0	−4
Does he sit in a better position?		4	2	0	−4
Does he walk better (straighter, with less limp, or					
with less support)?		4	2	0	−4
Does he walk farther, faster, or easier?		4	2	0	−4
Are his joints straighter (less contractures)?		4	2	0	−4
hip?		4	2	0	−4
knee?		4	2	0	−4
ankle?		4	2	0	−4
Can the child do things he could not do before?		4	2	0	−4
feeding?		4	2	0	−4
bathing?		4	2	0	−4
dressing?		4	2	0	−4
toileting?		4	2	0	−4
Does he play with things better?		4	2	0	−4
Does he speak or communicate better?		4	2	0	−4
Does he get along with other children better?		4	2	0	−4
Does he seem happier or more self-confident?		20	8	0	−4
Has he improved or got worse in other ways?		4	2	0	−4
In what ways? _____		4	2	0	−4
_____			Total_____		

Guide for Identifying Disabilities

This chapter has a chart, 7 pages long, to help you find out **what disability a child possibly has,** and **where to look up that disability in this book.**

In the **first column** of the chart, we list the more noticeable signs of different disabilities. Some of these signs are found in more than one disability. So in the **second column** we add other signs that can help you tell apart similar disabilities. The **third column** names the disability or disabilities that are most likely to have these signs. And the **fourth column** gives the page numbers where you should look in this book. (Where it says *WTND* and then a number, this refers to the page in *Where There Is No Doctor.*)

If you do not find the sign you are looking for in the first column, look for another sign. Or check the signs in the second column.

This chart will help you find out which disabilities a child might have. It is wise to look up each possibility. **The first page of each chapter on a disability describes the signs in more detail.**

> *IMPORTANT:* Some disabilities can easily be confused. Others are not included in this book. When you are not sure, try to get help from someone with more experience. At times, special tests or X-rays may be needed to be sure what the problem is.

Fortunately, **it is not always necessary to know exactly what disability a child has.** For example, if a child has developed weakness in his legs and you are not sure of the cause, you can still do a lot to help him. Read the chapters on disabilities that cause similar weakness, and the chapters on other problems that the child may have. For this child, you might find useful information in the chapters on polio, *contractures,* exercises, braces, walking aids or wheelchairs, and many others.

Sometimes it is important to identify the specific disability. Some disabilities require specific medicines or foods—for example, night blindness, rickets, or cretinism. Others urgently need surgery—for example, spina bifida or cleft lip and palate. Others require special ways of doing *therapy* or exercises—for example, cerebral palsy. And others need specific precautions to avoid additional problems—for example, spinal cord injury and leprosy. For this reason, it helps to learn as much about the disability as you can. Whenever possible, seek information and advice from more experienced persons. (However, even experts are not always right. Do not follow anyone's advice without understanding the reasons for doing something, and considering *if* and *why* the advice applies to the individual child.)

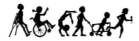

In addition to this chart, 2 other guides for identifying disabilities are in this book:

GUIDE FOR IDENTIFYING CAUSES OF JOINT PAIN, p. 130.
GUIDE FOR IDENTIFYING AND TREATING DIFFERENT FORMS OF FITS (EPILEPSY), p. 240.

GUIDE FOR IDENTIFYING DISABILITIES

SIGNS PRESENT AT OR SOON AFTER BIRTH

IF THE CHILD HAS THIS	AND ALSO THIS	HE MAY HAVE	SEE PAGE
born weak or 'floppy'	• often a difficult birth • delayed breathing • born blue and limp • or born before 9 months and very small	• cerebral palsy • developmental delay	87 277
slow to begin to lift head or move arms	• round face • slant eyes • thick tongue	• Down syndrome (mongolism) • cretinism	279 282
	small head, or small top part of head	microcephalia (small brain) mental retardation	278
	none of above	developmental delay for other reasons	289
does not suck well or chokes on milk or food	• pushes milk back out with tongue • or will not suck	cerebral palsy	87
	• cannot suck well • chokes or milk comes out nose	• check for cleft palate • possibly severe retardation	120 277
one or both feet turned in or back	no other signs	club foot	114
	• hands weak, stiff or clubbed • some joints stiff, in bent or straight positions	arthrogryposis	122
	dark lump on back	spina bifida	167
'bag' or dark lump on back	• clubbed feet • or feet bend up too far • or feet lack movement and feeling	spina bifida (sometimes no 'bag' is seen, but foot signs may be present)	167
head too big; keeps growing	may develop:	hydrocephalus (water on the brain)	169
	• eyes like 'setting sun' • increasing mental and/or physical disability • blindness	At birth, this is usually a sign of spina bifida.	167
		in an older child, possibly tapeworm in brain, or a brain tumor	*WTND* 143
upper lip and/or roof of mouth incomplete	• difficulty feeding • later, speech difficulties	cleft lip (hare lip) and cleft palate	120
birth deformities, defects, or missing parts	(may or may not be associated with other problems)	See • birth defects • amputations • Down syndrome • developmental delay	119 227 279 287
abnormal stiffness or position	• from birth • some muscles weak • some joints stiff • head control and mind normal	arthrogryposis	122
	• Muscles tighten more in certain positions. • may grip thumb tightly	spastic cerebral palsy *Note:* muscle tightness (spasticity) usually does not appear until weeks or months after birth.	89

IF THE CHILD HAS THIS	AND ALSO THIS	HE MAY HAVE	SEE PAGE
one arm weak or in strange position	does not move the arm much holds it like this	Erb's palsy (weakness from damage to nerves in shoulder during birth)	127
	leg on same side often affected	hemiplegic (one-sided) cerebral palsy	90
dislocated hip at birth leg held differently, shorter; flap covers part of vulva	On opening legs like this, leg 'pops' into place or does not open as far.	dislocated hip from birth (often both hips) may be present with: • spina bifida • Down syndrome • arthrogryposis Also see p. 156.	155 167 279 122
slow to respond to sound or to look at things	(may be due to one or a combination of problems)	Check for signs of: • developmental delay • cerebral palsy • blindness • deafness	290 87 243 257

SIGNS IN CHILDREN

slower than other children to do things (roll, sit, use hands, show interest, walk, talk)	slow in most or all areas:	Developmental delay, check for signs of:	287
	• round face • slant eyes • single deep crease in hand	Down syndrome (mongolism)	279
	• movements and response slow • skin dry and cool • hair often low on forehead • puffy eyelids	cretinism	282
	has continuous strange movements or positions, and/or stiffness	cerebral palsy also check for: • blindness • deafness • malnutrition	87 243 257 320
does not respond to sounds, does not begin to speak by age 3	may respond to some sounds but not others Check for ear infection (pus).	Check for: • deafness • severe developmental delay (with or without deafness) • severe cerebral palsy	257 283 87
does not turn head to look at things, or reach for things until they touch her	Eyes may or may not look normal.	• blindness and/or • severe mental retardation • severe cerebral palsy	243 277 87
Eyelids or eyes make quick, jerky, or strange movements.	Check for one or a combination of these.	• blindness • fits • too much medicine • cerebral palsy • other problems affecting or damaging the brain	243 233 15 87 14

IF THE CHILD HAS THIS	AND ALSO THIS	HE MAY HAVE	SEE PAGE
All or part of body makes strange, uncontrolled movements.	• begins suddenly, child may fall or lose consciousness • child is normal (or more normal) between 'fits'	epileptic fits (Pattern varies a lot in different children—or even in the same child.)	233
	slow, sudden, or rhythmic movements; fairly continuous (except in sleep); no loss of consciousness	athetoid cerebral palsy (*Note:* Fits and cerebral palsy may occur in the same child.)	89
Body, or parts of it, stiffens when in certain positions: poor control of some or all movements.	• different positions in different children • Body may stiffen backward and legs cross.	spastic cerebral palsy	89

PARTS OF BODY WEAK OR PARALYZED

IF THE CHILD HAS THIS	AND ALSO THIS	HE MAY HAVE	SEE PAGE
floppy or limp weakness in part or all of body **no loss of feeling** in affected parts **no spasticity** (muscles that tighten without control) **normal at birth**	• usually began with a 'bad cold' and fever before age 2 • irregular pattern of parts weakened. Often one or both legs—sometimes arm, shoulder, hand, etc.	polio	59
	• begins little by little and steadily gets worse • about the same on both sides of body • often others in the family also have it	• muscular dystrophy • muscular atrophy	109 112
		tick paralysis	not in book
	• Paralysis starts in legs and moves up; may affect whole body. • or, pattern of paralysis variable	Guillain-Barré paralysis (usually temporary)	62
		paralysis from pesticides, chemicals, foods (lathyrism)	15
	lump on back (See p. 57.)	tuberculosis of spine	165
floppy or limp weakness usually **some loss of feeling**	• one or both hands or feet • develops slowly in older child. Gets worse and worse.	leprosy	215
	• born with bag on back (Look for scar.) • feet weak, often without feeling	spina bifida	167
	• usually from back or neck injury • weakness, loss of feeling below level of injury • may or may not have muscle spasms • loss of bladder and bowel control	spinal cord injury paraplegia (lower body) quadriplegia (upper and lower body)	175
	injury to nerves going to one part of body	hand weakness sometimes caused by using crutches wrongly	393

IF THE CHILD HAS THIS	AND ALSO THIS	HE MAY HAVE	SEE PAGE
weakness usually **with stiffness or spasticity of muscles** **no loss of feeling**	usually affects body in one of these patterns 1. one side 2. both legs 3. whole body	• 1: cerebral palsy (or stroke, usually older persons) • 2 and 3: cerebral palsy • occasional other causes	87
	Muscles tighten and resist movement because of joint pain.	JOINT PAIN (many causes—see below)	130

JOINT PAIN

one or more painful joints	• begins with or without fever • gradually gets worse, but there are better and worse periods	juvenile arthritis	135
		other causes of joint pain See chart on joint pain.	130

WALKS WITH DIFFICULTY OR LIMPS

dips to one side with each step	one leg often weaker and shorter	Check for: • polio • cerebral palsy • dislocated hip	59 87 155
	• usually begins age 4 to 8 • may complain of knee pain	damaged hip joint	157
walks with knees pressed together	• muscle spasm and tightness • upper body little affected	spastic diplegic or paraplegic cerebral palsy	87
stands and walks with knees together and feet apart	feet less than 3" apart at age 3	normal from ages 2 to 12	113
no other problems	feet more than 3" apart at age 3	knock-kneed	114
walks awkwardly with one foot tiptoe	muscle spasms and poor control on that side. Hand on that side often affected.	hemiplegic cerebral palsy	90
		(stroke in older persons)	not in book
walks awkwardly with knees bent and legs usually separated	• jerky steps, poor balance • sudden, uncontrolled movements that may cause falling	athetoid cerebral palsy	89
	• slow 'drunken' way of walking • learns to walk late and falls often	• poor balance (ataxia)— often with cerebral palsy • Down syndrome (mongolism) • cretinism	90 279 282
walks with both feet tiptoe	• weakness, especially in legs and feet • gradually gets worse and worse	muscular dystrophy	109
	legs and feet stiffen (spasticity of muscle)	spastic cerebral palsy	89
	no other problems	normal? (some normal children at first walk on tiptoes)	292

IF THE CHILD HAS THIS	AND ALSO THIS	HE MAY HAVE	SEE PAGE
walks with hand(s) pushing thigh(s) or with knee(s) bent back	weak thigh muscle / difficulty lifting leg	• polio • muscular dystrophy • arthritis (joint pain) • other causes of muscle weakness	59 109 135 112
Foot hangs down weakly (foot drop).	Child lifts foot high with each step so that it will not drag.	• polio • spina bifida • muscular dystrophy • muscular atrophy • nerve or muscle injury • other cause of weakness	59 167 109 112 35 139
dips from side to side with each step	due to muscle weakness at side of hips, or double dislocated hips, or both	• polio • cerebral palsy • spina bifida • Down syndrome • muscular dystrophy • child who stays small • arthrogryposis • dislocated hips (may occur with any of the above)	59 87 167 279 109 126 122 155
walks with one (or both) hip, knee, or ankle that stays bent	joints **cannot** be slowly straightened when child relaxes (see page 79).	• contractures (shortened muscles) • joined or fused joints may be secondary to: • polio • joint infection • other causes	77 80 59 131 231
	Joints **can** gradually be straightened when child relaxes.	spasticity, often cerebral palsy	89
Knees wide apart when feet together (bow legs). Waddles or dips from side to side (if he walks).	under 18 months old	often normal	113
	Any combination of these: • Joints look big or thick. • Child is short for age. • Bones weak, bent, or break easily. • Arms and legs may seem too short for body, or 'out of proportion'. • Belly and butt stick out a lot.	Consider: • rickets (lack of vitamin D and sunlight) • brittle bone disease • children who stay very short (dwarfism) • cretinism • Down syndrome • dislocated hips	125 125 126 282 279 155
flat feet	no pain or other problems	normal in many children	113
	• Pain may occur in arch of foot. • Deformity may get worse.	may be problems in: • cerebral palsy • polio • spina bifida • Down syndrome	87 59 167 279

BACK CURVES AND DEFORMITIES

sideways curve of backbone	When child bends over, look for a lump on one side.	'scoliosis'—may occur alone or as complication of: • polio • cerebral palsy • muscular dystrophy • spina bifida • other physical disability	59 87 109 167 162

IF THE CHILD HAS THIS	AND ALSO THIS	HE MAY HAVE	SEE PAGE
swayback	• belly often sticks out • may be due to contractures here, or weak stomach muscles	'lordosis'—may occur in: • polio • spina bifida • cerebral palsy • muscular dystrophy • Down syndrome • cretinism • child who stays small • many other disabilities	 59 167 87 109 279 282 126 161
rounded back		'kyphosis'—often occurs with: • arthritis • spinal cord injury • severe polio • brittle bone disease	 136 175 59 125
hard, sharp bend of or bump in backbone	• starts slowly and without pain • often family history of tuberculosis • may lead to paralysis of lower body	tuberculosis of the spine	165
dark soft lump over backbone	• present at birth • sometimes only a soft or slightly swollen area over spine • weakness and loss of feeling in feet or lower body	spina bifida ('sack on the back')	167

OTHER DEFORMITIES

missing body parts	born that way	born with missing or incomplete parts	121
	accidental or surgical loss of limbs (amputation)	amputations	227
	gradual loss of fingers, toes, hands, or feet, often in persons who lack feeling	• osteomyelitis (bone infections) sometimes seen with: • leprosy (hands or feet) • spina bifida (feet only)	159 215 167
hand problems (For hand problems from birth, see p. 305.)	• floppy paralysis (no spasticity) • without care may lead to contractures so that fingers cannot be opened	may occur with: • polio • muscular dystrophy • muscular atrophy • spinal cord injury (at neck level) • leprosy • damage to nerves or cords of arms All may lead to contractures.	 59 109 112 175 215 127
	• uncontrolled muscle tightness (spasticity) • strange movements • or hand in tight fist	spastic cerebral palsy may lead to contractures	89
	burn scars and deformities	burns	231
clubbing or bending of feet (For club feet from birth, see p. 114.)	may begin as floppy weakness and become stiff from contractures, if not prevented	may occur with many physical disabilities, including: • polio • cerebral palsy • spina bifida • muscular dystrophy • arthritis • spinal cord injury	 59 87 167 109 139 175

DISABILITIES THAT OFTEN OCCUR WITH
OR ARE SECONDARY TO OTHER DISABILITIES

Developmental delay: child slow to learn to use her body or develop basic skills	caused by slow or incomplete brain function or by severe physical disability, or both	often seen in: • mental retardation • cerebral palsy • severely or multiply disabled children	277 87 283
	caused by overprotection: treating children like babies when they could do more for themselves	some delay can occur with almost any disability	287
Contractures joints that no longer straighten because muscles have shortened Joints will not straighten.	• usually due to muscle weakness or spasticity • Often, muscles that pull a joint one way are much weaker than those that pull it the other way (muscle imbalance).	often secondary to: • polio • cerebral palsy • spina bifida • arthritis • muscular dystrophy • Erb's palsy • amputations • leprosy	59 87 167 135 109 127 227 215
	sometimes due to scarring from burns or injuries	burns	231
Behavior problems	may come from: • brain damage • difficulty understanding things • overprotection • difficult home situation (Some children with epilepsy from brain damage may pull out hair, bite themselves, etc.)	behavior problems common with: • mental retardation • fits (epilepsy) • cerebral palsy and for emotional reasons, with: • spinal cord injury • muscular dystrophy • deafness • learning disability	277 233 87 175 109 257 365
Slow to learn certain things only; otherwise intelligent.	• often over-active or nervous • sometimes behavior problems	learning disability	365
Speech and communication problems	• often, but not always, due to deafness or retardation (or both) • Some children can hear well and are INTELLIGENT but still cannot speak.	may occur with: • deafness • developmental delay • cerebral palsy • Down syndrome • cretinism • children who stay small • brittle bone disease • cleft lip and palate (Deafness may occur together with these and other disabilities.)	257 287 87 279 282 126 125 120
other problems that sometimes occur *secondary* to other disabilities (Some of these we have already included in this chart.)	**Main disability** • cerebral palsy _____ • many disabilities with paralysis _____ • persons who have lost feeling: leprosy, spinal cord injury, spina bifida	**Common secondary disabilities** • blindness • deafness • fits _____ • spinal curve _____ • pressure sores • osteomyelitis (bone infection) • loss of urine and bowel control	 243 257 233 161 195 159 203

Polio

CHAPTER 7

Infantile Paralysis

HOW TO RECOGNIZE PARALYSIS CAUSED BY POLIO

- *Paralysis* (muscle weakness) usually begins when the child is small, often during an illness like a bad cold with fever and sometimes diarrhea.

- Paralysis may affect any *muscles* of the body, but is most common in the legs. Muscles most often affected are shown in the drawing.

- Paralysis is of the **'floppy'** type (not stiff). Some muscles may be only partly weakened, others limp or floppy.

- In time the affected limb may not be able to straighten all the way, due to shortening, or *'contractures'*, of certain muscles.

- The muscles and bones of the affected limb become thinner than the other limb. The affected limb does not grow as fast, and so is shorter.

MUSCLES COMMONLY WEAKENED BY POLIO

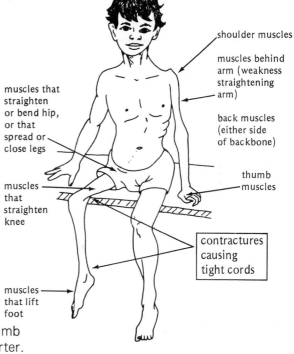

shoulder muscles

muscles behind arm (weakness straightening arm)

back muscles (either side of backbone)

muscles that straighten or bend hip, or that spread or close legs

thumb muscles

muscles that straighten knee

contractures causing tight cords

muscles that lift foot

- Unaffected arms or legs often become extra strong to make up for parts that are weak.

- **Intelligence** and the mind are not affected.

- **Feeling** is not affected.

- 'Knee jerks' and other *tendon* reflexes in the affected limb are reduced or absent. (In cerebral palsy, 'knee jerks' often jump more than normal. See p. 88.) Also, the paralysis of polio is 'floppy'; limbs affected by cerebral palsy often are tense and resist when straightened or bent (see p. 102).

reduced tendon jerks

- The paralysis does not get worse with time. However, secondary problems like contractures, curve of the backbone and *dislocations* may occur.

Of children who become paralyzed by polio:

30% recover completely in the first weeks or months.

30% have mild paralysis.

30% have moderate or severe paralysis.

10% die (often because of difficulty breathing or swallowing).

BASIC QUESTIONS AND ANSWERS ABOUT POLIO

How common is it? In many countries, polio—or 'poliomyelitis'—was for many years the most common cause of physical disability in children. In some areas, one of every 100 persons may have some paralysis from polio. Where *vaccination* programs are effective, polio has been greatly reduced.

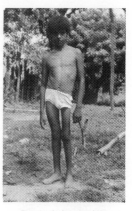

What causes it? A *virus (infection).* The infection attacks parts of the *spinal cord,* where it damages only the *nerves* that control movement. In areas with poor hygiene and lack of latrines, the polio infection spreads when the stool (shit) of a sick child reaches the mouth of a healthy child. Where sanitation is better, polio spreads mostly through coughing and sneezing.

Paralysis in one leg

Do all children who become infected with the polio virus become paralyzed? No, only a small percentage become paralyzed, about 1 out of every 100 to 150 children who are exposed to the virus. Most only get what looks like a bad cold, with fever, vomiting or diarrhea.

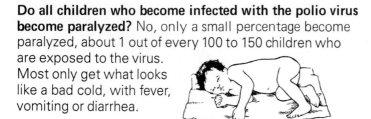

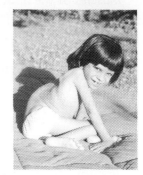

Is the paralysis contagious? No, not after 2 weeks from when a child first gets sick with polio. In fact, most polio is spread through the *stool* of non-paralyzed children who have 'only a cold' caused by the polio virus.

Severe paralysis

At what age do children get polio? In areas with poor sanitation, polio most often attacks babies **from 8 to 24 months** old, but occasionally children up to age 4 or 5. As sanitation improves, polio tends to strike older children and even young adults.

Who does it most often affect? Boys, a little more than girls. Unvaccinated children much more often than vaccinated children, especially those living in crowded, unsanitary conditions.

How does the paralysis begin? It begins after signs of a cold and fever, sometimes with diarrhea or vomiting. After a few days the neck becomes stiff and painful and parts of the body become limp. Parents may notice the weakness right away, or only after the child recovers from the acute illness.

Once a child is paralyzed, what changes or improvements can be expected? Often the paralysis will gradually go away, partly or completely. Any paralysis left after 7 months is usually permanent. The paralysis will not get worse. However, certain secondary problems may develop—especially if precautions are not taken to prevent them.

What are the child's chances of leading a happy, productive life? Usually very good—provided the child is encouraged to do things for himself, to get the most out of school, and to learn useful skills within his physical limitations (see p. 497).

Can persons with polio marry and have normal children? Yes. Polio is not inherited (familial) and does not affect ability to have children.

SECONDARY PROBLEMS TO LOOK FOR WITH POLIO

By **secondary** problems, we mean further disabilities or complications that can appear after, and because of, the original disability.

CONTRACTURES OF JOINTS

A contracture is a shortening of muscles and tendons (cords) so that the full range of limb movement is prevented.

Unless preventive steps are taken, joint contractures will form in many paralyzed children. Once formed, often they must be corrected before braces can be fitted and walking is possible. Correction of advanced contractures, whether through exercises, casts, or surgery (or a combination), is costly, takes time and causes discomfort. Therefore **early prevention of contractures is very important.**

A full discussion of contractures, their causes, prevention, and treatment is in the next chapter (Chapter 8). Methods and aids for correcting contractures are described in Chapter 59.

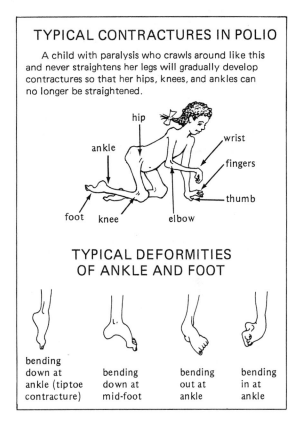

TYPICAL CONTRACTURES IN POLIO

A child with paralysis who crawls around like this and never straightens her legs will gradually develop contractures so that her hips, knees, and ankles can no longer be straightened.

TYPICAL DEFORMITIES OF ANKLE AND FOOT

bending down at ankle (tiptoe contracture)

bending down at mid-foot

bending out at ankle

bending in at ankle

OTHER COMMON DEFORMITIES

Weight bearing (supporting the body's weight) on weak joints can cause deformities, including:

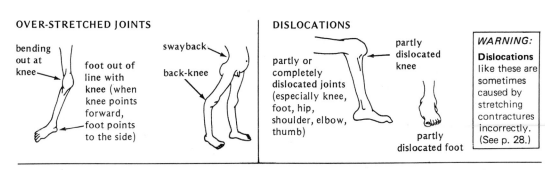

OVER-STRETCHED JOINTS

bending out at knee

foot out of line with knee (when knee points forward, foot points to the side)

swayback

back-knee

DISLOCATIONS

partly or completely dislocated joints (especially knee, foot, hip, shoulder, elbow, thumb)

partly dislocated knee

partly dislocated foot

WARNING:

Dislocations like these are sometimes caused by stretching contractures incorrectly. (See p. 28.)

SPINAL CURVE

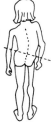

Minor curve of spine can be caused by tilted hips, as a result of a short leg.

More serious curve of the *spine* is caused by muscle weakness of the back or body muscles. The curve can become so severe that it endangers life by leaving too little room for the lungs and heart.

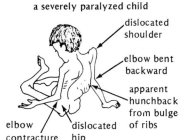

a severely paralyzed child

dislocated shoulder

elbow bent backward

apparent hunchback from bulge of ribs

elbow contracture

dislocated hip

At first, the spinal curve straightens when the child is positioned better. But in time the curve becomes more fixed (will not straighten any more). For information on spinal curves, see Chapter 20.

WHAT OTHER DISABILITIES CAN BE CONFUSED WITH POLIO?

- Sometimes **cerebral palsy** can be mistaken for polio—especially cerebral palsy of the 'floppy' type.

However, **cerebral palsy** usually affects the body in typical patterns:

Polio has a more irregular pattern of paralysis:

CEREBRAL PALSY all 4 limbs  arm and leg on same side both legs

POLIO

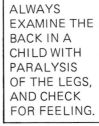

In cerebral palsy, usually you can find other signs of brain damage: over-active knee jerks and abnormal reflexes (see p. 88), developmental delay, awkward or uncontrolled movement, or at least some muscle tenseness (*spasticity*).

- In **muscular dystrophy,** paralysis begins little by little and steadily gets worse (see p. 109).

- **Hip problems** (see p. 155) can cause limping, and muscles may become thin and weak. Check hips for pain or dislocations. (*Note:* Dislocated hip may also occur secondary to polio.)

> *Note:* Polio can occur before or after a child has any of these other problems. Check carefully.

- **Clubbed foot** is present from birth (see p. 114).

- **'Erb's palsy'**, or partial paralysis in one arm and hand, comes from birth injury to the shoulder (see p. 127).

- **Leprosy.** Foot and hand paralysis begins gradually in older child. Often there are skin patches and loss of feeling (see p. 215).

- **Spina bifida** is present from birth. There is reduced feeling in the feet, and often a lump (or scar from surgery) on the back (see p. 167).

> ALWAYS EXAMINE THE BACK IN A CHILD WITH PARALYSIS OF THE LEGS, AND CHECK FOR FEELING.

- **Injuries to the spinal cord** (see p. 175) or to particular nerves going to the arms or legs. There is usually a history of a severe back or neck injury, and loss of feeling in the paralyzed part.

- **Tuberculosis of the spine** can cause gradual or suddenly increasing paralysis of the lower body. Look for typical bump on spine (see p. 165).

- **Other causes of paralysis or muscle weakness.** There are many causes of floppy paralysis similar to polio. One of the most common is **'Guillain-Barré' paralysis.** This can result from a virus infection, from poisoning, or from unknown causes. It usually begins without warning in the legs, and may spread within a few days to paralyze the whole body. Sometimes feeling is also reduced. Usually strength slowly returns, partly or completely, in several weeks or months. *Rehabilitation* and prevention of secondary problems are basically the same as for polio.

WHAT CAN BE DONE?

DURING THE ORIGINAL ILLNESS, when the child first becomes paralyzed:

- **No medicines** help, either during the first illness, or later.

- **Rest** is important. **Avoid forceful exercise** because this may increase paralysis. **Avoid injections.**

- **Good food** during recovery helps the child become stronger. (But take care that the child does not eat too much and get fat. An overweight child will have more problems with walking and other movements.) For suggestions about good food, see *Where There Is No Doctor,* Chapter 11.

- **Position** the child to be comfortable and to avoid contractures. At first the muscles will be painful, and the child will not want to straighten his joints. Slowly and gently try to straighten his arms and legs so that the child lies in as good a position as possible. (See Chapter 8.)

GOOD POSITION

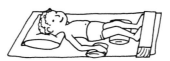

Arms, hips, and legs as straight as possible. Feet supported.

BAD POSITION

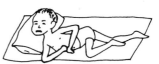

Bent arms, hips, and legs. Feet in tiptoe position.

Note: To reduce pain, you may need to put cushions under the knees, but try to keep the knees as straight as you can.

FOLLOWING THE ORIGINAL ILLNESS:

- Continue with **good food** and **good positions.**

- As soon as the fever drops, start **exercises** to prevent contractures and return strength. **Range-of-motion exercises** are described in Chapter 42. Whenever possible, make exercises fun. **Active games, swimming,** and other **activities to keep limbs moving as much as they can** are important throughout the child's rehabilitation.

- **Crutches, leg braces** *(calipers),* and other aids may help the child to move better and may prevent contractures or deformities.

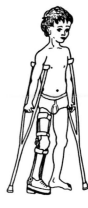

- In special cases, **surgery** may be needed to correct contractures, or to change the place where strong muscles attach, so that they help do the work of weak ones. When a foot is very floppy or bends to one side, surgery to join certain bones of the foot may help. But because bone surgery stops the growth of the foot, usually it should not be done before age 12 or 13.

- Encourage the child to **use his body and mind** as much as possible, to play actively with other children, to **take care of his daily needs,** to **help with work,** and to **go to school.** As much as possible, **treat him like any other child.**

REHABILITATION OF THE CHILD WITH PARALYSIS

All children paralyzed by polio can be helped by certain basic rehabilitation measures—such as exercise to keep a full range of motion in the affected limbs.

However, **each child will have a different combination and severity of paralyzed muscles, and therefore will have his own special needs.**

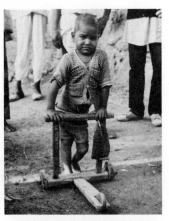

For some children, normal exercise and play may be all that are needed. Others may require special exercises and playthings. Still others may need braces or other aids to help them move about better, do things more easily, or keep their bodies in healthier, more useful positions. Those who are severely paralyzed may be helped most by a wheelboard (trolley) or wheelchair.

For this child, walking provides exercise that stretches his legs and feet, and prevents contractures. (Tilonia, India)

Every child needs to be carefully examined and evaluated in order to best meet his or her particular needs. The earlier you evaluate a child's needs, and take steps to meet them, the better.

Unfortunately, in most areas where polio is still common, village rehabilitation programs do not exist or are just beginning. Many children (and adults) who have been paralyzed for a long time already have severe deformities or joint contractures. Often these must be corrected before a child can use braces or begin to walk.

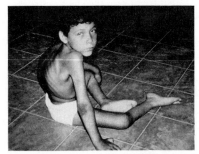

This child, who had polio as a baby, already had severe contractures in the hips, knees, and feet. (PROJIMO)

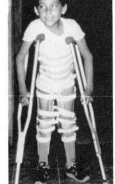

It took several months of exercises at home and then a series of plaster casts in the village rehabilitation center to straighten the contractures so he could walk with braces.

Because contractures are such a common problem, not only with polio but with many other disabilities, we discuss them separately in the next chapter. **Before evaluating a child with polio, we strongly suggest you read Chapter 8 on contractures.**

WARNING: Before deciding on any aid or procedure, carefully consider its advantages and disadvantages. For example, some deformities may be best left uncorrected because they actually help the paralyzed child stand straighter or walk better (see p. 530). And some aids or braces may prevent a child from developing strength to walk without aids (see p. 526). **Before deciding what aid or procedure to use, we suggest you read Chapter 56, "Making Sure Aids and Procedures Do More Good Than Harm."**

PROGRESS OF A CHILD WITH POLIO:
THE CHANGING NEEDS FOR AIDS AND ASSISTANCE

1. **exercises to keep full range of motion,** starting within days after paralysis appears and continuing throughout rehabilitation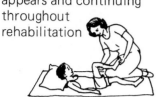

2. **supported sitting** in positions that help prevent contractures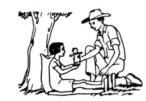

3. **active exercises** with limbs supported, to gain strength and maintain full motion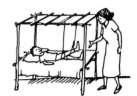

4. **exercise in water—walking, floating, and swimming, with the weight of the limbs supported by the water**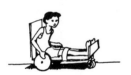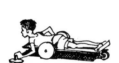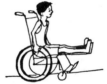

5. **wheelboard or wheelchair** with supports to prevent or correct early contractures.

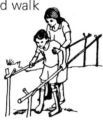 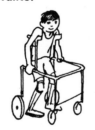 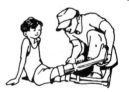

Note: These also provide good arm exercise in preparation for walking with crutches.

6. **braces** to prevent contractures and prepare for walking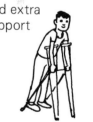

7. **parallel bars** for beginning to balance and walk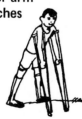

8. **walking machine or 'walker'**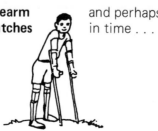

9. **crutches modified as walker** for balance and extra support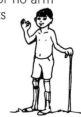

10. **under arm crutches**

11. **forearm crutches** and perhaps in time . . .

12. **a cane** or no arm supports at all

Note: These pictures are only an example—but most of the steps are necessary for many children. Children who begin rehabilitation late may also have contractures or deformities requiring corrective steps not shown here.

EVALUATING A CHILD'S NEEDS FOR AIDS AND PROCEDURES

Step 1: Start by learning what you can through talking with the child and family (see Child's History, p. 37 to 38). As you do this, **watch the child move about.** Observe carefully which parts of the body seem strong, and which seem weak. Look for any differences between one side of the body and the other—such as differences in the length or thickness of the legs. Are there any obvious deformities, or joints that do not seem to straighten all the way? If the child walks, what is unusual about the way she does it? Does she dip forward or to one side? Does she help support one leg with her hand? Is one hip lower than the other? Or one shoulder? Does she have a humpback, a swayback, or a sideways curve of the back?

These early observations will help you know what parts of the body you most need to check for strength and range of motion. Often, by watching a child you can begin to get an idea about what kind of aids or assistance may help. For example:

Carmen appears to have severe paralysis affecting both legs and her right arm. Weakness in her *trunk* (main part of the body) appears to have caused a severe S-shaped curve of the spine.

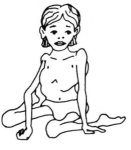

She will probably never walk, and will need a wheelchair or wheelboard.

You may want also to make her a body brace, or help her in other ways to sit more upright and try to keep the spine from bending more.

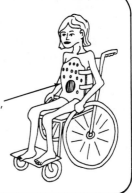

Pedro appears to have severe paralysis in his legs and hips. It looks as if his hips, knees, and feet cannot straighten (contractures). Weak stomach muscles and severe hip contractures may be the cause of his swayback.

Because his arms look strong, Pedro will probably be able to walk with crutches and leg braces. But first his contractures must be straightened.

If the contractures cannot be straightened by gradual stretching, he may need surgery.

strap to gradually straighten hips

casts to straighten knees and ankles

Because of hip weakness, he may need long leg braces with a hip band.

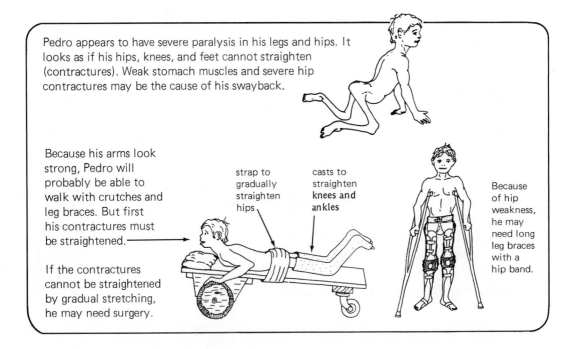

Manuel walks with the help of a stick. He appears to have paralysis mainly in his right leg and foot. Because of weak thigh muscles, he 'locks' his knee backward in order to bear weight on it. This 'back-kneeing' has become more and more extreme as the cords behind the knee stretch. The foot is very unstable and flops to one side. The weaker leg looks somewhat shorter—and for walking is much shorter because of the bent-back knee and bent-over foot.

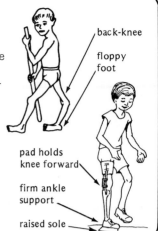

back-knee

floppy foot

pad holds knee forward

firm ankle support

raised sole

He might be able to walk without the stick if he uses a below-knee brace to stabilize his foot. (See p. 550.)

But the back-knee would become worse and worse until he could not walk. So probably he should have a long-leg brace. The brace might allow his knee to bend backward just a little for stability—so that no knee lock is needed.

Afia leans forward and pushes her weak left thigh with her hand when she walks. Her left knee cannot quite straighten. Her weak leg looks a little shorter than the other.

Or she may need an above-knee brace with a strap to pull the knee back.

Or she may only need a below-knee brace that helps push her knee back.

Exercises to get her knee straighter or so it can bend very slightly backward may be all that is needed for Afia to walk without using her hand.

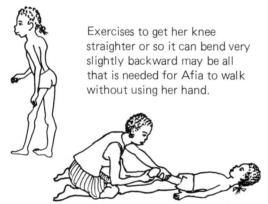

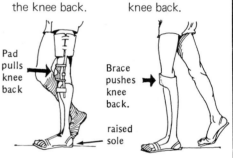

Pad pulls knee back

Brace pushes knee back.

raised sole

The brace bends the foot down just a little, so that by bearing weight on toes (rather than heel) her knee is pushed back.

To get a better idea about which of the three solutions may work best for Afia, you will need to do a careful physical examination, testing range of motion and muscle strength of the hip, knee, and ankle joints.

Step. 2: This is the **physical examination.** It should usually include:

1. **Range-of-motion testing,** especially where you think there might be contractures. (See "Physical Examination," p. 27 to 29, and "Contractures," p. 79 and 80.)

2. **Muscle testing,** especially of muscles that you think may be weak. Also test muscles that need to be strong to make up for weak ones (such as arm and shoulder strength for crutch use). (See p. 27 and p. 30 to 33.)

3. **Check for deformities:** contractures; dislocations (hip, knee, foot, shoulder, elbow); difference in leg length; tilt of hips; and curve or abnormal shape of the back. (See p. 34.)

Step 3: After the physical exam, **again observe how the child moves or walks.** Try to **relate her particular way of moving and walking with your physical findings** (such as weakness of certain muscles, contractures, and leg length). (For an example, see p. 70.)

Step 4: Based on your observations and tests, try to **figure out what kind of exercises, aids, or assistance might help the child most.** Consider the advantages of different possibilities: benefit, cost, comfort, appearance, availability of materials, and whether the child is likely to use the aid you make. Ask the child and parents for their opinions and suggestions.

Step 5: Before making a final brace or aid to fit the child, if possible **test to see how well it may work** by using a temporary aid or old brace from another child. For example,

If a child's ankle bends over to the outside like this . . .

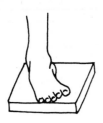

. . . a lift on the outer side of the sole like this, may help to keep the foot straighter.

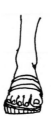

But *before* nailing and glueing in the lift, quickly make a trial one of cardboard or something else and fasten it temporarily to the sandal or shoe with tape or string. Then have the child walk.

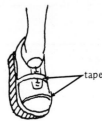
tape

Note: For a few children, a lift like this will help. For many it will not.

> **Ask the child what she thinks.**

Step 6: After the child, her parents, and you have decided what kind of brace or aid might work best, **take the necessary measurements and make the brace or aid.** When making it, once again it is wise to put it together temporarily so that you can make adjustments before you rivet, glue, or nail it into its final form. (See p. 540.)

Step 7: Have the child **try the brace or aid for a few days** to get used to it and to see how well it works. Ask the child and parents if it seems to help. Does it hurt? Are there any problems? How could it be improved? Is there something that might work better? Make what adjustments are necessary. But remember that no brace or aid is likely to meet the needs of a child perfectly. Do the best you can.

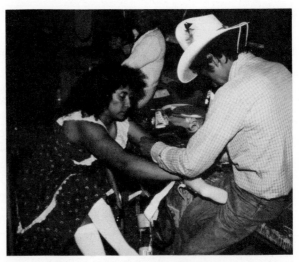

Mari and Chelo making a child's brace

Here is a story of how workers in a small village rehabilitation program figured out what kind of aids a child needed. **How many of the steps we have just discussed did they follow? Was each step important?**

A STORY: A BRACE FOR SAUL

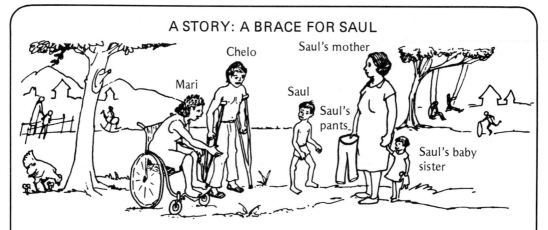

One day a mother from a neighboring village arrived at the village center with her 6 year old son, Saul. Mari and Chelo, 2 of the village rehabilitation workers, welcomed them warmly. Learning that Saul had polio as a baby, they asked him to walk, and then to run, while they watched carefully. Saul limped a lot and one leg looked thinner and shorter. With each step it bent back at the knee.

"He walks quite well, really," said Mari. "But he has to 'lock' his knee back in order to put weight on it. That knee is going to keep stretching back and some day it will give out."

"A long-leg brace would protect his knee," suggested Chelo.

"Oh, please, no!" said Saul's mother. "A year ago we took Saul to the city and the doctors had a big metal brace made for him. It cost so much we are still in debt! Saul hated it! He would always take it off and hide it. We tried and tried to get him to use it, but he wouldn't."

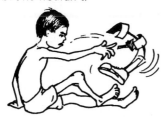

"That's not surprising," said Mari. "Often a child who can walk without a brace will refuse to use one—even if he walks better with it. We could make him a long-leg brace out of plastic. It would be much lighter. What do you say, Saul?" Saul began to cry.

"Don't worry, Saul. Maybe we can do something simpler," said Mari. "But first let's examine you, okay?" Saul nodded.

On muscle testing Saul, they found he could not straighten his knee at all. But he had fair strength for bending his knee back

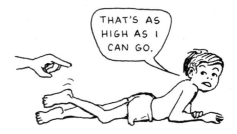

and his hip forward,

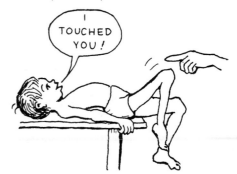

and good strength for bending his hip back.

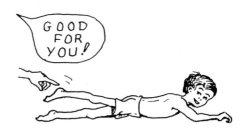

"With the hip and thigh strength he has, he should almost be able to stand on that leg without the knee bending back," said Mari. "Saul, let's see you try it like this. Pretend you're a stork!" For a moment Saul could do it. "Good!" said Mari. "Every day stand like that and see how high you can count without letting your knee go back. Every day try to beat your old record! Okay?"

"Okay," said Saul. Sounds like fun!"

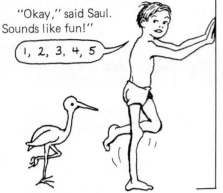

1, 2, 3, 4, 5

"The stork exercises may help," said Chelo. "But I still think he needs a brace. At least at first."

We must weigh the advantages against the disadvantages," said Mari. "A long-leg brace would keep his knee straight. But it could weaken the muscles he needs to strengthen. Since the brace would keep his leg from bending back, he wouldn't have to use his muscles to do it.

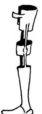

A long-leg brace might weaken the muscles Saul needs to strengthen.

"On the other hand, we might try a short-leg brace that holds his foot at almost a right angle. Then, to step flat he will have to keep his knee nearly straight. It could help him strengthen his behind-the-thigh muscles."

"Let's try it!" Everyone agreed, except Saul.

short-leg plastic brace

Chelo brought someone's old, lower-leg plastic brace and showed it to Saul. "See how it will fit right around your leg. It isn't heavy at all. Lift it! And no metal joints to get in the way! What do you say? Do you want to try it?"

"I guess so," said Saul.

When the brace was made, they tested it. Saul said he liked it. At first, when he tried hard, he could walk without bending his knee back. But after a few days, his mother complained that often he would walk, or even stand, with his knee bent way back as before, and his toes in the air, like this.

"WE THOUGHT IT WOULD WORK LIKE THIS . . ."

"BUT IN FACT IT WORKED LIKE THIS."

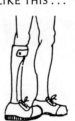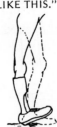

"I have an idea," said Chelo. "Why don't we let the heel stick out behind the shoe. That way, when he steps, his weight will come well forward of the back of his heel. This should help bring his foot down and his knee forward."

They tried it, and most of the time (especially when he was reminded) Saul walked without letting his knee bend back much.

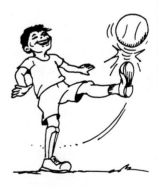

"THIS WORKED BETTER."

Heel extended backward helps prevent back-kneeing.

rounded front of sole to avoid pushing knee back at end of step

At home Saul's mother encouraged him to do his stork exercises. As his muscles grew stronger, he began to walk without bending his knee far back—even in active play!

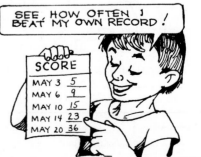

SEE, HOW OFTEN I BEAT MY OWN RECORD!

SCORE

MAY 3 5
MAY 6 9
MAY 10 15
MAY 14 23
MAY 20 36

"WILL MY CHILD EVER BE ABLE TO WALK?"

This is often one of the first questions asked by the parents of a disabled child. It is an important question. However, we must help parents realize that other things in life can be more important than walking (see p. 93).

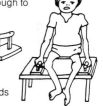

If the child whose legs are severely paralyzed by polio is to walk, generally she will need at least 2 things:

1. **fairly strong shoulders and arms** for crutch use
2. **fairly straight legs** (hips, knees, and feet). (It is important to correct contractures so that the legs are straight or nearly straight before trying to adapt braces for walking.)

To evaluate a child's possibility for walking, always **test arm and shoulder strength:**

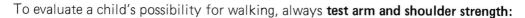

Have her try to lift her body weight off the ground with her arms, like this.

If she can easily lift up and down several times, she has a GOOD chance of being able to walk using crutches.

If her arms and shoulders are so weak she cannot begin to lift herself, her chances for crutch-walking are POOR.

If her shoulder and arm strength is FAIR, and the child can almost lift herself, daily exercise lifting her weight like this may increase strength enough to make crutch use possible.

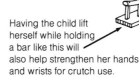

Having the child lift herself while holding a bar like this will also help strengthen her hands and wrists for crutch use.

Pushing herself in a wheelchair or wheelboard (trolley) is a practical way to strengthen shoulders, arms, and hands.

If the child cannot lift herself because of weak elbows, put simple splints on her arms to see if she can lift herself with these.

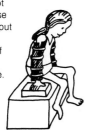

If she can lift herself with the elbow splints, maybe she can use crutches that give elbow support.

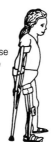

If she is fat, she should lose weight. This will make walking on weak limbs much easier.

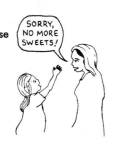

SORRY, NO MORE SWEETS!

Now check how straight the legs will go. (See range-of-motion testing, p. 27.)

If the hips, knees, and feet can be placed in fairly straight positions, chances for walking soon with braces are good (if arm strength is good).

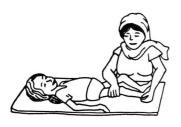

But if the child has much contracture of the hips, knees, or feet, these will need to be straightened before she will be able to walk.

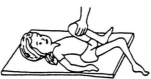

For correction of contractures, see Chapters 8 and 59.

Sometimes, if contractures are severe in one leg only, the child can learn to walk on the other leg only, with crutches. But it is best with both legs, whenever possible.

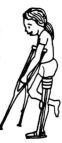

After checking arm strength and leg straightness, the next thing to **check is the strength in the ankles, knees, and hips.** This will help you decide if the child needs braces, and what kind.

A child with a foot that hangs down (foot drop), **or flops to one side** may be helped by a below-knee brace of plastic or metal.

For foot drop, you can make a brace that lifts the foot with a spring or rubber band. (See p. 545.)

PLASTIC   METAL

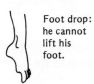

Foot drop: he cannot lift his foot.

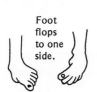

Foot flops to one side.

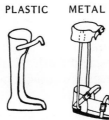

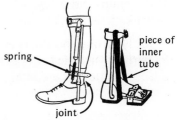

spring

joint

piece of inner tube

The kind of brace you choose will depend on various factors, including cost, available skills and materials, and what seems to work best for the particular child. **Advantages and disadvantages of different kinds of braces, and how to make them, are discussed in Chapter 58.**

A child with a weak knee may need a long-leg brace of plastic or metal.

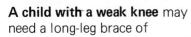

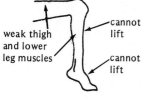

weak thigh and lower leg muscles

cannot lift

cannot lift

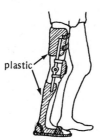

plastic

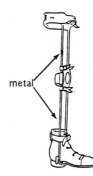

metal

Upper-leg braces may be made with or without a knee joint that locks straight for walking and bends for sitting. Different models are discussed in Chapter 58.

Note: **Not all children with no strength to straighten the knee need long-leg braces:** A child with strong butt muscles may be able to walk without a brace.

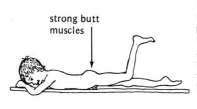

strong butt muscles

STRONG butt muscles pull the thigh back and keep the knee from bending.

A child who has FAIR butt strength and a straight knee may be helped enough by a lower-leg brace that pushes the knee back.

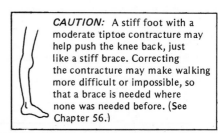

brace pushes knee back

Slightly downward angle of a stiff brace causes it to push the knee backward when weight bearing.

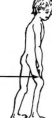

A child with weak butt muscles may walk with one hand pushing on the weak thigh.

Or he may walk by bending the knee back to 'lock' it for weight bearing.

> *CAUTION:* A stiff foot with a moderate tiptoe contracture may help push the knee back, just like a stiff brace. Correcting the contracture may make walking more difficult or impossible, so that a brace is needed where none was needed before. (See Chapter 56.)

If a child has a contracture and cannot walk with his knee straight, correcting the contracture until his knee bends very slightly backward may allow him to walk better.

A child with very weak hip muscles may find his leg flops or twists about too much with a long-leg brace.

He may need a brace with a hip band to help stabilize the leg at the hip.

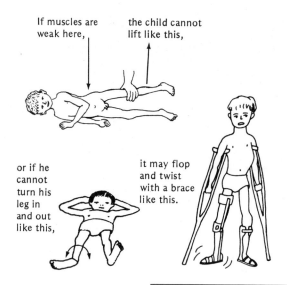

If muscles are weak here,

the child cannot lift like this,

or if he cannot turn his leg in and out like this,

it may flop and twist with a brace like this.

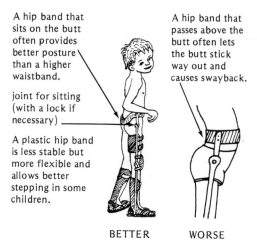

A hip band that sits on the butt often provides better posture than a higher waistband.

joint for sitting (with a lock if necessary)

A plastic hip band is less stable but more flexible and allows better stepping in some children.

A hip band that passes above the butt often lets the butt stick way out and causes swayback.

BETTER   WORSE

A child with weak body and back muscles, who cannot hold up her body well, may need long-leg braces attached to a body brace or body jacket.

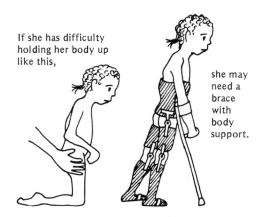

If she has difficulty holding her body up like this,

she may need a brace with body support.

Note: Often a child at first may need a hip band or body jacket to help stabilize her for walking. A few weeks or months later she may no longer need it. Removing it may help the child gain more strength and control. It is **important to re-evaluate the child's needs for bracing periodically.**

> **Take care to use no more bracing than is needed.**

A child whose backbone is becoming seriously curved may benefit from a body brace (or in severe cases, she may need surgery).

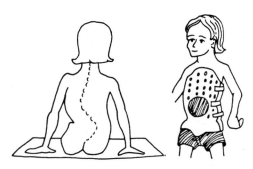

If necessary, the body brace can be attached to long-leg braces as shown above.

More information on spinal curve can be found in Chapter 20. For information on how to make body braces and jackets, see Chapter 58.

PREVENTION OF POLIO

- **Vaccinate** babies with polio vaccine. It is usually best to give the first polio vaccination around 3 months of age. Be sure they get the vaccine 4 times by the time they are 18 months old. They should get a 5th dose when they are 5 years old.

POLIO VACCINE, the best protection–IF it has been kept cold continuously!

- **Vaccinate as many children as possible.** The vaccine given by mouth is alive. So, if most of the children are vaccinated, the live vaccine will spread to children who have not been vaccinated, and protect them also.

- **Try to keep the live polio vaccine frozen** until shortly before it is used. For up to 3 months it can be thawed and refrozen. But it must be kept cold or it will spoil.

- **Seek community help** with vaccination and in keeping vaccines cold. Sometimes vaccines do not reach villages because health posts lack refrigeration. But often storekeepers and a few families have refrigerators. Win their interest and cooperation.

WHY IS IT THAT YOU ALWAYS HAVE ICES FOR SALE AND WE CAN'T FIND A WAY TO KEEP VACCINES COLD?

LACK OF TRUE COMMUNITY PARTICIPATION, MA'AM!

ICE STICKS FROZEN POP

- To give best protection, **vaccinate the child when she does not have a fever or a cold or diarrhea.** But if by 6 months of age, the child still has not been vaccinated, give her the polio vaccine even if she is a little sick. However, there is a chance that the vaccine may not work if it is given when the child is sick (with a virus infection). Therefore, still try to give the complete series of 3 vaccinations and one booster later, when the child is not sick.

It is estimated that in poor countries **at least one-third of vaccines are spoiled by the time they reach the children.** Therefore, **even in children who have been vaccinated, additional precautions are needed:**

- **Breast feed** your baby as long as possible. Breast milk contains 'antibodies' that may help protect against polio. (Babies rarely get polio before 8 months old because they still have their mothers' antibodies. Breast feeding may make this protection last longer.)

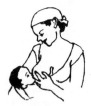

BREAST MILK PROTECTS AGAINST INFECTIONS– INCLUDING POLIO

- **Organize the people** and help out in popular campaigns to encourage vaccination and breast feeding. **Community theater** and **puppet shows** are good ways to raise awareness on these issues. See Chapter 48.

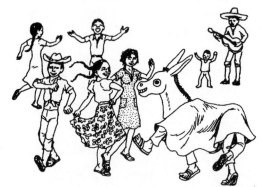

PREVENTION of secondary problems

We have already discussed some ways to prevent new problems or complications in a child with paralysis. In summary, important measures include:

- **Prevent contractures and deformities.** Begin appropriate **range-of-motion** exercises as soon as the paralysis appears.

- At the first sign of a joint contracture, do **stretching exercises** 2 or 3 times a day— every day.

Stretching exercises work better if you stretch the joint firmly and continuously for a few moments, instead of 'pumping' the limb back and forth.

We emphasize this point because in many countries parents are taught the pumping method— which does very little good.

CORRECT

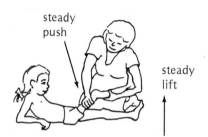

steady push

steady lift

WRONG

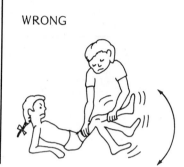

For more details, see "Contractures," Chapter 8.

- **Evaluate the child's needs regularly,** and **change or adapt aids, braces, and exercises to meet her changing needs.** Too little or too much bracing can hold the child back or create new problems.

- **Be sure crutches do not press hard under the arms;** this can cause paralysis of the hands (see p. 393).

- **Try not to let the child's physical disability hold back her overall physical, mental, and social development.** Provide opportunities for her to lead an active life and take part in games, activities, school, and work with other children. PART 2 of this book discusses ways to help the community meet the needs of disabled children.

OTHER PARTS OF THIS BOOK THAT MAY BE USEFUL
IN MEETING NEEDS OF A CHILD AFFECTED BY POLIO
Especially important chapters are marked with a star:

For more information on polio, see References p. 637.

A BOY WITH POLIO BECOMES AN OUTSTANDING HEALTH AND REHABILITATION WORKER

Marcelo Acevedo was disabled by polio. He and his family lived in a village 2 days from the closest road. Village health workers from Project Piaxtla helped Marcelo get surgery for his knee contractures. After surgery he got braces and went to school. Then they trained him as a village health worker, and he returned to serve his village.

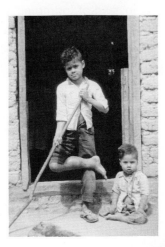

Marcelo at age 4, sitting with his older brother who was temporarily disabled when a tree fell on his leg.

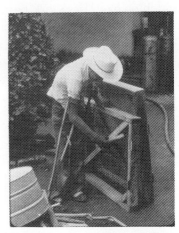

Marcelo training at Project Piaxtla.

When PROJIMO was formed, Marcelo joined as a village rehabilitation worker. He studied brace-making as an apprentice in 2 brace shops in Mexico City.

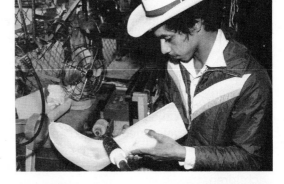

Marcelo making a plastic leg brace.

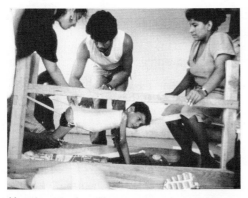

Marcelo and other villagers make a plaster body mold of a young boy's chest. The child had polio and has a severe curve of the spine.

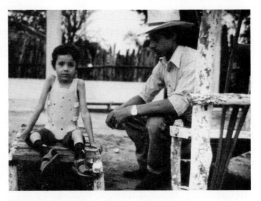

With his plastic body brace, made by Marcelo, the child can sit much straighter. (See p. 558.)

Marcelo is now one of the leaders in PROJIMO, and has gained the respect of the whole village. He has recently married a village woman.

Contractures

CHAPTER **8**

Limbs That No Longer Straighten

WHAT ARE CONTRACTURES?

When an arm or leg is in a bent position for a long time, some of the muscles become shorter, so that the limb cannot fully straighten. Or shortened muscles may hold a joint straight, so it cannot bend. We say the joint has a 'contracture'. Contractures can develop in any joint of the body. For example:

1. Miguel spent the first years of his life crawling because one leg was paralyzed.

   Because he could not stand, he kept his hip and knee bent and his foot in a tiptoe position, like this.

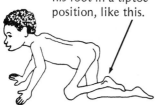

2. In time, he could not straighten his hip or knee, or bend his foot up. He had developed a:

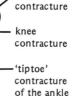

hip contracture

knee contracture

'tiptoe' contracture of the ankle

You can feel the tight *cord* here,

when you push here.

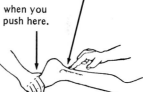

3. Because of the contractures, Miguel could not stand or walk, even with a brace.

shortened muscles causing hip contracture

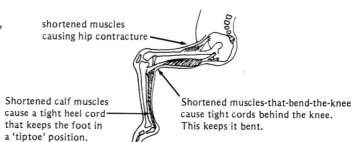

Shortened calf muscles cause a tight heel cord that keeps the foot in a 'tiptoe' position.

Shortened muscles-that-bend-the-knee cause tight cords behind the knee. This keeps it bent.

Contractures develop whenever a limb or joint is not moved regularly through its full range of motion. This is likely when:

- a very weak or sick child is in bed for a long time.

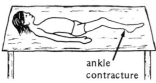

ankle contracture

- a child with an amputation keeps joints bent.

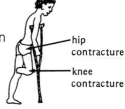

hip contracture

knee contracture

- a paralyzed limb is kept bent or hanging.

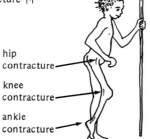

hip contracture

knee contracture

ankle contracture

- a child has joint pain that prevents her from straightening her joints.

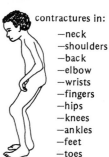

contractures in:
—neck
—shoulders
—back
—elbow
—wrists
—fingers
—hips
—knees
—ankles
—feet
—toes

Why is it important to know about contractures?

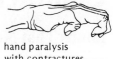

hand paralysis
with contractures

- Most contractures can be prevented through exercise and other measures. Yet **in many communities, at least half of the physically disabled children already have contractures.**

- Contractures make rehabilitation more difficult. **Often they must be corrected before a child can walk or care for himself.**

- Correction of contractures is **slow, costly, and often very uncomfortable or painful.**

- It is best not to let contractures develop, and if they do begin to develop, to correct them as soon as possible. Early contractures often can be easily corrected at home, with **exercises** and **positioning.** Advanced, old contractures are much more difficult to correct, and may require gradual stretching with plaster casts, or surgery.

For all these reasons . . .

> **Every family with a disabled child should understand how contractures develop, how to prevent them, and how to recognize and correct them when they first begin.**

Muscle imbalance—a major cause of contractures

CP When the muscles that bend or pull a limb in one direction are much stronger than those that pull it in the opposite direction, we say there is a 'muscle imbalance'. When paralysis, painful joints, or spasticity (see p. 89) cause a muscle imbalance, contractures are much more likely to develop.

CP

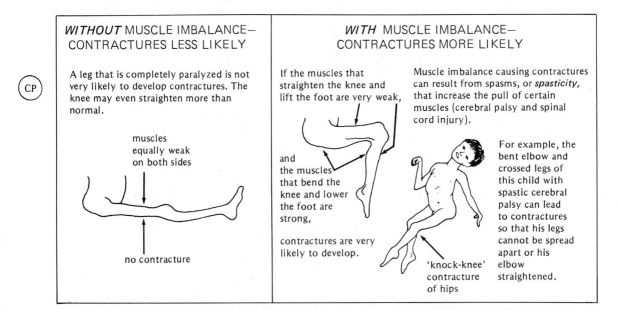

WITHOUT MUSCLE IMBALANCE— CONTRACTURES LESS LIKELY

A leg that is completely paralyzed is not very likely to develop contractures. The knee may even straighten more than normal.

muscles equally weak on both sides

no contracture

WITH MUSCLE IMBALANCE— CONTRACTURES MORE LIKELY

If the muscles that straighten the knee and lift the foot are very weak,

and the muscles that bend the knee and lower the foot are strong,

contractures are very likely to develop.

Muscle imbalance causing contractures can result from spasms, or *spasticity,* that increase the pull of certain muscles (cerebral palsy and spinal cord injury).

For example, the bent elbow and crossed legs of this child with spastic cerebral palsy can lead to contractures so that his legs cannot be spread apart or his elbow straightened.

'knock-knee' contracture of hips

To check for muscle imbalance, test and compare the strength of the muscles that bend a joint, and of the muscles that straighten it. (See muscle testing, p. 30.)

EXAMINING THE CHILD FOR CONTRACTURES

This is done through testing the **'range of motion'** of different joints, as described on p. 27 to 29. Most contractures will be obvious when you test for them. But hip contractures can easily be missed.

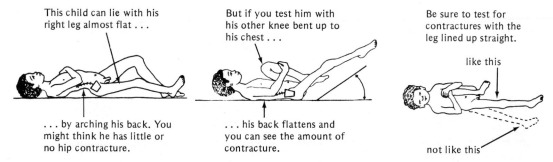

This child can lie with his right leg almost flat . . .

. . . by arching his back. You might think he has little or no hip contracture.

But if you test him with his other knee bent up to his chest . . .

. . . his back flattens and you can see the amount of contracture.

Be sure to test for contractures with the leg lined up straight.

like this

not like this

Also **be sure joints do not dislocate** when you test for contractures, because this can fool you, too. For example:

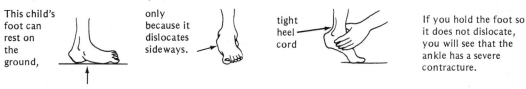

This child's foot can rest on the ground,

only because it dislocates sideways. →

tight heel cord →

If you hold the foot so it does not dislocate, you will see that the ankle has a severe contracture.

How to tell contractures from spasticity

Spasticity (muscle tightening that the child does not control) is common when there is damage to the brain or spinal cord. (See p. 89.) It is sometimes mistaken for contractures. It is important to know the difference.

(CP)

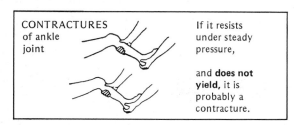

SPASTICITY of ankle joint	If at first it resists under steady pressure, and then it **slowly yields,** it is probably spasticity.

CONTRACTURES of ankle joint	If it resists under steady pressure, and **does not yield,** it is probably a contracture.

Spasticity often leads to contractures. For details, see p. 102 and 103.

MEASURING CONTRACTURES

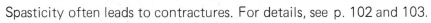

This can be done by folding a paper and measuring the angle, as shown here,

and then tracing that angle onto a record sheet.

Or use a 'compass'.

Or make a simple instrument of 2 thin pieces of wood joined by a bolt or rivet, tight enough so that they move stiffly.

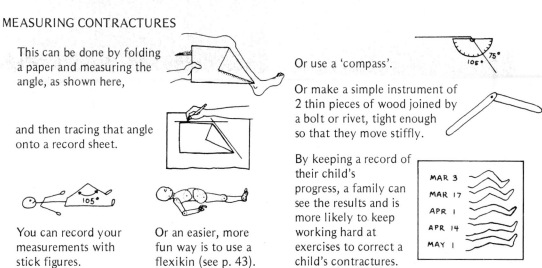

You can record your measurements with stick figures.

Or an easier, more fun way is to use a flexikin (see p. 43).

By keeping a record of their child's progress, a family can see the results and is more likely to keep working hard at exercises to correct a child's contractures.

MAR 3
MAR 17
APR 1
APR 14
MAY 1

Can a contracture be straightened in the village?

Contractures usually begin with shortening of muscles, causing tight cords (tendons). Later, the *nerves*, skin, and 'joint capsule' also can become tight. (A 'joint capsule' is the tough covering around a joint.)

When a contracture is only in the muscles and cords, it can usually be straightened by exercises and casts at a village rehab center, although sometimes this may take months. But if the contracture also involves the joint capsule, it is often much more difficult or impossible to correct, even with many months of using casts. Surgery may be needed.

> *Note:* If you find the information on this page hard to understand, do not worry. Come back to it later, when you meet very stubborn contractures.

TO TEST THE KNEE JOINT:

Check the range of motion of the knee with the hip straight and then bent.

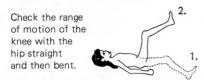

Explanation: One of the main muscles that causes a knee contracture is the 'hamstring muscle', which runs all the way from the hip bone to the bone of the lower leg. This means that when the hip is bent, the tight muscles will bend the knee more.

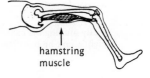

hamstring muscle

If the knee straightens more when the hip is straight

than when the hip is bent,

probably this is a **muscle contracture** (a short hamstring muscle).

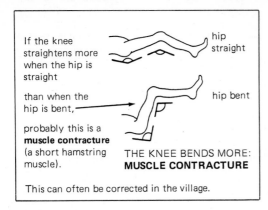

hip straight

hip bent

THE KNEE BENDS MORE: **MUSCLE CONTRACTURE**

This can often be corrected in the village.

But if the knee straightens equally when the hip is straight or bent,

probably there is contracture of the **joint capsule.**

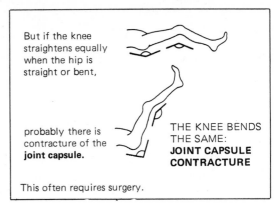

THE KNEE BENDS THE SAME: **JOINT CAPSULE CONTRACTURE**

This often requires surgery.

TO TEST THE ANKLE JOINT:

Check the range of motion of the ankle with the knee straight and then bent.

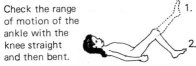

Explanation: One of the main muscles that pulls the foot to a tiptoe position runs from the thigh bone all the way to the heel. This causes the heel cord to pull more when the knee is straight than when the knee is bent.

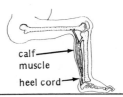

calf muscle

heel cord

If the foot pushes down more when the knee is straight

than when the knee is bent, it is a **muscle contracture.**

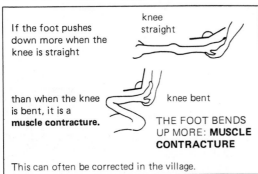

knee straight

knee bent

THE FOOT BENDS UP MORE: **MUSCLE CONTRACTURE**

This can often be corrected in the village.

But if the foot angle is the same when the knee is straight or bent,

there probably is a contracture of the **joint capsule.**

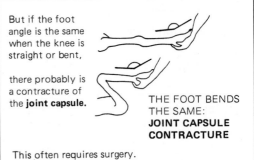

THE FOOT BENDS THE SAME: **JOINT CAPSULE CONTRACTURE**

This often requires surgery.

JOINTS THAT DO NOT MOVE AT ALL

If a joint moves only a little, the joint capsule may be very tight, or there may be a deformity in the bones. With exercises, try to gradually increase the movement.

If a joint does not move at all, the bones may be 'fused' (joined together). This often happens when there is a lot of pain and damage in the joint. When a joint has fused, exercise will usually not bring back motion. The only surgery that might help return joint motion is to put in an 'artificial joint' of metal or plastic. This surgery is very costly, and if the person is very active, the joint may not last more than a few years.

PREVENTION AND EARLY MANAGEMENT OF CONTRACTURES

Contractures can often be prevented by (1) positioning, and (2) range-of-motion exercises.

POSITIONING

If a child is likely to develop contractures or has begun to develop them, try to position her to stretch the affected joints. Look for ways to do this during day-to-day activities: lying, sitting, being carried, playing, studying, bathing, and moving about.

During a severe illness (such as acute polio), or a recent spinal cord injury, contractures can develop quickly. Therefore, early preventive positioning is very important:

CORRECT	CORRECT	WRONG
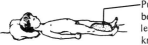 Put a pillow between legs to hold knees apart.	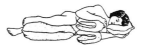	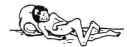
Lying and sleeping straight helps prevent contractures.	Also use pillows for side-lying to keep a good position.	Lying and sleeping with the legs in a twisted or bent position causes contractures.

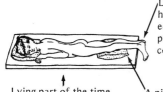 Letting feet hang over edge helps prevent ankle contractures.		
Lying part of the time face down helps stretch hips backward. A pillow here helps stretch knees.	A foot board helps to prevent ankle contractures.	The foot support can be leaned forward a little so that the child can stretch his feet by pushing against it. (Be sure to pad it.)

Support feet at right angles.	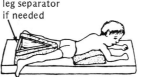 leg separator if needed	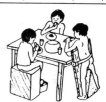
If knee contractures might develop, keep the knees straight as much as possible.	A child who spends most of the time sitting should spend part of the day lying or standing (on a frame if necessary). This will help prevent contractures of the hips and knees.	

WRONG	BETTER	BEST
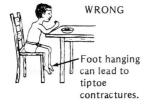 Foot hanging can lead to tiptoe contractures.	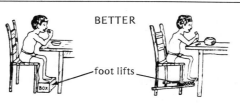 foot lifts	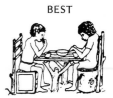
	Figure out ways to help the child stay in contracture-preventing positions.	child-sized furniture

For a child with spasticity whose legs press together or cross, look for ways to sit, lie, or carry him with his legs separated. Here are a few examples.   For more examples of ways to prevent 'knock-knee' contractures, see p. 100.

For more ideas about special seating and positioning, see Chapter 65.

Exercises to prevent contractures

Just as cats, dogs, and many other animals stretch their bodies after they wake up, children often enjoy stretching their limbs and testing their strength. This is one of the purposes of play.

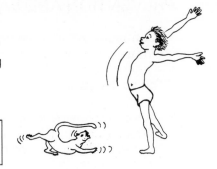

> **Daily stretching keeps the joints able to move smoothly and freely through their full range of motion.**

Unfortunately, some children, because of illness, paralysis or weakness, are not able to stretch all parts of their bodies easily during their play and daily activities. If some part of their body is not regularly stretched or moved through its full range, contractures may develop.

To maintain full, easy movement of their joints and limbs, these children therefore need daily exercises that move the affected parts of their bodies through their full range of motion.

Range-of-motion exercises for the shoulder.

Range-of-motion exercises for each body joint are discussed in Chapter 42.

As much as possible, the child herself should try to move the affected part through its range of motion. Often the limb will be too weak and help is needed. But **be sure the child moves it as much as she can herself.**

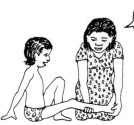

BEND YOUR FOOT UP AS FAR AS YOU CAN. I'LL HELP YOU.

Have the child move the part as far as she can without help. Then help her to move it the rest of the way.

Where there is muscle imbalance, strengthening the weaker muscles can help prevent contractures. **Examples of muscle strengthening exercises are on pages 138 to 143 and 388 to 392.**

As much as possible, try to **make exercises fun.**

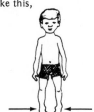 A child whose feet tend to bend *inward* like this,

may benefit from exercises that bend them *outward,* like this.

Walking on boards in a V-shape may provide similar stretching and be more fun.

But going with father on the V-shaped paths to the bean fields may be even more fun—and it stretches his ankles more, because it is a long way.

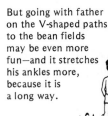

FOUR WAYS TO APPROACH STRETCHING EXERCISES: To prevent (or help correct) contractures, exercises can be done in 4 different ways, depending on the needs and ability of the child. These 4 ways, shown on the next page, progress from **exercises where the child depends completely on help, to exercises that she does on her own as a part of everyday activity.**

FOUR WAYS TO DO EXERCISES THAT STRETCH A TIGHT HEEL CORD

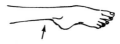

1. Someone else moves the limb.

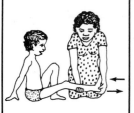

Often necessary—but not much fun.

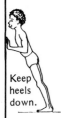

Keep heels down.

Leaning against a wall stretches the feet more than standing upright does.

2. The child does his own exercises, but without using the muscles in the affected part.

(This may help to prevent a contracture but will not help much to correct it.)

Here the child does his own stretching with some help from his mother.

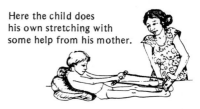

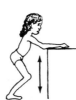

If the child is strong enough, bending the knees or touching the toes is a good way to stretch the muscles that cause a tight heel cord.

CAUTION: When doing these exercises, carefully **check to see that the foot is not dislocating to the side.** If so, you should use Method 1, being careful to hold the foot in such a way that it does not 'cave in' to the side.

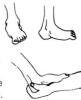

3. The child does the exercise—using muscles of the affected part.

WITH ASSISTANCE:

If the child has some strength to raise his foot, have him raise it as far as he can. Then help him to raise it as far as it will stretch.

Developing the muscles that lift the foot may help prevent contracture.

NOW PULL YOUR FOOT UP. I'LL HELP!

I'M TRYING!

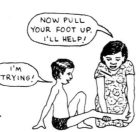

AGAINST RESISTANCE:

If the child has enough strength to raise his foot against resistance, he should do so. But be sure that the foot comes **all the way up.**

sand bag tied to foot

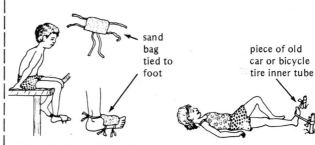

piece of old car or bicycle tire inner tube

4. The child does the exercise—during normal daily activities.

Figure out ways or aids so that the child can take part in ordinary activities that stretch muscles and prevent contractures.

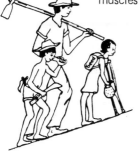

standing and walking uphill to stretch heel cords

picking vegetables

chest band that hooks over crutch top

strong wire

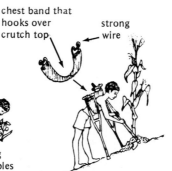

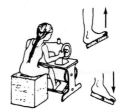

Sewing on a machine can exercise foot and combat contractures.

bar that permits child to squat and bend ankles

DIFFERENT METHODS TO CORRECT CONTRACTURES

- When contractures are just **beginning** to develop, **stretching exercises** and **simple positioning** may be all that is needed to correct them.

- When contractures are **more advanced,** stretching must be done steadily over a long time, using **fixed positions, casts, braces,** or **special equipment** that keep a continuous pull on the affected joints.

- When contractures are **old and severe,** correction by **surgery** may be needed.

Even when contractures are advanced, it is usually best to try to correct them as much as possible using simpler, less harsh methods first.

If a contracture is advanced:

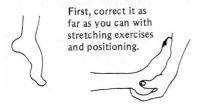 First, correct it as far as you can with stretching exercises and positioning.

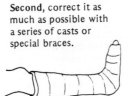 Second, correct it as much as possible with a series of casts or special braces.

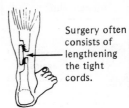 Third, if more correction is still needed, consider surgery. Surgery often consists of lengthening the tight cords.

**Instructions for correcting contractures
using plaster casts or braces are in Chapter 59.**

CAUTION: Some **orthopedic** surgeons are quick to recommend surgery. However, we have found that many contractures often said to need surgery can be corrected in the village or home by exercise and casting or braces. In any case, **stretching exercises and bracing are often needed for a long time after surgery (or forever) to prevent the contractures from coming back.**

Also, some contractures are best left uncorrected (see Chapters 42 and 56). When in doubt, consult an experienced physical therapist.

Exercises to correct contractures—'stretching exercises'

These are similar to the range-of-motion exercises used to prevent contractures, except that steady, gentle but firm stretching is required:

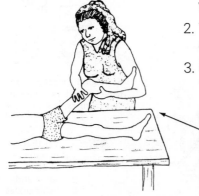

1. Hold the limb in a steady, stretched position while you count slowly to 25.

2. Then gradually stretch the joint a little more, and again count slowly to 25.

3. Continue increasing the stretch in this way, steadily for 5 or 10 minutes. Repeat several times a day.

CAUTION: **To avoid damaging the limb, hold it near the joint,** as shown. It is acceptable if the stretching hurts the child a little, but it should not hurt him a lot. **If you want faster results, do not apply more force. Stretch the limb for longer and more times each day.**

In children who do not feel in their legs, take special care not to stretch forcefully. You could cause injuries.

STRETCHING EXERCISE INSTRUCTION SHEETS

Some stretching exercises are done best using special techniques. Often they need to be done at home for weeks or months. You will find instruction sheets for the most frequently needed stretching exercises in Chapter 42, "Range-of-motion and Other Exercises." They include:

Stretching exercise for a **tight heel cord.** See p. 383.	Stretching exercise for a **bent knee.** See p. 384.	Stretching exercise for a **bent hip.** See p. 385.

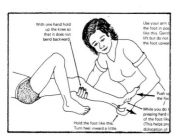 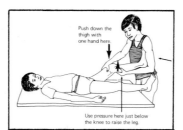 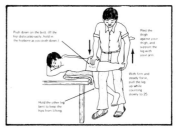

HOLDING A CONTRACTED JOINT IN A STRETCHED POSITION FOR LONG PERIODS

Chapter 59 discusses the use of casts, braces, and other aids to stretch difficult contractures. These include:

a series of plaster casts and wedges	**adjustable braces**	**elastic stretching devices**
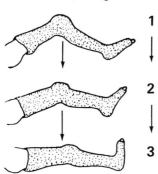	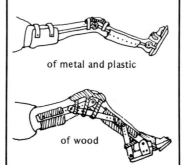 of metal and plastic — of wood	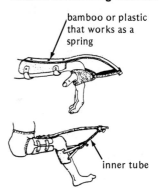 bamboo or plastic that works as a spring — inner tube

Advantages:

- Holds leg in exactly the position you want it.
- Child (or parents) cannot easily remove it.
- Especially useful for difficult deformities that bend in different directions.

Disadvantages:

- Cannot be easily removed to check for sores, to bathe, and to exercise. (Therefore, casts should usually not be used on children with arthritis or children without feeling in their legs.)
- Hot in warm weather.
- Expensive (plaster bandage).
- Adjustments require trip to clinic or rehabilitation center.

Advantages:

- Can be adjusted by family at home.
- Can be easily removed to check for sores, for bathing, and exercise.

Disadvantages:

- More difficult to make and to fit well.
- Difficult to use on child with various deformities that go in different directions.
- Child (or parents) may remove and not use it.

Advantages:

- Same as for adjustable braces, and also:
- Does not need frequent adjustment because it keeps pulling as joint stretches.

Disadvantages:

- Clumsy—gets in the way.
- Difficult to make so they work well.
- Often not good with spasticity.

HIP CONTRACTURES

Hip 'flexion' contractures (in which the thighs stay bent forward at the hips) are often difficult to straighten and require special techniques.

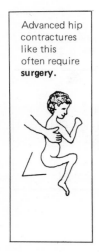

Advanced hip contractures like this often require **surgery.**

Less advanced hip contractures like this can sometimes be straightened using **positioning and straps.**

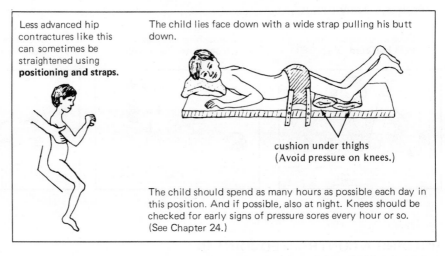

The child lies face down with a wide strap pulling his butt down.

cushion under thighs
(Avoid pressure on knees.)

The child should spend as many hours as possible each day in this position. And if possible, also at night. Knees should be checked for early signs of pressure sores every hour or so. (See Chapter 24.)

Life can be made more interesting for the child during the weeks or months of stretching by using a lying frame on which she can move about.

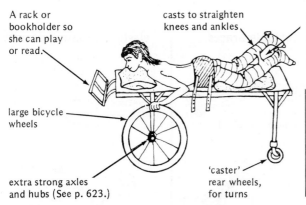

A rack or bookholder so she can play or read.

casts to straighten knees and ankles

A bar fastened between the 2 leg casts helps keep them in a stable position (and also helps prevent contractures that pull the legs together).

For other designs see p. 618.

large bicycle wheels

extra strong axles and hubs (See p. 623.)

'caster' rear wheels, for turns

CAUTION: When stretching contractures this way, be careful to prevent pressure sores (bed sores), especially on the knees. If the child complains a lot, loosen the strap a little. For eating, bathing, toilet, and exercise she can be unfastened and moved into convenient positions. But it is best that she remain strapped down about 20 out of each 24 hours.

The child with more severe contractures at the hips may need to be strapped on an angled frame.

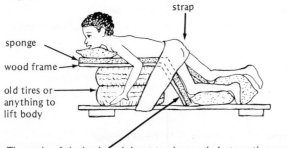

strap

sponge

wood frame

old tires or anything to lift body

The angle of the leg boards is set to give gentle but continuous pressure against the thighs. As the contracture is gradually corrected, the angle is changed by raising the leg boards or by lowering the body board.

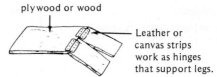

plywood or wood

Leather or canvas strips work as hinges that support legs.

For children with different angles of contracture in each hip, the 2 leg boards can be adjusted differently.

For additional information on contractures relating to different disabilities, aids, and equipment, see the INDEX under 'Contractures'. For methods to correct contractures, see Chapter 59.

CHAPTER **9**

Cerebral Palsy

WHAT IS CEREBRAL PALSY?

Cerebral palsy means 'brain *paralysis*'. It is a *disability* that affects movement and body position. It comes from brain damage that happened before the baby was born, at birth, or as a baby. The whole brain is not damaged, only parts of it, mainly parts that control movements. Once damaged, the parts of the brain do not recover, nor do they get worse. However, the movements, body positions, and related problems can be improved or made worse depending on how we treat the child and how damaged his or her brain happens to be. **The earlier we start, the more improvement can be made.**

In many countries cerebral palsy is the most frequent cause of physical disability. In other countries it is second only to polio. About 1 of every 300 babies is born with or develops cerebral palsy.

How to recognize cerebral palsy

EARLY SIGNS:

- **At birth** a baby with cerebral palsy is often **limp** and **floppy,** or may even seem normal.

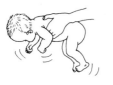

NORMAL   FLOPPY

Child hangs in upside down 'U' with little or no movement.

- Baby may or may not breathe right away at birth, and may turn blue and floppy. Delayed breathing is a common cause of brain damage.

- **Slow development**
  Compared to other children in the village, the child is slow to hold up his head, to sit, or to move around.

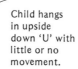

- He may not use his hands. Or he only uses one hand and does not begin to use both.

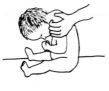

- **Feeding problems**
  The baby may have difficulties with sucking, swallowing and chewing. She may choke or gag often. Even as the child gets bigger, these and other feeding problems may continue.

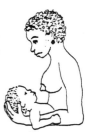

- **Difficulties in taking care of the baby or young child.** Her body may stiffen when she is carried, dressed, or washed, or during play. Later she may not learn to feed or dress herself, to wash, use the toilet, or to play with others. This may be due to sudden stiffening of the body, or to being so floppy she 'falls all over the place'.

The baby may be so limp that her head seems as if it will fall off. Or she may suddenly stiffen like a board, so that no one feels able to carry or hug her.

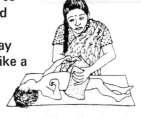

Body stiffens like a board.

- The baby may cry a lot and seem very fussy or 'irritable'. Or she may be very quiet (passive) and almost never cry or smile.

- **Communication difficulties**   The baby may not respond or react as other babies do. This may partly be due to floppiness, stiffness, or lack of arm gestures, or control of face *muscles.* Also, the child may be slow in beginning to speak. Later some children develop unclear speech or other speaking difficulties.

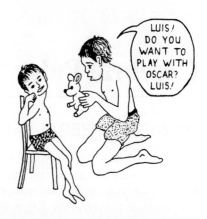

  Although parents find it hard to know exactly what the child wants, they gradually find ways of understanding many of his needs. At first the child cries a lot to show what he wants. Later he may point with his arm, foot or eyes.

- **Intelligence**   Some children may seem dull because they are so limp and slow moving. Others move so much and awkwardly they may appear stupid. Their faces twist, or they may drool because of weak face muscles or difficulty swallowing. This can make an intelligent child appear mentally slow.

  About half of the children with cerebral palsy are mentally retarded, but this should not be decided too soon. The child needs to be given help and training to show what she is really like. Parents can often tell that she understands more than she can show.

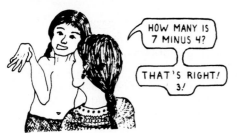

With help and training, some children who have been considered retarded prove to be quite intelligent.

- **Hearing and sight** are sometimes affected. If this problem is not recognized, the family may think that the child lacks intelligence. Observe the child carefully and test him to find out how well he can hear and see. (See p. 450 to 453.)

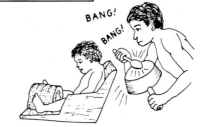

Even if a child can hear loud banging, he may not hear well enough to understand words.

- **Fits** (epilepsy, seizures, convulsions) occur in some children with cerebral palsy. (See Chapter 29.)

- **Restless behavior**   Sudden changes of mood from laughing to crying, fears, fits of anger, and other difficult behavior may be present. This may partly be due to the child's frustration of not being able to do what he wants with his body. If there is too much noise and activity the child can become frightened or upset. The brain damage may also affect behavior. These children need a lot of help and patience to overcome their fears and other unusual behavior. (See Chapter 40.)

- **Sense of touch, pain, heat, cold, and body position** are not lost. However, the children may have trouble controlling movements of their bodies and trouble with **balance.** Because of their damaged brains they may have difficulty learning these things. Patient teaching with lots of repetition can help.

- **Abnormal reflexes**   Babies have certain 'early reflexes' or automatic body movements that normally go away in the first weeks or months of life. In children with brain damage, they may last much longer. However, these are only important if they affect how the child moves. **'Knee jerk' and other tendon-jump reflexes are usually over-active** (jump higher than normal). If you are not sure, testing for abnormal reflexes may help you tell cerebral palsy from polio. (See p. 40.)

TYPES OF CEREBRAL PALSY

Cerebral palsy is different in every child. Different experts have worked out different ways of describing it. But do not worry about labeling a child's particular type of cerebral palsy. This does not usually help his treatment.

It is helpful, however, to recognize 3 main ways that cerebral palsy can appear. In a particular child, it may appear in one or another of these ways—but usually in some sort of combination.

1. MUSCLE STIFFNESS OR 'SPASTICITY'

The child who is *'spastic'* has **muscle stiffness,** or 'muscle tension'. This causes part of his body to be rigid, or stiff. Movements are slow and awkward. Often the position of the head triggers abnormal positions of the whole body. The stiffness increases when the child is upset or excited, or when his body is in certain positions. **The pattern of stiffness varies greatly from child to child.**

TYPICAL SPASTIC POSITIONS WHEN LYING ON THE BACK:

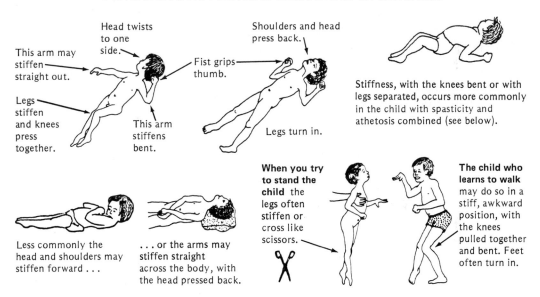

This arm may stiffen straight out.

Head twists to one side.

Legs stiffen and knees press together.

This arm stiffens bent.

Fist grips thumb.

Shoulders and head press back.

Legs turn in.

Stiffness, with the knees bent or with legs separated, occurs more commonly in the child with spasticity and athetosis combined (see below).

Less commonly the head and shoulders may stiffen forward . . .

. . . or the arms may stiffen straight across the body, with the head pressed back.

When you try to stand the child the legs often stiffen or cross like scissors.

The child who learns to walk may do so in a stiff, awkward position, with the knees pulled together and bent. Feet often turn in.

2. UNCONTROLLED MOVEMENTS OR 'ATHETOSIS'

These are slow, wriggly, or sudden quick movements of the child's feet, arms, hands, or face muscles. The arms and legs may seem jumpy and move nervously, or just a hand or the toes may move for no reason. When he moves by choice, body parts move too fast and too far. Spastic movements or positions like those shown above may continually come and go (constantly changing muscle tension). His balance is poor and he falls over easily.

Most children with athetosis have normal intelligence, but if the muscles needed for speech are affected, it may be hard for them to communicate their thoughts and needs.

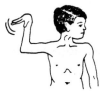

Typical athetoid arm and hand movements may be as a regular shake or as sudden 'spasms'. Uncontrolled movements are often worse when the child is excited or tries to do something.

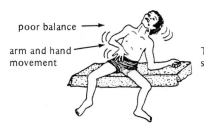

poor balance

arm and hand movement

This child has severe athetosis.

3. POOR BALANCE OR 'ATAXIA'

The child who has 'ataxia', or poor balance, has difficulty beginning to sit and stand. She falls often, and has very clumsy use of her hands. All this is normal in small children, but in the child with ataxia it is a bigger problem and lasts longer (sometimes for life).

Because children who have mainly a balance problem often appear more clumsy than disabled, other children are sometimes cruel and make fun of them.

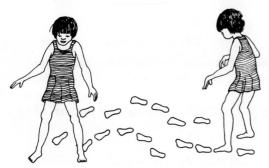

To keep her balance the child with ataxia walks bent forward with feet wide apart. She takes irregular steps, like a sailor on a rough sea or someone who is drunk.

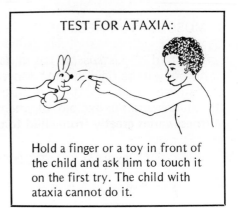

TEST FOR ATAXIA:

Hold a finger or a toy in front of the child and ask him to touch it on the first try. The child with ataxia cannot do it.

Many children who have spasticity or athetosis also have problems with balance. This may be a major obstacle in learning to walk. However, much can often be done to help a child improve her balance.

NOTE: Children with any type of cerebral palsy as **babies are often mainly limp or floppy.** Stiffness or uncontrolled movements begin little by little. Or the child may be limp in some positions and stiff in others.

Parts of the body affected

DEPENDING ON WHICH LIMBS ARE INVOLVED, THERE ARE 3 TYPICAL PATTERNS:

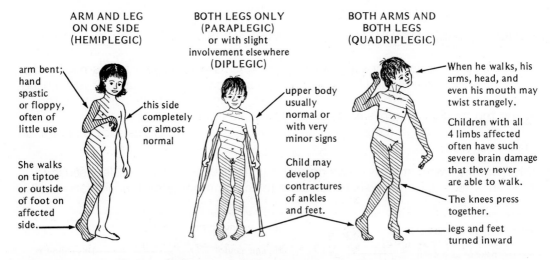

ARM AND LEG ON ONE SIDE (HEMIPLEGIC)

BOTH LEGS ONLY (PARAPLEGIC) or with slight involvement elsewhere (DIPLEGIC)

BOTH ARMS AND BOTH LEGS (QUADRIPLEGIC)

arm bent; hand spastic or floppy, often of little use

this side completely or almost normal

She walks on tiptoe or outside of foot on affected side.

upper body usually normal or with very minor signs

Child may develop contractures of ankles and feet.

When he walks, his arms, head, and even his mouth may twist strangely.

Children with all 4 limbs affected often have such severe brain damage that they never are able to walk.

The knees press together.

legs and feet turned inward

Although most cerebral palsy children fit one or another of these patterns, check also for minor problems in other parts of the body.

QUESTIONS ABOUT CEREBRAL PALSY

1. What causes it?

In each child with cerebral palsy, the parts of the brain that are damaged are different. The causes are often difficult to find.

- **Causes before birth:**
  - **Infections** of the mother while she is pregnant. These include **German measles** and shingles (herpes zoster).
  - Differences between the blood of mother and child **(Rh incompatibility).**
  - Problems of the mother, such as **diabetes** or **toxemia of pregnancy.**
  - **Inherited.** This is rare, but there is a 'familial spastic paraplegia'.
  - **No cause can be found** in about 30% of the children.

- **Causes around the time of birth:**
  - **Lack of oxygen (air)** at birth. The baby does not breathe soon enough and becomes blue and limp. In some areas, misuse of hormones (oxytocics) to speed up birth narrows the blood vessels in the womb so much that the baby does not get enough oxygen. In other cases, the baby may have the cord wrapped around her neck. The baby is born blue and limp—with brain damage.
  - **Birth injuries** from difficult births. These are mostly large babies of mothers who are small or very young. The baby's head may be pushed out of shape, blood vessels torn, and the brain damaged.
  - **Prematurity.** Babies born before 9 months and who weigh under 2 kilos (5 pounds) are much more likely to have cerebral palsy. In rich countries, over half the cases of cerebral palsy happen in babies that are born early.

- **Causes after birth:**
  - **Very high fever** due to infection or dehydration (water loss from diarrhea). It is more common in bottle-fed babies.
  - **Brain infections** *(meningitis, encephalitis).* There are many causes, including malaria and tuberculosis.
  - **Head injuries.**
  - **Lack of oxygen** from drowning, gas poisoning, or other causes.
  - **Poisoning** from lead glazes on pottery, pesticides sprayed on crops, and other poisons.
  - **Bleeding or blood clots in the brain,** often from unknown cause.
  - **Brain tumors.** These cause progressive brain damage in which the signs are similar to cerebral palsy but steadily get worse.

2. Is cerebral palsy contagious? No! It cannot be passed from one child to another.

3. Can persons with cerebral palsy marry and have children? Yes. And the children will not have the condition (except maybe in a very rare type of cerebral palsy).

4. What medical or surgical treatment is there?

Except for drugs to control fits, medicines usually do not help. (Although medicines to reduce spasticity are often prescribed, they usually do no good, and may cause problems.) Surgery is sometimes useful for correcting severe, stubborn contractures. However, surgery to weaken or release spastic muscles is less often effective and sometimes makes things worse. Careful evaluation is needed. Surgery usually should be considered only **if the child is already walking** and has increasing difficulty because of contractures. In a child who cannot balance well enough to stand, surgery usually will not help. Sometimes surgery to separate the legs can help make cleaning and bathing easier.

5. What can be done?

The damaged parts of the brain cannot be repaired, but often the child can learn to use the undamaged parts to do what she wants to do. It is important for parents to know more or less what to expect:

> **The child with cerebral palsy will become an adult with cerebral palsy. Searching for cures will only bring disappointment. Instead, help the child become an adult who can live with her disability and be as independent as possible.**

Families can do a lot to help these children learn to function better. Generally, **the child who is more intelligent will learn to adapt successfully to her condition.** However, intelligence is not always necessary. In fact, some intelligent children become more easily frustrated and discouraged, so they stop trying. Extra effort is needed to find new and interesting ways to keep them progressing. **Even severely retarded children can often learn important basic skills.** Only when mental damage is so great that the child does not respond at all to people and things is there little hope for much progress. However, before judging the child who does not respond, be sure to check for deafness or loss of eyesight.

> *IMPORTANT:* Rather than try to treat the symptoms of cerebral palsy, we can do more for the child if we **help her with development of movement, communication, self-care and relationships with others.** Sometimes we can partly correct the symptoms through helping the child develop basic skills.

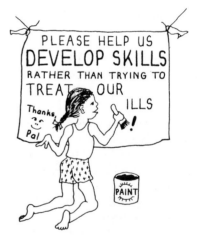

By standing on her knees as she paints a sign, this girl is improving her balance to help her (possibly) stand and walk.

Family members can learn to play and do daily activities with the child in ways that help her both to function better and to prevent secondary problems such as *contractures.*

Most important is that the parents (and grand-parents!) **learn not to do everything for the child. Help her just enough that she can learn to do more for herself.**

For example, if your child is beginning to hold up her head, and to take things to her mouth,

instead of always feeding her yourself

look for ways to help her begin to feed herself (see p. 329).

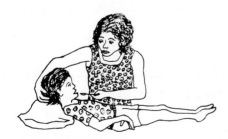

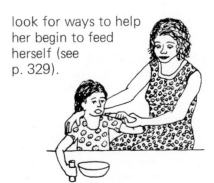

6. Will my child ever be able to walk?

This is often one of the biggest concerns of parents. Walking is important both *functionally* and socially. But in terms of the child's needs, other skills may be more important. For the child to lead as happy, independent a life as possible, necessary skills and accomplishments (in order of importance) are:

1. Having confidence in yourself and liking yourself
2. Communication and relationship with others
3. Self-care activities such as eating, dressing, toileting
4. Getting from place to place
5. (And if possible) walking

We all need to realize that **walking is not the most important skill a child needs**—and it is certainly not the first. Before a child can walk he needs reasonable head control, needs to be able to sit without help, and to be able to keep his balance while standing.

Most children with cerebral palsy do learn to walk, although often **much later than normal.** In general, the less severely affected the child is and the earlier she is able to sit without help, the more likely she is to walk. If she can sit without assistance by age 2, her chances for walking may be good—although many other factors are involved. Some children begin to walk at age 7, 10, or even older.

Hemiplegic and diplegic children usually do learn to walk, although some may need crutches, braces, or other aids.

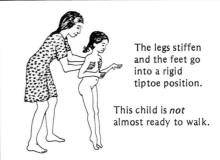

The legs stiffen and the feet go into a rigid tiptoe position.

This child is *not* almost ready to walk.

A COMMON MISTAKE

When a child with severe brain damage is held like this, her legs may automatically stiffen and her feet point down—the so-called 'tiptoe reflex'. Because the feet sometimes take jerky 'steps', parents think the child is 'almost ready to walk'. This is not so. The tiptoe reflex must be overcome before the child can begin to learn to walk. Do not hold the child in this position or make her try to walk. It will only strengthen this disabling reaction. (See p. 291.)

Many severely affected children may never walk. We need to accept this, and aim for other important goals. **Whether or not the child may someday walk, he needs some way to get from place to place.** Here is a true situation that helped us to realize that other things are more important than walking.

In a Mexican village, we know 2 brothers, both with cerebral palsy.

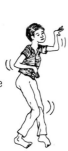

Petronio walks but with great difficulty. Walking tires him and makes him feel so awkward that he stays at home and does not play or work. He is unhappy.

His brother, Luis, cannot walk. But since he was small, he has loved to ride a donkey. He uses a wall to get off and on by himself. He goes long distances and earns money carrying water. He is happy.

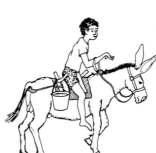

(Not only does the donkey take Luis where he wants to go, but by keeping his legs apart, it helps prevent knock-knee contractures. This way *'therapy'* is built into daily activity.)

There are many different ways to help children who cannot walk, or who walk with difficulty, get where they want to go. These include **wheelboards, wagons, wheelchairs, special walkers,** and **hand-pedal tricycles.** Many of these are described in PART 3 of this book (see the Index).

How can we help?

First, with the help of parents and family we observe the child carefully to see:

- what the child *can* do.
- what he looks like when he moves and when he is in different positions.
- what he *cannot* do, and what prevents him from doing it.

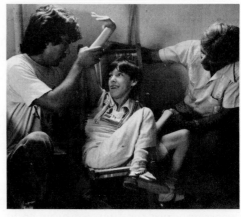

A village worker and father examine a child with severe cerebral palsy.

WHAT THE CHILD CAN DO

Can the child:

- lift her head? hold it up? sit? roll over?
- pull herself along the floor in any way possible? crawl? walk?

How does the child use her **hands?**

- Can she grasp things and hold on; let go; use both hands together (or only one at a time)?
- Can she use her fingers to pick up small stones or pieces of food?

How much can the child do for herself?

- Can she feed herself; wash herself; dress herself? Is she 'toilet trained'?

What can the child do in the home or in the fields to help the family?

After observing and discussing what the child **can do,** we must **expect him to do these things.** If the parents are used to doing almost everything for the child, at first this may be difficult (for both parents and child). But soon it will help the child have more confidence. The parents, also, will be encouraged by seeing what he can do for himself, and they will think less about what he cannot do. Here a grandmother helps her grandchild became more self-reliant:

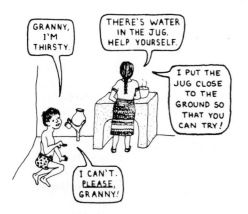
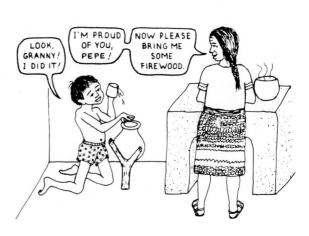

It was difficult for the grandmother not to bring her grandson a cup of water—especially when he begged her. But she understood that in the long run it would do him more good to manage for himself. For more ideas about how a family can help a child with cerebral palsy, read the story of Maricela on pages 5 to 7 and the story of Enrique on page 288.

HELPING THE CHILD ACHIEVE BETTER POSITIONS

Due to abnormal pull of muscles, children with cerebral palsy often spend a lot of time in abnormal positions. These abnormal positions of the limbs and body should be avoided as much as possible, or the child can become deformed. For example,

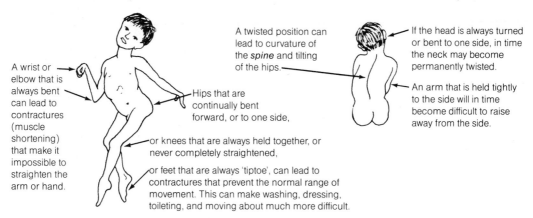

A twisted position can lead to curvature of the *spine* and tilting of the hips.

If the head is always turned or bent to one side, in time the neck may become permanently twisted.

A wrist or elbow that is always bent can lead to contractures (muscle shortening) that make it impossible to straighten the arm or hand.

Hips that are continually bent forward, or to one side,

An arm that is held tightly to the side will in time become difficult to raise away from the side.

or knees that are always held together, or never completely straightened,

or feet that are always 'tiptoe', can lead to contractures that prevent the normal range of movement. This can make washing, dressing, toileting, and moving about much more difficult.

Whenever possible the child should be in positions that prevent rather than cause these problems. Whatever the child is doing (lying, sitting, crawling, standing) try to encourage positions so that:

- her head is straight up and down.
- her body is straight (not bent, bowed, or twisted).
- both arms are straight and kept away from the sides.
- both hands are in use, in front of her eyes.
- she bears weight equally on both sides of her body—through both hips, both knees, both feet or both arms.

Encourage positions that the child can manage at her stage of development. Play with her, talk with her, give her interesting things to do in these positions.

Not all children will be able to stay in these positions without some kind of support. Special chairs, tables, wedges, pads, or bags of clean sand may be needed to keep a good position.

For example, the child at the top of the page might need a chair like this.

sitting

crawling

standing

lying

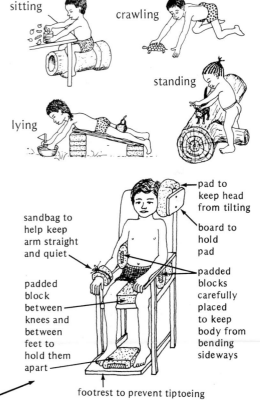

pad to keep head from tilting

board to hold pad

sandbag to help keep arm straight and quiet

padded blocks carefully placed to keep body from bending sideways

padded block between knees and between feet to hold them apart

footrest to prevent tiptoeing

Note: Remove straps and supports as soon as the child is able to stay in a good position.

> **WARNING:** Do not leave a child in any one position for many hours as his body may gradually stiffen into that position. Change his position often. Or better, encourage him to change it. If he can change his own position effectively, then chairs, seats, and other aids must not prevent him from moving.
>
> AIDS SHOULD RESTRICT A CHILD'S MOVEMENT AS LITTLE AS POSSIBLE.

When the child with cerebral palsy moves she may do so in a very strange or abnormal way. To some extent this should be allowed, as long as the child is able to do things as best she can. But also show the child other ways to move in order to correct some of the abnormal positions that she repeats again and again. For example,

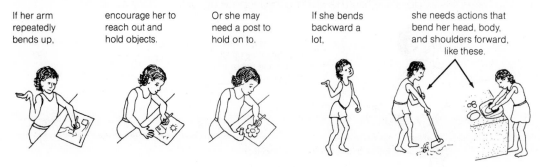

If her arm repeatedly bends up,

encourage her to reach out and hold objects.

Or she may need a post to hold on to.

If she bends backward a lot,

she needs actions that bend her head, body, and shoulders forward, like these.

Corrective actions and positions can be found while working in the fields, in the home, or while playing with brothers and sisters. Here are some more suggestions for corrective positions (from physical therapists Nancy Finnie and Sophie Levitt).

Lying and sleeping

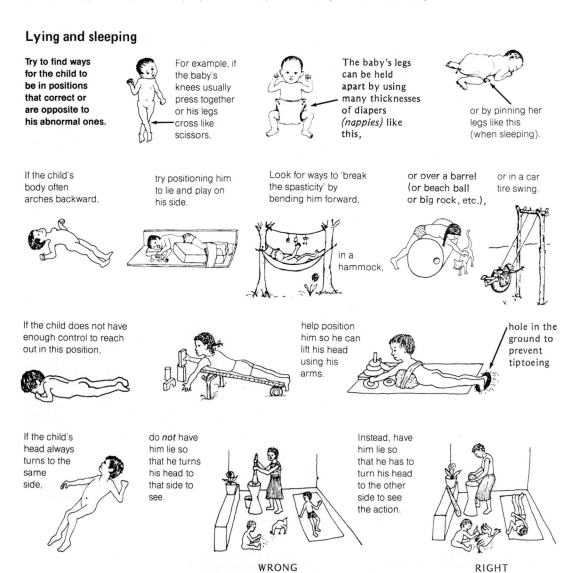

Try to find ways for the child to be in positions that correct or are opposite to his abnormal ones.

For example, if the baby's knees usually press together or his legs cross like scissors,

The baby's legs can be held apart by using many thicknesses of diapers (nappies) like this,

or by pinning her legs like this (when sleeping).

If the child's body often arches backward,

try positioning him to lie and play on his side.

Look for ways to 'break the spasticity' by bending him forward,

in a hammock,

or over a barrel (or beach ball or big rock, etc.),

or in a car tire swing.

If the child does not have enough control to reach out in this position,

help position him so he can lift his head using his arms.

hole in the ground to prevent tiptoeing

If the child's head always turns to the same side,

do *not* have him lie so that he turns his head to that side to see.

Instead, have him lie so that he has to turn his head to the other side to see the action.

WRONG

RIGHT

For more suggestions on head control, see p. 302.

Rolling and twisting

A child with cerebral palsy is often very stiff when it comes to twisting or rotating the main part of her body. However, such twisting is necessary for learning to walk. Rolling also helps develop body twisting.

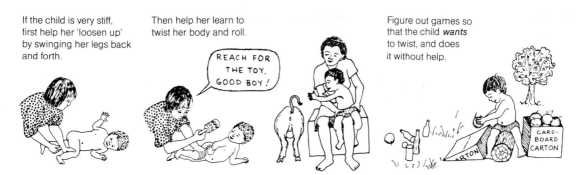

If the child is very stiff, first help her 'loosen up' by swinging her legs back and forth.

Then help her learn to twist her body and roll.

REACH FOR THE TOY. GOOD BOY!

Figure out games so that the child *wants* to twist, and does it without help.

For more ideas to develop twisting and rolling, see p. 304.

Sitting

The way that you help position a child for sitting also depends on the type of abnormal body positions he has. For example,

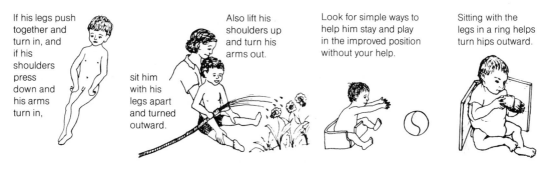

If his legs push together and turn in, and if his shoulders press down and his arms turn in,

sit him with his legs apart and turned outward.

Also lift his shoulders up and turn his arms out.

Look for simple ways to help him stay and play in the improved position without your help.

Sitting with the legs in a ring helps turn hips outward.

For the child with spasticity who has trouble sitting, you can control his legs like this. This leaves your hands free to help him control and use his arms and hands. Help the child feel and grasp parts of his face.

Sit the child on your belly with his legs spread and feet flat. Give support with your knees as needed. As he begins to reach for his face, help his shoulders, arms, and hands take more natural positions. Make a game out of touching or holding parts of his face. MAKE IT FUN!

NOW TOUCH YOUR NOSE.   GOOD BOY.

As the child develops, encourage her to put her arms and body in more normal positions through play and *imitation.*

Children who have trouble with balance (from cerebral palsy, polio, or other disability) often sit with their legs in a 'W' in order not to fall over.

Sitting in a "W" should usually be discouraged because it can increase contractures and loosen or damage hips and knees. However, if it is the only way a child can sit and use her hands, it should be allowed.

Look for ways for the child to sit with legs spread forward. Here are 2 examples.

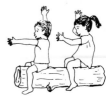

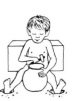

The pot or log keeps the knees apart. The holes for heels help too.

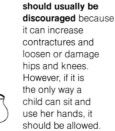

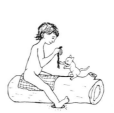

If the child's legs stay apart, his butt sticks out, and his shoulders are pulled back,

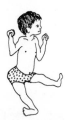

first sit him with his body bent forward and his legs together. Then bend his shoulders forward and turn them in.

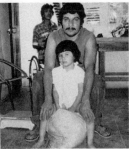

A sack of grain provides a roll to hold this child's legs apart. Her father pushes down on her knees. This helps her to hold her feet flat and sit up straighter. (PROJIMO)

Look for ways that the child will sit and play in the improved position without help.

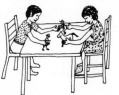

Play with her at a table. Sit across from her to have her reach forward for toys with both hands.

Be sure her feet are on a flat surface.

For ideas on special seats and sitting positions to prevent 'knock-knee' contractures, see below. Other ideas on special seats for children with cerebral palsy are on pages 308, 573, 607 to 612, 621 and 624.

Moving about

Because children with cerebral palsy are usually delayed in walking, they need other ways to get from place to place. The methods used will depend on both the needs and abilities of the child—also the resources, skills, and imagination of family, friends, and local craftspersons.

Aids for ways to get from place to place should provide corrective positions. The following examples are all designed to help prevent 'knock-knee' contractures. They also provide other types of corrective positioning.

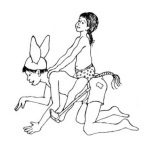

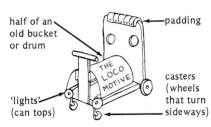

half of an old bucket or drum — padding

THE LOCO MOTIVE

'lights' (can tops)

casters (wheels that turn sideways)

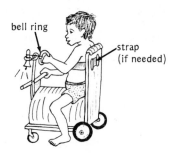

bell ring

strap (if needed)

Wheelboards

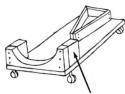

Pad or put a pillow over this support. (Some children will not need this support.)

Adapting wheelboards for travel on rough surfaces

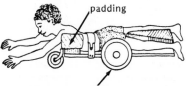

padding

By placing large wheels near the middle, if the smaller front caster gets stuck, the child can lift with his arms and go on. Or if a fixed front wheel is used, he can lift it off the ground to make turns.

For dirt or bamboo floors, larger wheels will be needed.

Some children will need wheelchairs. **For wheelchair designs, see Chapters 64, 65 and 66.**

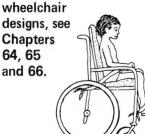

For special cushions, to help hold a child's hips back and her knees apart, see p. 609.

For other wheelboard designs, see p. 618.

Standing

Many children with cerebral palsy stand and walk in strange positions. A child's unsure balance often increases the uncontrolled tightening of certain muscles and makes balance even more difficult.

As a result the child stands in an awkward position that can lead to deformities and contractures.

When you help the child keep her balance, she is less tense and can stand straighter.

Look for ways to provide similar assistance during play and other activities.

Here a cart provides easier balance and keeps the arms straight.

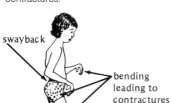

swayback

bending leading to contractures

tiptoeing

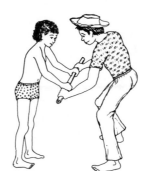

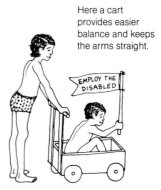

EMPLOY THE DISABLED

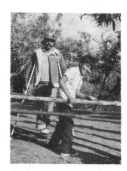

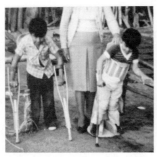

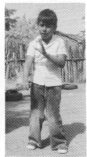

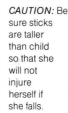

Miguelito began to walk at age 8 —first on parallel bars.

Soon he learned to use crutches. Here he races another child who is learning to walk.

And now he can walk alone.

Two sticks can help the child once she develops some standing balance. At first you can hold the tops of the sticks. But let go as soon as possible.

CAUTION: Be sure sticks are taller than child so that she will not injure herself if she falls.

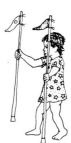

The child who cannot yet stand alone can be placed in a standing frame for an hour or 2 each day.

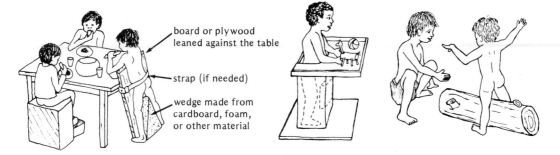

board or plywood leaned against the table

strap (if needed)

wedge made from cardboard, foam, or other material

Even for the child who may never stand alone or walk, standing in a frame helps prevent deformities. It also helps the leg bones grow and stay strong. Start at about the age normal children begin to stand—around one year old.

For ideas on 'standing frames' see p. 574 and 575.

Hand use

Try to find ways that the child can play or do things using her hands while she is in the corrective positions of sitting, standing or lying.

Encourage her to touch, feel, and handle as many different shapes and surfaces as possible: things that are big, small, hot, cold, sticky, smooth, prickly, hard, soft, thin, and thick.

This girl in the rehabilitation center of the Khao-i-dang refugee camp in Thailand develops hand control by sliding colored rings on a pole.

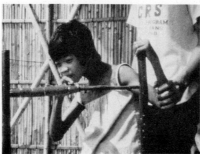

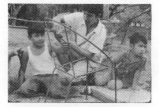

A boy with cerebral palsy at the PROJIMO rehabilitation center helps paint a chair frame.

For more ideas of developing use of the hands, see p. 305.

CORRECTIVE CARRYING POSITIONS

As in other activities, try to carry a child in positions that work to correct abnormal positions.

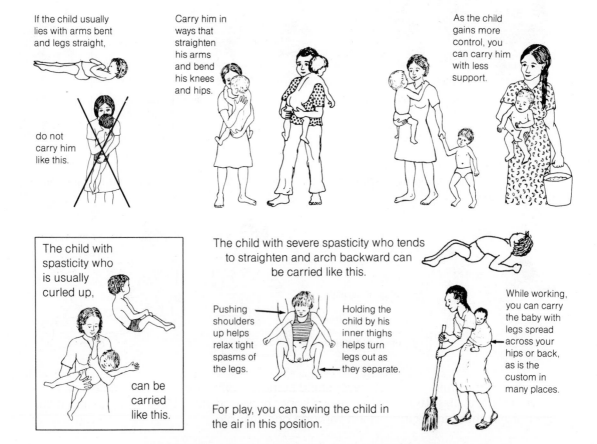

If the child usually lies with arms bent and legs straight,

do not carry him like this.

Carry him in ways that straighten his arms and bend his knees and hips.

As the child gains more control, you can carry him with less support.

The child with spasticity who is usually curled up,

can be carried like this.

The child with severe spasticity who tends to straighten and arch backward can be carried like this.

Pushing shoulders up helps relax tight spasms of the legs.

Holding the child by his inner thighs helps turn legs out as they separate.

For play, you can swing the child in the air in this position.

While working, you can carry the baby with legs spread across your hips or back, as is the custom in many places.

For other good carrying positions, see p. 303.

CONTRACTURES IN CEREBRAL PALSY

Abnormal muscle tightness often leads to contractures (muscle shortening and reduced motion of joints, see Chapter 8). In time, the muscles that keep a limb bent become shortened so that the limb cannot straighten even when the muscles relax. But with care, contractures can often be prevented.

Without care to prevent it:

SPASTICITY (Uncontrolled tightening of muscles)	leads to	CONTRACTURE (Fixed shortening of muscles)

The **typical contractures of cerebral palsy** are similar to the abnormal positions of cerebral palsy. They can include:

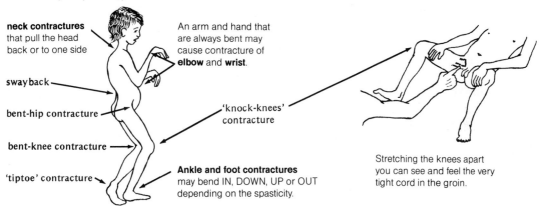

neck contractures that pull the head back or to one side

An arm and hand that are always bent may cause contracture of **elbow** and **wrist**.

swayback

bent-hip contracture

'knock-knees' contracture

bent-knee contracture

'tiptoe' contracture

Ankle and foot contractures may bend IN, DOWN, UP or OUT depending on the spasticity.

Stretching the knees apart you can see and feel the very tight cord in the groin.

Chapter 8 discusses contractures, and ways to prevent and correct them. Page 79 explains how to tell spasticity from contractures.

Spasticity and contractures combined

Decreased range of motion may be caused partly by spasticity and partly by contractures. Therefore, whenever a child has spasticity, check to see if contractures are also forming, and if so, how much.

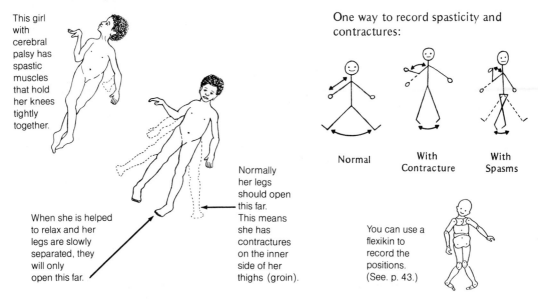

This girl with cerebral palsy has spastic muscles that hold her knees tightly together.

When she is helped to relax and her legs are slowly separated, they will only open this far.

Normally her legs should open this far. This means she has contractures on the inner side of her thighs (groin).

One way to record spasticity and contractures:

Normal

With Contracture

With Spasms

You can use a flexikin to record the positions. (See. p. 43.)

PREVENTING CONTRACTURES

In cerebral palsy, it is important that steps to prevent contractures be included in activities that help the total development of the child. Many of the **corrective positions** we have already suggested for activities such as lying, sitting, standing, and moving about are helpful in preventing contractures. When there are signs of developing contractures, give even more time and care to corrective positions.

Range-of-motion exercises

Although the reasons contractures form in cerebral palsy and polio are different, many of the stretching and holding exercises discussed in Chapter 8, "Contractures," and in Chapter 42, "Range-of-Motion and Other Exercises," will be helpful. However, in cerebral palsy, take care to **do exercises in ways that do not increase spasticity, but help to relax the spastic muscles.**

RELAXING SPASTIC MUSCLES

To help relax spastic muscles, before beginning range-of-motion exercises try the following to see what works best for your child:

1. Apply warm soaks (see p. 132) to spastic muscles or have the child sit or lie in warm water.

2. Slowly twist or help the child to twist his body from side to side. This reduces spasticity throughout the body, and is a good first stretching exercise. Make it into a game. (See p. 304.)

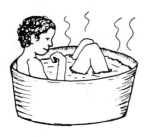

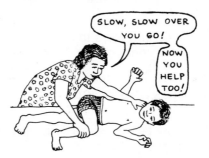

SLOW, SLOW OVER YOU GO!

NOW YOU HELP TOO!

> **CAUTION**
> ABOUT MASSAGE
>
> In some countries, people and even therapists use massage, or rubbing, to try to relax spastic muscles. Although massage often helps relax muscle spasms, cramps, or tight muscles from other causes, in spasticity, massage usually increases the muscle tightness. As a general rule, DO NOT MASSAGE SPASTIC MUSCLES.

Pulling or pushing directly against spastic muscles causes them to tighten more. To correct abnormal positions, sometimes you can use 'tricks' to release or 'break' the muscle spasms.

Muscle tension in any part of the body is affected by the position of the head and body. Spasms that straighten the legs and pull the knees together can be partly relaxed by bending the head and back forward.

Do not pick up the child like this. Her head will bend back and her whole body and legs stiffen more.

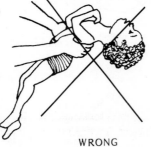

WRONG

If you roll her a little to one side, it will be easier to bend her head and back forward. This relaxes her hips and legs so that they also bend.

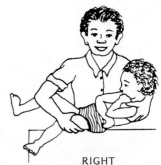

RIGHT

Whatever you do with the child, look for ways that will help relax and stretch the tight muscles. Here are some examples.

Rosa's body stiffens backward, while her knees straighten stiffly and press together.

To wash between her legs, *do not* try to pull her legs apart at the ankles.

This will make her legs pull together more tightly.

Instead, put something under her head and shoulders to bend them forward. This helps to relax the stiffness in her whole body.

Then bend the legs and slowly separate them. If you hold them above the knees, they will open more easily.

Washing will be easier with her knees bent. After washing her (with warm water, if possible) you can help stretch the tight muscles.

Slowly open her legs as wide as they will go, and then gradually straighten her knees.

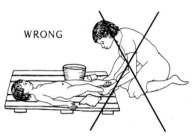

WRONG

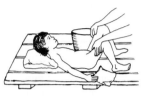

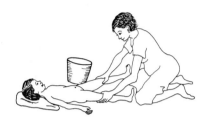

When you try to feed the child, if her head and shoulders stiffen backward,

do *not* try to pull her head forward. It will push back more.

You may find that her head relaxes more if you put your arm across the back of her neck and push her shoulders forward.

Or, you may find that raising the front of the chair seat keeps her hips bent, relaxes her in general, and gives her much more control.

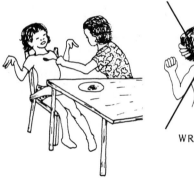

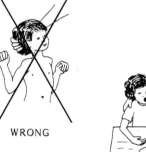

WRONG

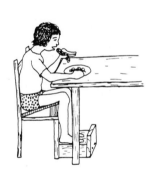

When you want to help your child dress, if her arms press against her chest,

do *not* try to pull them straight. They will stiffen more.

Try holding her arms above her elbows, and gently turning her arms out and straighten them at the same time.

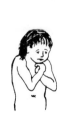

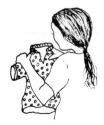

WRONG

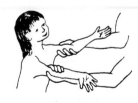

Note: **These suggestions will work for some children but not for others. Keep trying different ways until you find what works best.**

DEVELOPING EARLY SKILLS

Most children with cerebral palsy develop basic skills and abilities more slowly than other children. This is partly because of their difficulty with balance and movement. Also, in some children, mental slowness or problems with seeing or hearing make learning more difficult. Because slow development occurs with many different disabilities, we discuss activities for child development in a separate section of this book.

In this chapter, therefore, we give only a few suggestions for assisting a child with cerebral palsy to learn new skills.

VERY IMPORTANT:

To understand better how to help a child with cerebral palsy develop early skills, **you also need to read other chapters.** Chapters 34 and 35 are about **helping the child whose mind and/or body are slow to develop.** Chapters 36 to 41 discuss ways of **helping children develop and become more self-reliant.**

Although Chapters 34 to 41 are written to help any children who are slow to develop, many suggestions are included for the specific needs of the child with cerebral palsy. These are marked with (CP) in the margin.

To help a child develop new skills, first observe all the things that she can and cannot do. Like a normal baby who progresses stage by stage in a certain order, the child with cerebral palsy must do the same. Charts showing the normal 'developmental milestones' are on pages 292 and 293. You can use them to help decide the next steps or skills that the child may be ready to learn.

Help the child advance slowly, at her own speed, in small steps. If we try to go too fast because of her age, she can become discouraged by failure. Also, her progress can be held back. This happens when we stand a child and try to make him walk before he is ready. (See p. 291.)

Move ahead at a speed that fits your child — not too fast and not too slow.

To help a child with cerebral palsy develop skills takes a lot of time, energy, patience, and love. The whole family needs to help, and also, if possible, others in the community. (See Chapter 33.)

Remember that **positioning is very important.** When the child has been helped to lie, sit, and stand in ways that give him better positions and control, he will start learning to do things he could not do before.

Good balance is one of the most important goals for the development of the child with cerebral palsy. It is important to help a child improve her balance from as young an age as possible. At each stage of the child's development—lying, sitting, creeping, standing, and walking—better balance is needed to progress to the next stage.

Helping improve balance

Detailed suggestions of activities to improve balance are included in Chapter 35, "Early Stimulation Activities," especially pages 306 to 312. Here we give you a brief look at some of the basic suggestions explained in more detail in that chapter.

TESTING A CHILD'S BALANCE

POOR BALANCE	BETTER BALANCE	GOOD BALANCE
If when you sit a child over 10 months old, she falls stiffly to one side with no effort to 'catch' herself, her balance is poor.	If she can balance using her arms when you gently push her, her balance is fair.	If she can do it by bending her body, without using her arms, her balance is good.

When lying

Encourage the child to shift weight from one arm to the other by reaching for objects, 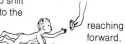 reaching forward, and reaching sideways.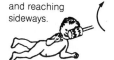

Lie him on your body and tip a little from side to side so that he begins to catch himself.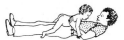

When sitting

Let her start to fall so that she begins to catch herself.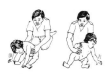

Sit her across your knees. Raise one knee so she has to balance. Then lower your hands. Start with hands high.

As the child improves, use a tilting board.

Encourage the child to twist and reach to the side.

Use as little sitting support as needed. Often low back support is enough for a child who straightens stiffly.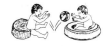

For creeping and crawling

Note: Some children advance to standing without ever crawling.

Shift weight from one arm to the other. Provide support as needed, and gradually take it away.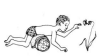

Shift weight from one leg to the other.

Play trying to balance on a tipping surface.

Crawl forward, sideways, and backward.

crawling scooter

For standing and walking

Stand and balance on knees.

CAUTION: Not for a child with bent-knee spasticity.

Pull to stand.

(Often the child will stand better when he pulls himself up than when someone helps him.)

Stand while holding on, and reaching.

Help with standing and then walking.

Give less and less support while he walks with only a 'safety-belt'—and then alone.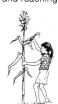

Have the child practice stepping forward, backward, and sideways.

Whenever possible, **turn these activities into games. Talk to the child** a lot while you do them to help develop language skills at the same time (see p. 313).

Skills for daily living and self care

A child with cerebral palsy will get abilities later than other children—but **she will get them!** Of course, the child may not achieve everything, and may not always walk. But **make sure the child achieves what she can in each important area of development:**

The child will often need a lot of help with **language and communication skills.** Develop these skills in whatever way seems possible: using words, gestures, pointing (with hand, foot, head, or eyes), or with communication boards. (See Chapter 31 and p. 578.)

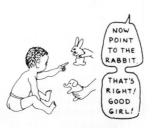
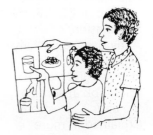

Help the child become as independent as possible in **eating, dressing, washing, toileting,** and in meeting other **daily needs.** Do this by guided practice, imitation, and step-by-step learning. These self-care skills are discussed in Chapters 36 to 39.

Develop some form of. **moving about** and, if necessary, use wheel-boards, wheelchairs, pedal tricycles, walkers, crutches, or other aids. (See Chapters 63, 64, 65, and 66.)

Keep experimenting until you find what works best.

For example, this girl, with poor body and hip control, tends to 'fall through' the space between her arms when the handgrips on the walker are upright.

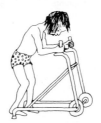

She does much better on a higher walker with a handgrip that runs from one side to the other.

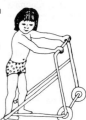

Often leg braces *do not* help a child with cerebral palsy walk better. But sometimes they do. When in doubt, try low-cost braces first, to look for possible problems. For example:

Carla walks in a very crouched position.

She may be helped by below-knee braces that hold her feet at nearly a right angle (90°)

or by above-knee braces that keep her knees almost straight . . .

But it is possible that the below-knee braces will throw her badly off balance,

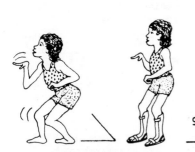
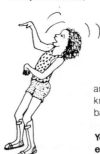

and that the above-knee braces will make balancing even harder.

You will need to experiment!

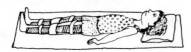

Even if braces for walking do not work, Carla may be helped to walk straighter by using 'night splints' to hold her knees straight and prevent contractures. (See p. 540.)

IMPORTANT: Practice in learning skills should take place with family and friends so that the child develops skills in relating to others. However, the **child will also need time to practice her skills alone** and with the person who is mainly responsible for treating or teaching her.

CAUTION: Many suggestions for developing basic skills are discussed in Chapter 34, "Child Development and Developmental Delay," and Chapters 36 through 39 on developing skills for self-care. However, **for the child with cerebral palsy, some of these activities will need to be done differently** to help reduce and not increase muscle spasms. **If any activity increases spasticity, try it differently until you find a way that reduces muscle tension and improves position.**

PREVENTION

With these precautions, children will be less likely to have cerebral palsy:

- **Good nutrition of the mother,** both before and during pregnancy, reduces the chance of premature birth-and of cerebral palsy.

- If possible, girls should **avoid pregnancy until full grown** (16 or 17 years old).

- **Avoid unnecessary medicines during pregnancy.**

- Try to **avoid** getting near persons with **German measles** during pregnancy. Or get vaccinated against German measles before becoming pregnant.

- Go for regular **health check-ups during pregnancy** (prenatal care). If there are any signs that giving birth may be difficult, try to arrange for a skilled midwife or doctor to attend the birth—if possible, in a hospital. (See the list of "Signs of Special Risk," *Where There Is No Doctor,* p. 256.)

- During labor, do not let the midwife try to speed things up by

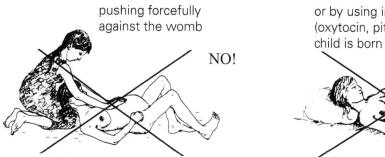

pushing forcefully against the womb — NO!

or by using injections or hormones (oxytocin, pituitrin, etc.) before the child is born — NO!

- Be familiar with, and be sure your midwife is familiar with, all the precautions and **emergency measures** of childbirth. Learn what to do if the baby is born blue and limp and does not breathe right away, or has the cord wrapped around the neck. Plan for emergency transport to the nearest clinic or hospital. (See *Where Women Have No Doctor,* pages 88 to 95.)

- **Breast feed** the baby (breast milk helps prevent and fight infection), and make sure the baby gets enough to eat. (See *Where There Is No Doctor,* p. 121 and 271.)

- **Vaccinate** the baby (especially for measles).

- When the baby has a **fever,**

uncover him completely.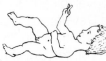

Never wrap the baby up in clothing or blankets.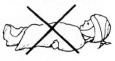

If the fever is high, wet the child and fan him until he is cooler.

This can make the fever worse and cause fits or permanent brain damage.

Be sure the child with fever drinks a lot of liquids, and follow the other instructions on pages 75 to 76 of *Where There Is No Doctor.*

- Know the signs of **meningitis** and get (or begin) treatment quickly.

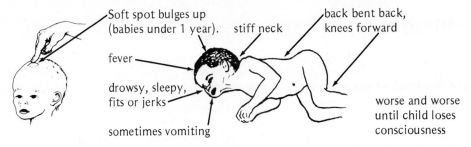

Soft spot bulges up (babies under 1 year).

stiff neck

back bent back, knees forward

fever

drowsy, sleepy, fits or jerks

sometimes vomiting

worse and worse until child loses consciousness

- When your baby has **diarrhea,** prepare Rehydration Drink and give it to him every few minutes to prevent or correct dehydration. See *Where There Is No Doctor,* p. 151 to 161.

> **Preventing dehydration helps prevent fits and brain damage (cerebral palsy).**

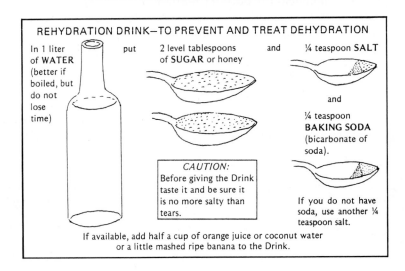

REHYDRATION DRINK—TO PREVENT AND TREAT DEHYDRATION

In 1 liter of WATER (better if boiled, but do not lose time)   put   2 level tablespoons of SUGAR or honey   and   ¼ teaspoon SALT

and

¼ teaspoon BAKING SODA (bicarbonate of soda).

CAUTION: Before giving the Drink taste it and be sure it is no more salty than tears.

If you do not have soda, use another ¼ teaspoon salt.

If available, add half a cup of orange juice or coconut water or a little mashed ripe banana to the Drink.

OTHER PARTS OF THIS BOOK WITH INFORMATION CONCERNING CEREBRAL PALSY

Cerebral palsy is a complex disability that involves many problems and needs. Therefore much of the basic information you will need is in other chapters. It is essential that you read Chapters 4, 8, 33 to 43, and 62 to 66.

Throughout the book, important information about cerebral palsy has been marked with a (CP) in the margin. Many references to cerebral palsy are also included in the INDEX.

Muscular Dystrophy

CHAPTER **10**

Gradual, Progressive Muscle Loss

Muscular dystrophy is a condition in which *muscles,* month by month and year by year, get weaker and weaker. Because the *disability* gradually gets worse, we say it is 'progressive'.

HOW TO RECOGNIZE IF MUSCLE WEAKNESS IS CAUSED BY MUSCULAR DYSTROPHY

- Mostly affects boys (rarely girls).

- Often brothers or male relatives have same problem.

- First signs appear around ages 3 to 5: the child may seem awkward or clumsy, or he begins to walk 'tiptoe' because he cannot put his feet flat. Runs strangely. Falls often.

- Problem gets steadily worse over the next several years.

- Muscle weakness first affects feet, fronts of thighs, hips, belly, shoulders, and elbows. Later, it affects hands, face, and neck muscles.

- Most children become unable to walk by age 10.

- May develop a severe curve of the spine.

- Heart and breathing muscles also get weak. Child usually dies before age 20 from heart failure or pneumonia.

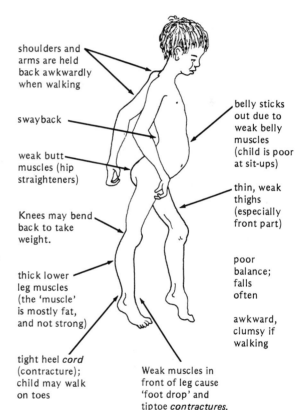

shoulders and arms are held back awkwardly when walking

swayback

weak butt muscles (hip straighteners)

Knees may bend back to take weight.

thick lower leg muscles (the 'muscle' is mostly fat, and not strong)

tight heel *cord* (contracture); child may walk on toes

belly sticks out due to weak belly muscles (child is poor at sit-ups)

thin, weak thighs (especially front part)

poor balance; falls often

awkward, clumsy if walking

Weak muscles in front of leg cause 'foot drop' and tiptoe *contractures.*

Early common sign of muscular dystrophy

- To get up from the ground, the child 'walks up' his thighs with his hands.

  This is mainly because of weak thigh muscles.

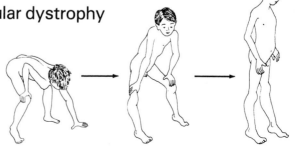

QUESTIONS ABOUT MUSCULAR DYSTROPHY

How common is it? It is not very common. *Rehabilitation* centers may see one child with muscular dystrophy for every 30 or 40 with cerebral palsy or polio.

What causes it? Nobody knows. But in 2 out of 3 families with muscular dystrophy, there is a history of it among male relatives of the mother. Though the parents are usually normal, the mother carries the 'gene' that produces dystrophy in her sons. Her daughters will develop normally, but they may have sons with muscular dystrophy.

What treatment is there? None. No medicines help. Special therapy or exercises will not stop the weakness from increasing. Surgery to release tiptoe contractures is at best of temporary benefit.

The family can, however, do much to help the child make the best of his life and adapt to his limitations as they progress.

Also, activities, exercises and braces to prevent contractures may help the child to keep walking longer (see p. 111). If the child sits in a bad position, pillows or supports to help him sit straighter can help prevent deformities.

Is the child's mind affected? About half of these children are somewhat mentally retarded (slow learners); some are very intelligent.

What can be done? The family can do many things to help the child live more fully and happily. The child should remain active and continue normal activities for as long as possible. Play with other children is important. So are learning and exploring. The child should go to school. Encourage other children to help him with learning and play. The teacher should realize that some—but not all—children with dystrophy learn a little more slowly than normal. Try to include the child in as many family and community activities as possible.

The steadily increasing weakness and the lack of effective treatment will be hard for both the family and child to accept. Friendly assistance, advice, and encouragement from health workers and friends can be a big help. Help the family to look at the situation honestly, and to do their best.

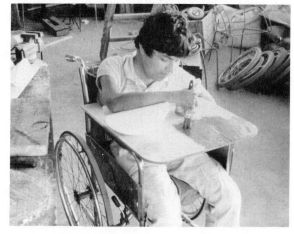

A boy with muscular dystrophy paints the top of his wheelchair table. Although he cannot lift his arm without help, a simple 'arm rocker' made of foam plastic lets him move it in all directions. It also allows him to feed himself. (See p. 331.)

> **The goal of the family is to help the child be as active and happy as possible, and to adjust to his increasing limitations.**

Helping the child to keep walking for as long as possible

Exercise. To keep as strong as possible and prevent contractures, probably the best therapy, at least at first, is to stay active, to walk, run, and play. While range-of-motion and stretching exercises may help (see Chapter 42), it is even better to involve the child in games, work, and other activities that keep his joints flexible. Even though he is slow and awkward, encourage him to take part. Feeling sorry for him and just letting him sit is the worst thing you can do.

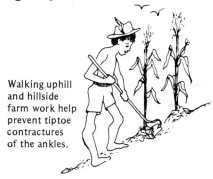

Walking uphill and hillside farm work help prevent tiptoe contractures of the ankles.

Braces. Long-leg braces should not be used until absolutely necessary, as they will let the child's legs grow weaker faster. Sometimes lightweight plastic ankle splints, worn day and night, will help delay ankle contractures and keep him walking better. (See Chapter 58.)

If **contractures of the knees and hips** begin to develop, try resting or sleeping with 'sand bags' to press down the legs and help straighten them.

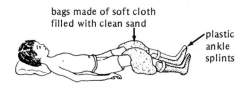

bags made of soft cloth filled with clean sand

plastic ankle splints

sand bag

cushion

CAUTION: Balance your efforts to provide therapy or surgery against the need of the child (and his family) to lead as full, happy, and normal a life as possible. His weakness will increase and his life will be short regardless of all efforts. The goal of all care for the child with muscular dystrophy should be to help him get the most out of living *NOW.* The temporary benefits of surgery should be weighed against the pain and hardships it would involve.

Other aids. The child will reach a point where he needs to use **crutches.** Later, (often by age 10) he will not be able to walk. Do not force him when it becomes too hard. Instead, try to obtain or make a **wheelchair.** (See Chapters 64 to 66.) At first, the child may be able to roll it himself. But as his weakness progresses, he may need to be pushed.

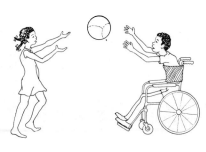

A wide cloth or canvas strap across his belly and chest may allow the child to play, to lean forward, and to use his arms more freely.

Breathing deeply is important, especially when the muscles that move the lungs begin to weaken. Encourage the child to sing loudly, to shout, to blow whistles, and to blow up balloons.

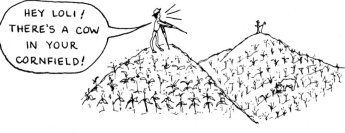

HEY LOLI! THERE'S A COW IN YOUR CORNFIELD!

Shouting and climbing are both good exercises for the lungs.

Other problems

- **Getting fat** is a common problem in children with dystrophy. The child needs to eat a healthy balanced diet. But take care not to let him eat too much—especially sweet things. Extra body weight will make walking, breathing, and other activities more difficult for his weakening body, and will make it harder for family members to lift him.
- **Constipation (hard, difficult stools)** may become a problem. Drinking lots of liquid helps. So does eating fruits and vegetables, and foods with lots of fiber (see p. 212).
- **Spinal curve** can become severe (see picture of Tito drawing, below). A corset or body brace may help hold the child in a straighter position so he can use his arms better and breathe better (see p. 164).
- **Arm weakness** in time may become a problem for self-care and eating.

You can make a simple aid to help get the hand to the mouth. More ideas of aids for eating and reaching are on p. 330 and 331.

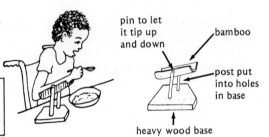

pin to let it tip up and down — bamboo — post put into holes in base — heavy wood base

CAUTION: If elbow contractures develop, it is probably better to leave them, as a bent elbow is more useful than a stiff, straight one. (See p. 122.)

It is important to help the child gain interests and skills that he can continue to develop even as he becomes very weak. He should stay in school, if possible, even when he has to go in a wheelchair.

Learning to draw and paint can be fulfilling. In Los Pargos, an organization of families of disabled children in Mexico (see p. 517), 4 brothers with muscular dystrophy have all become very good artists. Their paintings have won prizes in contests and are sold to raise money for the group. The best artist of all was the oldest brother, Tito. He took pride in his paintings and enjoyed teaching the other children. He did one of his best paintings, a sea turtle with wings, a week before he died, at age 17.

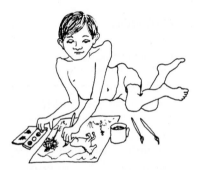

Even when he was so weak he could barely move, Tito continued to create beautiful pictures.

PREVENTION: The only way to prevent muscular dystrophy is for women who may have the dystrophy gene not to have children. This mostly means sisters of affected boys and close relatives on the mother's side. If you have one son with dystrophy, other sons will be likely to have it too. You might consider not having more children.

OTHER MUSCULAR DYSTROPHIES AND MUSCULAR ATROPHIES

The type of dystrophy just described—also called progressive, pseudohypertrophic, or Duchenne's muscular dystrophy—is the most common. But there are many different types of muscular dystrophy and muscular atrophy. All start little by little: some in early childhood, some between ages 13 to 19, and some in adults. All steadily get worse and worse. Some types, however, almost stop after a certain age, and the person may live to active old age, although handicapped.

Club Feet, Flat Feet, Bow Legs, and Knock-Knees

CHAPTER **11**

WHAT IS A DEFORMITY AND WHAT IS NORMAL?

Sometimes parents worry because they think a part of their child's body is abnormal or deformed. But **in small children, often what seems unusual is within what is normal,** and will get better as the child grows. For this reason, it is important to know what variations are normal and which may be problems.

Note: For children born with parts of their bodies missing or shortened, see Chapter 12 on birth defects.

1. Many children are born with their **feet somewhat bent or crooked.** To learn the difference between a normal bend caused by the baby's position in the womb, and true club feet, see the next page.

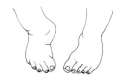

CURVED FEET:
NORMAL in the first weeks or months of life

'FLAT' FEET:
NORMAL until age 2

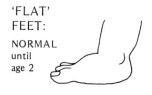

2. 'Fat' or 'flat'?—When most babies begin to walk, they walk on the insides of their feet, with their legs wide apart. Also their feet still have baby fat on the bottom. As a result, the feet look very flat. In nearly all cases, they will get better by themselves. (See p. 117.)

3. A baby's legs often bend outward ('bow legs'), like this. → This bending starts to disappear at the age of 18 months. Then the legs slowly straighten until they actually bend inward a little, like this.

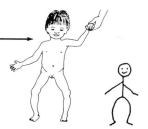

BOW LEGS:
NORMAL until about 18 months

KNOCK-KNEES:
NORMAL between 2 and 12 years

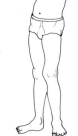

4. This 'knock-kneed' position generally develops around age 2. By age 5 or 6 the knees begin to straighten.

Note: Children with brain damage sometimes develop a 'knock-knee' way of standing or walking. If the child with knock-knees also moves or walks in a stiff or jerky way, or shows other problems, check for signs of brain damage. (See p. 35 and Chapter 9 on cerebral palsy.)

(CP)

IMPORTANT: **In any child who develops bow legs or knock-knees, check for signs of rickets and other problems. See Chapter 13.**

SEVERE KNOCK-KNEES

To check for severe knock-knees, have the child stand with her knees touching. If the distance between the ankle bones is more than **3 inches** in a 3 year old, or **4 inches** in a 4 year old, the problem is probably severe enough to need attention.

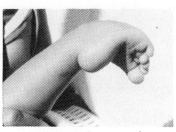

Sign of a problem

3 years old

4 years old

more than 3 inches (7½ cm.)

more than 4 inches (10 cm.)

If the knock-knees are severe, braces may help straighten the knees and keep the condition from getting worse (see p. 539). In a child over 6 or 7 years old, braces usually do not help. In extreme cases, surgery may be needed. Knock-knees may also lead to flat feet.

CLUB FEET

About 3 out of 1,000 children are born with a club foot (or feet). Sometimes it runs in the family, but usually the cause is unknown.

Sometimes a newborn baby's feet turn inward, just because they were in that position in the mother's womb.

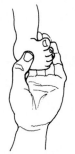

club foot before correction

If the front part of a baby's foot is turned inward, it will often straighten out by itself before she is 2 years old.

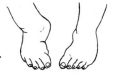

front part only bent

back part straight

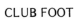

To find out whether the condition is likely to correct itself, or if it is a true deformity (club foot) that needs special attention, try to put the foot in a normal position.

Bent foot straightens:

NORMAL

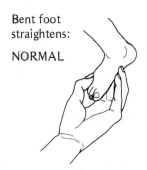

If you can easily straighten the foot, and bend it into a position opposite to the way it was turned, the foot probably does not have a bone deformity and will get better by itself. Also, if you scratch the foot lightly, the child often will move it into a normal position.

Bent foot does not straighten:

CLUB FOOT

If you cannot put the foot in a normal position, it will need to be straightened with strapping or casts (see Chapter 60).

Are club feet a sign of some other problem? Although club foot often occurs without any other problem, occasionally it is a complication of spina bifida (problem in the *spinal cord,* see Chapter 22). Always check the child's spine and test if he has feeling in his feet (see p. 39).

The feet may also gradually become deformed into a 'club foot' position, because of cerebral palsy, polio, arthritis, or spinal cord damage.

Rarely, club feet occur together with a 'clubbed hand' or other weakness and deformities of the body. See Arthrogryposis, p. 122.

Correcting club feet (For details, see Chapter 60.)

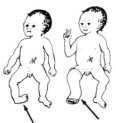

A club foot should be held
in a cast, or strapped in
a straighter position,
soon after birth—until it
is corrected past normal.

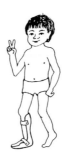

After correcting the
foot, daily stretching
exercises are often
needed to help keep
the foot straight.

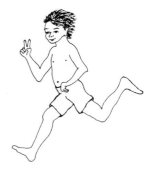

A brace is used
(day and night if
necessary) to keep
the foot from
bending in again,

until finally,
normal use and
exercise keeps
the foot straight.

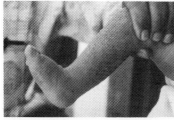

club foot after correction with casts,
by village workers (PROJIMO)

About 60% of club feet can be effectively
straightened without surgery in 6 to 8 weeks, using
either **strapping** or **casts. These methods are described in
Chapter 60.**

**Correction of club feet should begin soon after the child is born—if possible, in the
first 2 days.** At birth, a baby's bones and joints are still soft. As the child gets older, his
bones get harder and become less flexible.

Usually, good correction without surgery is only possible in the first year of life. If
the deformity is not severe, however, a club foot can sometimes be corrected with
casts, even if the child is already 2, 3, or even 5 years old or more. But in an older
child, it takes longer, and surgery is more often needed for good, lasting results.

Some children with very deformed feet will need surgery, even if strapping or casting
is done early. However, we have found that some children for whom surgeons have
recommended surgery can have their feet straightened with **casts** at a village center.

Keeping the feet straight once they are corrected

Once a club foot has been straightened, great care must be taken to keep it straight.
The whole family must make sure that the following precautions are taken:

- An ankle brace should be worn **night** and **day** at least until the child is
walking, and often until the child is 15 or 18 years old.

- Foot-stretching exercises will be needed,
especially if there is any sign that the foot
is clubbing again. Gently and steadily
stretch the foot **past** its normal position in
the opposite direction of the deformity.
Do this exercise 2 or more times a day.

Bend foot out.

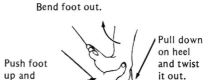

Push foot
up and
twist it out.

Pull down
on heel
and twist
it out.

- Check the foot regularly. Return quickly to the *rehabilitation* center for
an *evaluation* if there is any sign that the clubbing is coming back.

How long will it take?

How difficult it is to straighten a club foot, how long it takes, and how long braces and special exercises will be needed depends on a number of factors:

- **The severity of clubbing.** A severely deformed foot with abnormal bones is much harder to correct.

- **Abnormal muscle balance,** if present, will keep pulling the foot to the inside, even after it is corrected. (See muscle testing, p. 30.)

- Generally, correction is more difficult if both feet are clubbed.

- Club feet in **girls** (although less common) are likely to be more difficult to correct than in boys.

- If there are any **other abnormalities** (such as a clubbed hand or stiffness in the knees or elbows), club feet may be especially difficult to correct. Usually surgery is needed.

- **The older the child,** the harder it is to correct a club foot. Past the age of 2 years, it is often not possible without surgery.

- **Children without feeling in their feet** (spina bifida) require special precautions and slower correction to avoid pressure sores (see p. 173). Casts, if used, must not apply much pressure, and must be changed often.

If a child's foot shows little or no improvement after 4 weeks of casting, or if improvement stops in spite of continued casting, surgery is probably needed for more complete correction.

BRACES FOR USE AFTER CORRECTING CLUB FEET

For some feet, a plastic ankle brace may work well.

For more difficult feet, a metal brace may be needed, with an ankle strap that pulls the ankle inward.

A slight build-up on the outer edge of the sandal or shoe may also help.

For instructions on making braces, see Chapter 58.

For babies under one year, or small children at night, feet can be held in a good position using a bar that joins the 2 feet. For a simple design, see p. 539.

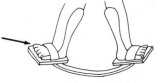

For the child whose feet bend mostly at the middle or front

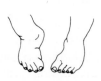

wearing shoes in reverse may help keep the feet corrected.

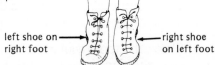

left shoe on right foot

right shoe on left foot

FLAT FEET

Most children whose only problem is flat feet really have no problem at all—except that poorly informed doctors or greedy special-shoe salesmen make their parents think so!

Most babies have naturally *fat* feet, which can look *flat*.

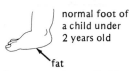

normal foot of a child under 2 years old

fat

Do not confuse a FAT foot with a FLAT foot!

In older children and adults there is a lot of natural variation in people's arches.

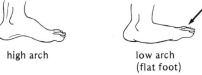

high arch

low arch (flat foot)

foot print

Even a foot as flat as this, if it causes the child no pain, need not be considered a problem. Often flat feet run in families. If parents or relatives have similar feet but no pain, or if the child can move his feet strongly in all directions, do not worry about it.

Do not worry about flat feet if there is no pain, obvious weakness, or loss of movement.

Children who are late beginning to walk often have weak arches with flat feet, until their feet get stronger.

Even children with very flat feet seldom develop a problem or have more than average pain or discomfort when they do a lot of standing or walking. **Usually flat feet are a problem only when paralysis or brain damage is the cause**—as in some children with polio, cerebral palsy, or spina bifida. Also, children with **Down syndrome** sometimes have flat feet that may lead to pain or discomfort.

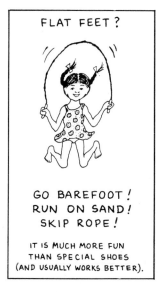

FLAT FEET ?

GO BAREFOOT!
RUN ON SAND!
SKIP ROPE!

IT IS MUCH MORE FUN THAN SPECIAL SHOES (AND USUALLY WORKS BETTER).

Correcting flat feet

The best treatment to help the child with flat feet and no other problem may be to **go barefoot.** Walking barefoot on sand or rough ground helps the feet get stronger and form a natural arch. Walking on tiptoe, skipping rope, and picking things up with the toes may also help.

BEWARE of going barefoot where hookworm is common.

CAUTION: Special exercises, training in 'foot posture', shoe adaptations, heel wedges and shoe inserts (heel cups and insoles) are often prescribed to correct flat feet. However, studies show that usually **none of these help.** Use of insoles to support the arches may even cause weaker arches. Usually insoles should be tried only when pain is a problem, or in some severe flat feet caused by polio, cerebral palsy, or Down syndrome.

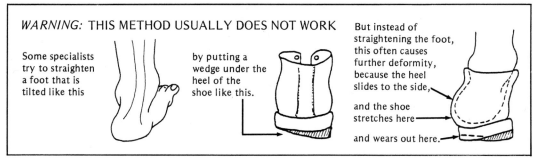

WARNING: THIS METHOD USUALLY DOES NOT WORK

Some specialists try to straighten a foot that is tilted like this

by putting a wedge under the heel of the shoe like this.

But instead of straightening the foot, this often causes further deformity, because the heel slides to the side,

and the shoe stretches here

and wears out here.

INSOLES AND OTHER FOOT SUPPORTS

An insole is a firm pad that is put inside a shoe or sandal to support the arch.

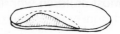

Some children with flat feet resulting from polio, cerebral palsy, or Down syndrome may be helped by insoles or other foot supports. But other children will not be helped. Each child's needs should be carefully considered. If after trying an insole for 2 weeks, the child walks with more difficulty, change the insole or stop using it.

Insoles can be made of leather, porous rubber, or a piece of a car tire, shaping it with care so that it will support the foot comfortably.

Before making the final insole, put a piece of cardboard, wood or some other material shaped like the insole, under the child's foot. Try different heights to find what seems to work best. **Make sure the heel is in a straight line with the leg.**

After making the insole, check the position of the foot. Do this with the child standing on just the insole, and then with the insole inside the shoe. Watch him walk, and ask him how it feels. If everything seems right, check it again in 2 weeks.

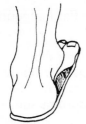 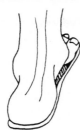 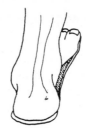

CORRECT—The heel is in a straight line with the leg.

TOO LOW—The heel tilts outward. The insole should be thicker.

TOO HIGH—The heel tilts inward. The insole is probably too thick.

CAUTION: A person who has a weak ankle and low arch sometimes cannot use an insole, because it lets his ankle turn outward as he walks. He may have learned to walk in a way that keeps his ankle from turning out. For such a person, an insole may make walking more difficult, or may force him to use a brace to keep his foot straight.

IMPORTANT: The thickest part of an insole should be directly under the ankle bone, just in front of the heel, like this. ——

CORRECT

It should *not* be in the middle of the arch, like this. This can deform the foot more without correcting the problem. ——

WRONG

WARNING: Many commercial insoles, and even orthopedic shoes, have the arches in this incorrect position. Check them carefully. If they are like this, do not use them. Also be sure shoes are not so wide that the heel slips to the side.

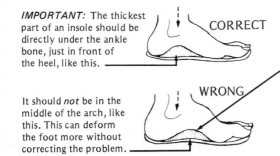

If the child's foot is flat or very floppy due to paralysis, often an insole is not enough. He may need a short plastic brace that supports the foot like this,

built-in sole

or a brace that supports the foot and ankle, like this. ——

For instructions on making plastic braces, see Chapter 58.

There is probably only one shoe or sandal alteration that does any good. A small metal plate on the inner edge of the heel stops uneven wear—and may help prevent foot pain.

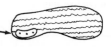

CHAPTER **12**

Common Birth Defects

TYPES OF BIRTH DEFECTS

One out of every 100 or so babies is born with some kind of obvious defect or deformity. There are many different types. In this chapter we describe a few of the most common: **cleft lip** and **cleft palate, extra or joined fingers or toes,** and **short, missing, or deformed limbs.** We also discuss children born with multiple *contractures* **(arthrogryposis).** Please also refer to the chapters on **club feet** (Chapter 11), and **spina bifida** (Chapter 22).

CAUSES

In many cases, the cause of a birth defect is not known. But sometimes a defect may be caused by one of the following:

- **Poor nutrition during early pregnancy.** This is thought to be one cause of cleft lip and palate.

The mother of this girl with cleft lip and palate did not get enough to eat while she was pregnant.

- **Genetic (hereditary).** Sometimes certain defects run in families. For example, if one parent was born with an extra thumb, there is a greater chance that a child will be born with a similar defect. One or both parents may be 'carriers' of the factor that causes a defect, without having it themselves. However, it may be present in relatives. Often both parents must have a 'defect factor' for a child to be born with the defect. For this reason, **birth defects are more common in children whose parents are closely related,** and who therefore carry the same defect factors.

- **Medicines, pesticides, chemicals, and poisons.** Especially during the first 3 months of development, a baby in the womb can easily be harmed by chemicals and poisons. **Many medicines, drugs, and pesticides** (plant, insect, and rat poisons) can cause birth defects if a pregnant mother is exposed to them.

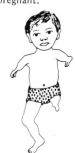

A doctor gave this boy's mother a medicine for 'morning sickness'.

- **German measles.** If the mother gets German measles during the first 3 months of pregnancy, it can cause defects in the baby. These usually affect the senses (hearing and seeing), the brain (cerebral palsy and *retardation*), or organs inside the body (heart, liver). Sometimes the baby is born with 'rubber band-like' grooves on the limbs and deformed or missing fingers or limbs.

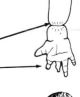

- Children born to **mothers 40 years of age or older** are more likely to have Down syndrome and defects of the hands, feet, or organs inside the body (heart, liver). In this age group, about 1 mother in 50 will have a child born with Down syndrome or defects.

This boy's mother was 45 years old when he was born.

For ways to prevent birth defects, see p. 124.

CLEFT LIP AND CLEFT PALATE

A cleft lip (or 'hare lip') is an opening or gap in the upper lip, often connecting to the nostril.

A 'cleft palate' is an opening in the roof of the mouth connecting with the canal of the nose.

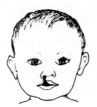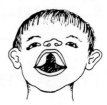

simple cleft lip   double cleft lip   cleft palate

Usually 1 in about 800 children is born with a cleft lip, cleft palate, or both.

Babies with these conditions often have trouble sucking, and may choke or gag on food that gets into their nose. Usually breast feeding is the best way to feed these children.

Put the breast deep into the mouth so that the milk comes out on the back of the baby's tongue.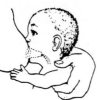

Occasionally the mother may need to get milk from her breasts by squeezing them, and then feed the milk to her baby with a spoon.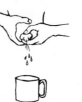

To prevent choking, feed the baby while he is sitting up with his head tilted forward a little.

Make every effort to have the defects corrected by surgery since this can greatly improve the child's looks, eating ability, and speech. **The best age for surgery** is usually at **4 to 6 months for the lip** and about **18 months for the palate.**

To prepare for surgery, parents should frequently stretch **the deformed lip,** so that the 2 sides meet in the middle.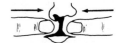

Even after the cleft lip and palate have been successfully repaired, speech problems often occur. The family should gently encourage the child to speak as clearly as she can. Lip and tongue exercises may help (see p. 314). The child who cannot get surgery may need to learn sign language, using her hands to help people understand her (see p. 266).

JOINED FINGERS AND EXTRA OR DEFORMED FINGERS OR TOES

Some children are born with 2 or more fingers joined together. This does not cause much difficulty in use of the hand. However, special surgery can often separate the joined fingers.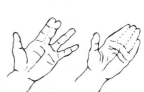

When a child is born with a small extra finger or toe that has no bone in it, you can tie a string tightly around it, like this. In a few days the finger will dry out and fall off.

Larger extra fingers or toes, if they get in the way, can be removed by a surgeon.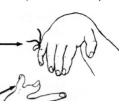

A child who is born
with a toe that sticks
out may need surgery in
order to wear shoes.
The toe can sometimes
be put straight. At
other times it may be
simpler to remove it.

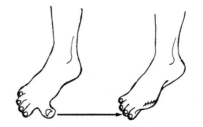

To get the best
results, the
surgery should be
done by a specially
trained *orthopedic*
or plastic surgeon.

INCOMPLETE OR MISSING ARMS OR LEGS

Sometimes medicines a mother takes early in pregnancy
cause a child to be born with missing or incomplete arms or legs,
or both.

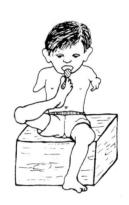

A child born without arms but with normal legs and feet can
often learn to use his feet almost as if they were hands: for
eating, writing, drawing, playing games, and doing many kinds
of work.

**It is important to encourage the child to use her feet, or
whatever part of her body possible, to do everything she can for
herself.**

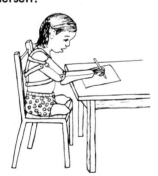

The child who is born with incomplete arms and legs
can be helped a lot by **artificial arms with hooks for
grasping** (see p. 230).

We do not give instructions for making these arms in
this book, as they are fairly complicated. However, try
every possibility to get artificial arms for the child.
They can make a very big difference in her life. If
possible, the child should get her first limbs by age 3.

For ideas about aids and artificial limbs for children born with missing or defective
hands and feet, see Chapter 27, "Amputations," and Chapter 67, "Artificial Legs."

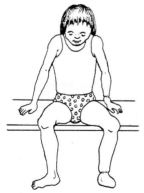

This little girl was born with 'rubber
band-like' constrictions in her hand and
leg, and with parts of her fingers and
foot missing. The deformities happened
because her mother had German measles
when pregnant.

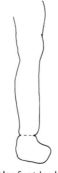

Her foot looked
like this.

Village
rehabilitation
workers made her
a plastic brace
with a partial
foot built into
it, so she could
wear a regular
shoe or sandal.

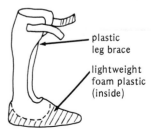

plastic
leg brace

lightweight
foam plastic
(inside)

A firm foam-plastic foot was shaped and
attached to a plaster mold of the foot (see
Chapter 58). The plastic brace was heat molded
over this.

ARTHROGRYPOSIS (Multiple contractures from birth)

Arthrogryposis means 'curved joints'. Children with this *disability* are born with stiff joints and weak *muscles.* The strange position of arms and/or legs may give a child the look of a wooden puppet.

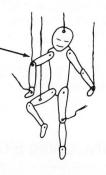

In some children, both arms and legs may be severely affected. In others, only the legs or feet, or hands or arms may be affected.

A child born with clubbed feet and with one or both arms stiff with hands turned out, may have arthrogryposis.

TYPICAL BABY WITH ARTHROGRYPOSIS

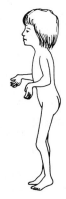

mind completely normal

Sometimes the face is long and the jaw large.

shoulders sometimes turned in

often arms are stiff at elbows and weak

wrist often bent up or out stiffly

hands and fingers often very weak

hips often bent upward or outward stiffly; may be dislocated

spine often curved but *trunk* strength usually normal

club foot common

contractures with 'webbing' of skin behind joints (at knees, hips, elbows, or shoulders)

knees bent or straight, in a stiff position

The **cause** of arthrogryposis is not known. It may be a *virus infection* of the mother, during pregnancy. Arthrogryposis is a **rare condition** in most of the world, but for unknown reasons, in parts of Central and South America it occurs more frequently. (In PROJIMO, in Mexico, 1 of every 100 disabled children seen has arthrogryposis.)

Rehabilitation of the child with arthrogryposis aims at helping the child do as much for herself as possible.

Some children with arthrogryposis are able to walk, especially if contractures are corrected. Correction of club feet (see p. 115) and hip and knee contractures should begin gradually, and without forcing, soon after birth, with casting (see p. 565), positioning, and/or range-of-motion exercises (see p. 115).

TYPICAL STANDING POSITION OF A CHILD WITH ARTHROGRYPOSIS

If both hips are dislocated, surgery to put the bones back into their sockets is not usually helpful. The child walks as well without surgery. If only one hip is dislocated, surgery may help.

Often, however, contractures of arthrogryposis can only be corrected by surgery. The possible benefits—and losses—which surgery may bring should be carefully evaluated. For example, a stiff elbow in a bent (contracted) position may be much better for eating than an elbow that has been straightened, and will not bend.

MORE USEFUL   LESS USEFUL

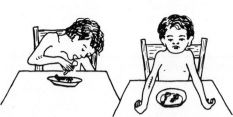

WARNING: A STIFF ELBOW IS OFTEN MORE USEFUL LEFT BENT

Most children with arthrogryposis are very intelligent. If given a chance, many can learn to do a lot of things for themselves, even with *severe disability*. Often they try hard and are eager to learn. **It is very important that these children be encouraged and helped to do as much as they can for themselves, and that they go to school.** The following story may help give you an idea of the possibilities of a child with arthrogryposis.

SIMPLE STEPS TOWARD INDEPENDENCE—A true story

Gabriel is 7 years old. He lives with his family in Mazatlán, Mexico. He was born with arthrogryposis. Some of his joints are stiff and straight, others are stiff and bent. He lacks most of the muscles in his arms, legs, and hands. He cannot sit alone or lift a hand to his mouth.

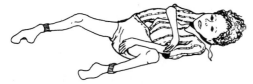

Gabriel's parents love him dearly and care for him tenderly. However, when he was born, doctors told them that nothing could be done for him. So his parents grew used to doing everything for him. As he grew older, they carried him in their arms, changed his *diapers* when he dirtied them, and gave him food in his mouth. They treated him like a baby—though he no longer was one.

When his mother learned of PROJIMO, she took Gabriel there, hoping that with surgery or special medicine, he might improve. The village *rehabilitation* workers at PROJIMO investigated all possibilities. They even took him to a famous hospital for disabled children. But the specialists said they could do nothing for Gabriel.

Fortunately, therapists who were visiting PROJIMO as instructors explained to the team that in fact there was a lot that could be done, not to help Gabriel walk, but to help him do more for himself—within his possibilities. The team began to work with the family, to help Gabriel become more independent.

Now, with the help of the village rehabilitation workers and his family, Gabriel is able to meet some of his basic needs for himself. He feels less like a baby and more like a young man. He has stopped using diapers; he asks when he needs to go to the toilet. He has learned to use his mouth like a hand, to hold and do things.

He has learned to feed himself. He swings his arm onto the table using his neck muscles, and hooks his hand over a spoon. Using the edge of the table and the rim of the dish to push against, he see-saws the spoon to his mouth. To drink he uses a straw with a bend in it.

Gabriel's family has joined Los Pargos, an organized group of families of disabled children. He attends school in a specially-adapted wheelchair that he can move himself. He is learning to read, write, paint pictures, and to play with other children.

There is much more that Gabriel and his family will be able to achieve, now that they all see how much he can do for himself. Gabriel is happy and eager to learn more.

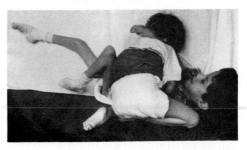

Gabriel wrestling with another disabled child.

Various aids and *adaptations* can help children with arthrogryposis or similar disabilities become more independent:

Eating aids are described on p. 330 to 332.

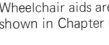

Wheelchair aids are shown in Chapter 64.

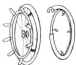

Writing aids are shown on p. 5, p. 230, and p. 501.

PREVENTION OF BIRTH DEFECTS

It is not possible to prevent all birth defects. Some babies form differently inside the womb and no one knows why. But many birth defects can be prevented. For ways to make it less likely that children will be born with birth defects, see Chapter 3. To reduce the chances of having birth defects, pregnant women must stay in good health and avoid certain dangers:

- **Eat well during pregnancy.** Eating enough good food gives strength, prevents infection, builds a healthy baby and helps prevent too much bleeding during birth. Be sure to eat food that has enough folic acid. (See *Where There Is No Doctor*, Chapter 11 and *Where Women Have No Doctor*, Chapter 11.)

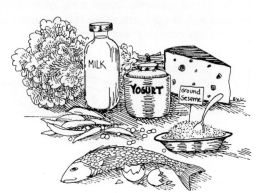

- **Avoid all medicines and drugs during pregnancy** unless you are sure they will not damage the baby. (Vitamins, some antacids, and iron in the correct dose are alright.) Alcohol and tobacco during pregnancy can also damage the developing child.

- **Avoid any contact with pesticides and other poisons**. If a pregnant woman's husband or family members must use pesticides or poisons, they should wash their own clothes, and protect the pregnant woman from the chemicals.

- **Avoid marrying close relatives.** When close family members have children together, the children are much more likely to have birth defects.

- **If you already have one or more children with a serious birth defect,** it is more likely you may have another, so you might consider not having more.

- While pregnant, stay far away from anyone with German measles (rubella) if you have never had it. If you are not pregnant, try to catch it before you get pregnant. *Vaccines* give protection against German measles but you should not become pregnant for 1 month after rubella immunization.

- Getting syphilis or herpes when you are pregnant can cause the baby to be born with birth defects. Make sure to be tested and treated early for sexually transmitted diseases.

- Consider not having more children after age 35 or 40, or if you have had one child with Down syndrome, since the chance of having another is increased.

Most birth defects can be prevented when women can afford good food to eat, when they do not have to work with toxic chemicals, and when they have good health care.

Birth defects should not be treated as a problem for families to deal with on their own. The causes of birth defects affect the whole community. To prevent birth defects, we must change the world we live in so that it is safer for women and families.

Children Who Stay Small or Have Weak Bones

In this chapter we look at children whose bones are weak and deformed, and at children who do not grow as tall as other children. We include **rickets, brittle bone disease,** and **children who stay very short** (dwarfism). In all of these conditions, **the legs may become bowed,** and the shape or proportions of the bones are often not normal.

RICKETS

Rickets is weakness and deformity of the bones that occurs from lack of vitamin D. Vitamin D occurs in whole milk, butter, egg yolks, animal fats, and liver, especially fish liver oil. The body also makes its own vitamin D when sunlight shines on the skin. Children who do not eat enough foods with vitamin D, and who do not get enough sunlight, gradually develop signs of rickets.

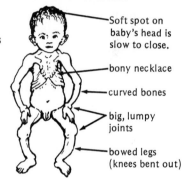

SIGNS OF RICKETS

Soft spot on baby's head is slow to close.

bony necklace

curved bones

big, lumpy joints

bowed legs (knees bent out)

Rickets is fairly common in some countries, especially in cool mountain areas of Asia and Latin America where babies are kept inside and wrapped up. Rickets is also increasing in crowded cities where children are seldom taken into the sunlight.

Treatment for rickets is to give fish liver oil, and to spend time in the sunlight. The best and cheapest form of **prevention** is to be sure sunlight reaches the child's skin. Foods that contain vitamin D also help.

BRITTLE BONE DISEASE

The child is born with bent or twisted limbs, or with broken bones. (Or he may seem normal at birth, and the bones begin to break later.) He may start to walk at near the normal age, but increasing deformities due to breaks may soon make walking impossible. Because of the many broken and bent bones, these children stay very short. Parents sometimes do not realize when their child breaks a bone.

Brittle bone disease is not common. Sometimes it is *inherited,* and someone else in the family will have the same problem.

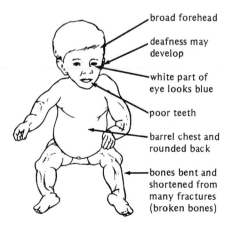

SIGNS OF BRITTLE BONE DISEASE

broad forehead

deafness may develop

white part of eye looks blue

poor teeth

barrel chest and rounded back

bones bent and shortened from many fractures (broken bones)

There is no medical treatment. However, sometimes surgery can be done to straighten and strengthen the leg bones by putting a metal rod down the middle of them. This may help the child walk for longer, but he may eventually need a wheelchair to move about. Back problems increase with age; a body brace may help (see p. 164).

Children with brittle bone disease are often intelligent and do well in school. Increasing deafness may become a problem. Help them to develop their minds and learn skills that do not require physical strength. The child must learn how to protect his body from breaks. It helps to sleep on a firm bed.

CHILDREN WHO STAY SHORT (Dwarfism)

Parents often worry when a child does not grow as quickly as other children. Shortness has many causes. Here we discuss only a few.

- **Normal slow growth.** Some children normally grow more slowly and mature sexually later than others. If the child is normal and healthy in other ways, do not worry. He will probably grow quickly when he begins to grow up sexually, even if this happens as late as 15, 16, or 17 years old.

- **Normal short size.** When one or both parents are shorter than average, they may have children who are also short. Shortness 'runs in the family' and this is normal. Make sure the child is healthy and eats well.

- **Poor nutrition.** Some children do not grow normally because they do not get enough to eat, or do not eat the food their bodies need. They may seem normal except that they are thin, small, have big bellies, and get sick often. Or they may lack energy, seem very unhappy, or develop swollen feet, hands, and faces. These children need more and better food (see p. 321). They may also need more stimulation, play, love, and attention in order to grow and develop more quickly (see Chapter 35).

- **Long-term illness or medication.** Severe long illness often slows down a child's growth. Also, certain medicines such as cortisone or steroids for arthritis, if given for a long time, can slow down growth and weaken bones.

- **Dwarfism.** Some children are born with a condition in which the body does not grow normally. There are many different patterns and causes. In 1 of 5 children it is inherited, and certain relatives will also be very short.

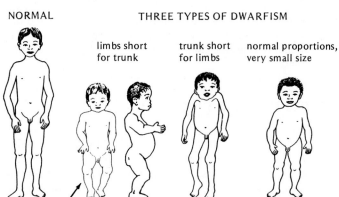

NORMAL   THREE TYPES OF DWARFISM

limbs short for trunk   trunk short for limbs   normal proportions, very small size

In the **most common type of dwarfism,** the arms and legs are short for the body. The head is big, the forehead bulges, and the bridge of the nose is flat. The child often has a swayback, pot belly, and bowlegs. Hip problems, club feet, or eye problems and hearing loss may occur.

TREATMENT

There is no medical treatment for most children who are short, including those with dwarfism. In many countries, doctors prescribe 'growth' hormones to short children to make them grow faster. These may cause some growth at first, but they soon make the bones mature and stop growing, so that the child stays smaller than he would have without treatment. **Do not give hormones to speed growth.**

Children who are very short for their age sometimes are made fun of by other children, or get treated as though they are younger than they really are. Life can be difficult for them and they may feel unhappy or unsure of themselves. It is important that everyone treat them just like other children their age. CHILD-to-child activities can help other children become more understanding (see Chapter 47).

Erb's Palsy

CHAPTER 14

Arm Paralysis from Birth Injury

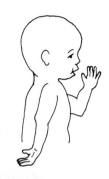

WHAT IS IT?

Erb's palsy is a *paralysis* of the *muscles* in a baby's arm, caused by injury of the *nerves* in the shoulder at birth (during delivery).

The baby lies with one arm and hand twisted backward and does not move the arm as much as the other.

If the full range of motion of the arm is not kept through regular exercise, *contractures* will develop that may prevent lifting the arm above the shoulder or turning the hand palm up.

HOW COMMON IS IT?

Nerve damage causing Erb's palsy occurs in approximately 1 out of every 400 births. It is much more common in babies who are born butt first (breech) because the shoulder is easily stretched and the nerves injured.

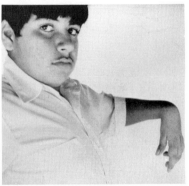

Severe Erb's palsy in 14 year old boy. This is as high as he can lift his arm.

WHAT CAN BE DONE ABOUT IT?

With the baby, start range-of-motion exercises 2 times a day.

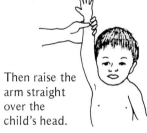

Extend the child's arm and turn the hand upwards.

Then raise the arm straight over the child's head.

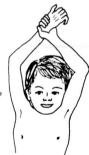

When the child is old enough, have him do exercises himself, for range of motion and to increase strength.

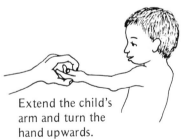

Ask him to lift his arm as high as he can, turning the palm up as far as he can,

and then lift it with the other hand as high as he can, with the palm up.

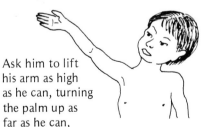

Note: If contractures have already formed, do exercises more often, for a longer time. Each time try to turn the hand up and lift the arm as high as possible. Hold it in the stretched position while you count to 25, or sing a song.

Other helpful exercises

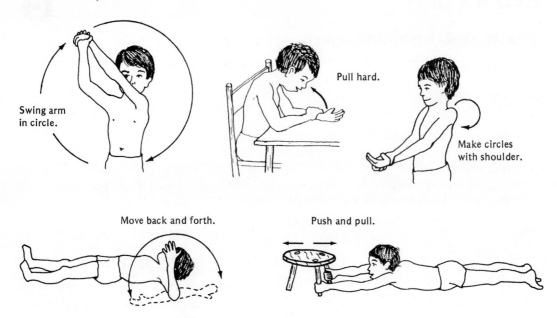

Swing arm in circle.

Pull hard.

Make circles with shoulder.

Move back and forth.

Push and pull.

Look for ways to include these exercises in work and play.

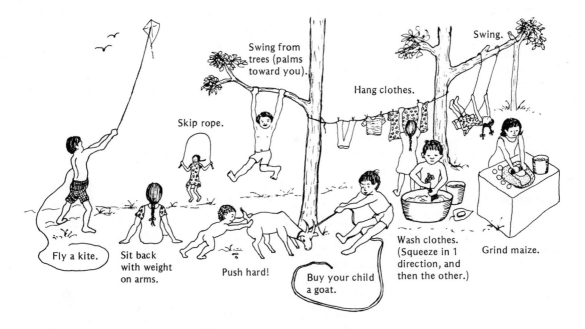

Fly a kite.

Skip rope.

Swing from trees (palms toward you).

Hang clothes.

Swing.

Sit back with weight on arms.

Push hard!

Buy your child a goat.

Wash clothes. (Squeeze in 1 direction, and then the other.)

Grind maize.

PREVENTION

Erb's palsy can sometimes be prevented if the midwife or doctor takes care not to strain or force the baby's shoulder when being born. Examination of the mother's belly before birth should let the midwife know if the baby is likely to be born breech. In this case a hospital delivery by a skilled doctor or midwife may reduce the chance of injury.

Contractures and significant *disability* from Erb's palsy can largely be prevented by exercises. Some weakness may last throughout life.

CHAPTER **15**

Painful Joints

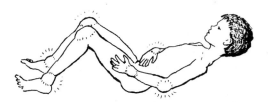

Joint pain in children has many causes. Depending on the cause, different treatments may be needed. The chart that follows will help you decide what the cause of **chronic** (long-lasting) joint pain in a child might be. However, other less common causes may also be possible. Sometimes laboratory tests may be needed to be more certain.

Specific treatment is needed for certain kinds of joint pain—especially those caused by *infection.* However, some basic principles of care and *therapy* apply to most joint pain, regardless of the cause. Following the chart of causes, you will find some general guidelines for the care of joint pain. These guidelines are described in more detail in Chapter 16 on juvenile arthritis.

Three chapters on disabilities with joint pain are "Juvenile Arthritis" (Chapter 16), "Rheumatic Fever" (Chapter 17), and "Hip Problems" (Chapter 18). However, arthritis (joint pain and damage) can occur with any *disability* where paralysis or *muscle imbalance* cause abnormal positions or twisting of joints. Many children with polio develop painful *dislocations* or, when they are older, arthritis.

NOTE: The chart does not include the many *infectious* diseases that may cause *temporary* joint pain. These do not usually lead to long-term disabilities. For details of diagnosis and treatment of illnesses that cause temporary joint pain, consult a health worker or see a medical text such as *Where There Is No Doctor.*

CAUTION: **Try not to confuse similar illnesses.** Two of the most common causes of joint pain in children are **rheumatic fever** and **juvenile arthritis.** Even some doctors and health workers get them mixed up and diagnose juvenile arthritis as rheumatic fever. The two illnesses do have similarities. However, rheumatic fever almost always follows a period of sore throat with fever. **If the child did not have a sore throat, probably the joint pain is not due to rheumatic fever.** When in doubt, however, 10 days of penicillin may be a wise precaution. See p. 154 for information on doses of penicillin.

Carefully study the differences between the common causes of joint pain. If you are not sure, seek help from someone with more experience.

COMMON CAUSES OF CHRONIC JOINT PAIN IN CHILDREN (pain that lasts more than 2 weeks or keeps coming back)

Problem	Age it often begins	Pain in **one** or in **several** joints	Fever	Other signs	Treatment and therapy
rheumatic fever (See Chapter 17.)	5 to 15 years old	Usually pain is in **several** joints. (Rarely it begins with severe pain and swelling in only one joint, but often there is also some pain in other joints.) Often pain starts in ankles and wrists, then knees and elbows. Pain may change from some joints to others.	High fever is typical (usually starts suddenly).	• Joint pain and fever usually begin 1–3 weeks after severe sore throat with fever (strep throat). • Small lumps may appear under the skin over joints. • sometimes wiggly reddish circles on skin • in severe or advanced cases, heart problems ('heart murmur', difficulty breathing, or chest pain) • usually gets better in 6 weeks to 3 months—but likely to come back	• pencillin V for 10 days each time throat gets sore (or continuously if heart is affected) • aspirin or ibuprofen in high doses with **precautions (See p. 134.)** • rest • range-of-motion (ROM) exercises • Apply heat or cold to painful joints.
juvenile arthritis (also called juvenile rheumatoid arthritis or Still's disease) (See Chapter 16.)	Any age, but often begins between 2–7 or 9–12 years old Lasts for years (Often the arthritis gets better when child becomes sexually developed)	May affect **few** joints, **many** joints, or almost **all** joints. (In 1/3 of children it begins in only **one** joint—later it may affect others.)	Often some fever when pain is worst. (Rarely, it begins with high fever.)	• usually no history of sore throat • severely painful, hot, swollen joints often leading to muscle weakness, contractures and deformities • sometimes a rash that comes and goes • may begin little by little, or suddenly and severely • one or both eyes may become red and sore (iritis) and become damaged • usually lasts for years with periods when it gets better and then worse	• aspirin or ibuprofen in high doses with **precautions to avoid stomach upset (See p. 134.)** • Apply heat or cold to painful joints. • ROM exercises • exercises without motion to strengthen muscles • lots of rest, but also moderate activity • lots of understanding and support
destruction or slipping of cap of thigh bone at the hip (See Chapter 18.)	Destruction: mostly boys 4–8 years old Slip: mostly boys 11–16 years old	pain in **one hip** (rarely both) Destruction: Cap of head of thigh bone breaks into pieces and gradually re-forms in 2 to 3 years X-ray needed to make definite diagnosis normal	no fever	• child begins to limp—often without complaining of pain • may complain of pain in knee or thigh (or sometimes hip); gradually develops weakness for raising leg like this	• For destruction: it may be best to do nothing, although many specialists still recommend casting, braces or surgery. • For slip: surgery to pin the cap into the right place may be needed.
below-knee pain (Osgood-Slater's problem)	Boys 11–18 years old	usually **one** knee only knee cap ligament painful swelling over bone here due to loosening of bone surface loosening of bone surface (seen on X-ray)	no fever	• especially in very active, strong boys • may begin with pain after jumping, running, or forceful exercise	• Avoid forceful exercises or activities until pain goes away (usually in 2 to 3 years). • aspirin or ibuprofen and hot (or cold) soaks for pain. • The problem may last for years but in time will go away, although the bony bump remains.

Condition	Age	Joint affected	Fever	Signs	Treatment
'hot' infection of a joint (bacterial infection: staphylococcus, streptococcus, typhoid, etc.)	any age, but rarely in very young children	**one** hip, knee or ankle joint rarely more than one joint	often low fever, sometimes high fever, at least at first	• sometimes follows injury to joint or illness such as typhoid • usually begins suddenly • joint often red, hot, swollen • joint destruction may be severe—leading in time to a fused or 'frozen' joint, or dislocation	• Identify cause of infection (lab tests needed). • Treat with appropriate antibiotic. • Apply splint to avoid motion and activity during early stage.
'cold' or 'slow' infection of a joint tuberculosis (TB), (or less commonly, syphilis, gonorrhea, or fungus—which are not discussed here)	any age, but mostly in older children and young adults	**one** hip or knee, or in backbone (See TB of spine, p. 165.) Joint may gradually become large or deformed, but not very hot or red. often much pain (sometimes no pain until the bone or joint damage is severe) warm, soft, swelling	no fever	• often history of TB in family • Only half of these children have signs of lung TB. • strongly positive TB skin test (test has meaning only in children not vaccinated against TB) • child often quite thin or sickly (but not always) • Pain usually begins little by little and may become so bad that the child cannot move his leg.	• anti-tuberculosis medicines (2 or 3) for at least 1 year (See *Where There Is No Doctor*, p. 180.) • daily ROM exercises • **aspirin or ibuprofen and hot soaks for pain** • 'exercises-without-motion' to keep muscle strength
sprains and torn ligaments	older child or adult	**one** joint only hot and swollen at first	no fever	• Ankles and knees are common sites. • often results from forceful twisting • Joint may be loose or floppy, and remain weak for months or years. It may easily be twisted or injured again.	• Apply cold during first day after sprain; following days, apply heat. • Avoid motion but keep joint in good position. • **aspirin or ibuprofen for pain** • Provide temporary support with elastic or adhesive bandage or (in severe cases) a cast or ankle brace.
injury to joint surface (for example: torn meniscus, bursitis)	older child or adult	usually **one** joint only, often the knee	no fever	• usually after twist or strain or injury • may hurt suddenly or go weak at certain times but not at others • Swelling or 'liquid' under skin may form behind knee or on the edge of joint.	• Provide support with elastic bandage. • rest, moderate activity • gentle ROM exercises • **aspirin or ibuprofen for pain** • If problem continues, seek help of a specialist.
dislocated joint due to injury (dislocation is when a bone comes out of its socket)	at birth or in older child	**one** joint. Hips, shoulder, and elbows are most common.	no fever	• at first, very painful and weak • In weeks or months (if uncorrected) pain becomes less but weakness often remains. • Joint looks deformed.	• Have an experienced person try to put the bone back in its socket (the same day or soon after the dislocation occurs). Older dislocations and some new ones may need surgery. • Provide support for a few weeks with elastic bandage (especially shoulders and knees). • Gently do ROM exercises every day.
dislocated joint due to muscle weakness or muscle imbalance	occurs in older child with polio, other paralysis, or arthritis	usually **one** joint weak shoulder dislocated from weight bearing pain mild to severe, often occurs with weight bearing and increases with time	no fever	• deformed (strangely shaped) joints • Knees, shoulders, hips, feet, elbows may gradually dislocate because muscles pulling them in one direction are stronger, or because muscles surrounding the joint are so weak. • Careless stretching exercises may cause or increase dislocation.	• Try to put dislocated joint back into place. • Avoid positions that force joint out again. • For partial dislocations of knee, careful stretching exercises may help—but take care to avoid further dislocation. (See p. 374.)

How to care for painful joints

1. REST THE JOINTS

The more painful the joint, the more it needs rest. Some movement is important, but no forceful exercise or heavy use of the joint.

If joints are swollen, it helps to keep them lifted up.

2. HEAT AND COLD

Applying heat (see side box) or cold to the joint often reduces pain and makes motion easier. For cold, use packs of ice wrapped in a cloth or towel for 10 or 15 minutes. Experiment to see which works better. **Usually cold works better on hot, inflamed joints** and **heat on sore, stiff joints.**

Hot wax can be used instead of hot water. Some specialists say that it does not do more good than hot water, but persons with arthritis find it very soothing.

Heat beeswax or paraffin until it just melts (but not too hot—test it first on a finger).	Dip the hand or painful joints into the hot wax.	Take it out. The wax will quickly harden.

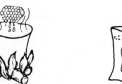

When it cools, dip it in again.

3. PAINKILLERS

Usually aspirin or ibuprofen work best, because they **reduce both pain and inflammation**. For doses and precautions, see p. 134.

Note: For severe pain, **splints to prevent motion** help reduce pain and prevent contractures.

4. RANGE-OF-MOTION (ROM) EXERCISES

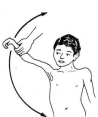

It is important to move the joints through their full range of motion at least twice a day (especially if splints are used). If it hurts, apply heat or cold first, and move them very slowly. Do not force! (See Chapters 16 and 42.)

5. EXERCISES WITHOUT MOTION

These are exercises to strengthen muscles without bending the painful joints. For example, a child with a painful knee can keep her thighs strong by tightening her thigh muscles while her leg is straight. She should hold the muscles tight until they get tired and begin to tremble. This will strengthen them and keep them strong. (See p. 140 and p. 368.)

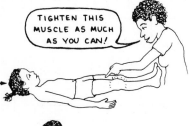

TIGHTEN THIS MUSCLE AS MUCH AS YOU CAN!

6. CONTINUE DAILY ACTIVITIES

With most joint pain, it is important that the child remain fairly active. She should try to continue with all daily activities that do not strain or overwork the painful joints. Moderate activity is usually recommended (except for acute infections or injuries, when complete rest may be needed for several days).

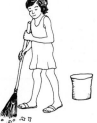

HOT SOAKS

1. Boil water. Let it cool until you can hold your hand in it comfortably.

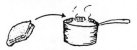

2. Wet a thick cloth or towel in hot water and squeeze out the extra.

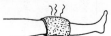

3. Wrap the cloth around the joint.

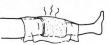

4. Cover the cloth with a piece of thin plastic.

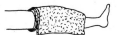

5. Wrap with a dry towel to hold in the heat.

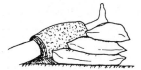

6. Keep the joint raised.

7. When the cloth starts to cool, put it back in the hot water and repeat.

Designs for therapy baths

Floating and playing in water provide exercise and therapy for many kinds of physical disabilities—especially those in which movement is limited because of pain or muscle spasms.

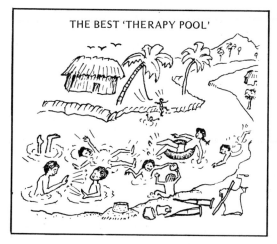

THE BEST 'THERAPY POOL'

For children who have the opportunity, bathing, swimming, and playing in rivers and ponds with other children is good—but only when the rivers or pools are not dangerous and do not transmit diseases.

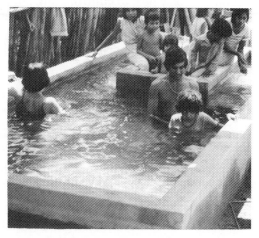

This 'therapy pool' at PROJIMO has one large deep tank for standing, swimming, and play. And it has 2 narrow 'water lanes' at different depths for children to learn to walk while supported by water. Disabled and non-disabled children play here together.

TUBS OR TANKS OF SUN-HEATED WATER (solar heating)

Bathing in warm water is especially helpful. The penetrating heat of the water helps to improve blood flow, calm pain, and relax the muscles.

You can dig a hole in the ground and cover its sides with plastic sheets or cement to prevent the water from leaking out. So that the sunlight heats the water faster, use black plastic, or paint the cement a dark color. (Green is friendlier than black.)

sheet of strong, black plastic

layer of sand or soft mud (or use cement)

A sheet of clear (see-through) plastic stretched over the water when not in use will make it heat faster in the sunlight.

TUB WITH A SELF-CIRCULATING SUN HEATER

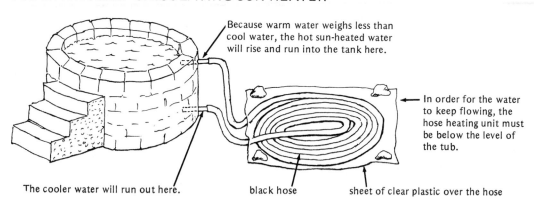

Because warm water weighs less than cool water, the hot sun-heated water will rise and run into the tank here.

In order for the water to keep flowing, the hose heating unit must be below the level of the tub.

The cooler water will run out here.

black hose

sheet of clear plastic over the hose

INFORMATION ON ASPIRIN AND IBUPROFEN FOR SWOLLEN JOINTS IN PERSONS WITH ARTHRITIS OR RHEUMATIC FEVER

Aspirin and ibuprofen are usually the best medicines for joint pain:

- They not only help to **control pain,** but also **reduce inflammation** (swelling and damage to joint surfaces). Thus they help stop destruction of the joints. Many other painkillers such as paracetamol do not do this.
- Aspirin is **not expensive**. Ibuprofen is a little bit more expensive.

In order for aspirin to work well without causing problems:
- Take the correct dose at the right times **every day**.
- Keep taking the same amount of medicine even after the pain has lessened. This will control swelling and let the joints begin to heal.

PRECAUTIONS

A. Aspirin and ibuprofen can cause stomach-ache, chest pain (so-called 'heartburn'), or even make holes (ulcers) in the stomach. To avoid these problems:

- **Always take these medicines with food or a large glass of water.**
- If this does not prevent stomach pain, take the medicine not only with food and lots of water, but also with a spoonful of an antacid such as Maalox, or Gelusil.

Stop taking aspirin if:

- stomach pain still occurs after following the above precautions
- you start to vomit or shit blood, or if your shit looks like black tar (digested blood)

B. **The dose of aspirin to reduce swelling is almost as much as the dose that can poison.** An early sign of poisoning is ringing in the ears. **If the ears begin to ring, stop taking aspirin until it stops**. Then take it again, but in a slightly lower dose.

C. **Keep aspirin out of the reach of children.**

CAUTION: **To prevent choking do not give medicine to a child while she is lying on her back, or if her head is pressed back. Always make sure her head is lifted forward.**

DOSES OF ASPIRIN AND IBUPROFEN FOR ARTHRITIS AND RHEUMATIC FEVER

The dosage given here is the anti-inflammatory dosage, which is double the normal dosage for reducing pain and lowering fever.

Aspirin

Aspirin for adults usually comes in 300 mg. or 500 mg. tablets. Children's aspirin usually comes in 75 mg. tablets. Be sure to figure out the dose correctly for the tablets you have.

The aspirin dosage is 80 to 100 mg./kg./day in 4 to 6 divided doses. For example, a child weighing 25 kilos would take 2000 to 2500 mg. each day, or 1 tablet of 500 mg. 4 to 5 times a day (always with meals or lots of water). You can give up to 130 mg./kg./day, divided in 5 to 6 doses, in acute cases.

When using 500 mg. tablets, the doses are:

Adults: 2 to 3 tablets, 4 to 5 times a day

Children, 8 to 12 years: 1 tablet, 4 to 5 times a day

Children, 3 to 7 years: half a tablet, 4 to 5 times a day

Children, 1 to 2 years: one-quarter tablet, 4 to 5 times a day

The dose of aspirin for your child is: _____

Ibuprofen

Ibuprofen usually comes in 200 mg. tablets. The dose for a child over 7 kg, is 20 to 40 mg. of ibuprofen for each kg. of body weight in divided doses 3 to 4 times a day.

For example, a child weighing 30 kilos could take 600 to 1200 mg. each day, or 1 to 2 tablets of 200 mg. 3 times a day (always with meals or lots of water).

The dose of ibuprofen for your child is:

_____

If there are no swollen joints, use acetaminophen (tylenol, paracetamol) just for pain. Both **aspirin and ibuprofen should not be given to children under 1 year old**. For other medicines for pain, see the Green Pages in *Where There Is No Doctor*.

Juvenile Arthritis

CHAPTER **16**

Chronic Arthritis in Children

HOW TO RECOGNIZE IT

- The arthritis (joint pain) often begins between the ages of 5 and 10, but may begin in very young children or teenagers.
- Usually it keeps getting worse for several years.
- There are times when the pain and other signs get better, and times when they get worse.
- It affects different children in different ways. It can be mild or very disabling.

Signs

JOINTS THAT MAY BE AFFECTED

First, these joints   Later, these joints

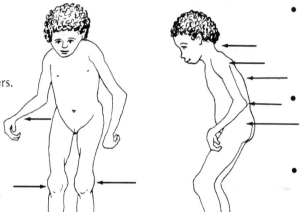

- **Joint pain.** Often begins in the knees, ankles, and wrists. Later it affects the neck, fingers, toes, elbows, and shoulders. Still later, the hips and back may be affected.

- Joints are especially painful and **stiff in the morning** (morning stiffness).

- **Fevers and rash** that come and go. (In some children these are the first signs.)

- The knees become large and may turn inward.

- Pain may make it difficult to straighten the knees, hips, and other joints. The *cords* may tighten, forming *contractures,* and the bones may gradually become *dislocated.*

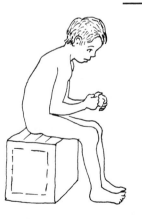

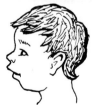

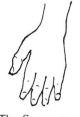

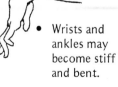

- A child with severe arthritis often sits with his arms and legs bent in the least painful position. Without exercise and good positioning, contractures may form so that he cannot walk or even stand up.

- Children with severe arthritis in the neck and jaw may have a small, short chin.

- The fingers may become very thin and deformed, or thick, with slender tips.

- Wrists and ankles may become stiff and bent.

- Contractures may develop in the fingers or toes, and with time the bones may fuse (stick together).

More information about JUVENILE ARTHRITIS

There are 3 types of juvenile arthritis:

1. Fever type: There are times during the day when the child has a high fever, a rash, and feels ill and tired. He looks very sick. The joint pain seems less important, and it begins days or months after the other signs. There may be severe anemia (child looks pale).

2. Many-joints type: More than 5 joints with pain. The child hurts a lot, and moves very little. Often severe contractures develop. The child does not grow much, and his sexual development is delayed.

3. Few-joints type: Fewer than 5 joints affected. It can affect more joints after months or years. If the back is affected, it is more likely that severe arthritis will continue when he is adult. It may affect the eyes, causing iritis and blindness.

iritis

What causes it?

The exact cause of juvenile arthritis is not known, but it has something to do with the body's 'immune system' (defenses against disease). This begins to attack not only germs, but parts of the body itself. The problem is usually not *hereditary,* and is not related to climate, diet, or the child's way of life. It is not caused by anything the parents may have done. It cannot spread from one child to another. It does not affect the child's intelligence.

Will the child get worse, or better? What about her future?

The progress of the disease varies a lot. Typically, there are times when the joints become very painful, and times when they hurt less. Often the joint pain and *disability* will get worse and worse for several years, then gradually start to improve. Two out of 3 children will stop having active arthritis after 10 years, although the damage already done to the joints may cause some permanent disability. Some children will continue to have arthritis when they are adults, but it is usually milder.

> **Most children with arthritis will become adults who walk, work, and have full and happy lives.**

How does it affect the child and her family?

A child with severe arthritis suffers a lot. After a night of being kept awake by the pain, the child may be irritable, sad, and dull. But when the pain is less, she may be friendly and lively.

Since the arthritis often continues to get worse for years, even with all efforts to cure it, both the child and her family may lose hope and stop trying.

Also, the family may not understand how much the child is suffering, because the cause of the pain does not show. (In children's arthritis the joints do not usually get red, as they do in adults.) So the family sometimes calls the child a 'cry-baby' or a trouble-maker. The child may feel abandoned or guilty. The situation is very hard on the whole family.

The family needs the help and support of understanding neighbors, health workers, and, if possible, a rehabilitation worker. They need to understand that by continuing exercises, *therapy,* and medicines—often for years—**the child does have hopes of getting better.** If therapy takes the form of games with other children and family members, it may help both her body and spirit.

SECONDARY PROBLEMS

When parts of the body do not get enough movement or exercises, joint contractures are common. With time, the bones may become fused (joined together) or dislocated. Also, the *muscles* that straighten the arms and legs become very weak. However, with exercises and with enough movement and good positioning, all these problems can be prevented or made less severe.

Managing juvenile arthritis

The child will need:

1. **medicine** to relieve the pain and help prevent damage to the joints
2. plenty of **rest,** keeping the body in **good positions**
3. **exercises** and **movement** to prevent contractures and deformities, and to keep the muscles strong
4. **mental, physical, and social activities,** so that the child's life is full and satisfying
5. if necessary, **aids,** and **braces** or **casts** to correct contractures and to help the child to move about

---

MEDICINE

Aspirin and ibuprofen are usually the safest and best medicines. They not only help the pain, but also reduce swelling and damage in the joints. For precautions and doses, see the INFORMATION SHEET on p. 134.

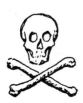

WARNING : **Indomethacin (Indocin), phenylbutazone**, and related medicines should not be given to children. They cause holes in the stomach (ulcers) and are not more effective than aspirin or ibuprofen. If a doctor prescribes one of these medicines for a child, get advice from other doctors.

For patients who have not responded to aspirin and ibuprofen completely, other medicines such as sulfasalazine, gold, hydroxychloroquine, methotrexate and leflunomide are available. These medicines should be used only by experts who treat arthritis.

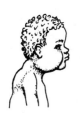

'moon face' and hump of fat on the back of the neck caused by steroids

Corticosteroids have a strong anti-inflammatory effect but they are dangerous. Steroids make the child's body less able to fight *infection*, stop his growth, and weaken his bones so that they break easily. If the child takes a lot of steroids, his face becomes round and a hump of fat forms on the back of his neck and shoulder. As a rule, **steroids should be used only when the child's life or eyesight is in danger**. Steroid eyedrops at the first signs of iritis can prevent blindness.

REST AND POSITION

Children with arthritis need a lot of rest. They tire easily, and should have a chance to rest often. **Help the child to be in positions that keep the arms, wrists, hips, and legs as straight as possible.**

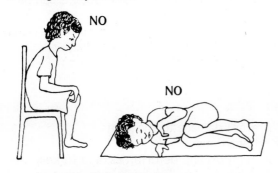

NO

NO

In these positions, contractures develop more easily.

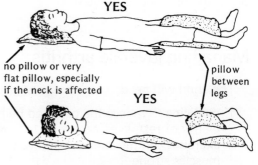

YES

no pillow or very flat pillow, especially if the neck is affected

pillow between legs

YES

In these positions, contractures are less likely to develop.

Although it may hurt more, it is better for the child to lie on her back or stomach, **not** on her side with her legs bent.

When pain is worst, alternate rest with legs straight and slightly bent.

Rest and sleep with the arms and legs as straight as possible. Use pillows only in a way that gently helps the joints straighten more. Let the legs slowly straighten under their own weight.

EXERCISES AND MOVEMENT

Our goal is to prevent contractures and dislocations, and to maintain the fullest possible range of motion for the body. So exercises are needed to **strengthen the muscles that straighten the joints.**

HOW PAIN CAUSES CONTRACTURES

When these muscles are tightened, they straighten the knee,

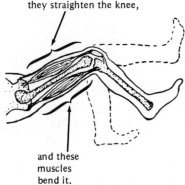

and these muscles bend it.

Because it hurts to straighten the knee, the child with arthritis does not use these muscles much. So they become very weak.

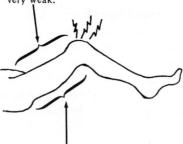

But these muscles stay tightened to keep the knee bent and guard against pain. So they stay stronger.

Since the muscles on top are weaker than those below, the uneven muscle strength keeps bending the leg more and more, even during sleep.

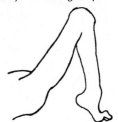

NOTE: This kind of uneven muscle strength is called *muscle imbalance.*

Because contractures from arthritis result mainly from unequal muscle strength, it is important that the child **do all exercises and activities in ways that will strengthen the weak muscles that straighten the joints,** not the muscles that bend them. For example:

Do exercises that work this muscle.

But do **not** do exercises that work this muscle.

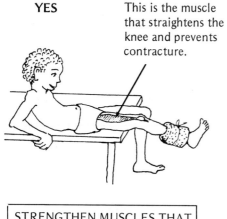

YES   This is the muscle that straightens the knee and prevents contracture.

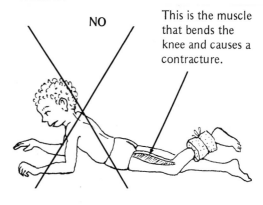

NO   This is the muscle that bends the knee and causes a contracture.

> STRENGTHEN MUSCLES THAT STRAIGHTEN THE JOINT.

> DO NOT STRENGTHEN MUSCLES THAT BEND THE JOINT.

Follow this same logic with all exercises and activities. And **look for ways to make the exercises useful and fun.**

For example, Alicia has arthritis and can no longer walk by herself or straighten her arms and legs completely. As a way of moving herself about and getting some exercise, she can sit on a chair with *casters,* as shown here. But she should be careful to move in a way that helps prevent contractures.

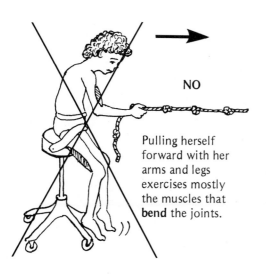

NO

Pulling herself forward with her arms and legs exercises mostly the muscles that **bend** the joints.

This can make contractures worse.

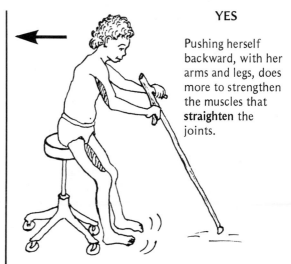

YES

Pushing herself backward, with her arms and legs, does more to strengthen the muscles that **straighten** the joints.

This helps prevent contractures.

Helping the child to strengthen the right muscles

One problem with exercises is that, when either you or the child try to straighten a joint, pain—or the fear of pain—can cause her to tighten the muscles that bend it. For example:

If you pull like this, the muscles that bend the elbow will pull against you—and get stronger.

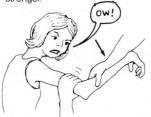

OW!

The muscles that straighten the elbow will not be used—and will get weaker.

Even if the child herself tries to straighten her elbow, the pain will cause the stronger, bending muscles to tighten.

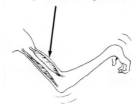

As a result, these exercises may strengthen the bending muscles instead of the weaker straightening muscles. This means that these exercises can actually make contractures get worse!

EXERCISES WITHOUT MOTION

So it is important that the child learn to do exercises that strengthen the muscles that pull against contractures, not those that make them worse. This will be easiest and least painful if she does **exercises without motion.**

First help her to learn which muscles move parts of her body in different directions.

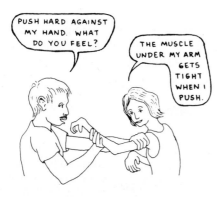

PUSH HARD AGAINST MY HAND. WHAT DO YOU FEEL?

THE MUSCLE UNDER MY ARM GETS TIGHT WHEN I PUSH.

Have her exercise these muscles by relaxing and tightening them, **without moving her arm.**

Then help her find interesting ways to strengthen the muscles that need it without moving them. For example, she can lean on a fence like this.

Everyday she can step a little farther back from the fence, to take more weight on her arms.

Notice that this exercise also strengthens her knee-straightening muscles and helps stretch her heel cords, wrists, hips, back, and neck, in order to look the llama in the eye.

Note: **We have shown these exercises in a girl who already has contractures. But it is best to start them before contractures begin.**

You can figure out similar exercises without motion for all the weak muscles that need strengthening to help prevent or correct contractures.

For example, to strengthen the knee-straightening muscles, the child can lie on her back with her leg as straight as possible. Have her tighten the muscles on top of her thigh (*without* tightening those underneath) and count to 25. Then relax and repeat 10 times. She should do this 3 or 4 times a day. Again, look for ways to make it more fun.

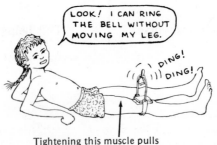

LOOK! I CAN RING THE BELL WITHOUT MOVING MY LEG.

DING! DING!

Tightening this muscle pulls the kneecap and rings the bell.

You can strap a small bell or flag to the leg, so that it will ring or move when the knee bone moves.

Progression of exercises for the child with an ARTHRITIC KNEE

(Arthritis often starts in the knee and later affects other joints.)

CONCEPTS:

1. Strengthen the muscles that straighten the knee (without strengthening those that bend it).
2. Do not move the knee when doing exercises.
3. Keep changing the position in which you do the exercise, and add weights to make the exercises harder as the child's strength increases.

First exercise: leg on ground

First do the exercise without motion lying down.

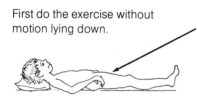

Tighten here without moving and count to 25. Relax and repeat 10 times. Do it 3 or 4 times a day.

After a few days, do it sitting up.

Tighten here without moving.

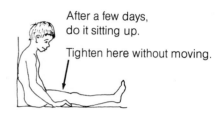

Second exercise: straight leg raise

1. With the leg straight, tighten the muscles on top of the thigh (as in the first exercise).

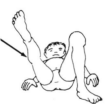

2. Then lift the leg without bending the knee, and slowly count to 5 or 10.
3. Lower the leg slowly.
4. Rest.

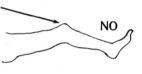

When you lift the leg, be sure that the knee points up or slightly out to the side.

Do not let knee bend at all. (If the knee bends even a little when you lift the leg, it means that the muscles here are still too weak. Go back to first exercise.)

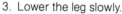

NO

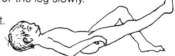

When the child can do this exercise lying down **without bending his knee,** begin putting weights on his leg:

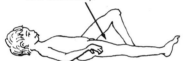

first 1/2 kilo

Gradually increase the weight to 1 kilo,

and 1 1/2 kilos.

For the weight, you can use a small bag full of sand.

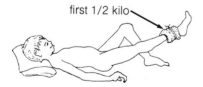

After a few days, have him do the same exercise sitting up:*

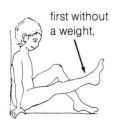

first without a weight,

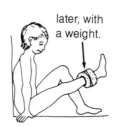

later, with a weight.

Again, gradually increase the weight. Begin with half a kilo, and build up to 5 kilos. But do not increase the weight until the child can do the exercise at the first weight without bending his knee.

CAUTION: **Do not do this sitting exercise if the child has arthritis in the hip, or hip contractures. It uses the hip-bending muscles that will make the contractures worse.**

When the child can do the exercise at 2 kilos without bending her knee, she can begin doing the following variation. Keep the leg raised the whole time.

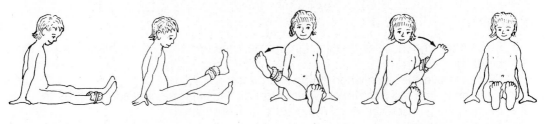

1. Tighten the muscle on top of the thigh.

2. Lift the leg, keeping it straight.

3. Move the leg to the side and turn it outward.

4. Move the leg back in and turn it inward.

5. Lower the leg and relax.

IMPORTANT: **If there is also arthritis in the hip, or hip contractures, do these exercises lying down, not sitting up.**

Third exercise: knee slightly bent

1. Lie down with a rolled towel or blanket under the knee.

2. Turn the leg out to the side.

3. Lift the foot and slowly count to 5 or 10.

4. Lower it slowly.
5. Rest.
6. Repeat the exercise 10 to 30 times.

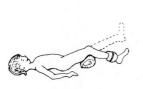

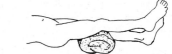

Make sure that only the foot is raised, not the thigh, and that the knee is lifted as straight as possible.

As the child gains strength, continue with the same series of steps as for the second exercise.

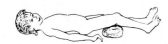

strips of inner tube (or use sandbag)

1. Lying down, lift the foot with a weight on it. Build weight up slowly to 5 kilos.

2. Sitting up, lift the foot without a weight.

3. Sitting up, lift the foot with a weight. (Build up to 5 kilos.)

If arthritis or contractures have begun in her hip, it is best to do the exercise lying down with the hip as straight as possible (nothing under the knee).

Do these 2 exercises only if there is no danger of hip contractures.

To strengthen the muscles, continue the exercise until the child can no longer hold the leg straight or it begins to shake slightly. The more often the child does these exercises the faster the muscles will get stronger. These exercises can be done even when the joint is swollen and painful. However, if the joint hurts more during or after the exercise, use less weight and repeat fewer times.

Exercising an ARTHRITIC KNEE through daily activities

WALKING. Walking is one of the best exercises for strengthening the thigh—**if** the child puts some weight on the leg.

For arthritis, try to **use canes, not crutches. A crutch can cause contractures.**

NO   YES

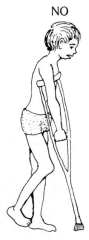

A cane helps strengthen weak muscles and prevent contractures.

WARNING: If a child uses a crutch and does not step down with his leg, this strengthens only the muscles that bend the leg.

If he uses a cane, he must put some weight on the leg. This strengthens the muscles that straighten the leg.

During the times when the child's arthritis is less painful, she should be active. It is fine for her to run, ride a bicycle, or take long walks—as long as this does not cause much joint pain.

After the child can walk fairly well without aids, a good exercise is walking on the heels. (If the arthritis also affects the ankles, this may not be possible. But try.)

These activities strengthen weak thighs.

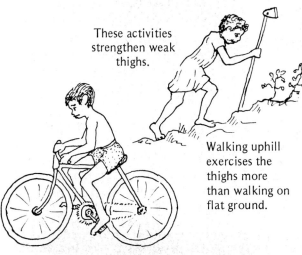

Walking uphill exercises the thighs more than walking on flat ground.

SWIMMING. Swimming is one of the best exercises for a person with arthritis.

Floating and play in water also is good exercise. The water holds up the body and allows movement of the arms and legs without weight, yet against the gentle resistance of the water.

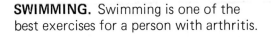
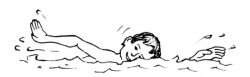

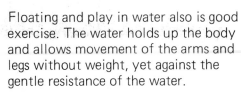
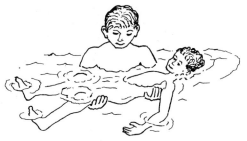

Range-of-motion exercises for children with arthritis

For a child with arthritis, it is important that **every day he move his body, arms, and legs through as full a range of motion as possible.**

But this is not always easy. Pain and stiffness make straightening of joints difficult. So before starting to exercise, take steps to calm the pain and relax the tense muscles. **Aspirin** helps do this. Take it half an hour before beginning exercise (or before getting up to help morning stiffness).

> *Note:* **Range-of-motion exercises for different joints are described in Chapter 42. Here we discuss ways to make them easier for children with arthritis.**

Heat helps relax muscles and calm pain. Suggestions for applying hot soaks and hot wax are on p. 132. If many joints are painful, it helps to lie in warm water (a little warmer than body temperature).

If possible, get or make a tub large enough for the child to lie straight and to stretch his arms and legs in all directions.

Warm water not only helps calm pain, but gently lifts and takes the weight off body parts. This makes motion easier. Support the child only as much as needed so that his arms and legs are loose and held up by the water. Ask him to relax completely. Let him begin to move his arms and legs. The more he relaxes, the more they will straighten as he moves.

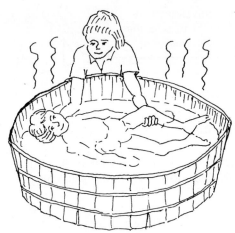

Ideas for making tubs or water pits heated by the sun are on p. 133.

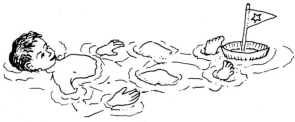

Find ways for the child to play in the water. This will help him forget his pain and make straightening the joints easier.

In moments when she has her leg or arm most straight, ask her to hold that position a moment without bending.

This way, little by little, she will find she can straighten her joints more and more.

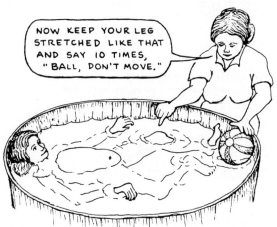

NOW KEEP YOUR LEG STRETCHED LIKE THAT AND SAY 10 TIMES, "BALL, DON'T MOVE."

'Floating-in-air' devices for relaxing and moving painful joints

The best way for relaxing and reducing weight to exercise arthritic joints is to float in warm water. When this is not possible, after applying hot soaks (see p. 132), the leg or arm can be hung in a simple device—loosely, as if floating in water.

'FLOATING' AN ARTHRITIC LEG

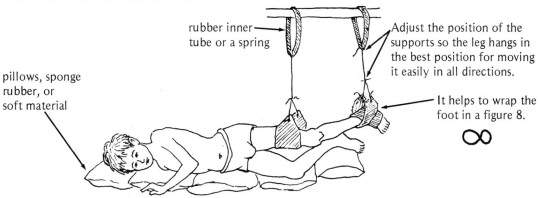

rubber inner tube or a spring

Adjust the position of the supports so the leg hangs in the best position for moving it easily in all directions.

pillows, sponge rubber, or soft material

It helps to wrap the foot in a figure 8.

∞

After hanging the limb, wait until the child relaxes, then have him swing it gently this way and that.

Let the leg move with its own weight as in a swing. Increase the swinging until the knee and hip bend and straighten completely (or as much as possible).

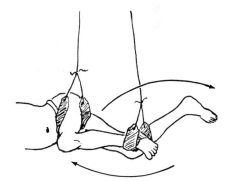

Look for ways to turn the exercise into a game.

For example, the child might knock gourds or blocks down while another child tries quickly to set them up again, and see who wins.

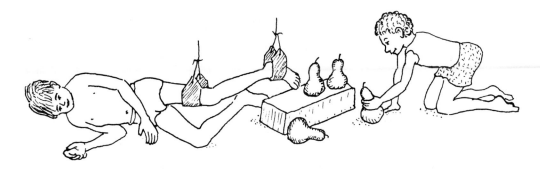

The gourds can be put farther and farther away so that he has to stretch more each time to knock them down. When his leg is most stretched, ask him to hold it that way a moment before letting it bend.

Also have the child do exercises lying on his back and swinging his leg outward (to one side). This helps prevent knock-knee contractures.

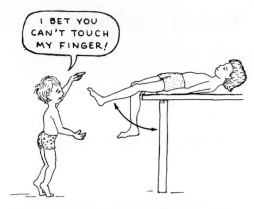

The child can also swing her leg while sitting or lying on a table edge. Encourage her to swing the leg as far up and back as possible. Turn it into a game.

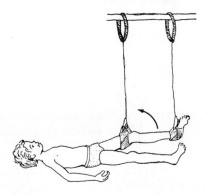

A device like this helps strengthen the muscles that straighten the knee. This way works better than a weight tied to the ankle because the pull continues even when the knee is bent.

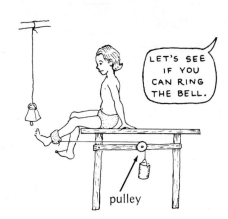

pulley

Put stones or pieces of metal in an old can. Use only as much weight as will let the child straighten her knee completely. As the leg becomes stronger, add more weight.

Movement of the arms. This is done much like the legs:

LYING FACE UP

Swing the arm away from the body.

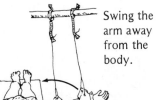

LYING ON THE SIDE

Swing the arm forward and back.

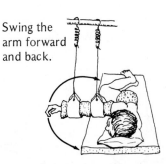

These movements can be done keeping the hot soaks on the arm.

AND SITTING

Swing the shoulder and elbow through their full range of motion.

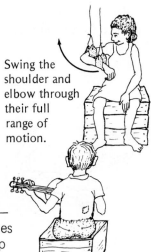

Encourage the child to move her limb in a rhythmic manner— perhaps to music. Try to help her forget the pain. If she becomes interested in something else—a game or the music—this will help reduce the tightness of her muscles.

Look for ways to do these movements as part of daily activities.

CORRECTING CONTRACTURES CAUSED BY ARTHRITIS

For general information on the **cause, prevention, and correction of contractures,** see Chapter 8. **Range-of-motion and strengthening exercises** will help prevent or correct early contractures (see Chapter 42). For severe contractures, **stretching aids or casts** may be needed (see Chapter 59). However, when using casts or other aids to straighten contractures, **it is very important to continue exercises without motion** to strengthen the muscles that straighten the limb.

PRECAUTIONS FOR CASTING AN ARTHRITIC LIMB

1. First examine the joint for signs of dislocation. Try moving the bones forward and backward and from side to side.

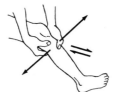

CAUTION: **If the joint is partly dislocated or very loose, it is best not to use casts or stretching devices, as these can increase the dislocation.** It is better to continue with the exercises, taking care not to force the joint.

2. If there are no signs of dislocation, little by little straighten the joint as far as is possible without causing much pain.

CAUTION: **Do not pull like this, or you may dislocate the joint.**

LIKE THIS

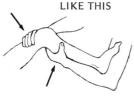

Lift with your hand behind the knee to keep the bones correctly in place, like this.

NOT LIKE THIS

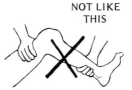

dislocated joint

3. With the joint as straight as you can get it without too much pain, carefully cast the leg (see p. 560).

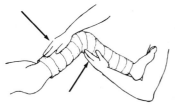

Until the cast dries, apply steady pressure here so that the bones keep their right locations and the joint stays straightened.

4. As long as the cast is in place, do **without-motion** exercises several times a day. This helps keep the straightening muscles strong.

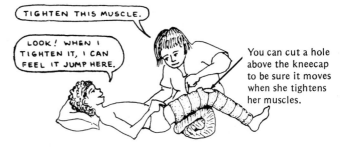

TIGHTEN THIS MUSCLE.

LOOK! WHEN I TIGHTEN IT, I CAN FEEL IT JUMP HERE.

You can cut a hole above the kneecap to be sure it moves when she tightens her muscles.

5. Every 2 days remove the cast, apply heat and do range-of-motion exercises, bending and straightening the leg little by little. Then gently stretch the leg a little more, and put on another cast.

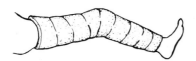

(*IMPORTANT:* It is best to replace the cast completely rather than to use wedges with the same cast, because of the risk of dislocation.)

6. Continue straightening the leg with new casts every 2 days until it is completely straight or does not straighten more.

Keep a record of the progress like this (see Chapter 5). This way you can tell when the leg is no longer getting straighter and it is time to stop using casts.

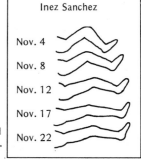

Inez Sanchez

Nov. 4

Nov. 8

Nov. 12

Nov. 17

Nov. 22

Homemade aids for stretching joints

Because daily movement of joints is so important with arthritis, casts should be avoided whenever possible. So try to figure out other ways to correct contractures. Use whatever materials you can find, such as plastic, bamboo, and inner tubes.

These are a few of the examples of aids invented in a Mexican village for a girl with arthritis.

CAUTION: **Make sure that the aids pull in a way that does not cause dislocations.**

KNEE

METHOD 1:

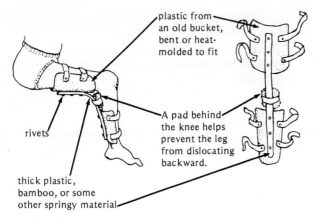

plastic from an old bucket, bent or heat-molded to fit

A pad behind the knee helps prevent the leg from dislocating backward.

rivets

thick plastic, bamboo, or some other springy material

METHOD 2:

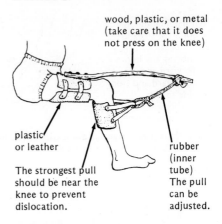

wood, plastic, or metal (take care that it does not press on the knee)

plastic or leather

The strongest pull should be near the knee to prevent dislocation.

rubber (inner tube) The pull can be adjusted.

Note: The behind-the-knee aid usually works the best. It is steadier and so causes less muscle tightening. Because it holds the leg more firmly, it is less likely to cause dislocations. It is also more comfortable and less awkward.

WRIST

Over-the-hand support

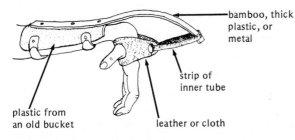

bamboo, thick plastic, or metal

strip of inner tube

plastic from an old bucket

leather or cloth

Under-the-hand support

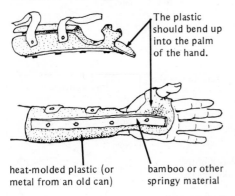

The plastic should bend up into the palm of the hand.

heat-molded plastic (or metal from an old can)

bamboo or other springy material

PRECAUTIONS in the use of aids for stretching contractures:

- They should be made in a way that will prevent dislocations. When using, **check often for early signs of dislocation.**

- The aids should not pull so much that they cause pain and defensive muscle tightening.

- Use them during most of the day and at night (about 20 of every 24 hours).

- Remove them 2 or 3 times a day in order to do exercises.

- Also do exercises without motion with the aids in place.

- Take care that the aid does not stop blood flow or press on nerves. If the hand or foot becomes cool, changes color, begins to hurt or becomes numb— remove the aid, and make the needed adjustments.

For other aids and devices for straightening contractures, see Chapter 59.

Correcting contractures of arthritic hips

Look for ways that the child can relax with her head as straight as possible. If she also has contractures in her knees, she can lie like this.

The child will relax and straighten her body more easily if she can play or read.

Place supports or cushions behind her back and head, but just enough so that she has to straighten herself some. As her hips and neck gradually straighten, keep lowering her back and head little by little.

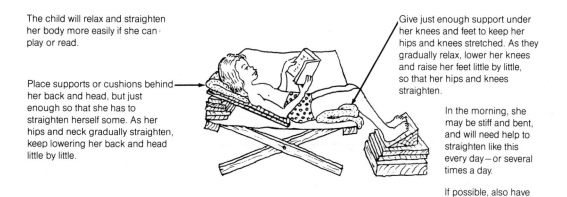

Give just enough support under her knees and feet to keep her hips and knees stretched. As they gradually relax, lower her knees and raise her feet little by little, so that her hips and knees straighten.

In the morning, she may be stiff and bent, and will need help to straighten like this every day—or several times a day.

If possible, also have her lie on her belly.

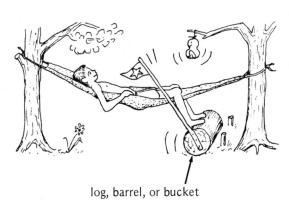

log, barrel, or bucket

Think of games or exercises in which the child will stretch his hips and knees. In this example, the boy rolls the log to lift the flag and hit the gourd. This helps strengthen the straightening muscles of his legs.

As the child's back, hips, and knees straighten more and he gains strength, the hammock can be stretched more tightly and a heavier weight put on the top of the stick, where the flag is.

A homemade walker similar to this can help a child with hip contractures begin to walk. It also provides exercise for the straightening muscles of both the arms and legs.

As the child's hips and knees straighten more and more, the crutches and seat can be raised.

It is best if she walks backward ("Pretend you're a crab!"). This way she will strengthen the straightening muscles in her legs. Walking forward would strengthen more the muscles that bend the legs, and this could increase contractures.

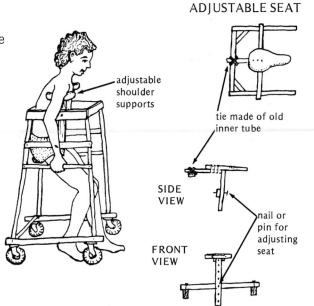

ADJUSTABLE SEAT

adjustable shoulder supports

tie made of old inner tube

SIDE VIEW

FRONT VIEW

nail or pin for adjusting seat

LEARNING TO MOVE AND TO SMILE—the story of Teresa

Teresa has had juvenile arthritis since age 7. When her mother first brought her to PROJIMO from a distant village at age 14, her body had stiffened into the shape of a chair. Her eyes were the only parts of her body she could move. Her joints hurt her so much that she spent every night crying. Years before, a doctor had prescribed aspirin for her pain. But the aspirin began to give her severe stomach pain, so she stopped taking it.

Once Teresa was a cheerful, active little girl. She had completed 3 years of school. Now she was sad and felt hopeless. She would cry out with pain each morning when her father carefully lifted her out of bed and sat her in a chair. She rarely spoke and never smiled.

When Teresa arrived at PROJIMO she had severe contractures of her wrists, fingers, elbows, hips, knees, ankles, and feet. The rehabilitation team had her start using aspirin again, but with care that she take it with meals, lots of water, and an antacid. They then began a long, slow process of therapy, part of which we show in the following photos.

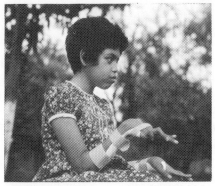

To help correct her wrist contractures, visiting therapists made these splints for her out of costly plastic.

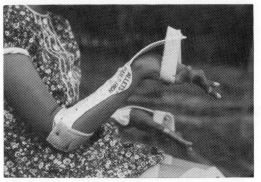

However, to the therapists' surprise, they found out that these low-cost splints made by villagers from a plastic bucket worked better (see p. 551).

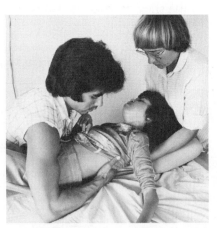

Every day the team spent several hours with Teresa, gently doing range-of-motion, stretching, and strengthening exercises. Here a visiting physical therapist teaches a village worker how to help Teresa increase movement in her stiff neck and back.

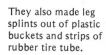

They also made leg splints out of plastic buckets and strips of rubber tire tube.

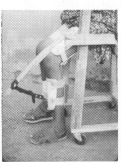

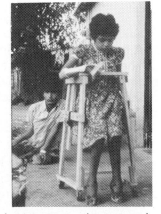

When Teresa could move her joints some, the team made her an adjustable walker. It had shoulder supports and a saddle seat that could be raised as her legs straightened. She learned to walk by pushing herself backward. This strengthened the muscles that straighten her legs.

Teresa was improving steadily. She began to talk, smile, and to take interest in things. An older brother came to visit for a few weeks. He learned about her exercises and therapy so he could help her when they returned to their village.

Unfortunately, soon after Teresa went home she became ill with dengue (break bone fever) and nearly died. Her family stopped both exercises and medicines. When she returned to PROJIMO 6 weeks later, she was as stiff and bent as when she first came. She was so depressed she spoke to no one. The team began her rehabilitation all over again.

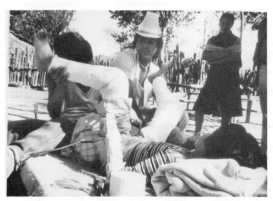

This time they straightened her legs and arms with plaster casts (see Chapter 59). They changed the casts every 2 days. With each cast change her joints were exercised.

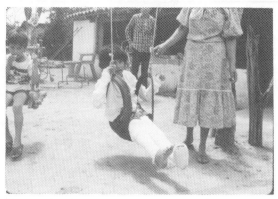

Finally, with the casts, Teresa's knees and wrists became fairly straight. She now had some hand movement and could play in the playground.

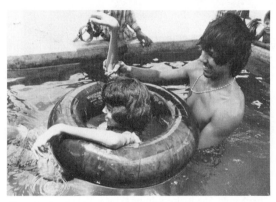

Exercise in the therapy pool at PROJIMO was fun and greatly improved her movement.

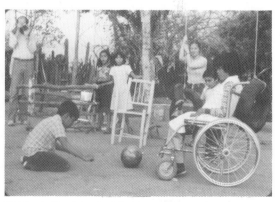

Kicking balls with other disabled children helped Teresa strengthen muscles that straighten legs.

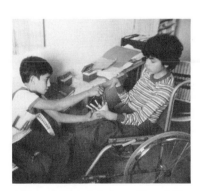

Village children help her with activities to use her hands. Here she weaves a basket.

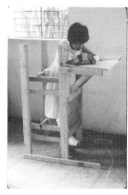

When her legs were stronger, the team made an adjustable standing frame for her.

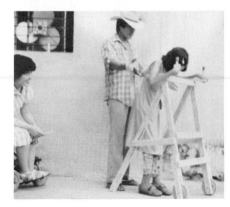

Later Teresa began to walk using a homemade walker with wood wheels. She wore leg braces for support.

As Teresa's legs and arms straightened, her neck bent forward more and more. She could not lift her chin from her chest. The village workers made her a head support, attached to a firm cloth around her chest. Over a period of months, the support gently brought up her head.

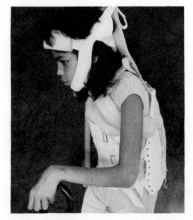
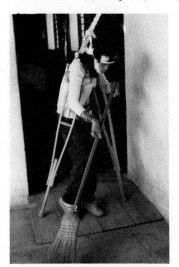
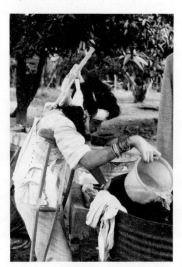

Teresa is now able to walk with crutches. Through daily work she gets much of the same therapy she gets doing her exercises.

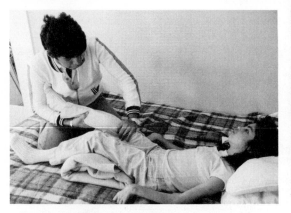
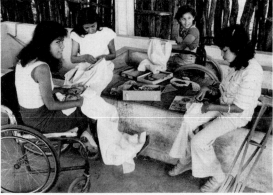

She also continues with her daily exercises to straighten and strengthen her arms and legs.

Sewing together with her friends helps Teresa improve the use of her hands. She is also gaining skills with her therapy.

(5 photos by Richard Parker)

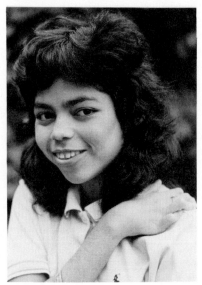

At home, Teresa now helps care for her younger brothers and sisters. She and her family share the household tasks. Before, others had to take care of her.

(photo by Andy Brown)

Rheumatic Fever

Rheumatic fever is a serious illness with **joint pain** and **fever.** It usually lasts about 6 weeks but may last up to 6 months (or rarely more). Then the joint pain usually goes away completely. But **heart damage,** if it has occurred, may be permanent or become *disabling* (shortness of breath; sickly child).

CAUSES

Rheumatic fever usually results **after a sore throat** caused by bacteria called 'streptococcus'. (The rheumatic fever is somewhat like an allergic reaction.) A 'strep throat' often starts suddenly with throat pain and fever and **without** signs of a cold. Rheumatic fever is most common where epidemics of strep throat are common—**in crowded communities with poor hygiene.**

PREVENTION

Rheumatic fever can often be prevented by giving penicillin to children who have signs of a strep throat. Keep giving penicillin for at least 3 days after all signs disappear. Long-term prevention involves improving hygiene and living conditions (a fairer society).

CAUTION: Most sore throats in children are not 'strep', but are caused by the common cold; these should **not** be treated with penicillin, or any other antibiotic and never injections (see p. 18). Typically, a **strep throat is quite painful and starts suddenly, with high fever,** and **without** a stuffy nose or other signs of a cold.

SIGNS OF THE TYPICAL CASE

- Child between the ages 5 to 15
- Began 1–3 weeks after the child had a severe sore throat
- **High fever**—child quite sick
- **Joint pain.** Pain often starts in one or more of the larger joints (especially wrists and ankles). Then it changes to other joints, often knees and elbows. The painful joints may swell and become red and hot.

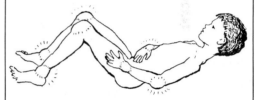

- Child gets well in about 6 weeks to 3 months, but **may get the same illness again after another sore throat.**

OTHER SIGNS (not always present)

- **Reddish curved lines** on skin
- **Lumps** (the size of peas) under the skin over or near the joints
- **Heart problems.** You may hear a 'murmur' if you put your ear over the child's chest. Instead of the typical 'lub-dub . . . lub-dub' of the heartbeat, you will hear a soft, long 'whoosh' for one of the sounds: 'whoosh-dub . . . whoosh-dub . . . whoosh-dub'. The 'whoosh' sound means a valve to the heart has been damaged so that it does not close completely. In extreme cases this can lead to heart failure (see *Where There Is No Doctor,* p. 325).
- Nosebleed, belly pain, chest pain, or signs of pneumonia occur in only a few cases.

Treatment

- If you think a child might have rheumatic fever, get medical advice quickly. Early treatment may help prevent heart damage. (After fever and joint pain have begun, treatment does not seem to shorten the length of the illness.)
- Give penicillin V by mouth for 10 days; or give a single injection of benzathine benzylpenicillin into the buttock *muscles* (one-half in each buttock); or inject procaine penicillin daily for 10 days. For children allergic to penicillin, use erythromycin. See box for doses. (For cautions in the use of penicillin, see *Where There Is No Doctor*, p. 351.)
- Give aspirin or ibuprofen in high dosage. See INFORMATION SHEET on page 134. Continue giving the medicines until a few days after all signs are gone.
- Apply heat or cold packs to painful joints to help reduce pain and swelling (see p. 132).
- Do full range-of-motion exercises of painful joints gently every day (see Chapter 42).
- Do 'exercises without motion' to maintain strength (see p. 140).
- The child should stay in bed or rest quietly most of the time until all signs are gone (about 6 weeks). Then he can begin activities little by little.

ANTIBIOTIC TREATMENT OF RHEUMATIC FEVER

Name of medicine	Age or weight	Dose	How to take
Penicillin V (by mouth)	up to 1 year . . . . 1 to 5 years . . . . 6 to12 years . . . . over 12 years	62.5 mg. 125 mg. 250 mg. 500 mg.	4 times a day for 10 days, by mouth
OR			
Benzathine benzylpenicillin (by injection)	up to 30 kg. . . . . over 30 kg.	450 to 675 mg. (600,000 to 900,000 units) 900 mg. (1,200,000 units)	single deep injection into the muscle, once every 3 to 4 weeks (give one-half into each buttock)
OR			
Procaine penicillin G (by injection)	all children	50 mg./kg./day or 50,000 units/kg./day up to a maximum of 1,200,000 units	daily, for 10 days, by deep injection into the muscle (give one-half into each buttock)
OR for persons allergic to penicillin:			
Erythromycin tablets (by mouth)	up to 2 years . . . . 2 to 8 years . . . . over 8 years	125 mg. 250 mg. 250 to 500 mg.	4 times a day for 10 days, by mouth

NOTE: It is safer to give children medicines by mouth rather than by injection whenever possible. For precautions in giving medicines to children, see p. 236.

PREVENTION of repeat attacks

Persons who have once had rheumatic fever have a risk of getting it again. For these persons, take care to treat any sore throat quickly with penicillin. If the person shows signs of heart damage (murmur) with the first attack, there is a high risk of further damage with repeat attacks. These persons would be wise to take a preventive dose of penicillin regularly for at least one attack-free year or until they are 17 years old (after which the risk of strep throat is lower). **Long-term prevention is especially important in persons who already have serious rheumatic heart damage.**

> PREVENTIVE DOSAGES:
> - or 1 injection of 1.2 million units of benzathine penicillin G, once a month,
> - or 1 tablet of 500 mg. of sulfadiazine 2 times a day,
> - or 1 tablet of 250 mg. of penicillin V, 2 times a day with an empty stomach.
> - For children allergic to penicillin, give 1 tablet of 250 mg. of erythromycin, 2 times a day.
>
> Before using these medicines, read the precautions. See the GREEN PAGES of *Where There Is No Doctor.*

CHAPTER **18**

Hip Problems

DISLOCATED HIPS

A hip is *dislocated* when the thigh bone is out of its socket at the hip. Some babies are born with one or both hips already dislocated. Sometimes these babies have no other problem. With early treatment, the problem can often be corrected easily, and the child will not be *disabled* or have a limp.

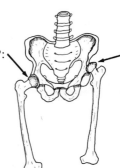

NORMAL HIP: The round head of the thigh bone is *inside* the hip socket.

DISLOCATED HIP: The head of the thigh bone often lies *above* the socket.

For this reason it is important to **examine all babies when they are 10 days old** to see whether they have dislocated hips.

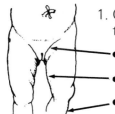

1. Compare the 2 legs. If one hip is dislocated, that side may show these signs:

- the upper leg partly covers this part of the body
- there are fewer skin folds
- the leg may seem shorter, or turn out at a strange angle

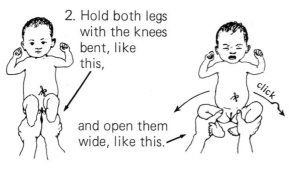

2. Hold both legs with the knees bent, like this,

and open them wide, like this.

If one leg stops early or makes a jump or click when you open it wide, the hip is dislocated.

3. To test a slightly older child, bend the knees and compare their height.

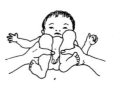

If one knee is lower, the hip on that side is probably dislocated.

Treatment

Keep the baby with his knees high and wide apart. To do this,

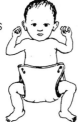

- use many thicknesses of *diapers (nappies)* like this,

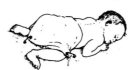

- or pin his legs like this (when the baby sleeps),

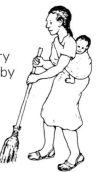

- or carry the baby like this.

In places where babies are traditionally carried with their legs spread on the woman's hips or back, usually no other treatment is necessary.

Dislocated hips with other orthopedic problems

Children with the *disabilities* listed here often are **born with dislocated hips.** Therefore, it is *essential* to examine these children carefully a few days after birth, to make sure there are no dislocations.

- **Down syndrome**
- **spina bifida**
- **arthrogryposis**
- **cerebral palsy**
- **club feet**

Many (but not all) dislocated hips can be corrected in the ways we described on page 155. Keeping the legs wide apart during the first months of the child's life helps to improve the shape of the socket.

If it is difficult to keep the legs apart, you may need to use casts or make special braces.

The casts should be used for 2 to 4 months or longer, depending on the child's age (longer for older children) and the amount of the deformity. (Use a cloth or bottle to catch the baby's pee, so it does not run inside the cast.)

Not all dislocations can be corrected in these ways. Some need surgery, and in some cases the hip is so deformed that the dislocation cannot be corrected, even with surgery.

With spina bifida, if one hip is dislocated, surgery may help. But if both hips are dislocated, hip surgery usually will not help the child to walk any better. (See p. 173.)

CAST

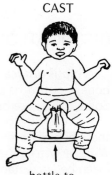

bottle to catch urine

BRACE

The stick here helps to keep the legs apart.

Dislocated hips can also occur **after the child is born,** either from an accident or as a complication of some other disability—especially **polio** (due to weakness in the muscles and cords that hold the hip joint together) or **cerebral palsy** (due to *spasticity* and *contractures*).

DISLOCATED HIP

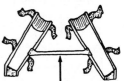

The spasticity and contracture of this muscle cause dislocation of the hip.

legs crossed like scissors

THE TELESCOPE TEST

To find out if the hip is dislocated or can easily be pulled out of joint, place the child on his back.

Pull up on his knee, and then push it down, like this.

At the same time, feel his hip with your other hand, like this.

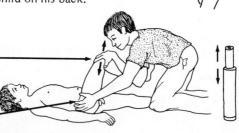

If the thigh bone moves in and out like a telescope, the hip is probably dislocated.

Dislocations that are complications of polio or cerebral palsy can seldom be corrected without surgery. **But often it is better not to operate,** because the operations do not always turn out well, and the children who have the possibility of walking will walk in spite of the dislocated hips.

HIP PROBLEMS DUE TO DESTRUCTION OR SLIPPING OF THE CAP OF THE THIGH BONE

There are 2 different hip problems that occur most often in active children, usually boys.

1. **Destruction** of the cap or 'growth center' on the 'head' of the thigh bone is called **Legg-Perthes disease**. It usually begins between **2 and 12 years of age**. It occurs in less than 1 of every 1,000 boys.

2. **Slipping** of the cap on the head of the thigh bone is less common. It happens, suddenly or little by little, usually between **11 and 16 years of age** (when the child is growing fast).

The cause in both cases is unknown.

Destruction of the growth center results from a temporary loss of blood supply. This causes death of the bone.

Destruction of the growth center is usually not related to other diseases. A similar kind of destruction of the growth center from loss of blood supply may be caused by tuberculosis of the hip, sickle cell anemia, HIV, cretinism, or use of corticosteroid medicines. A careful medical study is advisable.

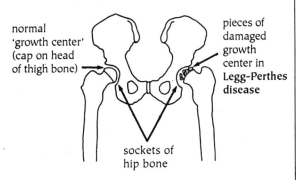

normal 'growth center' (cap on head of thigh bone)

pieces of damaged growth center in **Legg-Perthes disease**

sockets of hip bone

DIAGNOSIS: If a child has signs of one of these hip problems, try to get an X-ray to find out the cause.

SIGNS:

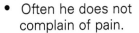

- Child begins to limp: body dips toward affected side.

- Often he does not complain of pain.

- Or he may feel some pain in the knee or thigh (or less often, hip)—although the problem is at the hip.

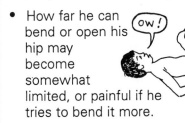

- How far he can bend or open his hip may become somewhat limited, or painful if he tries to bend it more. OW!

- In time the thigh becomes thinner and weakness develops in the muscles that lift the leg sideways.

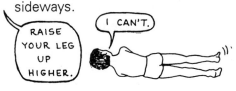

RAISE YOUR LEG UP HIGHER.   I CAN'T.

Treatment and progress of slipped growth center

When the growth center slips, if possible it should be put back into place surgically, and pinned. When surgery is impossible, the child should avoid all strenuous exercise, running, and jumping in the hope that the growth center will not slip farther until it becomes fused to the thigh bone (normally when the child is 16 to 18 years old). Without surgery, and especially if the slippage is severe, a progressive, destructive arthritis is likely to result.

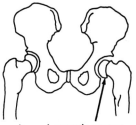

slipped growth center

Treatment and progress of Legg-Perthes disease

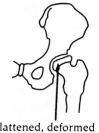

When the growth center has lost its blood supply, the bone dies and begins to break into pieces. At the same time, the body begins to make new bone. In 2 to 4 years, a new growth center is completely formed, and the child walks more or less normally again, usually without pain. However, the new growth center is usually flatter than before and does not fit into the hip socket as well. As a result, later in life, the hip joint begins to wear out and a *progressive*, destructive, painful arthritis may begin.

flattened, deformed
growth center

Many ways to treat Legg-Perthes have been tried. Most methods try to restrict movement and to keep the legs wide apart, a position that makes the growth center form a round and normal shape again.

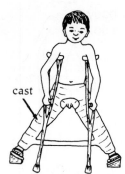

Casts or braces are kept on the child until the new growth center has formed completely—usually for 2 to 3 years! This is very hard on both the child and family.

cast

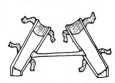

full-leg braces

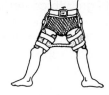

upper-leg braces only

Any of 3 different hip surgeries can make the head of the thigh bone fit more completely into the socket so the new growth center forms a rounder, normal shape.

Surgery is expensive and has more risks than casting or braces. But it is much quicker: only 6 weeks in bed with a cast. Then the child can lead a more or less normal life. But it still takes 2 years for the new growth center to form, and during this time the pain and/or limp may continue.

Sometimes crutches may be used to reduce pain, but they don't reduce damage to the bones as people used to think. **Moderate exercise, like swimming, can help to maintain and increase range of movement.**

There is a lot of debate about whether any of these methods—casts, braces, or surgery—are worth it. Especially for children under 6 years old, their pain and limp gradually go away with or without treatment. The best advice in these cases may be to do nothing. (This is a hard decision for parents to accept, but will make life happier for both the child and family.) Let the child remain active, but do not make him run, jump, or walk far if it bothers him. For older children, surgery may be the best option.

If the growth center heals to be rounded and fits well in the hip socket, the child will probably not have problems with arthritis later in life. But if the growth center does not reshape itself well, and especially if it doesn't fit well into the socket, he might develop arthritis earlier and more severely.

X-rays can help you decide what to do and what to expect when a child has Legg-Perthes.

Bone Infections

CHAPTER 19

Osteomyelitis

Bone *infections* are mostly a medical problem. Therefore we do not describe all of the many types of bone infections or details of medical and surgical treatment.

Chronic (long-lasting) bone infections are fairly common in villages where persons go barefoot and where injuries and illnesses that can lead to bone infections are frequent. They can be caused by fungus, or by many different kinds of bacteria (including typhoid, tuberculosis, and staphylococcus). Often these infections last for years, causing bone destruction and severe disability.

Bone infections are a very common complication of injuries, burns, and pressure sores in persons who have no feeling in their hands and feet. This includes persons with **spina bifida** (see p. 173), **spinal cord injury** (p. 196), and **leprosy** (p. 222). Because the person does not feel pain, often she does not rest, clean, or protect the injured area. As a result, it becomes infected. Gradually the infection gets deeper until it reaches the bone.

> THROUGH PROPER EARLY CARE OF SORES AND INJURIES, BONE INFECTIONS CAN USUALLY BE PREVENTED.

> *WARNING:* Deep pressure sores that do not heal, even after they are kept clean and no weight or pressure has been put on them for months, may have a bone infection. Bone infection is especially likely if the sore reaches the bone, or if a small hole at the bottom of the sore refuses to close and drains liquid or pus. If you think there might be a bone infection, get medical help if possible and go through all the steps to treat it adequately.

The loss of parts of the body sometimes seen in a person who has leprosy (Hansen's disease) is not caused by the leprosy germs. It is caused by other germs, which infect the bone because of injuries the person gets that are not cared for because they do not hurt.

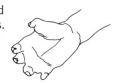

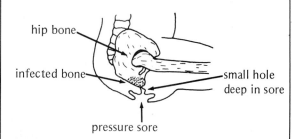

hip bone

infected bone

small hole deep in sore

pressure sore

Signs of chronic bone infection

- The skin near a bone has small, deep sores that heal and then open again to drain pus. Gradually the affected area gets bigger and new holes open.
- There may or may not be pain.
- The pus may or may not smell bad.
- Usually there is no fever—except sometimes at first or at times when the infection gets into the blood.
- Often the infection will get better with *antibiotics,* but keeps coming back.
- The affected bone may gradually become thicker as it is destroyed inside and forms a new bony covering.

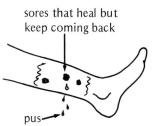

sores that heal but keep coming back

pus

Treatment

- Whenever possible get experienced medical help.

- If treated early with antibiotics such as penicillin or vancomycin in the right dosage, sometimes the infection will go away and not come back. If possible, a sample of the pus should be studied (cultured) by a medical laboratory to find out what kind of infection it is and what medicine is likely to work best. Usually the medicine must be given in the vein for a long time (months).

- If you cannot get the pus cultured, you might try treating the infection with penicillin V or dicloxacillin. Use relatively high doses. For dosage and precautions, see *Where There Is No Doctor*. Also seek medical help.

- Surgery may be needed to remove the dead, infected bone.

- Sometimes amputation is necessary (see p. 227).

- Even with excellent treatment, after months or years without problems, new sores may open and again begin to drain from the infected bone.

Rehabilitation and aids

What kind of *rehabilitation* or *orthopedic* aids may be needed will depend on the amount of destruction that has occurred. Sometimes surgery cannot be obtained or the person may prefer to live with the problem rather than with an amputated limb.

For prevention, rehabilitation, and aids, see Chapters 24, 26, and 58 on pressure sores, leprosy, and braces.

When there has been a lot of bone destruction, sometimes a brace can help make walking easier.

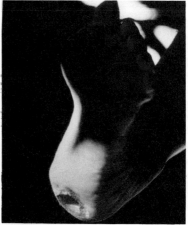

Large hole down to the bone in the foot of a woman with a bone infection (osteomyelitis). She has had this problem since childhood 30 years before.

WARNING: The pus from the infected bone may cause serious infections in other persons. Wash hands often. Wear gloves when handling anything with blood or body fluids on it. **Take great care with hygiene**.

Change bandages regularly. **Try to burn or bury used bandages**. Before burying bandages, put them in 2 plastic bags or wrap them in enough newspaper to stop any leaks.

If bandages are to be reused, soak them in cold water with a little bleach and then boil them before using them again. Mix just enough bleach solution for 1 day. Do not use it again the next day. It will not be strong enough to kill germs anymore.

Spinal Curve and Other Back Deformities

CHAPTER **20**

The backbone, or *'spine'*, is a chain of bones called 'vertebrae' that connect the head to the hipbone. Separating each of the vertebrae is a small cushion called a 'disk'. The backbone holds the body and head upright. It also encloses, in its hollow center, the *'spinal cord'* or trunk line of nerves connecting the brain to all parts of the body (see p. 35).

vertebrae

disks

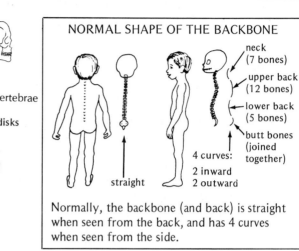

NORMAL SHAPE OF THE BACKBONE

neck (7 bones)

upper back (12 bones)

lower back (5 bones)

butt bones (joined together)

straight

4 curves:
2 inward
2 outward

Normally, the backbone (and back) is straight when seen from the back, and has 4 curves when seen from the side.

Sideways curve (scoliosis— S-shaped curve)

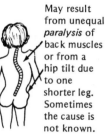

May result from unequal *paralysis* of back muscles or from a hip tilt due to one shorter leg. Sometimes the cause is not known.

Rounded back (kyphosis)

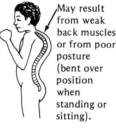

May result from weak back muscles or from poor posture (bent over position when standing or sitting).

Swayback (lordosis)

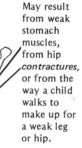

swayback

May result from weak stomach muscles, from hip *contractures*, or from the way a child walks to make up for a weak leg or hip.

Sharp bend or bump in spine (tuberculosis of the backbone)

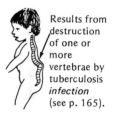

Results from destruction of one or more vertebrae by tuberculosis *infection* (see p. 165).

Of these different problems, scoliosis or a sideways curve is the most common serious problem. Often, however, rounded and/or swayback are seen together with scoliosis.

NON-FIXED AND FIXED SPINAL CURVES

With a non-fixed or *'functional'* curve there is no deformity of the vertebrae. This usually happens when the body tries to stand straight even though the hips tilt or there is other unevenness not in the spine.

Fixed or 'structural' curves are deformities in the bones of the back themselves.

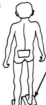

For example, a child with a shorter leg from polio will stand with his hips tilted. For him to stand straight, the spine has to curve.

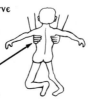

A non-fixed curve can usually be straightened by putting blocks under the foot, or by holding the child up under the arms.

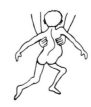

A fixed curve cannot be straightened by positioning or holding up the child.

Note: In some cases, with time a non-fixed curve may gradually become fixed.

CAUSES OF SPINAL CURVE (SCOLIOSIS)

Most **scoliosis** (about 80%) occurs in otherwise healthy children for no known reason. Sometimes it occurs in several members of the same family, so there may be a *hereditary* (familial) factor. Although about 1 of every 10 persons has some scoliosis (if looked for), only about 1 in 400 has enough of a curve to be a problem. **Curves of unknown cause are often first seen—and progress quickly—in children from 10–16 years old, during the period of rapid growth.**

Known causes of **fixed scoliosis** range from *infection* to tumor to rare disease. When possible, consult a doctor with experience in these problems.

Some children are born with fixed scoliosis, or develop it in early childhood, because of defects in the spine itself.

Sometimes one or more vertebrae are only partly formed and cause the spine to bend to one side.

Sometimes 2 or more vertebrae remain attached or 'fused' on one side. They can only grow on the unfused side, causing an increasing curve.

Non-fixed scoliosis always results secondary to other problems, such as uneven paralysis of the back muscles, or a hip tilt (often due to a shorter leg). Spinal curve often develops in children with **polio, cerebral palsy, muscular dystrophy, spina bifida, spinal cord injury, arthritis,** and **dislocated hip.** Be sure to examine all children with these *disabilities* for spinal curve. With time, non-fixed curves may gradually become fixed.

These problems can only be identified by X-rays.

Examining for spinal curve

This is discussed in the chapter on physical examination (Chapter 4).

a higher rib hump on one side

rib hump   vertebra

rib

Look along the line of the back with the child bent over.

The rib hump is formed because where the spine is curved, the vertebrae also are twisted to one side.

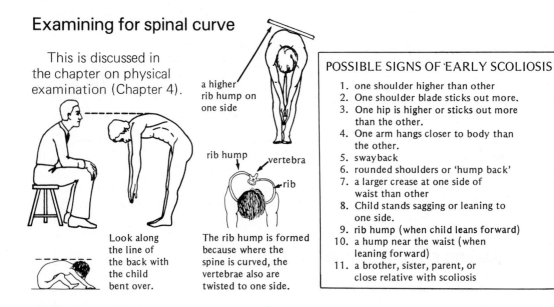

POSSIBLE SIGNS OF EARLY SCOLIOSIS
1. one shoulder higher than other
2. One shoulder blade sticks out more.
3. One hip is higher or sticks out more than the other.
4. One arm hangs closer to body than the other.
5. swayback
6. rounded shoulders or 'hump back'
7. a larger crease at one side of waist than other
8. Child stands sagging or leaning to one side.
9. rib hump (when child leans forward)
10. a hump near the waist (when leaning forward)
11. a brother, sister, parent, or close relative with scoliosis

CHECK FOR:

one shoulder lower than the other

hip tilt

To see the curve better, mark the tip of each vertebra.

The actual spinal curve is greater than the curve you have marked.

actual curve (as seen in X-rays)

overhead view of vertebrae

tips

When you examine for scoliosis, also check to see if the curve

can be straightened (non-fixed),

or cannot be straightened (fixed).

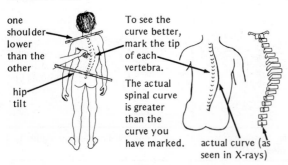
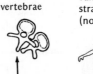

What to do

This will depend on:

- how severe the curve is.
- if it is getting worse—and if so, how quickly.
- whether the curve is fixed.
- the age of the child.

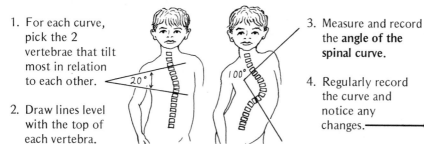

In a child who does not stand, check spinal curve while he is sitting. If one side of his butt is weaker and smaller, it may cause a **hip tilt.**

Put a book or board under the weaker butt, and see if this straightens his spine. If so, a cushion raised on one side may help him sit straighter.

How severe the curve is and whether it is getting worse can be best measured by X-rays.

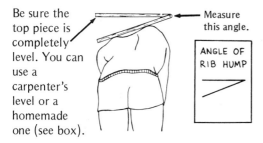

1. For each curve, pick the 2 vertebrae that tilt most in relation to each other.

2. Draw lines level with the top of each vertebra.

3. Measure and record the **angle of the spinal curve.**

4. Regularly record the curve and notice any changes.——————→

JUAN'S SPINE CURVE	
MAY 86	
JULY 86	
SEPT 86	
NOV 86	
JAN 87	
MAR 87	

Because X-rays are expensive and often hard to get, you can get some idea of whether the curve is getting worse by measuring the **angle of the rib hump.**

Be sure the top piece is completely level. You can use a carpenter's level or a homemade one (see box).

Measure this angle.

ANGLE OF RIB HUMP

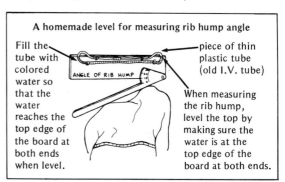

A homemade level for measuring rib hump angle

Fill the tube with colored water so that the water reaches the top edge of the board at both ends when level.

ANGLE OF RIB HUMP

piece of thin plastic tube (old I.V. tube)

When measuring the rib hump, level the top by making sure the water is at the top edge of the board at both ends.

Have the child stand or sit as straight as possible, while he bends forward.

If the rib hump angle stays about the same month after month, the curve is probably not getting worse. Keep checking it every few months. If the rib hump angle increases steadily, the curve is getting worse. X-rays should be taken and a decision made about what to do.

Non-fixed curves that are not getting worse should usually be treated only by doing something about the underlying problem.

For example, if the child's spinal curve is not fixed and comes from a hip tilt due to unequal leg length:

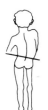

Measure the difference in leg length (see p. 34).

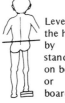

Level the hips by standing on books or boards.

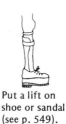

Put a lift on shoe or sandal (see p. 549).

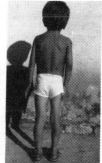

This child was developing a spinal curve due to hip tilt and short leg.

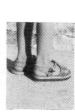

Village rehabilitation workers put a lift on his sandal.

This corrected his spinal curve and lop-sided posture.

Body jackets or bracing for a non-fixed curve usually do not help to correct the curve or even to prevent its getting worse. However, for a child with a curve so severe that it makes sitting or walking difficult, a body jacket or corset may help.

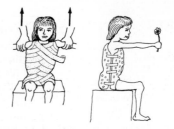

Instructions for making body jackets are on p. 558.

Spinal curves under 20° (fixed or non-fixed) usually need no special care—other than to be watched, and measured every few months to see if they are getting worse.

Some experts say that exercises to strengthen the back muscles, like this, help correct and slow down the curving of the spine. Other experts say it does no good. (We do not know.)

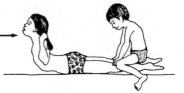

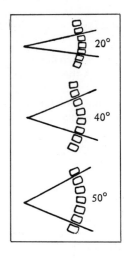

20°

40°

50°

Spinal curves over 20°, if they are fixed and getting worse, may get worse less quickly with a brace.

A brace like this (the Milwaukee brace) is often used. It works because it is so uncomfortable that the child must stretch his body as straight as possible to reduce the discomfort.

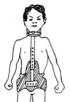

A plastic 'Boston brace' like this is more comfortable, can be completely hidden under the clothes, and probably does as much good.

SURGERY

For spinal curves over 50° which are quickly getting worse, surgery may be needed. Surgery 'fuses' (joins together) the most affected vertebrae. Usually it only partly straightens the spine. Except for very severe curves, surgery should be avoided in children under 12 years old because the fused part of the spine will not grow any more.

If the curve of the spine is less than 40° by the time the child stops growing, usually it will not progress further. If the curve is over 50°, it is likely to keep getting worse even after the child stops growing, and surgery is often recommended.

However, 'spinal fusion' surgery is very costly and requires an *orthopedic* surgeon specially trained in this operation. It can also be very hard on the child and family. When surgery cannot be obtained, a body jacket or brace should perhaps be used to help slow down the curve's progress. When a curve becomes too severe, there is no longer enough room in the chest for the lungs and heart to work well, and the child may get pneumonia and die.

EXERCISES FOR ROUNDED BACK AND SWAYBACK

Children with **rounded back** may benefit from exercises to help straighten it, like this.

These exercises are explained in the Exercise Sheet #5, p. 387.

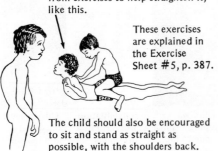

The child should also be encouraged to sit and stand as straight as possible, with the shoulders back.

Children with **swayback** may benefit from exercises to strengthen the stomach muscles, like this,

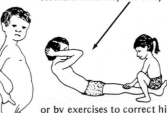

or by exercises to correct hip contractures (if the child has them). See Exercise Sheet #3, p. 385.

Tuberculosis of the Backbone

CHAPTER **21**

Pott's Disease

Tuberculosis (TB) of the backbone is not common, but is still seen in poor communities, especially in children. It is the most common form of tuberculosis of the bone.

It is important to recognize and treat it early, before damage to the backbone causes *nerve* damage and *paralysis.*

If a child begins to develop a sharp bend in the middle section of the backbone, with shortening and thickening of the chest, it is probably tuberculosis of the spine. You can almost be sure it is, if someone in the family has TB of the lungs.

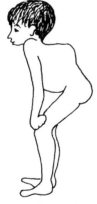

As the *spine* collapses forward, the child may have to hold himself up using his arms.

Seek medical help quickly. Skin test, X-rays (of the chest and spine), and microscope examination of pus from abscesses (pockets of pus) may help in the diagnosis. If the X-ray shows typical bone destruction, the child should be treated for tuberculosis even if no TB germs are found.

SIGNS

- It begins little by little—often without pain at first.

- A bump develops in the backbone. This is because the front part of one or more vertebrae is destroyed and collapses.

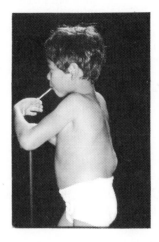
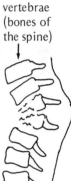

vertebrae (bones of the spine)

- The child has trouble bending over to pick things up.

- An abscess full of pus may form near the lump in the spine. It may open lower on the body and drain pus.

- As the condition gets worse, back pain may begin.

- Signs of **spinal cord** injury may develop: pain, numbness, weakness or paralysis in feet and legs, and loss of urine and bowel control. (See "Spinal Cord Injury," p. 175.)

- TB skin test is usually positive. (However, the skin test is of use only if the child has not been *vaccinated* against TB.)

- Often someone in the home has TB.

- Only half of children with TB of the spine also have TB of the lungs.

Treatment

- Use 2 to 3 **TB medicines** for at least a year, as for TB of the lungs. (See *Where There Is No Doctor,* p. 180.)

- A **back brace** may help keep the damaged spine straighter. It can be made of plaster, or of plastic using techniques similar to those used for making plastic leg braces (see p. 558).

Or make a very simple back brace from a metal tin or drum:

1. Cut an oval piece from a heavy tin.

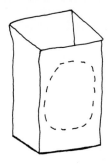

2. Hammer the tin to fit the child's back. Without forcing, try to put the back in the straightest position possible.

3. Pad the tin and wrap it with a soft cloth.

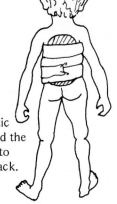

4. With an elastic bandage, bind the plate firmly to the child's back.

> *CAUTION:* Make sure the bandage does not hurt the child, damage his skin, or make it difficult for him to breathe.

The child in the photo on the previous page was effectively braced by a traditional bonesetter in this way.

- In severe or advanced cases, **surgery** may be needed to help straighten and stabilize the bones of the spine.

> *CAUTION:* Because of the risk of paralysis, an orthopedic surgeon should be consulted if possible.

Hopes for the future

With early, complete treatment the damaged bones will usually heal and the child may live normally, although often somewhat hunched over.

If nerve damage and paralysis have begun, sometimes surgery (or even bracing during treatment) can bring some improvement.

When nerve damage is severe, *rehabilitation* will be the same as for spinal cord injury (see Chapters 23, 24, and 25).

PREVENTION consists of early diagnosis and treatment of tuberculosis, and in the fight against poverty. Vaccination against TB may also help.

CHAPTER 22

Spina Bifida

WHAT IS IT?

Spina bifida (also called meningocele or myelomeningocele) is a defect that comes from a problem in the very early development of the unborn child. It happens when some of the back bones (vertebrae) do not close over the center tube of *nerves (spinal cord).* As a result, a soft unprotected area is left, which may bulge through the skin as a dark bag. This 'bag of nerves' is covered by a very thin layer (membrane) which may leak liquid from the spinal cord and brain. **Nobody knows what causes it.** But 1 of every 250 to 500 babies is born with spina bifida.

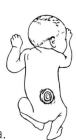

Problems that occur with spina bifida

- **High risk.** Without early surgery to cover the bag of nerves, it almost always gets *infected* and the child dies of meningitis.

- **Muscle weakness** and **loss of feeling.** The legs or feet may be **paralyzed** and have little or no feeling.

- **Hips.** One or both hips may be *dislocated.*

- **The feet** may turn down and in (club feet), or up and out.

- If the defect is relatively high up the back (L1 or above, see next page), there may be *muscle spasms (spasticity)* in the legs and feet (see p. 176).

- **Poor urine and bowel control.** The child may not feel when he pees or has a stool. When he gets older he may not develop control, and will pee or shit without knowing it.

- **Big head.** 'Hydrocephalus', which means 'water on the brain', develops in 4 out of 5 children with spina bifida. The liquid that forms inside the head cannot drain normally into the spinal cord, so it collects and puts pressure on the brain and skull bones. Although the child's head may look normal at birth, little by little it becomes swollen with liquid, like this.——————————————▶

- very big head

- big veins

- **The eyes** may turn downward because of pressure in the head. This 'setting sun sign' means **danger** of blindness and severe brain damage.

- **Brain damage.** Without early surgery to lower the pressure of the liquid in the head (and sometimes even if the surgery is done), some children become blind, mentally retarded, have fits (epileptic seizures, see p. 233), or develop cerebral palsy (see Chapter 9).

PROBLEMS THAT MAY OCCUR WHEN THE CHILD IS OLDER:

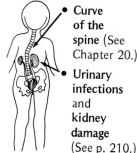

- **Curve of the spine** (See Chapter 20.)

- **Urinary infections and kidney damage** (See p. 210.)

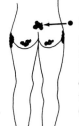

- **Pressure sores** may form over the bones, because the child cannot feel. (See Chapter 24.)

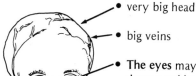

- **Foot injuries.** Children who can walk but have no feeling in their feet may easily develop sores or injuries. If neglected, these can lead to severe infections of the flesh, bone infection, and deformities or loss of the feet (see p. 222).

What is the future for a child with spina bifida?

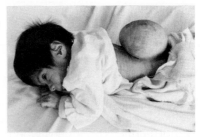

This will depend first on how serious the defect is, next on medical treatment and general care, and finally on special training and on family and community support.

The higher up the back the defect is or the more severely the spinal cord is affected, the worse the paralysis and other problems are likely to be. If the head is already very swollen, the child's chances are poor. The costs will usually be great, even for a rich family. Surgery to drain the liquid from the head is sometimes followed by infection. The operation may need to be repeated several times. In spite of the best medical attention, at least 1 of every 4 or 5 children born with severe spina bifida dies in the first months or years of life.

However, **the child with a defect that is low down on the back usually has less paralysis, and has a good chance of living a full and happy life.** With good family and community support, many children with spina bifida go to school, learn to do many kinds of work, get married, and have children.

Often these children are late in learning basic skills for self-care (getting dressed, eating, going to the bathroom). This is partly because of the *disability.* But it is also because their parents often overprotect them and do everything for them. **It is important for parents to help these children to do more for themselves.**

What are the chances that my child with spina bifida will walk?

This depends on many factors. However, the higher up the defect is on the spine, the more paralysis the child will probably have. The drawings below show how likely it is for the child to walk, based on the level of the defect. The shaded areas show the parts of the body affected by paralysis and loss of feeling.

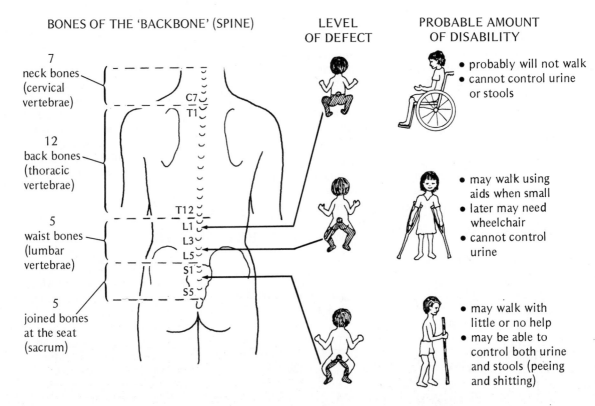

BONES OF THE 'BACKBONE' (SPINE)

7 neck bones (cervical vertebrae)

12 back bones (thoracic vertebrae)

5 waist bones (lumbar vertebrae)

5 joined bones at the seat (sacrum)

LEVEL OF DEFECT

PROBABLE AMOUNT OF DISABILITY

- probably will not walk
- cannot control urine or stools

- may walk using aids when small
- later may need wheelchair
- cannot control urine

- may walk with little or no help
- may be able to control both urine and stools (peeing and shitting)

CARING FOR THE CHILD WITH SPINA BIFIDA

Care of the defect. When there is a 'bag of nerves' on the spine of a newborn baby, his chances of living are much better if he has an operation within a few weeks. The surgery covers the defect with muscle and skin. Without this operation there is a high risk of injury and brain infection (meningitis); the child will probably not live very long.

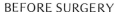
BEFORE SURGERY   AFTER SURGERY

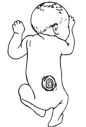 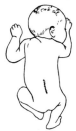

For children who cannot get an operation, try to protect the bag of nerves so that its thin covering is not injured or broken. (If it breaks, meningitis can occur.)

One way to protect the bag is to make a ring or 'donut' of soft cloth or foam rubber, and to tie it so that it surrounds the bag. Do not let the ring or clothing touch the bag.

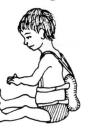 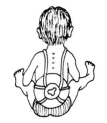

Hydrocephalus. It is important to measure the distance around the head of the child at birth, and every week or so afterward. If head size increases faster than normal (see chart on p. 41), or if you notice that the **head is swelling a lot,** the child probably has hydrocephalus.

A surgical operation called a 'shunt' may need to be done before the pressure of the liquid in the brain causes much damage. A tube is run from a liquid-filled hollow in the brain into the entrance to the heart or into the belly (abdominal cavity). This way the extra liquid is drained from the brain.

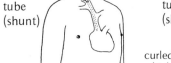
SHUNT—
BRAIN TO HEART

SHUNT—
BRAIN TO BELLY

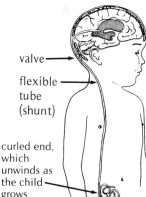

one-way valve →

flexible tube (shunt)

valve →

flexible tube (shunt)

curled end, which unwinds as the child grows

Not all children who have early signs of hydrocephalus need this operation. If the head is not very swollen and stops increasing rapidly in size, it may get better by itself.

CAUTION: 'Shunts' do not always give good results. Even with surgery, 1 out of 5 children with hydrocephalus dies before age 7, and more than half become mentally retarded. Others are intelligent, however, and develop normally. Before deciding on the operation, get advice from 2 or 3 specialists.

Note: We realize that, for many families, the operations described here will not be possible. Except where free hospital services are available, they are very costly.

Before deciding on surgery, there are several things to consider:

- What will the child's future be like, if he lives? Is he likely to suffer greatly, or might he have a chance to live a full and happy life, despite his limitations?
- If the family spends much money on operations, and then on daily care of the child, how will this affect the health and well-being of the other children in the family?

In short, before deciding whether to operate, it is important to consider carefully how this may affect the quality of life for both the child and the family.

Bladder and bowel management

A child with spina bifida usually does not develop the same control of peeing (bladder control) and shitting (bowel control) as other children do. The child may always dribble urine. Or, as she gets older, she may continue to empty her bladder or bowels without warning, perhaps without even knowing or feeling it. **Standard methods of toilet training will not work. Do not blame or scold her for her accidents.**

WARNING: In some children with spina bifida, the bladder does not empty completely. This is dangerous because if urine stays in the bladder for a long time, bacteria will grow in it and this can lead to infection of the bladder and kidneys. In children with spina bifida, urinary infections are a frequent cause of death.

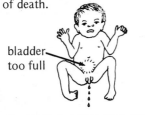

bladder too full

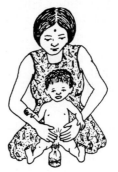

A mother can learn to feel how full the bladder is, and to tap on it gently to see if this makes the baby pee. If not, she can regularly press gently on the bladder to push out the urine.

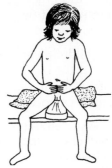

Later, some children can learn to empty their bladders by crying, rolling over, laughing, or sneezing. Others learn to do it by pressing on the stomach, like this, although this can also be risky (see p. 209).

Some children may need to use a 'catheter' or rubber tube to get the urine out. By age 5 they can often learn to 'catheterize' themselves. (See p. 206.)

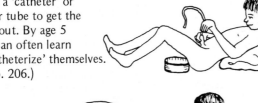

Girls often need to empty the bladder regularly with a catheter, and perhaps use diapers (nappies) to catch any urine that drips out in between.

As they grow older, boys are often able to use a 'condom' connected to a bag that collects the urine. (See p. 207.)

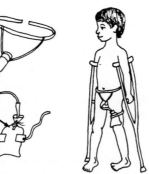

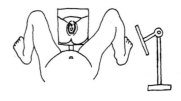

For girls, a mirror helps in finding the urine hole.

Most children with spina bifida can be helped to take care of both their bladder and bowel so that they stay relatively dry, clean, and healthy. Then they can go to school and do things outside the home with greater confidence. Therefore, **it is extremely important that rehabilitation workers and family members help the child work out a good bladder and bowel program.**

IMPORTANT INFORMATION on **urinary and bowel problems** and **prevention and treatment of urinary infections** is in Chapter 25, p. 203 to 214. Be sure to study this chapter!

PREVENTION and correction of contractures

Some children with spina bifida tend to develop *contractures* either because of muscle imbalance (see p. 78) or, less often, because of *spasticity* (abnormal muscle tightness). Contractures most often develop in the feet, hips, and knees. **Range-of-motion** and stretching exercises, as discussed in Chapter 42, can help prevent and correct early contractures.

CAUTION: Only do stretching exercises where there is stiffness or limited range of motion. When joints are floppy, **do not stretch them more** where they already bend too much. For example:

		YES			NO
If the foot is stiff in this position,	do exercises to gradually bring the foot up. (See p. 383.)		But if the foot is floppy or already bends up more than normal,	avoid exercises that would stretch it even more.	

Because children with spina bifida have stronger muscles for bending than for straightening the hips, they tend to develop **hip contractures,** like this child. Stretching exercises (p. 385) and lying on the belly (p. 86) may help.

Also, make sure walking aids help correct rather than increase the contractures.

angle of contracture

Tight tendons keep hip from straightening.

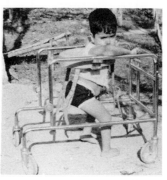

This expensive metal 'walker' lets this child with spina bifida 'walk' with hips bent. It can cause hip contractures and make walking without aids less possible.

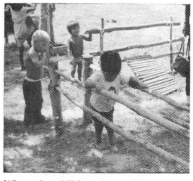

When the child is changed to parallel bars adjusted to the right height, he walks more upright. This helps prevent contractures and increases the possibility of walking without aids.

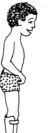

Sometimes a child stands with hips and knees bent, partly because his feet bend up too much.

This can lead to hip and knee contractures.

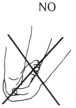

Lightweight below-knee braces that hold the feet in a more firm position may be all the child needs to stand straighter, walk better—and prevent contractures. (See p. 550.)

Do not let the child get fat. Because the legs and feet of a child with spina bifida are weak, it is important that she does not get too heavy. Even for a child who does not walk, moving will be easier if she is not fat. Encourage her to eat nutritious foods, but to avoid a lot of sweets, fatty foods, and sweetened drinks.

HELPING THE CHILD DEVELOP

Many children with spina bifida are paralyzed from the waist down. In spite of their disability, it is important for them to develop their bodies, their minds, and their social abilities as much as possible. Certain 'adaptive aids' can be used to help paralyzed children go through the same stages of development as able-bodied children, at close to the same age. (See the developmental chart on p. 292.)

For the child to progress through the early stages of development, it is important that he can

SEE STRAIGHT AHEAD	SIT WITH HIS HANDS FREE	EXPLORE HIS SURROUNDINGS	STAND WITH HIS HANDS FREE	SIT, STAND, AND WALK

NORMAL

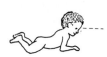 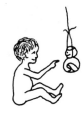 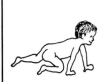 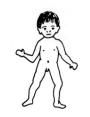 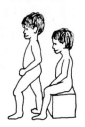

SPINA BIFIDA

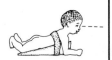 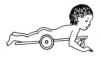 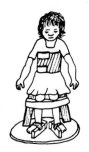 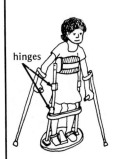

hinges

If she cannot get herself into a position where she can see what is happening in front of her, lie her on a 'wedge' or fix a carton or box so she can sit leaning back in it.	You can make a seat from an old bucket or some other object, so that she can sit and play.	You can make a little cart that helps her to move. The cart can have a handle so that another person can push it.	Make a standing frame that holds her in a standing position. Holding up the weight of her body on her legs will strengthen her bones, so they will not break as easily.	She can use a brace that holds her up, so that she can walk with crutches. It helps if the brace has hip and knee hinges so that she can sit down (see p. 575).

When adapting aids for children with spina bifida, remember that each child is different. Some children manage to walk without braces, perhaps with the aid of parallel bars like these, and later crutches. Others will need above-knee or below-knee braces (see Chapter 58). Other children will need wheelchairs.

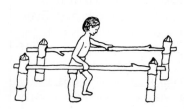

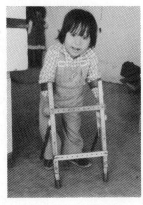

This child with spina bifida learned to walk using elbow crutches adapted to form a walker. As his balance and control improved, the supports on the crutches were gradually removed until he could walk with the crutches alone.

Surgery and orthopedic corrections

To prevent or correct **foot contractures** in many children, it may be necessary to straighten the feet in the same way as for club feet (see p. 565). So that the contractures do not come back, the children will need to do exercises (see p. 115 and 383) and perhaps use simple plastic braces (p. 550), at least at night.

For curving of the spine, if severe, some children need surgery or a body brace. (See p. 164.)

For children with spina bifida who have **one hip dislocated,** corrective surgery is sometimes helpful. But surgery generally is not recommended for those children with **both hips dislocated.** Usually they will walk just as well if the hips are left dislocated—and with fewer complications and less suffering. (See "Hip Problems," p. 156.)

> *CAUTION:* Before any orthopedic surgery is performed on a child with spina bifida, carefully evaluate the possibility she has of walking and whether the surgery will really help her.

PREVENTION of pressure sores and injuries

As a child who has no feeling in parts of his body grows older and heavier, there is increasing danger that pressure sores (bed sores) will form over bony areas that support his weight (mostly his butt or his feet). To prevent this:

- Have the child sleep and sit on a mattress or cushion that is soft (such as foam rubber), and **move or turn over often.**
- Examine the child's lower body daily for early signs of irritation or sores. Check especially the hips, knees, and feet.
- When he is a little older, the child can learn to check his own body each day for sores.

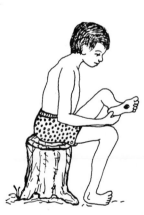

DANGER: Whether the cause is spina bifida or leprosy, children who walk but have no feeling in their feet run a high risk of cuts, burns, sores, and serious infections on their feet. Teach them to **check their feet every day.**

Also, **be sure that sandals, shoes, and orthopedic braces fit well and do not cause blisters or irritation.**

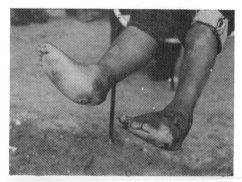

This child with spina bifida cut her feet on broken glass. Because the cuts did not hurt, they were neglected and became severely infected. In time, the infection spread to the bones in both her feet and began to destroy them. As a result, her feet are very deformed and she may lose them completely.

> *IMPORTANT INFORMATION* on prevention and treatment of pressure sores is in Chapter 24, p. 195 to 202. **Be sure to read it.** Also see Chapter 26 on Leprosy, p. 223 to 225 for special footwear and ways to protect the feet.

You will find other important information that relates to a child with spina bifida in other chapters of this book, especially:

Chapter 23, "Spinal Cord Injury"
Chapter 24, "Pressure Sores"
Chapter 25, "Urine and Bowel Management"

Also refer to the chapters on contractures, club feet, exercises, developmental delay, braces, wheelchairs, and special seating.

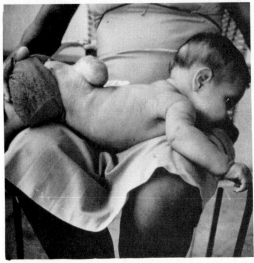

This child with spina bifida was born to a village family too poor to afford surgery.

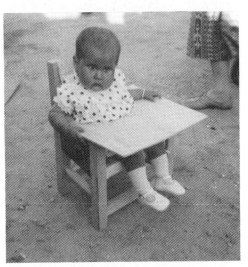

The PROJIMO team made her a special seat with a bowl attached to a hole in the back to protect her 'sack on the back'.

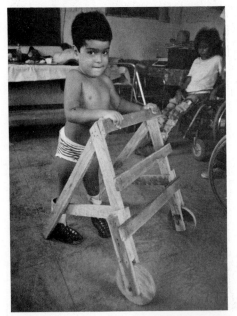

A child with spina bifida learns to walk with the help of a homemade walker. (PROJIMO)

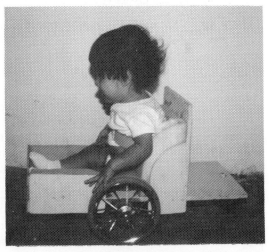

A one-year-old with spina bifida in a mini wheel-chair made by disabled workers (PROJIMO)

CHAPTER 23

Spinal Cord Injury

Spinal cord injury usually results from an accident that breaks or severely damages the central *nerve cord* in the neck or back: falls from trees or mules, automobile accidents, diving accidents, bullet wounds, and other injuries. Spinal cord injury is more common in adults and older children—and in many cultures it is twice as common in men as in women.

The *spinal cord* is the line of *nerves* that comes out of the brain and runs down the backbone (see p. 35). From the cord, nerves go out to the whole body. Feeling and movement are controlled by messages that travel back and forth to the brain through the spinal cord. When the cord is damaged, feeling and movement in the body below the level of the injury are lost or reduced.

Level of the injury

How much of the body is affected depends on the level of the injury along the backbone. The higher the injury is, the greater the area of the body that is affected.

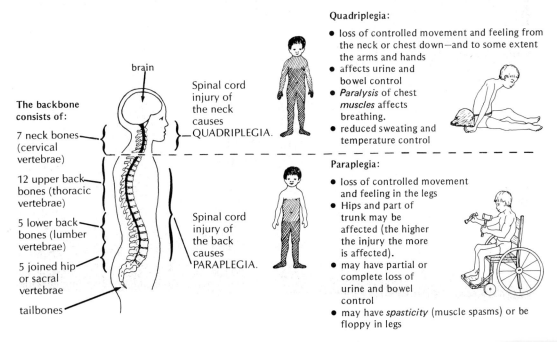

The backbone consists of:

7 neck bones (cervical vertebrae)

12 upper back bones (thoracic vertebrae)

5 lower back bones (lumber vertebrae)

5 joined hip or sacral vertebrae

tailbones

brain

Spinal cord injury of the neck causes QUADRIPLEGIA.

Spinal cord injury of the back causes PARAPLEGIA.

Quadriplegia:
- loss of controlled movement and feeling from the neck or chest down—and to some extent the arms and hands
- affects urine and bowel control
- *Paralysis* of chest *muscles* affects breathing.
- reduced sweating and temperature control

Paraplegia:
- loss of controlled movement and feeling in the legs
- Hips and part of trunk may be affected (the higher the injury the more is affected).
- may have partial or complete loss of urine and bowel control
- may have *spasticity* (muscle spasms) or be floppy in legs

Complete and incomplete injuries

When the spinal cord is damaged so completely that no nerve messages get through, the injury is said to be 'complete'. Feeling and controlled movement below the level of the injury are completely and permanently lost. If the injury is 'incomplete', some feeling and movement may remain. Or feeling and controlled movement may return (partly or entirely) little by little during several months. In incomplete injuries, one side may have less feeling and movement than the other.

X-rays often do not show how complete a spinal cord injury is. Sometimes the backbone may be badly broken, yet the spinal cord damage may be minor. And sometimes (especially in children) the X-ray may show no damage to the backbone, yet the spinal cord injury may be severe or complete. Often, only time will tell how complete the injury is.

EARLY QUESTIONS THAT A SPINAL CORD INJURED CHILD AND FAMILY MAY ASK

"Will my child always remain paralyzed?"

This will depend on how much the spinal cord has been damaged. If paralysis below the level of the injury is not complete (for example, if the child has some feeling and control of movement in her feet) there is a better chance of some improvement.

Usually the biggest improvement occurs in the first months. The more time goes by without improvement, the less likely it is that any major improvement in feeling or movement will occur.

Occasionally surgery to release pressure on the spinal cord or nerves, if done in the first hours or days following the injury, will bring back some movement or feeling. But surgery done more than a month after the injury almost never brings back any movement or feeling. Never agree to such surgery unless at least 3 independent and highly respected neurosurgeons recommend it.

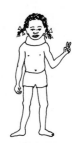

It is *very* unusual that a child who is paralyzed by a broken neck is walking with a neck collar in 6 weeks.

After one year, the paralysis that remains is almost certainly there to stay. As gently as you can, help both the child and parents accept this fact. It is important that they learn to live with the paralysis as best they can, and not wait for it to get better or go from clinic to clinic in search of a cure.

> **It is best to be honest with the child and the family. Explain the facts of the situation as clearly, truthfully, and kindly as possible.**

"My child's feet are beginning to move!"—spasticity

Immediately after a spinal cord injury the paralyzed parts are in 'spinal shock', and are loose or 'floppy'. Later (within a few days or weeks) the legs may begin to stiffen—especially when the hips or back are straightened. Also, when moved or touched, a leg may begin to 'jump' (a rapid series of jerks, called 'clonus').

This stiffening and jerking is an automatic reflex called 'spasticity'. It is not controlled by the child's mind, and often happens where spinal cord damage is complete. It is **not** a sign that the child has begun to feel where he is touched or is recovering control of movement.

CAUTION: Sudden jumping or stiffening of the legs when moved or touched does not mean feeling or controlled movement is returning. This is a spastic reflex.

Some children with spinal cord injury develop spasticity; others do not.

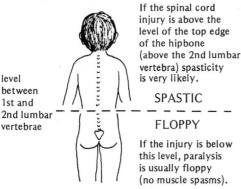

If the spinal cord injury is above the level of the top edge of the hipbone (above the 2nd lumbar vertebra) spasticity is very likely.

level between 1st and 2nd lumbar vertebrae

SPASTIC

FLOPPY

If the injury is below this level, paralysis is usually floppy (no muscle spasms).

Severe spasticity often makes moving and control more difficult. However, the child may learn to use both the reflex jerks and spastic stiffness to help her do things. For example,

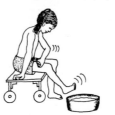

When the child wants to lift her foot, she hits her thigh, triggering the jerks that lift the leg.

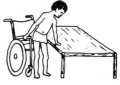

In lower back injuries, the spasticity or stiffness of the legs may actually help the child stand for *transfers*.

"Will my child be able to walk?"

This will depend mostly on how high or low in the back the injury is. The lower the injury, the better the chance of walking. A person with complete spinal cord injury in the neck has no chance of walking. She will need a wheelchair.

If the child's injury is in the lower back and if his arms are strong and he is not too fat, there is a chance he may learn to walk with crutches and braces. But he will probably still need a wheelchair to go long distances.

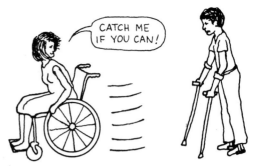

CATCH ME IF YOU CAN!

Many spinal cord injured persons prefer a wheelchair to walking with braces and crutches.

However, it is best not to place too much importance on learning to walk. Many children who do learn to walk find it so slow and tiring that they prefer using a wheelchair.

It probably makes sense to give most paraplegic children a chance to try walking. However, do not make the child feel guilty if he prefers a wheelchair. Let the child decide what is the easiest way for him to move about.

For independent living, other skills are more important than walking, and the family and child should place greater importance on these: skills like dressing, bathing, getting into and out of bed, and toileting. Self-care in toileting is especially important—and is more difficult because of the child's lack of bladder and bowel control.

"What are the hopes for my child's future?"

The chances of a paraplegic's leading a fairly normal life are good—provided that you:

1. avoid 3 big medical risks:

   - skin problems (pressure sores)
   - urinary infections
   - contractures (shortening of muscles, causing deformities)
     (*Contractures* are not a danger to life but can make moving about and doing things much more difficult.)

2. help the child to become more self-reliant:

   - home training and encouragement to master basic self-help skills such as moving about, dressing, and toileting
   - education: learning of skills that make keeping a household, helping other people, and earning a living more possible

A child who is paraplegic learns to walk with a plywood parapodium made by village rehabilitations workers. (PROJIMO)

It is more difficult for quadriplegic persons to lead a normal life because they are more dependent on physical assistance. However, in some countries many paraplegics and quadriplegics manage to lead full, rich lives, earn their own living, get married, and play an important role in the community. With effort and organization, the same possibilities can exist in all countries.

"Can anything be done about loss of bladder and bowel control?"

Yes. Although normal control rarely returns completely, the spinal cord injured child often can learn to be independent in his toilet, and to stay clean and dry (except for occasional accidents). Often he will need a special urine collecting device, will learn to use a catheter, and will learn to bring down a bowel movement with a finger or suppository. Management of bladder and bowels are discussed in Chapter 25.

VERY IMPORTANT INFORMATION ON URINE AND BOWEL CONTROL IS IN CHAPTER 25. BE SURE TO READ THIS CHAPTER!

"What about marriage, sex, and having children?"

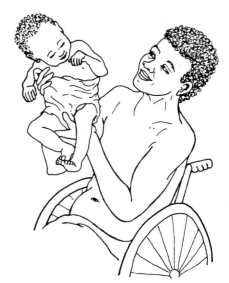

Many spinal cord injured persons marry and have loving, sexual relationships. Women with spinal cord injuries can become pregnant and have normal babies. Men may or may not be able to get a hard penis or ejaculate (release sperm). Paraplegic and quadriplegic men whose injuries are incomplete are more likely to have children. Some couples where the husband cannot release sperm decide to adopt children. Whether or not they can have children, male and female spinal cord injured persons often enjoy loving sexual relationships.

Especially for young men, fear of the loss of sexual ability is often one of the most fearful and depressing aspects of spinal cord injury. Honest, open discussion about this, and the possibilities that do exist, with a more experienced spinal cord injured person may help greatly. There is a good discussion of this in *Spinal Cord Injury Home Care Manual.* See reference, p. 639.

HELPING THE CHILD AND FAMILY ADJUST

Spinal cord injury, especially in the child, brings many of the same problems as does spina bifida. Also many aspects of rehabilitation are similar. (We suggest you read Chapter 22 on spina bifida to get additional ideas for the *rehabilitation* of young children with spinal cord injuries.)

Perhaps the biggest difference from spina bifida is that spinal cord injury begins later. One day the child is physically active and able, the next he is suddenly paralyzed and (at first) unable to do much for himself. He has lost all feeling and control in part of his body; it is like a dead weight.

This is very hard for the child—and family—to accept. Both have an enormous fear and uncertainty about the future. The child may become deeply depressed, or angry and uncooperative. He may refuse even to sit in a wheelchair because this means accepting not being able to walk.

There are no easy answers to the child's fear and depression, but here are some suggestions families have found helpful.

- Recognize that **the child's fear, depression, and anger are natural responses** and that with love, understanding and encouragement, he will little by little overcome them.

- **Be honest** to the child about her *disability.* Do not tell her, "We will find a cure for you," or, "Soon you will get well and be able to walk again." Very probably this is not true, and telling the child such things only makes it more difficult for the child to accept her disability and to begin shaping a new life. Also, as the promised 'cure' fails to happen, the child becomes more uncertain, distrustful, and afraid. In the end, it will be much easier for her if you gently tell the truth. Here is one example.————————————▶

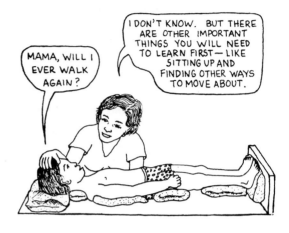

MAMA, WILL I EVER WALK AGAIN?

I DON'T KNOW. BUT THERE ARE OTHER IMPORTANT THINGS YOU WILL NEED TO LEARN FIRST—LIKE SITTING UP AND FINDING OTHER WAYS TO MOVE ABOUT.

- Provide opportunities to **keep the child's mind active: playing, working, exploring, learning** through stories, games, and studies. But at the same time **respect and be supportive of the child when he feels sad and frightened.** Let him cry, comfort him when he does, but do not tell him not to cry. Crying helps relieve fear and tension.

- **Start** the child with **exercises, activities, and relearning** to use her hands and body as soon as possible. Start with what the child can do, and build on that.

- Try to have the child **watch, talk with, and get to know other persons with spinal cord injury** (or children with spina bifida), especially those who are living full and happy lives.

- Invite the child's friends to come visit her, play with her, and let her know that they are eager for the day she will be back in school.

- **Encourage the child to do as much for herself as possible.** Let her do anything she can do for herself— even if it takes longer.

> **Help in ways that let the child do more for herself.**

- As much as possible, avoid 'tranquilizers' or other strong medicines. The child needs an alert mind and an ability to move actively all day.

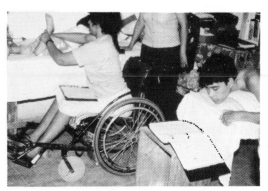

Look for ways to help spinal cord injured persons learn skills and play a useful, helpful role. Here 2 young, spinal cord injured persons in PROJIMO examine a disabled child, and give recommendations to the family, using an early draft of this book.

HOW TO PREVENT MORE SEVERE SPINAL CORD INJURY IN CASE OF ACCIDENT

When a person has just had an accident that may have injured the spinal cord, great care must be taken to prevent further damage.

After an accident, there may be spinal cord injury if:

- the person is unconscious, or

- the person cannot move, cannot feel, or has numbness in his legs or hands.

If you think the spinal cord might be injured:

- Do not move the person until a health worker with a large board or stretcher arrives. Especially **avoid bending the person's neck and back.**

- Lift the person without bending him, onto a board or stiff stretcher. (A stiff rack is better than a soft stretcher. Make one out of poles from trees or whatever is available.) Make ties of strips of clothing, or whatever you can.

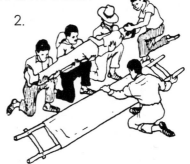

sandbags or rolls of clothing to hold head firmly

- Tie him down firmly and stabilize his head.

- Carry the person to a medical center or hospital. Try not to bounce or jiggle him.

HOW TO LIFT A SEVERELY INJURED PERSON ONTO A STRETCHER
from *Where There Is No Doctor*

1.

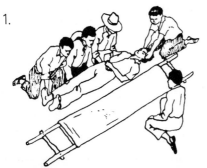

With great care, lift the injured person without bending him anywhere.

2.

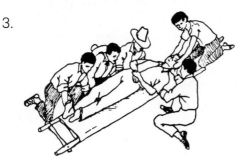

Make sure that the head and neck do not bend.

Have another person put the stretcher in place.

3.

With the help of everyone, place the injured person carefully on the stretcher.

4.

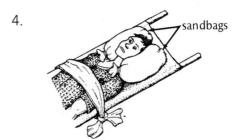

sandbags

If the neck is injured or broken, put bags of sand or tightly folded clothing on each side of the head to keep it from moving.

Common secondary problems in children with spinal cord injury

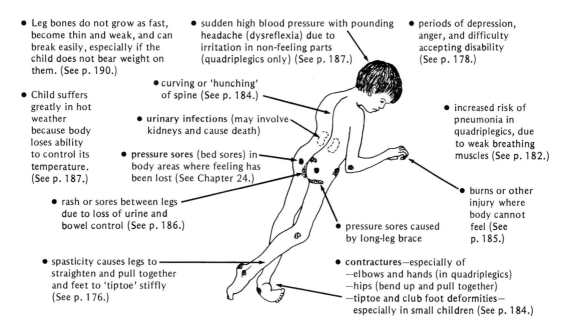

- Leg bones do not grow as fast, become thin and weak, and can break easily, especially if the child does not bear weight on them. (See p. 190.)
- Child suffers greatly in hot weather because body loses ability to control its temperature. (See p. 187.)
- rash or sores between legs due to loss of urine and bowel control (See p. 186.)
- spasticity causes legs to straighten and pull together and feet to 'tiptoe' stiffly (See p. 176.)
- curving or 'hunching' of spine (See p. 184.)
- urinary infections (may involve kidneys and cause death)
- pressure sores (bed sores) in body areas where feeling has been lost (See Chapter 24.)
- sudden high blood pressure with pounding headache (dysreflexia) due to irritation in non-feeling parts (quadriplegics only) (See p. 187.)
- periods of depression, anger, and difficulty accepting disability (See p. 178.)
- increased risk of pneumonia in quadriplegics, due to weak breathing muscles (See p. 182.)
- burns or other injury where body cannot feel (See p. 185.)
- pressure sores caused by long-leg brace
- contractures—especially of
  —elbows and hands (in quadriplegics)
  —hips (bend up and pull together)
  —tiptoe and club foot deformities—especially in small children (See p. 184.)

To prevent or reduce the harmful effects of these problems, **special precautions need to be taken early and continued throughout life.**

EARLY CARE FOR THE SPINAL CORD INJURED PERSON

Early care following spinal cord injury is best done in a hospital, especially if the child is likely to get **good nursing care.** Family members should stay with the child in the hospital to make sure the child is kept clean and turned regularly, so that bed sores and pneumonia are avoided. (Busy hospital staff with little experience treating spinal cord injuries sometimes let severe bed sores develop—which may threaten the child's life.)

CAUTION: During the first 6 weeks, or until any breaks in the bone have healed, **take great care when turning the child so that the angle of his back, neck, and head does not change.** Use the same methods and precautions used in lifting a newly injured person onto a stretcher (see p. 180). When the neck or back has healed, the child can start lying on his stomach, at first for 10 minutes and then longer if there are no problems.

Surgery of the spine may or may not be necessary. After surgery, the person must lie very still for at least 6 weeks. The main purpose of surgery is to prevent more damage—not to cure the paralysis. **The damage already done to the spinal cord cannot be corrected with surgery or medicine.**

Preventing pressure sores (bed sores)

When feeling has been lost, pressure sores can easily form on the skin over bony areas—especially on the hips and butt. The biggest risk of sores is in the first weeks after the injury. This is because the child must stay very still, and has not yet learned to move or turn over his body. Prevention of pressure sores is extremely important, and needs understanding and continuous care, both by the child and those caring for him.

**BE SURE TO READ CHAPTER 24 ON PREVENTION AND TREATMENT
OF PRESSURE SORES.**

Summary: early prevention of pressure sores (For details, see Chapter 24.)

- Lie on a soft mattress or thick, firm, foam rubber pad.
- Place pillows and pads to keep pressure off bony areas.
- Change position (turn over from front to back and side to side) every 2 to 3 hours. To avoid pressure sores, lying on the belly is the best position).
- Keep skin and bedclothes clean and dry.
- Eat good food rich in vitamins, iron, and protein.
- Move and exercise a lot to promote good flow of the blood.
- Check skin daily for earliest signs of pressure sores—and keep all pressure off beginning sores until the skin is healthy again.

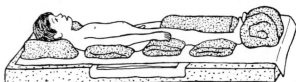

Avoiding contractures

In the first weeks following a spinal cord injury, when the child is in a lying position, joint contractures (muscles shortening) can easily develop, especially in the feet and elbows. Pillows and pads should be placed to keep the feet supported, the elbows straight, and the hands in a good position. Gentle range-of-motion exercises of the feet, hands, and arms should begin as early as possible, taking care not to move the back until the injury is healed. Further discussion on the prevention of contractures in the spinal cord injured is on p. 184.

PHYSICAL THERAPY FOLLOWING SPINAL CORD INJURY

ASSISTED BREATHING AND COUGHING

Persons with spinal cord injury in the neck or upper back often have part of their breathing muscles paralyzed. Slowly the remaining muscles become stronger and breathing improves. But breathing often stays weak. The person may not be able to cough well and can more easily get pneumonia.

To help the person cough, place hands as shown below. Ask him to cough, and as he does, push firmly inward on the chest. Be careful not to move the backbone.

TWO-PERSON
ASSISTED COUGH   (NOW COUGH.)

Do this several
times a day when
the person has a
cold, and more often
if the person
develops more trouble
breathing or seems to
have a lot of mucus in
his lungs or throat.

ONE-PERSON
ASSISTED COUGH   (BREATHE DEEP.)

To help the child breathe
deep and to stimulate the
breathing muscles, press
lightly here while the
child tries to breathe
deeply in and out.

Do this for a few
minutes, several
times a day.

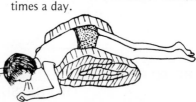

If the person has a lot of mucus in her
lungs, it also helps to lie her down, like this,——
and pat her back briskly. This helps loosen the
mucus so that it can be coughed out. Be sure she
drinks lots of water to help loosen the mucus.

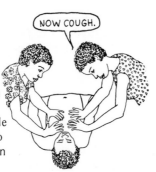

MOVEMENT AND EXERCISE

Do range-of-motion exercises for about 10 minutes for each arm and leg. In the first weeks, do the exercises twice a day. Later, once a day may be enough. If any signs of contracture develop, spend more time and effort on those parts of the body. From the start, exercises should be both *passive* (someone else moves the child's body parts) and whenever possible, *active* (the child does it himself).

Range-of-motion exercises should begin with great care the day after the spine is injured (see Chapter 42). The exercises will help to improve the flow of blood (which reduces the chance of bed sores), to prevent contractures, and to build the strength of the muscles that still work. Range-of-motion exercises should be **continued throughout life,** when possible as a part of day-to-day activity.

CAUTIONS:

- Until any breaks or tears in the spine have healed (6 weeks or more) exercise must be very gentle and limited, with smooth motions and no jerking.

  - Especially at first, take great care that exercises do not move the position of the back and neck. Start with feet, ankles, hands, wrists, and elbows.

  - If exercises trigger severe muscle spasms or jerking, do not do them until the break is healed.

- Do not use force in trying to get the full range of motion, as joints can easily be damaged.

- For quadriplegics often it is better to stretch the fingers only when the wrist is bent down like this,

  but not when it is bent back like this.

  This way enough contracture is left to be useful for taking hold of things. Although the fingers lack movement by muscles, they close around an object when the wrist is bent back.

If possible, get instructions from an experienced *physical therapist*.

- Try to keep the full range of motion of all parts of the body. But **work most with those joints that are likely to develop contractures,** especially:

  - paralyzed parts that tend to hang in one position, such as the feet,

    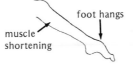

    muscle shortening — foot hangs

    Prevent this through exercises (see p. 383) and by supporting feet (p. 184).

  - or, joints that are kept straight or bent by spasticity or by muscle imbalance (see p. 78). For example:

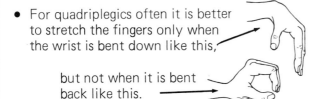

In quadriplegia the muscles that straighten the elbow are usually paralyzed, while the muscles that bend the elbow stay fairly strong. These muscles keep the elbow bent, and in time they shorten so that the arm can no longer straighten fully.

It is important that the arms can straighten until they bend backward a little — which is the only way he can lift himself with his arms.

For this reason, straight arm positioning and early range-of-motion exercises for the elbow are essential. While he is still kept lying down, teach him to straighten his elbows by turning his hands up and then lifting his arms.

MAINTAINING HEALTHY POSITIONS

The position that the body is in during the day and night is also important to prevent contractures.

Contractures that cause 'tiptoeing' of the feet can develop easily, especially when there is spasticity. **Keep the feet in a supported position** as much of the time as possible:

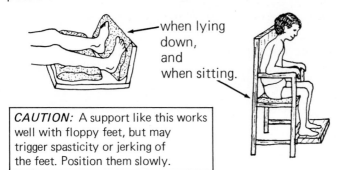

when lying down, and when sitting.

CAUTION: A support like this works well with floppy feet, but may trigger spasticity or jerking of the feet. Position them slowly.

Teach the child to make sure his feet are in a **good position.**

Even for the child who may never walk, maintaining the feet in a flat position makes moving from chair to bed, toilet or bath easier.

Another common problem for children with spasticity is that the knees pull together and in time contractures prevent the legs from separating. To prevent this, when the child lies on her side she should learn to

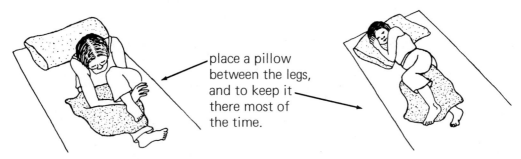

place a pillow between the legs, and to keep it there most of the time.

A common problem with wheelchair users is that they slump forward. In time this can deform the spine.

In a wheelchair with a straight-up back a person with spinal cord injury slumps like this in order to balance.

A chair can be designed (or adapted) so that it tilts back. This provides balance for a better position.

A special cushion also helps keep the butt from sliding forward (and helps prevent pressure sores).

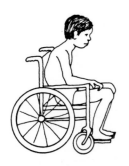

LESS APPROPRIATE

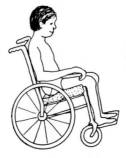

MORE APPROPRIATE

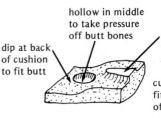

hollow in middle to take pressure off butt bones

dip at back of cushion to fit butt

raised sections to hold legs apart

curved bottom to fit sag in seat of wheelchair

If possible, make cushion out of 'micropore' foam rubber (foam with very tiny bubbles). Rubber-coated coconut fiber also works well.

For more suggestions for wheelchair adaptations, see Chapters 64 and 65. For more ideas on cushions, see p. 199 and 200.

EARLY PHYSICAL RE-EDUCATION

The goal for a spinal cord injured person is to become as independent as possible in doing what he or she wants and needs to do. But even before the skills of daily living are relearned, the person needs to **learn to protect the body where functions that used to be automatic have been lost.** The protective functions that may be lost or changed include:

1. Adjustment of blood pressure to changes in body position.
2. Feeling (including pain) that protects from injuries (such as bed sores).
3. Sense of body position and ability to keep balance.
4. Muscle strength and coordination.
5. Control of body temperature—especially keeping cool in hot weather.

1. **A sudden drop of blood pressure in the brain when the person rises** from lying to sitting, or sitting to standing, can cause dizziness or fainting. This is a common problem in spinal cord injury because the blood pressure adjustment mechanism is partly lost. Little by little the body can be helped to re-adapt, but precautions are needed. (These same precautions are for anyone who has been kept lying down a long time.)

Before beginning to sit, raise the head of the bed— a little more and a little longer each day.

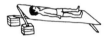

Start like this for 15 minutes.

In a week or 2 build up to this for 3 hours.

Lifting exercises help the body relearn to adjust blood pressure— and also prevent bed sores and strengthen arms.

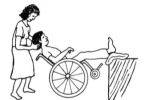

If the person begins to get dizzy or faint when sitting, tilt him back and lift his feet.

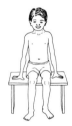

Before beginning to stand, make a standing board, and strap the child to it. Start at a low angle, and stand the board up more—and longer—each day.

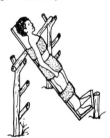

2. **The loss of feeling** in parts of the body can lead to **pressure sores and other injuries,** such as burns and cuts. This is because the body no longer feels pain and does not warn the child to change position or move away from danger.

It is important that the child learn to protect himself by changing positions often and avoiding injuries. This includes:

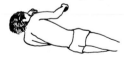

• learning to roll over

• turning at least every 4 hours when lying or sleeping

• lifting from sitting every 15 minutes (see p. 198)

• examining the whole body every day for signs of injuries or sores

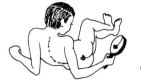

• washing daily

• learning to protect himself from burns and other injuries. For example,

NO!

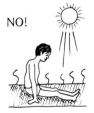

DO NOT sit on or touch hot objects (or roads).

NO!

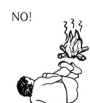

DO NOT sit, lie or sleep near an open fire.

Keeping clean is very important for persons with reduced feeling, especially if they lack bladder and bowel control. Take care to bathe daily. **Wash and dry the genitals, the butt, and between the legs as soon as possible each time they get wet or dirty.**

If redness, diaper rash, or sores develop, **wash more often** and **keep the sore area dry.** Keep the legs spread open and exposed to the air. When they must be covered, use soft absorbent cotton cloth. Putting a little vinegar in the rinse water after bathing the child, and after washing diapers and underclothes, helps prevent skin rash and *infection.*

For treatment of specific skin infections (fungus, yeast, bacteria) consult a health worker or a medical book (like *Where There Is No Doctor,* see Chapter 15).

3. **Loss of ability to sense what position the body is in** affects a person's sense of balance. So does loss of muscle control. The child needs to develop new ways to sense the position of his body and keep his balance. Start with the child sitting on a bench, if possible, in front of a mirror.

Help the child progress through these stages:

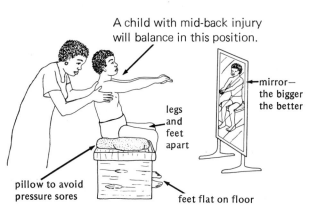

A child with mid-back injury will balance in this position.

mirror— the bigger the better

legs and feet apart

pillow to avoid pressure sores

feet flat on floor

- both hands on bench

- both hands on knees

- lift one arm sideways, forward, and back

- After doing this in front of a mirror, have him do it without the mirror.

- As the child gains better balance, start doing different movements with first one and then both arms, such as lifting weights or playing ball.

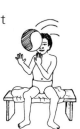

Note: Some children may have so much difficulty with balance that they may have to start in a wheelchair or a chair with high back and arm supports.

4. **Muscle re-education** All muscles that still work need to be as strong as possible to make up for those that are paralyzed. Most important are muscles around the shoulders, arms, and stomach.

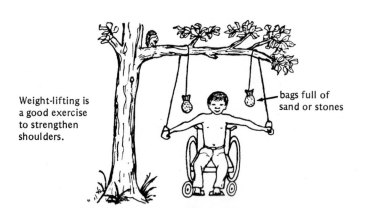

Weight-lifting is a good exercise to strengthen shoulders.

bags full of sand or stones

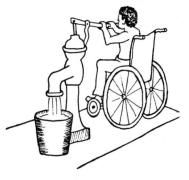

Look for ways to make the exercises useful and fun.

5. **Temperature control** Normally, when a person feels hot, he sweats and the blood vessels beneath the skin swell. This automatic cooling system is partly lost in persons with high spinal cord injury. In hot weather, they may get high fever or can even die of heat stroke.

For this reason they must learn (and be allowed) to rest quietly in the shade, in the coolest place possible, during the hottest part of the day.

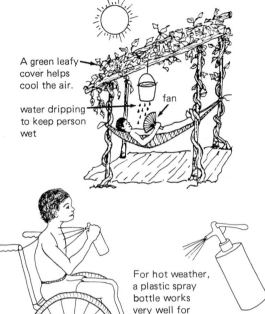

A green leafy cover helps cool the air.

water dripping to keep person wet

fan

For hot weather, a plastic spray bottle works very well for cooling the body.

Children with spinal cord injury can learn to paddle around very well in old tire tubes. They love it, and it is excellent arm and shoulder exercise. **However, it is very important that someone watches them.**

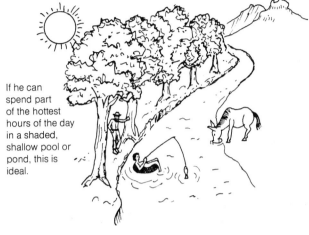

If he can spend part of the hottest hours of the day in a shaded, shallow pool or pond, this is ideal.

TAKE CARE also to **protect against cold.** Body temperature can also drop too low.

DYSREFLEXIA (Sudden high blood pressure with pounding headaches)

Persons with quadriplegia or very high paraplegia run the risk of 'dysreflexia'—or sudden, dangerous increase in blood pressure with severe pounding headaches.

Dysreflexia is the body's reaction to something that would normally cause pain or irritation, but which the person does not feel because of the spinal cord injury.

COMMON CAUSES OF DYSREFLEXIA

- **bladder problems**—especially when the bladder is too full, infected, or has bladder stones (This is by far the most common cause.)

- **stretching of the bowel**—from constipation, with a big ball of hard shit, or from finger pressure to remove the shit

- **pressure areas or sores**—or even irritation from lying on a small object without knowing it

- **burns**

- **spasm of the womb**—especially just before or in the first days of a woman's monthly period, or during childbirth

SIGNS (OF DYSREFLEXIA)

- severe pounding headache
- sweating of the head
- stuffy nose
- reddish skin patches on face and neck
- goose pimples above the level of injury
- slow pulse
- high blood pressure (up to 240/150)

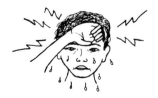

> **Dysreflexia is a medical emergency.** The high blood pressure could cause fits or deadly bleeding inside the brain.

What to do

Act quickly to remove the cause and lower the blood pressure.

- Quickly lower the blood pressure in the head.
  - If lying, sit up; stay sitting until the signs go away.

  - Change position, drop feet down, loosen belt or straps, remove tight stockings.

- Look for the cause of dysreflexia, and remove it if possible.
  - **Bladder.** Feel the lower belly to see if the bladder is full. **If a catheter is in place,** check for bends or kinks and straighten them to let urine flow. If the catheter is stopped up, open it by injecting 30 cc. of boiled and cooled water (or sterile saline solution) into the catheter. Or take the catheter out. **If a catheter is not in place** and the person cannot pee, put in a catheter and empty the bladder (see p. 206).

  - If a **urinary infection** appears to be the cause, inject an anesthetic solution into the bladder through a catheter. Use 10 cc. 1% lidocaine in 20 cc. of boiled water. Clamp the catheter for 20 minutes and then release. Treat the infection (see p. 210).

    Bowel. If the bladder does not seem to be the cause, check for a full bowel. How long has it been since the last bowel movement (shit)? Put some lidocaine *(Xylocaine)* jelly on your finger and check if the bowel is packed with hard shit. If it is, put in more lidocaine jelly. Wait 15 minutes, or until the headache becomes less. Then gently remove the shit with your finger.

  - **Pressure.** Change the child's position in order to relieve pressure over bony areas. (Sometimes just staying in the same position too long can bring on dysreflexia.)

- If the signs do not go away, get medical help as fast as possible.

- If the child has frequent or severe periods of dysreflexia, or you cannot find the cause, try to have him seen by a specialist on spinal cord injury, and possibly a 'urologist' (specialist of the urine system).

> *Suggestion:* For quadriplegics in villages, it is wise to have injectable 1% lidocaine (Xylocaine) and lidocaine gel available for dysreflexia emergencies.

Self-care

With help and encouragement of family, friends and *rehabilitation* workers, the child with spinal cord injury can learn to become as independent as possible in meeting his basic needs: **moving about, eating, bathing, dressing, toileting,** and in time **other skills for daily living.**

Progress toward self-care, especially at first, may be slow and frustrating. The child will need a lot of understanding and encouragement. Persons with low spinal cord injury will find it easier to relearn self-care skills than those with higher injuries who have less use of their hands and arms. Quadriplegics usually will remain at least partly dependent on others for some of their daily activities. To make activities easier both for themselves and their helper, it is important that they **avoid getting fat.**

Useful methods and techniques have been worked out for helping relearn basic skills. We cannot describe many of these in detail. However, much depends on determination, imagination, and common sense. Start with first things first—like rolling over and sitting up in bed.

A few **simple aids** can often help a person become more independent. For example,

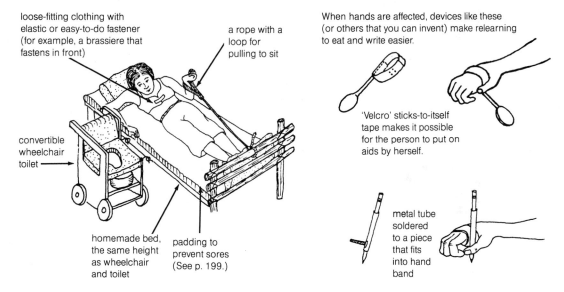

loose-fitting clothing with elastic or easy-to-do fastener (for example, a brassiere that fastens in front)

a rope with a loop for pulling to sit

When hands are affected, devices like these (or others that you can invent) make relearning to eat and write easier.

convertible wheelchair toilet →

'Velcro' sticks-to-itself tape makes it possible for the person to put on aids by herself.

homemade bed, the same height as wheelchair and toilet

padding to prevent sores (See p. 199.)

metal tube soldered to a piece that fits into hand band

For additional ideas of aids for self-care, see pages 571 to 578. Suggestions for getting in and out of wheelchairs and learning to walk with crutches are included in Chapter 43.

KEEPING ACTIVE

Many of the 'complications' of spinal cord injury happen because the person spends a lot of time just lying and sitting. To keep healthy, the body needs to keep active. Lack of movement and activity causes poor flow of the blood. This can lead to pressure sores, swollen feet, painful or dangerous blood clots (thrombosis) especially in the legs, increasing weakness of bones (osteoporosis) with risk of breaking them, stones in the bladder or kidneys, increased risk of urinary infections, and general physical weakness and poor health.

TO STAY HEALTHY
KEEP ACTIVE

It is important—both for the body and mind—that spinal cord injured persons keep physically active. Let your child do as much for herself as she can: pushing her own wheelchair, bathing, transferring, washing clothes, cleaning house, and helping with work.

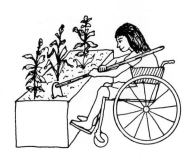

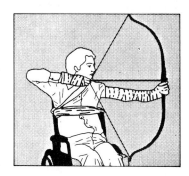

Active games and sports can also be encouraged. **Swimming, basketball,** and **archery** can be done well with upper body use only. Quadriplegics can become skillful with bow and arrow by using a straight-arm splint and a special hook, fastened to the hand, to pull the string.

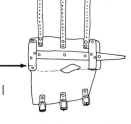

(*Note:* Archery may also help correct spinal curve. The arm that pulls the string should be on the side with bulge in the back.)

To keep leg bones growing well and to prevent them from becoming weak and breaking easily, even children who may always be wheelchair riders should stand for a while every day. Standing also helps the child's bowels move more often.

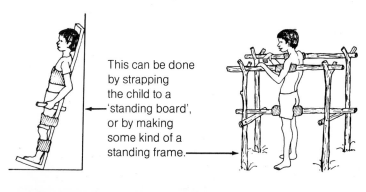

This can be done by strapping the child to a 'standing board', or by making some kind of a standing frame.

This standing frame was invented by a paraplegic youth and his father. The boy uses the spasticity in his legs to stand. When the muscles tire he hangs and sits on the padded poles.

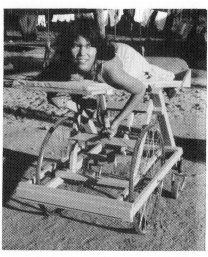

This design for a standing wheel-bed allows a spinal cord injured child with pressure sores on her butt to actively move about. The child can adjust it while on it, from a flat-lying position to a near-standing position. It can be made out of wood or metal.

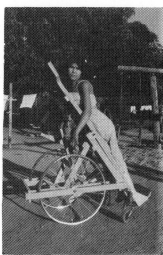

Spinal cord injured persons as leaders

Spinal cord injured persons in various countries are now taking the lead in making new lives for themselves and in getting their communities to recognize their abilities. Examples of 2 programs run primarily by spinal cord injured persons are included in Chapter 55. These are the Organization of Disabled Revolutionaries in Nicaragua (p. 519) and the Centre for the Rehabilitation of the Paralysed in Bangladesh (p. 518). Members of these and many similar organizations would be happy to share ideas and suggestions with any group of disabled persons interested in organizing their own program or shop.

OTHER PARTS OF THIS BOOK WITH INFORMATION USEFUL FOR SPINAL CORD INJURY

> *IMPORTANT:* In addition to this chapter, some essential information for spinal cord injury is in other parts of this book, especially Chapter 24, **"Pressure Sores,"** and Chapter 25, **"Urine and Bowel Management."** These chapters are a continuation of information on spinal cord injury. We have put them in separate chapters because the information they cover is also essential for other disabilities.

Chapters marked with a star (*) are **essential for basic care of spinal cord injury.**

For other references to spinal cord injury, see the INDEX, p. 652, and the books and reference materials listed on p. 638.

THE STORY OF JÉSICA

Jésica is a little girl who was paralyzed because of an unnecessary injection she received when she was 3 days old. Her mother does not know why or with what she was injected. This is the story of her rehabilitation at PROJIMO.

The injection resulted in an infection that reached her spine, and permanently paralyzed her legs.

scar from infection

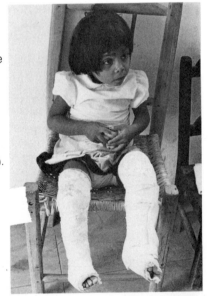

Misuse of medicines and especially injections is a common and preventable cause of disability. See Chapter 3.

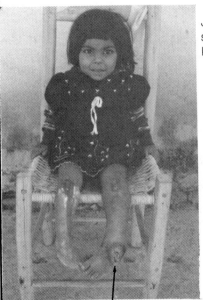

pressure sore

Jésica's feet became clubbed. When she tried to stand, she developed large, infected pressure sores on her knees and feet.

When Jésica first came to PROJIMO at age 4, the village team first treated the infected sores. Then they began to cast her feet to gradually straighten them (see Chapter 60).

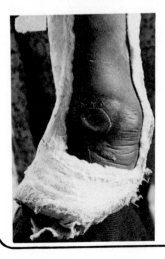

They left 'windows' in the casts to keep treating the sores.

Little by little the sores healed and Jésica's feet straightened. Here one of the workers changes her cast.

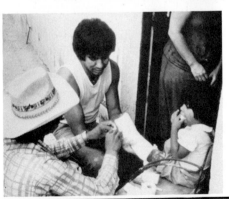

Jésica also lacks normal bowel and bladder control. From the uncontrolled loss of urine, she developed pressure sores in her genital area. Vania, an 8-year-old paraplegic girl, helped treat Jésica's sores. She also assisted Jésica with a 'bowel program', which helps her 'time' her bowel movements (see picture on p. 212). This makes daily activities and going to school much easier.

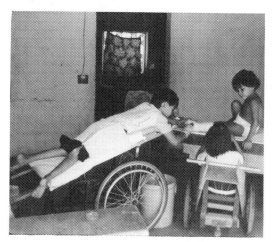

Vania treats the pressure sore on Jésica's foot.

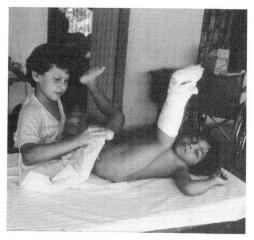

Here Vania cleans and dresses sores on Jésica's genital area.

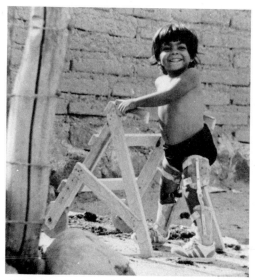

When her feet were straighter, the village workers made above-knee braces for her and a simple wood walker. In a few weeks Jésica was walking.

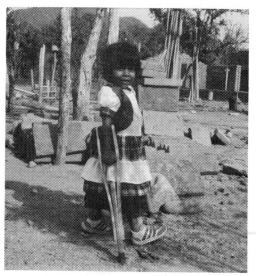

With practice Jésica was able to walk with crutches—and finally with only her braces.

Jesica now goes to school in the village. Seeing disabled persons at PROJIMO who were happy, active, and accepted in the community has given Jésica a more hopeful, confident, and adventurous outlook on life.

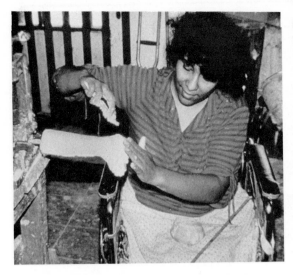

Mari, who is paraplegic, is one of the leaders of the PROJIMO team. Here she works on a cast for making a plastic brace. See her story on page 403.

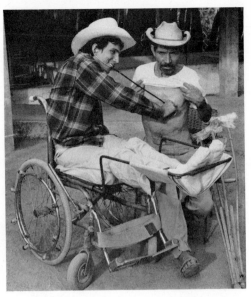

Victor, a young doctor, became quadriplegic in a traffic accident. He could do nothing for himself when he came to PROJIMO. The village workers helped him gain strength and develop many skills. Soon he became a member of the PROJIMO team and became the village doctor.

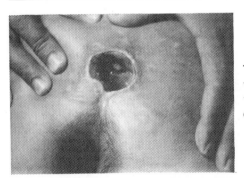

This pressure sore, at the base of the spine in a young man with quadriplegia, was present for 2 years. It was 15 cm across under the skin, and had completely destroyed the lower part of his spine.

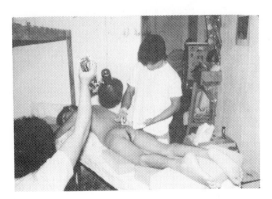

Village workers at PROJIMO clean and dress the pressure sore.

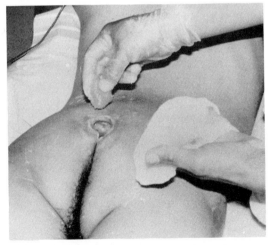

Here one of the workers packs the sore with a paste of sugar and honey. With this treatment 2 times each day, the sore stayed clean and free of infection, and healed rapidly (in about 6 months).

CHAPTER **24**

Pressure Sores

WHAT ARE THEY?

Pressure sores, or 'bed sores', are sores that form over bony parts of the body when a person lies or sits on that part of the body for too long without moving. Where

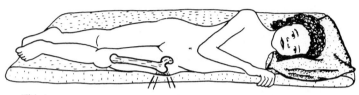

This is a common pressure sore point— over the top of the thigh bone.

the skin is pressed against the bed or chair, the blood vessels are squeezed shut so that the blood cannot bring air to the skin and flesh. If too much time passes without moving or rolling over, the skin and flesh in that spot can be injured or die. First a red or dark patch appears. And if the pressure continues, an open sore can form. The sore may start on the skin and work in. Or it may start in deep near the bone and gradually work its way to the surface.

Who is likely to get pressure sores?

When a normal healthy person lies or sits in one position for a long time, it begins to feel uncomfortable, or to hurt. So she moves or rolls over, and pressure sores are avoided. People most likely to get pressure sores are:

1. persons who are so **ill, weak,** or **disabled** that they cannot roll over by themselves. This includes persons *severely disabled* from **polio, brain damage, advanced muscular dystrophy,** or **a bad injury.**

2. persons who **have no feeling** in parts of their body, who do not feel the warnings of pain or discomfort when their body is being damaged. This includes persons with **spinal cord injury, spina bifida,** and **leprosy.**

> *WARNING:* **Because persons with spinal cord injury are at first unable to turn over, and also have lost the ability to feel in parts of their bodies, they are at very high risk for pressure sores.**

3. persons who have a **plaster cast** on an arm or leg (to correct a *contracture* or to heal a broken bone), when the plaster presses over a bony spot. At first the pressure will hurt and the child may cry or complain. But in time the spot will grow numb and the child will stop complaining—although a sore may be forming.

The risk is greater when using casts on children who have no feeling in their feet. On these children, even a corrective shoe or brace can easily cause a pressure sore— unless great care is taken.

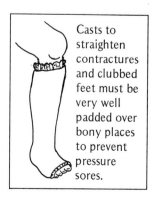

Casts to straighten contractures and clubbed feet must be very well padded over bony places to prevent pressure sores.

Where are pressure sores most likely to form?

They can form over any bony area. The places where they form most often are shown in the pictures.

The points of highest risk, all on the hips, are marked in CAPITAL LETTERS.

common sites of sores in feet that have lost feeling

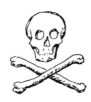

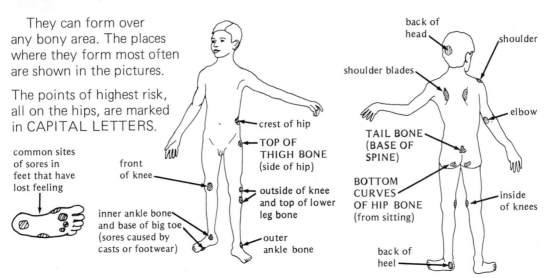

front of knee

crest of hip

TOP OF THIGH BONE (side of hip)

outside of knee and top of lower leg bone

inner ankle bone and base of big toe (sores caused by casts or footwear)

outer ankle bone

back of head

shoulder

shoulder blades

TAIL BONE (BASE OF SPINE)

elbow

BOTTOM CURVES OF HIP BONE (from sitting)

inside of knees

back of heel

How dangerous are they?

Pressure sores, if not very carefully cared for, can become large and deep. Because they contain dead skin and flesh, they easily become *infected.* If a sore reaches the bone, which it often does, the bone can also become infected. Bone infections are often very hard (and costly) to cure, may last for years, and may keep coming back, even after the original pressure sore has healed. (See "Bone Infections," Chapter 19.) Bone infections can lead to severe disabling deformities.

Infections in deep pressure sores often get into the blood and affect the whole body, causing fever and general illness. This can lead to death. In fact, **pressure sores are one of the main causes of death in persons with spinal cord injury.**

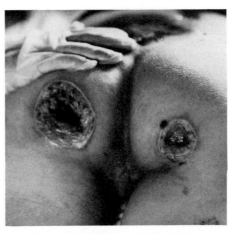

These pressure sores in a 15-year-old girl who is quadriplegic were treated with honey and sugar and healed in 2 months. (See p. 202.) PROJIMO

In persons with high spinal cord injuries (quadriplegia) the irritation from pressure sores can also bring about sudden severe headaches and high blood pressure (dysreflexia, see p. 187), which can also cause death.

How common are pressure sores?

In persons who have lost feeling in parts of their body, pressure sores are **very common.** Most spinal cord injured persons in rich countries, and nearly all in poor countries, develop pressure sores. Often the sores start in hospitals shortly after the back injury, due to **inadequate nursing care.** Therefore, **it is important that families of spinal cord injured persons, and the persons themselves, learn as early as possible about the prevention and early treatment of pressure sores, and take all the needed steps.**

PREVENTION OF PRESSURE SORES

> **It is important that both the child and family learn about the risk of pressure sores and how to prevent them.**

- **Avoid staying in the same position** for very long. **When lying down,** turn from side to side or front to back at least every 2 hours (or up to 4 hours if padding and cushioning are excellent). **When sitting,** lift body up and change position every 10 or 15 minutes.

- Use **thick, soft padding,** pillows, or other forms of cushion arranged so as to protect bony areas of the body. (For cushion designs, see p. 199 and 200.)

- Use **soft, clean, dry bed sheets.** Try to avoid wrinkles. Change bedding or clothing every day and each time the bedding gets wet or dirtied. **A person who stays wet gets pressure sores—especially if it is from urine.**

- **Bathe** the child daily. Dry the skin well by patting, not rubbing. It is probably best not to use body creams or oils, or talc, except on the hands and feet to prevent cracking, as these soften the skin and make it weaker. *Never* use heat-producing oils, lotions, or alcohol.

- **Examine the whole body** carefully every day, checking especially those areas where sores are most likely to occur. If any redness or darkness is present, take added care to prevent all pressure over this area until the skin returns to normal.

- **Good nutrition** is important for preventing pressure sores. Be sure the child gets enough to eat (but do not let her get fat). Give her plenty of fruits, vegetables, and foods with protein (beans, lentils, eggs, meat, fish, and milk products). If the child looks pale, check for signs of anemia (see p. 320) and be sure she gets iron-rich foods (meat, eggs, and dark green leafy vegetables) or takes iron pills (ferrous sulphate) and vitamin C (oranges, lemons, tomatoes, etc.)

- As much as is possible, the child should learn to examine her own body for pressure sores every day and take responsibility for all the necessary preventive measures herself.

Other precautions

- To avoid pressure sores or other injuries on feet that do not feel, use well-fitted, well-padded sandals or shoes. These and other precautions are discussed under "Spina Bifida" (p. 173) and "Leprosy" (p. 224).

- To avoid pressure sores when straightening limbs with casts, put extra padding over bony spots before casting and do not press on these spots as the cast hardens. Listen to the child when he says it hurts, and check *where* it hurts.

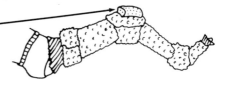

If it hurts in these spots, it is probably the tight *cord (tendon).* A little pain is normal with stretching, but if it hurts a lot, examine it.

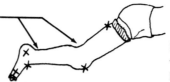

If it hurts in one of the spots marked with an X, it may be a pressure sore. Remove the cast and see.

Changing positions

When a child has recently had a spinal cord injury, he must be turned regularly, taking great care not to bend his back.

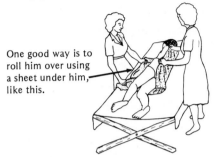

One good way is to roll him over using a sheet under him, like this.

As the child gets stronger, hang loops and provide other aids, if needed, so she can learn to turn herself.

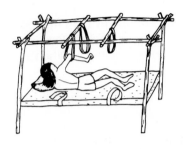

At first it is important that the person turn, or be turned, at least **every 2 hours,** day and night. Later, if there are no signs of pressure sores, the time between turns can gradually be lengthened to **4 hours.** To avoid sleeping through the night without turning, an alarm clock can be a big help.

When the child begins to sit or use a wheelchair, there is a new serious danger of pressure sores. **The child must get into the habit of taking the pressure off his butt every few minutes.**

Juan has strong arms. He can lift up his whole body and hold it up for a minute or two. This lets the blood circulate in the butt.

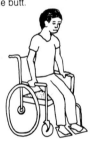

José's arms are weak. He takes the pressure off his butt by leaning his whole body over the armrest, first on one side, and then on the other.

When doing this, one buttock lifts in the air.

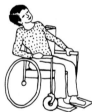

Carlota has a wheelchair with a low back, so she can lean back and lift her hips off the seat.

If the chair has no armrests, or they can be removed, the child can lie sideways over a pillow on a high bed. He can rest for 15 to 30 minutes like this.

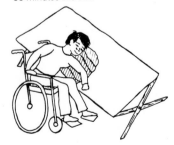

If he has very little arm and body control, he can put his feet on the floor (with help if needed) and lean forward with his chest on his knees. This takes the pressure off his butt.

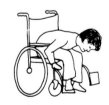

Or have someone tip his chair backward for one minute or more. For a longer 'nap' that rests the butt, someone can tip his chair backward onto a cot.

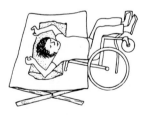

To prevent pressure sores when sitting, take the weight off your butt for one whole minute at least once every 15 minutes!

Padding and cushions for lying

To prevent pressure sores, it is essential that the person who has lost feeling lie and sit on a soft surface that reduces pressure on bony areas.

- It is best to lie on a flat surface with a **thick, spongy mattress.**

A thick **foam rubber** mattress often works well. However, some foam is so spongy that it sinks completely down under weight. Then the bony area is not protected from the hard board. A firm sponge with very small air bubbles **(microcell rubber)** works well, but is expensive.

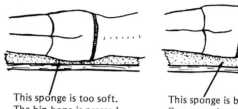

This sponge is too soft. The hip bone is pressed against the board below.

This sponge is better. It is firm enough to keep the hip bone off the board below.

A 'waterbed' (bag-like mattress filled with water) or air mattress also works well.

In some countries, an excellent mattress material is made of rubber-coated coconut fiber. Urine can be washed out by pouring water through it. Because this material is costly, a *rehabilitation* program in Bangladesh cuts a square out of a cheap mattress and fits in a square of the coconut fiber sponge.

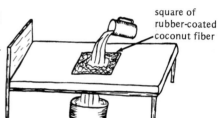

square of rubber-coated coconut fiber

- Careful placement of **pillows, pads,** or **soft, folded blankets** can also help prevent pressure sores. These are especially important in the first weeks or months after a spinal cord injury when the person must lie flat and be moved as little as possible. Pillows should be placed to avoid pressure on bony places, and to keep the person in a position that is healthy and that helps prevent contractures.

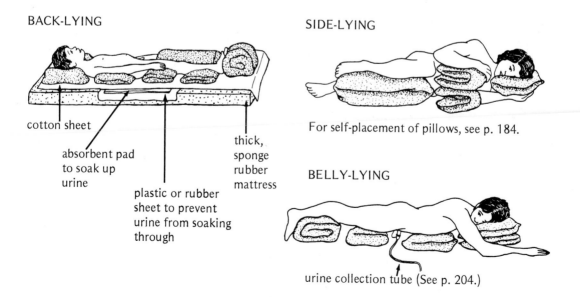

BACK-LYING

cotton sheet

absorbent pad to soak up urine

plastic or rubber sheet to prevent urine from soaking through

thick, sponge rubber mattress

SIDE-LYING

For self-placement of pillows, see p. 184.

BELLY-LYING

urine collection tube (See p. 204.)

Chair and wheelchair cushions

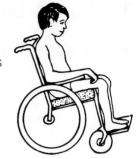

For the child who has lost feeling in his butt, the type of seat cushion he uses is very important—especially if his *paralysis* makes it difficult to lift up or change positions.

All spinal cord injured persons should use a good cushion. Sitting directly on a canvas or a poorly padded wood seat causes pressure sores.

Special cushions are made with 'soft spots' of an almost-liquid 'silicone gel' in the areas of greatest pressure. However, these cushions are very expensive. Also, the gel may get too soft and liquid in hot weather.

Good cushions can be made of **'microcell' rubber,** which is fairly firm. It works best if it is cut and shaped to reduce pressure on bony areas:

A good, low-cost way to make a fitted cushion is to build a base out of many layers of **thick cardboard** glued together. Cover it with a 2 or 3 cm.-thick layer of sponge rubber.

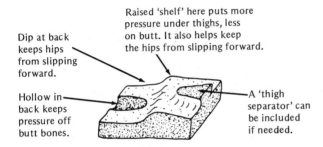

Dip at back keeps hips from slipping forward.

Raised 'shelf' here puts more pressure under thighs, less on butt. It also helps keep the hips from slipping forward.

Hollow in back keeps pressure off butt bones.

A 'thigh separator' can be included if needed.

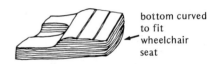

bottom curved to fit wheelchair seat

Wet the cardboard and sit on it wet for 2 hours, so it forms to the shape of the butt. Then let it dry, and varnish it.

Before making a specially-fitted cushion, you can make a 'mold' of the person's butt by having him sit in a shallow container of soft clay, mud, or plaster. Note the bony hollows and form the seat to fit them.

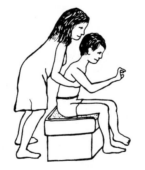

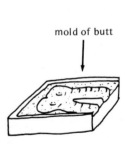

mold of butt

Air cushions made from **bicycle inner tubes** are excellent for prevention of pressure sores, and for bathing on a hard surface. Use 1, 2 or more tubes, depending on size of tube and size of child.

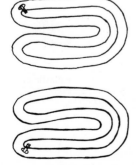

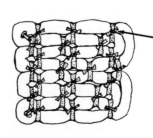

Bind loops of the tubes together with thin straps of inner tube.

Pump in enough air so that the whole butt is held up by air.

(Idea from wheelchair rider-builders at Tahanan Walang Hagdanang (House With No Stairs), Quezon City, Philippines)

TREATMENT OF PRESSURE SORES

Watch for the first signs of a pressure sore by examining the whole body every day. Teach the child to do this using a mirror.

If early signs of a sore appear (redness, darkness, swelling, or open skin), change body positions and use padding to protect that area from pressure.

For larger areas (like the bones near the base of the spine), you can try using a small (motor scooter) inner tube to keep weight off the sore area. Put a towel over the tube to soak up sweat. (Sweaty skin against the rubber can also cause sores.)

WARNING: For small areas such as heels, *never* use a ring or 'donut' of cloth to keep weight off the sore. This can cut off blood supply to the skin inside the ring and make the sore worse.   NO!

IF A PRESSURE SORE HAS ALREADY FORMED:

- **Keep pressure off the sore area** completely and continuously.

- **Keep the area completely clean.** Wash it gently with clean or boiled water twice a day. Do *not* use alcohol, iodine, merthiolate, or other strong antiseptics.

- **Eat well.** If lots of liquid comes out of the sore, a lot of protein and iron are lost with it. These must be replaced for quicker healing. Also take iron pills if signs of anemia are present. Eat foods rich in protein: beans, lentils, eggs, meat, fish, milk products.

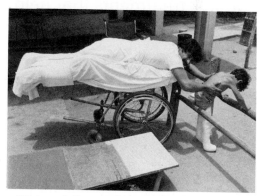

This paraplegic young man has a large pressure sore on his butt. Until it heals, he must not sit. Village rehabilitation workers made this wheel lying cart for him to move about on. Here he helps a boy learn to walk. (Photo, John Fago.)

- **Do not rub or massage** areas where pressure sores might be forming. This could tear weakened flesh and make the sore inside bigger.

IF A SORE IS DEEP AND HAS A LOT OF DEAD FLESH:

- Clean the sore 3 times a day.

- Each time, try to scrape and pick out more of the dead rotten flesh. Often, you will find the sore is much bigger inside than you first thought. It may go deep under the edges of the skin. Little by little remove the dead flesh until you come to healthy red flesh (or bone!).

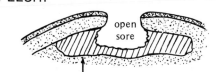

open sore

Dead flesh—may be gray, black, greenish, or yellowish. It may have a bad smell if infected.

- Each time after cleaning out the dead flesh, wash the sore out well with soapy water. Use liquid surgical soap if possible. Then rinse with clean (boiled and cooled) water.

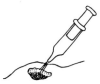

A large plastic or glass syringe works well for washing out the sore. Wash the syringe well with soap and water after each use.

If the sore is infected (pus, bad smell, swelling, redness, hot area around the sore, or the person has fevers and chills), get help from an experienced health worker and:

- Clean out the sore 3 times a day as described.
- If possible, take the person to a 'clinical laboratory' for a 'culture' to find out what germs are causing the infection and what medicine will fight it best.
- If a 'culture' is not possible, try treating the person with penicillin, tetracycline, or (if possible) dicloxacillin. (See WTND, p. 351.)

If the sore does not get better, or keeps draining liquid or pus from a deep hole, the bone may be infected. In this case, special studies, treatment, and possible surgery may be needed. Try to take the person to a capable medical center. (See Chapter 19.)

Things to remember when dressing a sore

Wear clean gloves while cleaning or filling the pressure sore, applying new bandages, and disposing of the used bandages. Put used bandages into a plastic bag and burn or bury it. See p. 160 for information on handling anything with blood or body fluids on it.

Two folk treatments that help in curing pressure sores

PAPAYA (PAW PAW)

Papaya has enzymes (chemicals) that digest dead flesh. Cooks use it to soften meat. The same enzymes can help soften the dead flesh in a pressure sore, and make it easier to remove. First clean and wash out a pressure sore that has dead flesh in it. Then soak a sterile cloth or gauze with 'milk' from the trunk or green fruit of a papaya plant and pack this into the sore. Repeat cleaning and repacking 3 times a day.

HONEY AND SUGAR

Once a pressure sore is free of dead flesh, filling it 2 to 3 times a day with honey or sugar helps prevent infection and speeds healing. This treatment, used by the ancient Egyptians and recently rediscovered by modern doctors, works remarkably well. It is now being used in some American and British hospitals.

To make filling the sore easier, mix honey with ordinary sugar until it forms a thick paste. This can easily be pressed deep into the sore. Cover the sore with a thick gauze bandage.

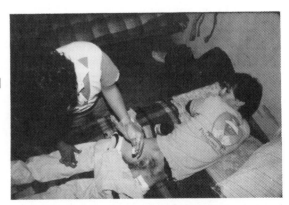

A village rehabilitation worker treats a young man's pressure sores with a paste made by mixing honey and sugar.

CAUTION: It is important to clean out and refill the sore at least 2 times a day. If the honey or sugar becomes too diluted with liquid from the sore, it will feed germs rather than kill them.

Molasses can also be used. In Colombia, South America, doctors shave thin pieces off blocks of raw sugar and put these into the sore.

Urine and Bowel Management

CHAPTER **25**

With Spinal Cord Injury and Spina Bifida

Most persons with *spinal cord* injury or spina bifida do not have normal *bladder* or *bowel* control (control for peeing and shitting). This loss of control can be inconvenient, embarrassing, and cause social and emotional difficulties. Also, the loss of control can cause skin problems and dangerous urinary *infections.* For these reasons, it is important to learn ways to stay clean, dry, and healthy. Most of the methods are not difficult, so children should be able to do it themselves. This will help them feel more self-reliant.

URINE MANAGEMENT

The main goals of urine management are:

1. to prevent urinary infection, and
2. self-care in staying as dry as possible.

Prevention of urinary infection is extremely important. **Infections of the urinary system (bladder and kidneys) are very common in both spinal cord injury and spina bifida, and are one of the main causes of early death.** Therefore, any method used for self-care or staying dry must also help prevent urinary infections. Make every effort to prevent germs from getting into the bladder. **Keeping clean is essential.** Also, it is important to empty the bladder regularly as completely as possible. If some urine stays in the bladder, bacteria will grow in it and cause infection.

> The ideal method of urine control empties the bladder completely and in a clean, regular, easy, and self-reliant way.

Different methods work best for different persons—depending mostly on what 'type' of bladder a person has. We discuss this on the next page.

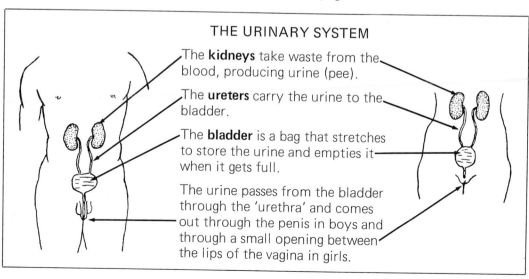

THE URINARY SYSTEM

The **kidneys** take waste from the blood, producing urine (pee).

The **ureters** carry the urine to the bladder.

The **bladder** is a bag that stretches to store the urine and empties it when it gets full.

The urine passes from the bladder through the 'urethra' and comes out through the penis in boys and through a small opening between the lips of the vagina in girls.

'Types' of bladder—in persons whose feeling and control have been partly or completely lost.

AUTOMATIC BLADDER: A person with *paralysis* whose legs have 'reflex spasms' (uncontrolled stiffening or jerking) usually also has reflex spasms in his bladder. As the bladder fills with urine, the walls of the bladder stretch and cause a reflex spasm. As the bladder squeezes, the muscles that hold back the urine relax, letting the urine flow out. This is called an 'automatic bladder' because it empties automatically when it gets full.

LIMP BLADDER (flaccid bladder): When a person's paralyzed legs are limp and do not have spasms, usually the bladder is also limp, or flaccid. No matter how much urine fills the bladder, it will not squeeze to empty. The bladder stretches until it cannot hold any more and the urine begins to drip out. The bladder does not completely empty this way. Some urine stays in the bladder, increasing the chance of infection.

The most simple methods of bladder management work well with an automatic bladder but do not work with a limp bladder. So **try to figure out which type of bladder a child has.**

For the first few days or weeks after the spinal cord has been injured, the bladder is almost always limp. Urine either drips out or does not come out at all. Then, as the 'spinal shock' wears off, persons with higher back injuries (above the 2nd lumbar vertebra, see p. 176) usually develop automatic bladders. In persons with lower back injuries, the bladder usually stays limp.

During the first weeks, usually a 'Foley catheter' is kept in the bladder all the time. However, after about 2 weeks, it is a good idea to test how the bladder works by removing the catheter and trying one of the methods described in this chapter. If the person is often wet, try another method for that type of bladder.

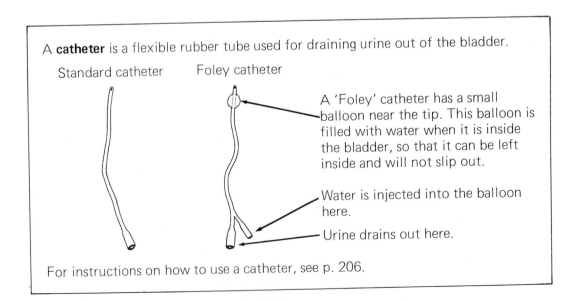

A **catheter** is a flexible rubber tube used for draining urine out of the bladder.

Standard catheter   Foley catheter

A 'Foley' catheter has a small balloon near the tip. This balloon is filled with water when it is inside the bladder, so that it can be left inside and will not slip out.

Water is injected into the balloon here.

Urine drains out here.

For instructions on how to use a catheter, see p. 206.

Methods for automatic bladder

1. **TRIGGERING:** This method usually causes the bladder-emptying reflex to work when the person is ready to pee. It can be done using a urinal, toilet, potty or jar. **This is the first method to try** because nothing is put into the bladder. It is easy, so a child can do it alone.

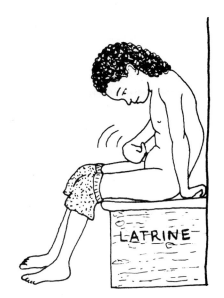

- Tap the lower belly (over the bladder) firmly with your hand for about 1 minute. Stop and wait for the urine to come.

- Tap again. Repeat several times until no more urine flows.

If possible, once a week after triggering use a catheter to see how much urine is left. If there is less than a cupful (150 cc.), continue the triggering program. If there is more than a cupful on several occasions, then the bladder is not emptying well enough. Try another method.

2. **PERIODIC USE OF A CATHETER:** This method allows the bladder to be emptied completely before becoming too full. Sometimes it can be used to prepare the body for triggering. Put a clean or sterile standard catheter into the bladder every 4 to 6 hours to empty the urine.

For instructions on how to put in a catheter, see the next page.

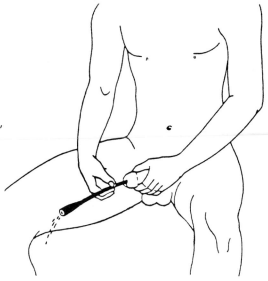

> *CAUTION:* If you drink more liquid than usual, put in the catheter more frequently to keep the bladder from stretching too much.

Note: To reduce risk of urinary infections, **regular frequent use of the catheter is more important than using a sterile catheter.** It is a mistake to stop using the catheter only because you don't have a chance to boil it (for example, when traveling, or at school). Just wash out the catheter with clean drinkable water after use, and keep it in a clean jar or towel. **(Do not go too long without catheterizing, and do not stop catheterizing altogether.** It is important for your bladder not to interrupt your program.

How to put in a catheter

Health workers and parents can easily be taught to put in a catheter. With a little practice, paraplegic and some quadriplegic children can also learn.

Note: The best catheter size is usually from #8 or #10 for a small child to #14 or #16 for a large child.

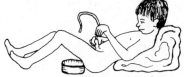

Children as young as age 5 can learn to catheterize themselves.

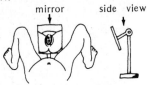

A mirror can help girls to find the urine hole.

Note: The great care with cleanliness shown here (boiling the catheter, wearing gloves) is important when using a fixed (Foley) catheter. However, for periodic use of a regular catheter, a *clean* rather than *sterile* technique is more practical (and therefore may be safer). Wash the catheter well with clean water after each use and keep it in a clean container. Wash your hands well before using it. See note on p. 205.

---

1. If possible boil the catheter (and any syringe or instrument you may be using) for 15 minutes, or at least wash them well and keep them clean.

2. Bathe well (at least daily). Wash well under foreskin or between vaginal lips and surrounding areas.

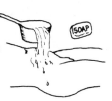

3. Wash hands with soap. After washing touch only things that are sterile or very clean.

4. Put very clean cloths under and around the area.

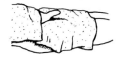

5. Put on sterile gloves— or rub hands well with alcohol or surgical soap.

6. Cover the catheter with a lubricant (slippery cream) like *K-Y Jelly* that dissolves in water (not oil or *Vaseline*).

7. **Pull back foreskin or open the vaginal lips,**

and wipe the urine opening with a sterile cotton soaked with surgical soap.

8. Holding the lips open or the foreskin back, gently put the catheter into the urine hole. Twist it as necessary but DO NOT FORCE IT.

Hold the penis straight at this angle.

9. Push the catheter in until urine starts coming out—then 3 cm. more.

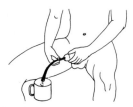

10A. If using a regular catheter, each time you pee tighten your stomach *muscles* or gently massage the lower belly to empty all urine. Then take out the catheter, wash it well, boil it, and store it in a clean jar or towel.

10B. If using a Foley (permanent) catheter, inject 5 cc. of sterile water into the little tube, to fill the balloon (or up to 10 cc. if it is a 30 cc. Foley), and connect the bigger tube to the collection tube or leg bag.

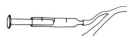

Change the catheter every 2 weeks (or more often if there is an infection).

To avoid infections when using a catheter, it is important to be very clean and to use only a catheter that is sterile, boiled, or very clean.

3. **FOLEY CATHETER** (fixed catheter): With this method, the catheter is left in all the time to drain the urine from the bladder continuously. A Foley is often used immediately after injury, and in some cases, for many months or years. The catheter connects to a collection bag that can be attached to the leg and worn under the clothes.

In many areas this is the easiest method because other supplies are difficult to get. However, a Foley can cause many problems, including:

- Bacteria can get into the bladder, causing a **high risk of infection.**

- **Continuous bladder irritation** can cause bladder stones to form.

- The catheter may cause a **sore on the underside of the penis** through which urine leaks. This may need surgery to correct.

If you have tried other methods unsuccessfully or no other equipment is available, a Foley catheter may be the only choice. To prevent complications it is **very important that it be used carefully:**

- Always wash your hands well before touching the catheter.

- Clean the skin around the catheter with soap and water at least twice a day and after each bowel movement.

- Do not disconnect the collection bag except to empty and wash it. Wash it out with soap or bleach *(Clorox)* and water once a day.

- If the catheter must be clamped, use a sterile plug, *never* a glass ampule (small bottle). It may break and cause injury.

- Keep the collection bag below the level of the bladder to keep the urine from flowing back.

- Tape the catheter to the leg when in a wheelchair. Boys should tape the catheter on belly when lying down.

- Check regularly to make sure the urine is emptying and that the catheter is not plugged up. Avoid sharp bends or folds in the tubing.

- When turning, lifting, or moving the person, remember to move the bag too. Do not let it pull at the catheter or stay under the person.

- If the catheter gets plugged up, take it out, squirt boiled water through it, and put it back. Or use a new one. In emergencies, you can squirt a little (cool) boiled water back through the catheter while it is in place. Use a sterile or very clean syringe.

4. **CONDOM CATHETER:** This is a practical method for men and boys who cannot control their urine. It can be used in combination with triggering, to avoid accidental wetting.

A condom catheter is a thin rubber bag that fits over the penis. It has a tube that connects to a collection bag. They come in different sizes.

If condom catheters are too costly or not available, a regular condom ('rubber', 'sheath', or 'prophylactic' for family planning) can be attached to the collection tube with a rubber band or tape.

Or a thin, very clean plastic bag can be used. Or, on a child, use the finger of a rubber glove (or a 'fingercot').

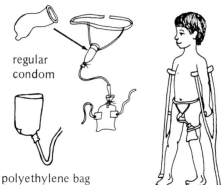

condom catheter

regular
condom

polyethylene bag

To hold the condom on the penis, a special very stretchy adhesive tape can be used as shown in this series of drawings.

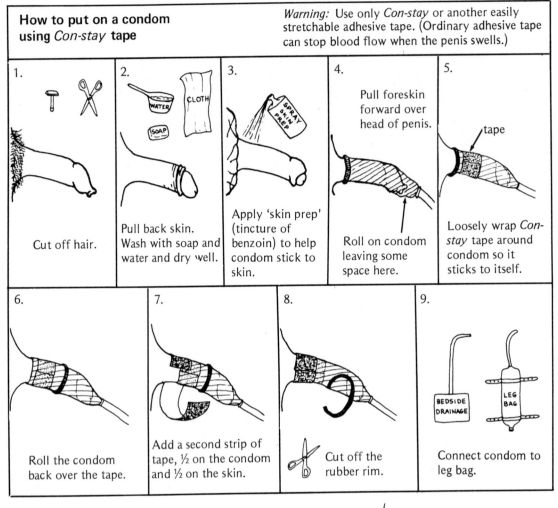

How to put on a condom using *Con-stay* tape	*Warning:* Use only *Con-stay* or another easily stretchable adhesive tape. (Ordinary adhesive tape can stop blood flow when the penis swells.)

1. Cut off hair.

2. Pull back skin. Wash with soap and water and dry well.

3. Apply 'skin prep' (tincture of benzoin) to help condom stick to skin.

4. Pull foreskin forward over head of penis. Roll on condom leaving some space here.

5. tape — Loosely wrap *Con-stay* tape around condom so it sticks to itself.

6. Roll the condom back over the tape.

7. Add a second strip of tape, ½ on the condom and ½ on the skin.

8. Cut off the rubber rim.

9. BEDSIDE DRAINAGE — LEG BAG — Connect condom to leg bag.

One of the safest and cheapest ways to hold a condom on the penis is to cut a ring → out of soft foam rubber. Pass the condom under the ring and turn it back over it.

 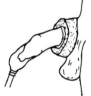

The ring can be used again and again. So can the condoms if they are carefully washed.

IMPORTANT PRECAUTIONS FOR CONDOM USE:

- Be sure it is **not too tight**—it could stop blood flow and severely harm the penis. Avoid non-stretch tape.

- If the penis has erections (gets hard and bigger), try to put on the condom when it is big.

- Remove the condom once a day and wash the penis well.

- If possible, remove it at night. Use a bottle or urinal to catch the urine.

- Check the condom and penis often to be sure everything is all right.

- If the penis becomes injured, swollen, or looks sore, remove the condom until the penis is healthy.

Methods for the limp bladder

If the person's bladder is limp (flaccid), it never empties by reflex. The bladder will constantly have urine sitting in it unless an effective emptying method is used.

Boys:

1. Put in a regular catheter every 4 to 6 hours to empty the bladder. Between catheter use, the boy can put on a condom to catch any leaking urine, as described on page 208.

2. A Foley catheter can be used, but may lead to problems (see p. 207).

3. Other alternatives include a surgical operation, which allows the urine to come out through a small opening on the belly into a bag. Or a special catheter is put into the bladder through a small hole in the lower belly.

Girls:

1. They can use a Foley catheter. This is often the simplest method, but can lead to urinary infections.

2. Or try an 'intermittent' (in and out) program, using a regular catheter every 4-6 hours. If there is leaking in between catheter times, use diapers, rags, or a thick sanitary pad to catch the urine. Change them often and wash often to protect the skin and prevent sores.

3. The surgical procedures mentioned for boys can also be done in girls.

OTHER SUGGESTIONS FOR THE LIMP BLADDER—BOTH SEXES

- The **push method:**

Push down over the bladder with the hands.

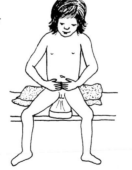

Or strain to push urine out by tightening the stomach muscles.

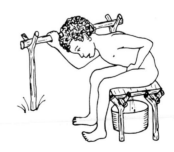

Or put a fist over the lower belly and gently press it by bending forward.

This method is recommended by many professionals, but it can cause problems. If the muscles do not relax to let the urine out, pushing on the bladder can force urine back into the kidneys—causing kidney infection and damage. Therefore, **the push method should only be used if the urine comes out easily with gentle pressure—or if there is no other way possible.**

- With boys with a limp bladder, the condom method can be used. But it is best to also use a regular catheter at least 3 times a day. This is because the bladder does not empty completely, which makes infection more likely.

URINARY INFECTIONS

Persons with spinal cord injury or spina bifida have a high risk of urinary (bladder) infections, for the reasons we have discussed. Long-term or untreated infections and kidney problems are a common cause of early death. Preventive measures are essential (see the bottom of the next page); but even when precautions are taken, some urinary infections are still likely to happen. Therefore, it is very important to recognize the signs and provide effective treatment.

Signs

When a person who has normal feeling has a urine infection, it burns when he pees. The person with spinal cord damage may not feel this burning and therefore has to use other signs to know when he has an infection. He may learn to recognize certain unpleasant feelings, or may only know that he does not feel as healthy as usual. Parents and health workers should learn to listen to the child and be aware of changes in behavior or other signs that might mean that he has an infection.

Possible urinary signs

- cloudy urine, possibly with pieces of mucus, pus, or blood specks
- dark or red urine
- strong or bad smelling urine
- increased bladder spasms (cramps)
- increased wetting or changes in bladder function
- pain in the mid-back (kidneys) or side (urine tubes)

Possible other signs

- body aches
- general discomfort
- increased muscle spasms
- fever
- dysreflexia (headache, goosebumps when sweating, high blood pressure, see p. 187.)

Treatment

At the first signs of infection, **drink even more water than usual.** *Antibiotics* (medicines that fight bacteria) may also be necessary. But avoid frequent use of antibiotics because they may become less effective (bacteria may become resistant).

If a person has had many urinary infections before, **take the person to a medical laboratory for a 'culture' and 'sensitivity test' of the urine. If possible, consult a specialist in urinary problems**. If this is not possible, start with the last medicine that was effective.

In patients with a first infection:

- Start with one of the medicines in **Group 1 on the next page.** After 2 days, if the person does not begin to improve, try another medicine in Group 1.
- If none of the medicines of Group 1 help, try the medicine in Group 2.
- If a medicine seems to help, continue taking it for at least a week, or for 4 days after the last signs have disappeared. Do not change from one medicine to another unless the medicine is not working or causes serious side effects.

TREATMENT FOR URINARY INFECTIONS				
	Medical name (and ***common brand***)	**Age**	**Dose**	**Repeat the dose**
GROUP 1	A. Co-trimoxazole (sulfamethoxazole 400 mg. with trimethoprim 80 mg.) ***(Bactrim*** or ***Septra)***	6 weeks to 5 months 6 months to 5 years 6 to 8 years 9 to 12 years	¼ tablet ½ tablet 1 tablet 2 tablets	2 times a day
	Note: This medicine can cause kidney damage unless the person **drinks lots of water.** The medicine also comes in double strength ***(Bactrim DS*** and ***Septra DS).*** Adjust tablet doses if using double strength tablets.			
	B. Amoxicillin (many brands) (100 mg./kg./day) ***Caution:*** **Do not use for persons allergic to penicillin**	up to 10 years over 10 years	125 mg. 250 mg.	3 times a day
	C. Nitrofurantoin ***(Furadantin, Macrodantin)*** (from 3 months: 5 to 7 mg./kg./day)	up to 5 years over 6 years	25 mg. 50 mg.	4 times a day
GROUP 2	Cephalexin ***(Keflex)*** (25 to 50 mg./kg./day)	under 1 year 1 to 5 years 6 to 12 years	100 mg. 125 mg. 250 mg.	4 times a day
All persons with a urinary infection should always drink lots of water, especially while they are taking medicine. After the infection is gone, continue drinking lots of water, and take all preventive measures.				

PREVENTION OF URINARY INFECTIONS

- Drink lots of liquid: adults, at least 2 liters (8 glasses) a day.
- Eat apples, grapes, or cranberries or drink their juices or take vitamin C tablets to make urine more acid. Bacteria grow with more difficulty in acid urine.
  (***Note:*** Orange or lemon juice and other citrus fruits and juices do not work! They make the urine *less* acid.)
- Keep hands, catheter, and collection bags very clean before, during, and after your bladder program.
- Do not lie in bed all day. Stay active.
- Do not clamp the Foley catheter or plug it with anything unless absolutely necessary, then use a sterile plug.
- Stick to your bladder program. Do not allow urine to sit in bladder.
- Do not let the catheter get bent or twisted so that urine cannot come out.
- If using a standard catheter periodically, be sure to put it in regularly, at least every 4 to 6 hours. To prevent infections, frequency of catheter use is even more important than cleanliness. It is safer to put in the catheter without boiling it than not to put it in. If infections are common, catheterize more often.

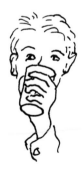

To prevent urinary infections, drink LOTS OF WATER

BOWEL MANAGEMENT IN SPINAL CORD INJURY AND SPINA BIFIDA

When there is damage to the spinal cord, almost always a person loses control over when he will have a bowel movement (pass stool or shit). This makes it hard to stay clean, which can be inconvenient or embarrassing. Although he can never get back complete control over the muscles that hold in or push out the stool, **a person can learn to help the stool come out, with assistance, at certain times of day.** This kind of 'bowel program' can greatly increase the person's self-confidence and freedom for school, work, and social activities.

Persons with spinal cord damage also often have problems with constipation, or the formation of hard stools that may wait days before coming out. Some constipation can be an advantage when a person lacks bowel control. But sometimes it can lead to serious problems, such as impaction (see p. 214) or dysreflexia (see p. 187). It is therefore important to **prevent serious constipation:**

- Drink lots of water.

- Eat foods high in fiber (such as bran, whole grain cereals, fruits, vegetables, cassava, beans, nuts).

- Stick to a scheduled bowel program.

- Keep active.

Planning a bowel program

Any bowel program will work better if you:

- Do the program **every day** (or every other day) and **at the same hour.** Do it even if the person has had an accidental bowel movement shortly before, or has diarrhea.

- Do the bowel program at the same time of day that the person usually had bowel movements before his injury. Often the bowels move best after a meal or a hot drink.

- If possible, do the program on a toilet or pot. The bowels work better sitting than lying.

- Be patient. The bowels sometimes take days or weeks to change their pattern.

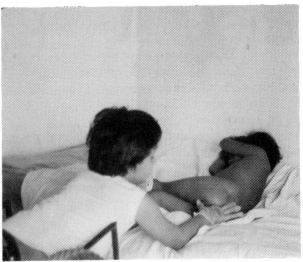

An 8-year-old paraplegic girl, Vania, helps a 5-year-old paraplegic girl with her daily bowel program. (See Story of Jésica on p. 192.)

Types of bowel

Different persons require different types of bowel programs, depending on whether their bowels are 'automatic', 'limp', or 'pull back'.

- **Automatic bowel** usually occurs in persons who have muscle spasms in their legs, and an 'automatic bladder'. The muscle or 'sphincter' in the anus (asshole) stays shut until there is a stimulation in the bowel to make it open, so that the stool can come out. An automatic bowel will 'move' in response to a suppository or stimulation by a finger.

- **Limp or 'flaccid' bowel** usually occurs in persons with low spinal cord damage who have limp (not spastic) legs and bladder. The sphincter muscle in the anus is also limp. So the person tends to 'ooze' or 'dribble' shit. A limp bowel does not respond to finger stimulation.

- **A bowel that pulls back** is neither automatic nor limp. When you put a finger up the anus, you can feel the stool move back up instead of coming out.

PROGRAM FOR AN AUTOMATIC BOWEL

- Start with a suppository if available. With a finger covered with a glove or plastic bag, and then oil, push the suppository about 2 cm. (1 in.) up the anus. Do not push it into the stool, but push it against the wall of the bowel. (Or try the program without a suppository; usually finger stimulation is enough.)

- Wait 5 or 10 minutes. Then help the person sit on a toilet or pot. If he cannot sit, have him lie on his left side (on top of old paper).

> SUPPLIES NEEDED
>
> - non-sterile glove, finger glove, or plastic bag
> - lubricant (vegetable or mineral oil works well)
> - old paper or newspaper
> - soap and water
> - if available, *suppositories* such as *Dulcolax* or glycerin. These are bullet-shaped pills that are pushed into the anus. They stimulate the bowel and cause it to push out the stool (shit).
>
> suppository

- Put an oiled finger into the anus about 2 cm. Gently move the finger in circles for about 1 minute, until the anus relaxes and the stool pushes out.

- Repeat the finger action 3 or 4 times, or until no more stool is felt.

- Clean the butt and anus well and wash your hands.

PROGRAM FOR A LIMP BOWEL

Since the bowel does not push, the stool must be taken out with a finger. It is best done after each meal, or at least once a day.

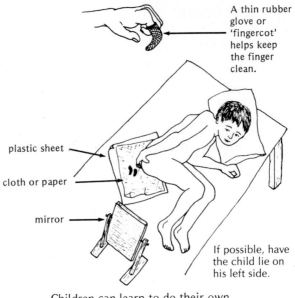

A thin rubber glove or 'fingercot' helps keep the finger clean.

plastic sheet

cloth or paper

mirror

If possible, have the child lie on his left side.

- If possible, do it sitting on a toilet or pot, or lying on your left side.

- With a gloved and oiled finger, remove as much stool as you can.

- Since a limp bowel tends to ooze stool, eat foods that make the stool firm or slightly constipated (not much stool-loosening foods).

Children can learn to do their own 'bowel program'. (See p. 212.)

PROGRAM FOR A BOWEL THAT PULLS BACK

For this kind of bowel, the bowel programs already described usually do not work. Finger stimulation makes the bowel act in the opposite direction, and pull the stool back in. The person will have 'accidents' during the day. Often it works better to,

- First, put some anesthetic jelly (such as *Xylocaine*) up the anus. If you cannot get the jelly, you can mix some liquid injectable *Xylocaine* (lidocaine) with *Vaseline* or any other jelly.

- Wait several minutes. Then do the automatic bowel program.

OTHER IMPORTANT POINTS

- Do not use enemas or strong laxatives regularly. They stretch the bowel, injure its muscles, and make following a regular program more difficult. A mild laxative may be taken occasionally, when needed. However, **drinking more liquid** and eating food high in fiber is usually enough.

- If there is bright red blood in the stool, probably a blood vessel was torn during the program. Be more gentle! If there is dark, old blood and the stools are black and tar-like, seek medical advice.

- A small amount of liquid stool (diarrhea) may be a sign of 'impaction' (a ball of hard stool stuck in the gut). Only liquid can leak around it. Do not give medicine to stop diarrhea; this could make the impaction worse. Try to get it out with a finger.

A bowel program may at first seem difficult and messy. But it soon becomes an easy habit. It is very important both for the person's health and his social well-being. Start now, do it regularly at the same hour, and DO NOT MISS A DAY.

Leprosy

CHAPTER 26

Hansen's Disease

What is leprosy? It is an *infectious* disease that develops very slowly. It is caused by germs (bacilli) that affect mostly the skin and *nerves.* It can cause a variety of skin problems, loss of feeling, and *paralysis* of the hands and feet:

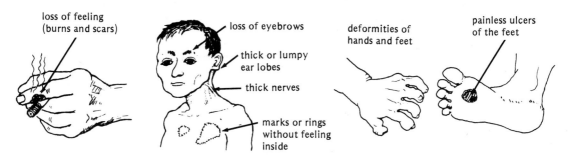

loss of feeling
(burns and scars)

loss of eyebrows

thick or lumpy
ear lobes

thick nerves

marks or rings
without feeling
inside

deformities of
hands and feet

painless ulcers
of the feet

How do people get leprosy? It can spread only from some persons who have untreated leprosy, and only to other persons who have 'low resistance' to the disease. It is probably spread either through sneezing or coughing, or through skin contact. Most persons who come into contact with leprosy have a natural ability to resist it. Either they do not get it at all, or they get a small unnoticeable infection that soon goes away completely.

From the time a person is first infected with leprosy germs, it often takes 3 or 4 years for the first signs of the disease to appear.

Leprosy is not caused by evil spirits, by doing something bad, by eating certain foods, or by bathing in river water, as some people believe. It is not *hereditary* and children of mothers with leprosy are not born with it. However, **children who live in close contact with someone who has untreated leprosy are more likely to get it.**

How common is leprosy? Leprosy is much more common in some parts of the world than others. It is more common where there are crowded living conditions and poor hygiene. But rich people can also get it.

More than 1 million people have leprosy. In some villages in Asia, Africa, and Central America, 1 person in 20 has leprosy.

Can leprosy be cured? Yes. There are medicines that kill leprosy germs. Usually within a few days of beginning treatment, a person can no longer spread the disease to others. (In fact, most persons, when their leprosy is first diagnosed, can no longer spread it.) However, **treatment in some persons must be continued for years to prevent the disease from coming back.**

Is early treatment important? Yes. Early treatment stops the spread of leprosy to others. Also, if treatment starts before loss of feeling, paralysis, and deformities have appeared, recovery is usually complete and the person is not physically or socially disabled.

> Persons receiving regular, effective treatment do not spread leprosy.

Checking children for signs of leprosy

In areas where leprosy is common, health and *rehabilitation* workers should work together with parents and schoolteachers to **check all children regularly for early signs of leprosy.** Most important are regular checkups of children in homes where persons are known to have leprosy. Checkups should be done every 6 to 12 months and should be continued for at least 3 years.

EARLY SIGNS

A slowly growing patch on the skin that does not itch or hurt. The patch may be somewhat different in color from the surrounding skin. (Patches of leprosy are never completely white, and are not scaly, except during a reaction—see p. 219.)

Note: In early skin patches, feeling is often normal, or nearly so. **If feeling is clearly reduced inside a patch, leprosy is almost certain.**

WHAT TO LOOK FOR

Examine the whole body for **skin patches,** especially the face, arms, back, butt, and legs.

If you find a slightly pale patch without a clear edge, keep watching the spot. Unless feeling is reduced inside the patch, look for other signs before deciding it is leprosy. (Many children have similar pale spots on cheeks and arms that are not leprosy.)

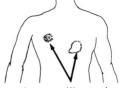

ringworm-like patches, with or without raised border

LATER SIGNS

1. **Tingling, numbness, or some loss of feeling in the hands and feet.**

   Or definite loss of feeling in skin patches.

TEST INSIDE THE SKIN PATCHES FOR REDUCED FEELING.

With the tip of a feather or stiff thread, lightly touch the skin inside and outside the patch and have the child tell you (without looking) where he feels the touch.

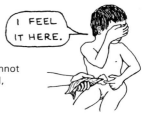

I FEEL IT HERE.

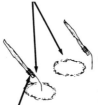

If the child cannot feel the thread, try pricking lightly with a sterile needle.

thread tied to stick

WARNING: Sterilize the needle in a flame before testing another child.

In a similar way, test for a numbness or reduced feeling in the hands and feet.

---

2. **Slight weakness or deformity in the hands and feet.**

   drop foot (Child cannot raise it.)

   weakness or clawing of toes.

Have the child straighten her fingers. If she cannot do this, it may be a sign of paralysis from leprosy.

Also have the child try to touch the base of her little finger with her thumb.

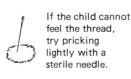

Muscle weakness here makes this movement difficult and may be a sign.

(*CAUTION:* These weaknesses may also be caused by polio, muscular dystrophy, or other problems.)

---

3. **Enlargement of certain nerves,** with or without pain or tenderness. The affected nerve feels like a thick cord under the skin. When they are quite thick, they may be easily seen.

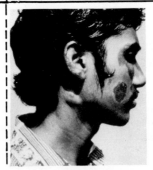

thickening nerve below the ear (From *A Manual of Leprosy;* see p. 638.)

Check for large nerves in these places.

Also check for large nerves in or near skin patches.

Diagnosing leprosy

Although skin patches are often the first sign of leprosy, many other diseases can cause similar patches. Only when there is a loss of feeling inside the skin patch, as compared with the skin outside the patch, can we be almost sure the person has leprosy. However, in some forms of leprosy, loss of feeling in skin patches may develop only years later, or not at all. Therefore, other evidence of leprosy must be looked for.

Another sign of leprosy—tingling, numbness, or loss of feeling in hands and feet—may also have other causes.

To make a fairly certain diagnosis of leprosy, the person should have at least 1 of these 3 major signs:

1. **definite loss or change of feeling in skin patches**

    Note: Leprosy patches on face often do not lose feeling as much as on other parts of the body.

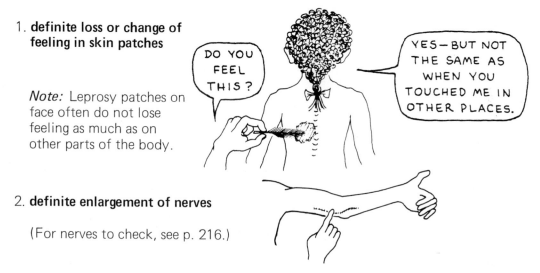

2. **definite enlargement of nerves**

    (For nerves to check, see p. 216.)

3. **presence of leprosy bacilli in a 'skin smear'**

    A 'split skin smear' is prepared by cutting a thin layer of skin from a skin patch. Less commonly it is taken from the moist skin deep inside the nose—an area that is often heavily infected. The skin sample is placed on a glass slide, colored with special stains, and examined with a microscope.

    The bacteria (bacilli) of leprosy, if present, can be seen under the microscope.

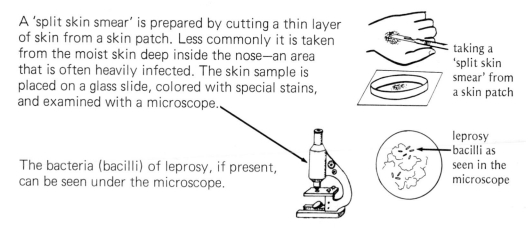

taking a 'split skin smear' from a skin patch

leprosy bacilli as seen in the microscope

> **Whenever you suspect leprosy but the diagnosis is uncertain, a 'skin smear' should be taken (by a trained worker).**

Note: Not many persons with leprosy show all 3 of these signs. Persons with loss of feeling in skin patches usually have no bacilli in their skin smears.

Types of leprosy

Depending on how much natural resistance a person has, leprosy appears in 2 different forms. You can count the number of skin patches to find out to find out the type of leprosy a person has—people with Pauci-Bacillary (PB) have up to 5 skin patches, while people with Multi-Bacillary (MB) leprosy have more than 5 skin patches.

PAUCI-BACILLARY (PB)

- **in persons with relatively high resistance**

- no bacilli in skin smear

- Person cannot pass leprosy on to others.

- Person may have up to 5 skin patches, variable in appearance, but often have raised margins and flat centers.

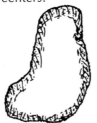

- Feeling is reduced or absent in centers of the skin patches.

- Skin on the face is **not** thickened.

- Nerve damage appears early, but usually only involves loss of feeling in skin patches. Usually it does not affect the eyes, hands, or feet. When it does, it often happens early and causes loss of feeling or strength in **only one hand or foot**.

MULTI-BACILLARY (MB)

- **in persons with low resistance**

- bacilli—few to many in skin smears

- Person can pass leprosy to others (until treated).

- more than 5 skin patches, raised or flat with irregular edges, and usually some loss of feeling; patches about the same on both sides of the body

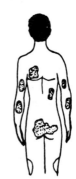

- The skin of the face may become thick, lumpy, reddish, especially over the eyebrows, cheeks, nose and ears.

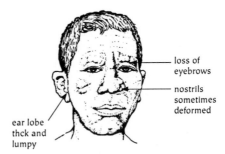

loss of eyebrows

nostrils sometimes deformed

ear lobe thck and lumpy

THE 'LION FACE' OF LEPROMATOUS LEPROSY

- Severe nerve damage often results, with loss of feeling and loss of strength in both hands and feet, with deformities.

Leprosy reactions

Sometimes persons with leprosy have sudden periods of increased problems. These may be something like an allergic reaction to the leprosy bacilli. Leprosy reactions can happen in untreated persons, during treatment, or after treatment has stopped. Reactions can occur when there are changes in the body, such as puberty in boys, in late pregnancy or following childbirth, during illness from other causes, after *vaccination,* or at times of emotional stress.

There are 2 types of leprosy reactions:

Type 1 reactions happen in persons with borderline leprosy when the body increases its fight against the leprosy germs. There is danger of new weakness and loss of feeling.

Signs to watch for are:

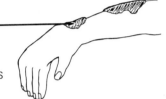

* skin patches may become swollen and red
* swollen hands and feet
* new tingling or weakness of hands and feet
* pain or discomfort along nerves (Rarely, lumps along the nerves form sores and drain pus.)

> *IMPORTANT:* Reactions sometimes cause new weakness and loss of feeling **without nerve pain.**

Type 2 reactions happen with lepromatous leprosy. The body is reacting against too many bacilli.

Signs may include:

* swollen, reddish, or dark lumps under the skin, especially on the face, arms, and legs
* fever
* pain in testicles, breasts, or fingers
* stuffiness or bleeding of the nose
* red eye, with or without pain.
  Danger: This may lead to **iritis** or loss of vision unless treated early.

Rarely, this reaction causes death due to swelling of the mouth, throat or lungs, or to kidney problems.

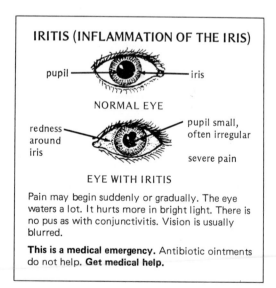

IRITIS (INFLAMMATION OF THE IRIS)

pupil — iris

NORMAL EYE

redness around iris — pupil small, often irregular — severe pain

EYE WITH IRITIS

Pain may begin suddenly or gradually. The eye waters a lot. It hurts more in bright light. There is no pus as with conjunctivitis. Vision is usually blurred.

This is a medical emergency. Antibiotic ointments do not help. **Get medical help.**

If untreated, leprosy reactions can quickly lead to permanent nerve damage with increased paralysis of the hands, feet, or eye muscles, or to permanent damage to the eyes.

> **Early treatment of leprosy reactions is very important to prevent paralysis, deformity, and blindness.**

Treatment of leprosy reaction is discussed on p. 221.

TREATMENT AND MANAGEMENT OF LEPROSY

Treatment and management of leprosy should include 4 areas:

1. **Long-term medical treatment** to control the leprosy infection should begin as early as possible.
2. **Emergency treatment** when necessary to control and **prevent further damage** from **leprosy reactions**.
3. **Safety measures**, aids, exercises, and education to prevent deformities (sores, burns, injuries, contractures).
4. **Social rehabilitation**: Work with the individual, parents, schools, and the community to create a better understanding of leprosy, to lessen people's fears, and to increase acceptance, so the child or adult with leprosy can lead a full, happy, meaningful life.

Medical Treatment

Multi-drug treatment (MDT) consisting of rifampin, DDS and clofazimine, is now recommended by the World Health Organization. MDT is usually supplied free. The treatment varies according to whether the patient is a child or an adult, and whether the patient has PB or MB leprosy.

For years, **DDS (dapsone)** was the main drug used. Unfortunately, in some areas the leprosy bacilli became 'resistant' to DDS (were not harmed by it).

Rifampin works much faster against leprosy. To prevent development of resistance, it is given in combination with other anti-leprosy medicines. Rifampin needs to be given only once a month. This reduces cost and side effects.

Clofazimine, although less effective in killing leprosy bacilli than rifampin, has the advantage that it also helps control leprosy Type 2 reaction.

Medicine for PB leprosy (Treatment is for 6 months.)	children under 10 years	children 10 to 14 years	adults	Take the monthly dose on the first day of treatment (day 1) and then every 28 days for 6 months. Take the daily dose every day for 6 months. Treatment must be completed within 9 months.
monthly dose rifampicin	300 mg.	450 mg.	600 mg.	
monthly dose dapsone	25 mg.	50 mg.	100 mg.	
daily dose dapsone	25 mg.	50 mg.	100 mg.	
Medicine for MB leprosy (Treatment is for 12 months.)	children under 10 years	children 10 to 14 years	adults	Take the monthly dose on the first day of treatment (day 1) and then every 28 days for 12 months. Take the daily dose every day, or as noted, for 12 months. Treatment must be completed within 18 months.
monthly dose rifampicin	300 mg.	450 mg.	600 mg.	
monthly dose clofazimine	100 mg.	150 mg.	300 mg.	
monthly dose dapsone	25 mg.	50 mg.	100 mg.	
daily dose dapsone	25 mg.	50 mg.	100 mg.	
daily dose clofazimine	50 mg twice a week	50 mg. every other day	50 mg.	

Check with your Ministry of Health and WHO for information about leprosy treatment.

Importance of long-term treatment

Treatment to cure leprosy takes a long time: from 6 months to 1 year or more depending on the type of leprosy. If treatment is stopped too soon or if the medicine is not taken at the right time, not only can leprosy return, but a sometimes a leprosy reaction may result which can cause even more nerve damage and paralysis or blindness.

It is therefore **essential that health and rehabilitation workers make sure the person with leprosy and her family understand the importance of taking the medicine regularly.** It is helpful if a health worker can be present when the child's monthly dose is taken. This way, he can check her for any complications of leprosy.

TREATED EARLY, LEPROSY NEED NOT BE A DEFORMING OR DISABLING DISEASE

Treatment of leprosy reactions

As we mentioned on p. 215, feeling loss, paralysis, and deformities need not happen to a person with leprosy. **Early diagnosis and treatment together with quick care of leprosy reactions should prevent the development of many deformities.**

Care of a leprosy reaction has 4 objectives:

- Prevent nerve damage that causes loss of feeling, paralysis, and contractures.

- Stop eye damage and prevent blindness.

- Control pain.

- Continue with medicine to kill leprosy bacilli and prevent the disease from getting worse.

Care includes:

1. **Medicine to reduce pain and inflammation**

   For mild reactions (skin inflammation but not pain or tenderness of nerves) use aspirin or ibuprofen. For dosage and precautions, see p. 134.

   For severe reactions (pain along nerves, increasing tingling, numbness or weakness, eye irritation, or painful testicles) **corticosteroids** (prednisolone) may be needed. Because this is a medical emergency and because **corticosteroids are dangerous and often misused medicines,** if at all possible **get experienced medical advice before using them.**

2. **Anti-leprosy medicine should be continued throughout the leprosy reaction.**

   Clofazimine helps to reduce Type 2 reactions and fights the leprosy bacilli. The dose of clofazimine can often be increased (to 200 mg. daily in adults) and later reduced as the reaction lessens. However, for severe reactions that damage nerves, prednisolone is needed.

3. **Splinting and exercise**

   Holding the affected limbs in splints during a severe reaction helps reduce pain and prevent nerve damage and contractures. (See Chapter 8.)

   Joints should be splinted in the most useful position. Splints can be made of plaster bandage or molded plastic (see p. 540). Very carefully pad splints for hands or feet that do not feel pain.

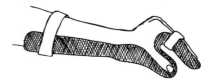

A good splint for the hand—to avoid contractures and maintain a useful position.

   Leave the splint on day and night until pain and inflammation are gone. Remove only for gentle range-of-motion exercise at least once a day. (See Chapter 42.)

Cause of deformities

When most people think of leprosy, they think of the severe deformities of the advanced case: deep open sores (ulcers), clawed fingers, gradual loss of fingers and toes, and eye damage leading to blindness. Actually, these deformities are not caused directly by leprosy germs, but result from damaged nerves. Nerve damage causes 3 levels of problems, one leading to the next:

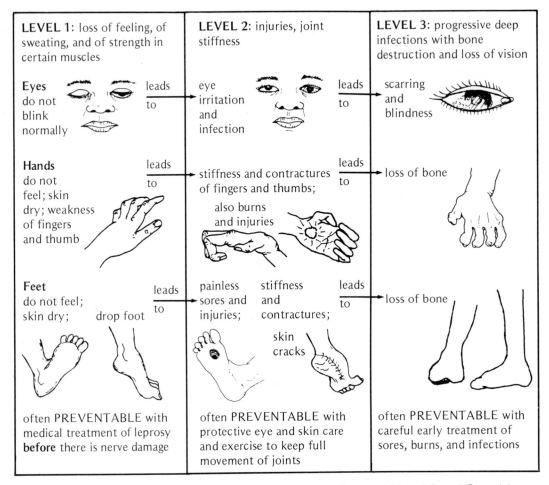

LEVEL 1: loss of feeling, of sweating, and of strength in certain muscles	LEVEL 2: injuries, joint stiffness	LEVEL 3: progressive deep infections with bone destruction and loss of vision
Eyes do not blink normally	leads to → eye irritation and infection	leads to → scarring and blindness
Hands do not feel; skin dry; weakness of fingers and thumb	leads to → stiffness and contractures of fingers and thumbs; also burns and injuries	leads to → loss of bone
Feet do not feel; skin dry; drop foot	leads to → painless sores and injuries; stiffness and contractures; skin cracks	leads to → loss of bone
often PREVENTABLE with medical treatment of leprosy **before** there is nerve damage	often PREVENTABLE with protective eye and skin care and exercise to keep full movement of joints	often PREVENTABLE with careful early treatment of sores, burns, and infections

When there are level 1 problems, there is a **lifelong danger** of level 2 and 3 problems. Because feeling has been lost, the person no longer protects herself automatically against cuts, sores, thorns, and other injuries. And because they do not hurt, these injuries are often neglected.

For example, if a person with normal feeling walks a long way and gets a blister, it hurts, so he stops walking or limps.

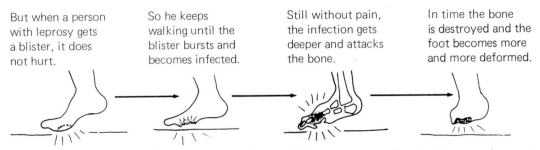

But when a person with leprosy gets a blister, it does not hurt.

So he keeps walking until the blister bursts and becomes infected.

Still without pain, the infection gets deeper and attacks the bone.

In time the bone is destroyed and the foot becomes more and more deformed.

Usually, leprosy bacilli cannot be found in these open sores. This is because the sores are not caused by the bacilli. Instead, they are caused by pressure, injury, and secondary infection.

PREVENTION OF INJURY for persons with loss of feeling and strength

Eyes: Much eye damage comes from not blinking enough, because of weakness or loss of feeling. Blinking keeps the eyes wet and clean. If the person does not blink well, or his eyes are red, teach him to:

- Wear sunglasses with side shades, and maybe a sun hat.

- Close the eyes tightly often during the day, especially when dust blows.

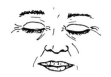

- Roll the eyeballs up as you try to close eyes tight.

- Keep eyes clean. Wash well around eyes, keep flies and dirty hands away.

Hands: When you work with your hands, or cook meals, take special care. Never pick up a pan or other object that *might* be hot without first **protecting your hand with a thick glove or folded cloth.** If possible, avoid work that involves handling sharp or hot objects. **Do not smoke.**

- **Use tools with smooth, wide handles,** or wrap cloth around handles.

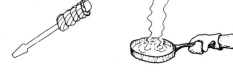

  To help the person with weak or deformed fingers hold a tool or utensil, you can mold a handle to the shape of the person's closed hand.

  Use epoxy putty, or plaster of Paris mixed with a strong glue. Have the person grip the handle while it is still soft. Then let it harden.

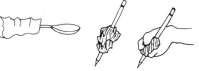

For more aids for gripping, see p. 230 and p. 577.

Feet:

- **Avoid going barefoot. Use shoes or sandals.** (For suggestions on appropriate footwear, see the next page.)

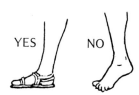

- **Learn to take short steps.** This helps protect the feet.

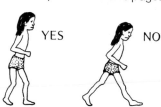

INJURY CARE

Eyes: Close eyes often. If necessary, use a simple eye patch. If eye gets infected (forms pus) use an antibiotic eye ointment. Put the ointment into lower lid without touching the eye.

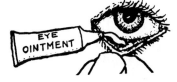

Hands and feet: If you have a cut or sore, keep the injured part very clean and at rest until it has healed completely. Take care not to injure the area again.

Things to do every day

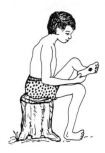

- **Checkups:** At the end of each day (or more often if you work hard or walk far) **examine your hands and feet carefully**—or have someone else examine them. Look for cuts, bruises, or thorns. Also look for spots or areas on the hands and feet that are red, hot, swollen, or show the start of blisters. If you find any of these, rest the hands or feet until the skin is completely normal again.

- If the skin gets dry and cracks, **soak the feet daily** in water for at least 20 minutes. Then rub cooking oil, *Vaseline,* or lanolin hand cream into them (not butter or animal fat. These attract insects and rats).

- As you rub oil into the hands and feet, do stretching exercises to keep the complete range of motion in the joints.

> **With continued daily care, most deformities of leprosy can be prevented.**

PREVENTION of contractures and deformities in persons with paralysis

Prevention of *contractures* from paralysis due to leprosy is similar to prevention of hand and foot contractures due to polio and other forms of paralysis. (See p. 81.) However, loss of feeling makes prevention more difficult.

Exercises to maintain full range of motion are covered in Chapter 42 (see especially p. 370 to 373).

- Exercises to prevent fixed clawing of the hands can be done by . . .

. . . gently straightening the fingers like this:

and like this:

Open your fingers as much as you can without help. Then use your other hand to open them the rest of the way. Close fingers and repeat.

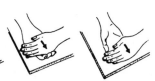

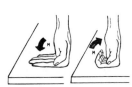

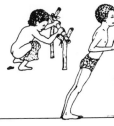

- A good exercise to prevent 'tiptoe' contractures with 'foot drop' is to stretch the heel *cords* by leaning forward against a wall or by squatting with heels on the ground.

Footwear for persons without feeling in their feet

The best footwear has:

- a well-fitted upper part that does not rub and has plenty of toe room (or leaves toes open).
- a soft innersole about 1 cm. thick.
- a tough under-sole so thorns, nails, and sharp rocks do not injure foot.
- Footwear should be acceptable (not look too strange or unusual) so that the person will use it.

AVOID:
- plastic shoes or sandals
- soft-soled sandals or thongs that thorns can pass through
- using nails to fasten heels and soles (These might poke through and injure the foot. Better to sew on soles or use glue.) NO!

Possible ways to get footwear

- Contact a leprosy hospital with a footwear workshop. They can make sandals if you send a tracing of the foot.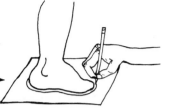

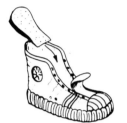

- Check the market. You may find a canvas shoe or tennis shoe that already has a good insole.

- Or you can put soft insoles into the shoes. But *CAUTION:* If you put an insole that is thick into a standard shoe, there may not be enough room for the toes—unless you cut out the part over the toes and leave them open.

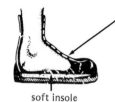

An insole that is thick may work if the foot is already short.

soft insole

- Make (or have a local shoemaker make) special footwear.

For the inner sole, you can use a soft sponge sandal or 'thong'. Or buy 'microcell' rubber, which is soft but firm.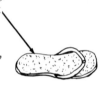

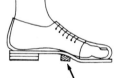 For the under-sole you can use a piece of old car tire.

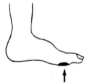

- For persons who have developed sores on their foot here,

a bar here or a   foot support here may help take pressure off the ball of the foot and prevent new sores.

- A very helpful lining for preventing sores is a soft, heat-moldable foam plastic called *'Plastazote'*. For instructions on making footwear with *Plastazote,* see *Insensitive Feet* on p. 638.

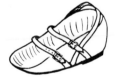

- For persons with a **'drop' foot,** a brace or 'lift' can help prevent sores and injuries.

You can get a brace or support at a rehabilitation workshop, or make a specially-fitted, well-padded plastic brace (see Chapter 58).

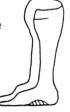

Or make a simple device to hold the foot up.

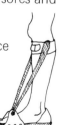

LEPROSY AND THE COMMUNITY

Historically, there has been a lot of fear and misunderstanding about leprosy. Persons with leprosy have often been thrown out of towns or treated with cruelty. Until recently, governments took persons with leprosy away from their families and locked them up in special institutions or 'leprosaria'. All this added to people's fears.

Today, leprosy can be cured—without any deformities or disabilities if treatment is begun early. It can be treated in the home. The person can continue going to school or to work. Having leprosy need not disable the person physically or socially.

But in many communities fear and misunderstanding remain. Persons still refuse to admit—even to themselves—the early signs of leprosy. They delay in getting treatment until permanent deformities appear. The disease continues to be spread to others by those who are not yet treated. And so the myth and the fear of leprosy are kept alive.

To correct this situation will require the efforts of all health and rehabilitation workers, schoolteachers, religious and community leaders, families of persons with leprosy, and organizations of the disabled. These steps are needed:

1. **Information and Education**   Schools, health centers, comics, radio, and television can be used to help educate the community about leprosy. Information should:
   - try to lessen the fears people have about leprosy and let them know it is curable.
   - stress the importance of early diagnosis and treatment.
   - tell people how to recognize early signs and where to get treated.
   - include popular stories of persons who think they might have leprosy, decide to get help, and are cured.

2. Integration of leprosy programs into general health care. Too often leprosy control is done as a separate program. It is important that people (and health workers) begin to see leprosy as 'just another serious health problem'— like diarrhea in children.

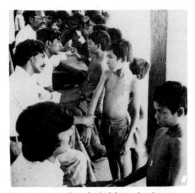

3. Regular screening (mass checkups) of children for skin patches and other early signs of leprosy. This can be part of a 'CHILD-to-child' program (see Chapter 47) in which school children learn first to examine each other, and then their younger brothers and sisters. A 'CHILD-to-child Activity Sheet on Leprosy' is available from TALC. (See p. 427.)

Screening school children for leprosy, India. (Photo, The Leprosy Mission.)

4. **Community pressure** and government orders to let children being treated for leprosy attend school, find work, attend festivals, and take part in public functions. (Organizations of disabled persons can help make this happen.)

5. **Self-help and community groups** of people affected by leprosy can raise awareness in the community and increase acceptance, care and respect. They can also organize to get medicines and treatment, and educate to prevent deformity. Where needed, community groups can advocate to get the schooling, health care, work, and social rights that persons with leprosy deserve.

> The example of a health worker who welcomes persons with leprosy and is not afraid to touch them can do much to calm needless fears and encourage acceptance.

Amputations

An amputation is the loss of some part of the body. Rarely, children are born without one or both hands or feet. More often, children lose an arm or leg because of accidents and increasingly because of war. Or limbs must be cut off because of advanced bone *infections* (see p. 160) or dangerous tumors (cancer).

Deciding what to do for a child with an amputation depends on a number of things, including the age of the child at the time of amputation, the amount of amputation, and above all, what the child (and parents) want and accept.

MISSING BOTH HANDS (any age)	He will probably want and accept hooks, or whatever can help him hold things better.	Until he can get gripping hooks, figure out ways to attach tools and utensils to his stumps so he can do more for himself.	A child with high arm amputations from birth often learns to use his feet almost as well as his hands.
MISSING ONE HAND	If she was born that way and is given an artificial limb early, she will usually accept it and keep using it.	But if her hand was amputated as an older child or she has gone for a long time without an artifical limb... 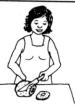	...she may prefer to keep using the stump, and refuse a limb even if one is made for her.
AN AMPUTATION BELOW THE KNEE (one or both legs) 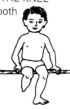	He should get an artificial leg as soon after the amputation as possible or by one year of age. 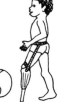	A growing child will often need a new, larger limb. Therefore, try to fit him with low cost limbs that are easy to replace. 	Limbs with detachable feet, although often expensive, can be lengthened
ONE LEG AMPUTATED ABOVE THE KNEE 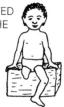	Up to age 10 (or more) she can walk well with a straight leg (no knee joint). 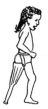	When older, she may prefer and will often walk better on a leg with a knee joint (if the family or program can pay for it and can keep replacing it as the child grows). 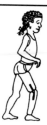	
BOTH LEGS AMPUTATED ABOVE THE KNEES	When very young, he may move about most easily on short 'stump' limbs. 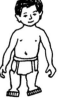	When older, he may prefer longer limbs that make him as tall as other children even if this means using crutches. 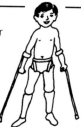	Children with very high amputation of the legs may do best in wheelchairs.

CARE OF THE AMPUTATED LIMB

The goals in caring for the stump are to maintain **a good shape** and **good position** for fitting an artificial limb. This means taking active steps to:

1. **avoid swelling,**
2. **keep the full range of motion** (prevent *contractures*), and
3. **maintain strength.**

WRAPPING THE STUMP

To prevent swelling and keep a good shape for fitting an artificial limb, it is important to wrap the newly amputated limb for a long time after it has been cut off.

The leg should be wrapped in a way that squeezes the liquid in the leg upward (rather than trapping it at the end). Use an elastic bandage in this manner:

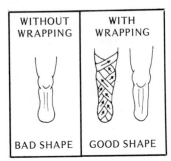

WITHOUT WRAPPING	WITH WRAPPING
BAD SHAPE	GOOD SHAPE

Below knee

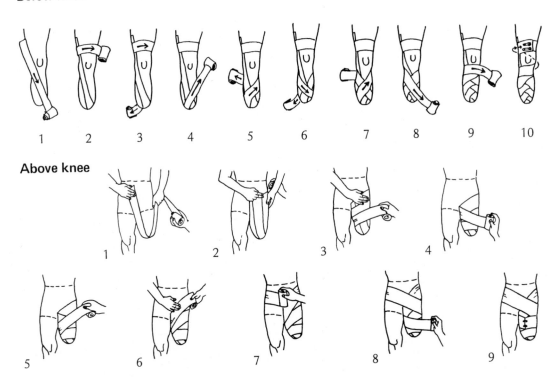

1   2   3   4   5   6   7   8   9   10

Above knee

1   2   3   4

5   6   7   8   9

ELEVATING THE STUMP

In addition to being wrapped, a newly amputated limb should be kept lifted high up most of the time. Avoid spending a lot of time with the arm or leg hanging down.

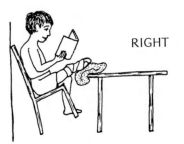

RIGHT

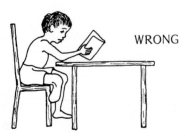

WRONG

PREVENTION of contractures

A child with an amputated leg does not use his leg normally. He usually keeps it bent, and he tends to develop contractures of the hip or knee (or both).

Therefore, special *positioning* and exercises are needed to prevent contractures and maintain full range of motion (see Chapter 42).

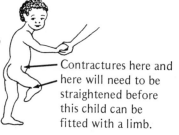

Contractures here and here will need to be straightened before this child can be fitted with a limb.

POSITIONS

Encourage positions that keep the joints stretched, and avoid those that keep the joint bent.

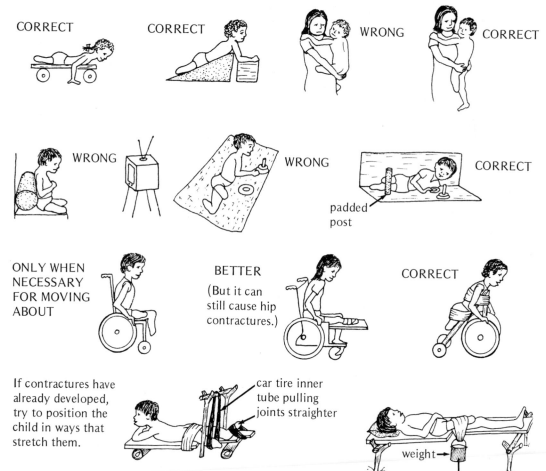

CORRECT

CORRECT

WRONG

CORRECT

WRONG

WRONG

CORRECT

padded post

ONLY WHEN NECESSARY FOR MOVING ABOUT

BETTER (But it can still cause hip contractures.)

CORRECT

If contractures have already developed, try to position the child in ways that stretch them.

car tire inner tube pulling joints straighter

weight→

STRETCHING EXERCISES

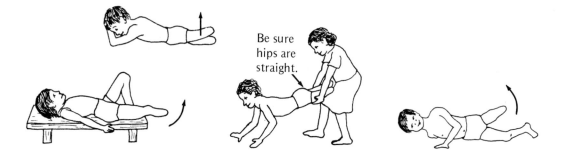

Be sure hips are straight.

STRENGTHENING EXERCISES

Try to strengthen especially those muscles that straighten the joints, and those muscles needed for walking.

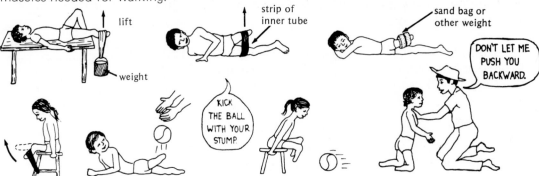

lift
weight

strip of
inner tube

sand bag or
other weight

DON'T LET ME
PUSH YOU
BACKWARD.

KICK
THE BALL
WITH YOUR
STUMP.

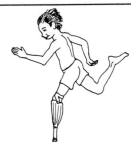

WARNING about walking aids

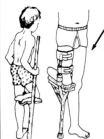

Walking aids or artificial limbs, like these, that keep the stump bent may be useful until the child can get a limb that keeps the joint straight.

However, it is very important that the child do **stretching and strengthening exercises daily** if he uses a bent-joint aid.

With a well-fitted stump-in-socket limb, normal activity usually provides all the stretching and exercise that are needed.

Instructions for making simple stump-in-socket limbs using bamboo and other local materials are in Chapter 67.

ALTERNATIVES FOR A CHILD WITH AMPUTATED HANDS

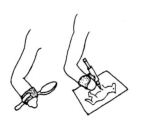

simple tool and utensil holders made of cloth, leather, or plastic (See p. 330.)

cuff with changeable tips

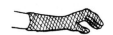

rubber or wood hand, not for use but for looks

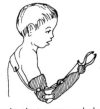

hooks that open and close to grip (operated by movements of shoulders and back)

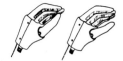

instead of hooks, an artificial hand with a thumb that opens and closes against 2 fingers (expensive and may not last)

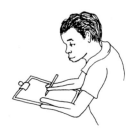

surgery that turns the 2 bones of the forearm into pinchers

This is a grasping aid for a child whose fingers have been lost but the base of the hand and wrist joint remain.

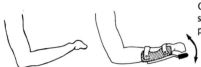

Child presses stump against post.

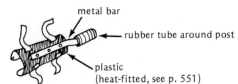

metal bar

rubber tube around post

plastic
(heat-fitted, see p. 551)

The type of aid a child and her parents choose for an amputation will depend on several things, such as **availability, cost, usefulness, looks,** and **local cultural factors.** For help in choosing an appropriate aid, see Chapter 56, "Making Sure Aids and Procedures Do More Good Than Harm," especially pages 531 and 532.

CHAPTER 28

Burns and Burn Deformities

Serious burns are common in villages where people cook, warm themselves, or sleep by open fires.

First aid for burns is discussed in health care manuals, including *Where There Is No Doctor.* Here we discuss only the precautions that can be taken to help prevent deformities and *disabilities* from burns.

The most common deformities resulting from severe burns are *contractures,* and the scarring, or sticking together, of skin around joints. For example:

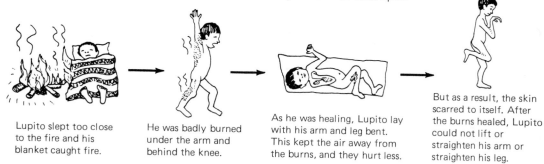

Lupito slept too close to the fire and his blanket caught fire.

He was badly burned under the arm and behind the knee.

As he was healing, Lupito lay with his arm and leg bent. This kept the air away from the burns, and they hurt less.

But as a result, the skin scarred to itself. After the burns healed, Lupito could not lift or straighten his arm or straighten his leg.

TO PREVENT SCARRING TOGETHER OF THE SKIN AT JOINTS:

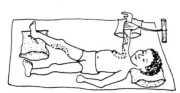

Keep the joints extended (straight) while the burns heal. You may have to support or tie the limbs so that the child does not bend them in his sleep.

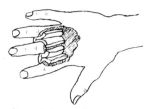

For burns between fingers or toes, keep them separated with sterile cloth pads with *Vaseline.*

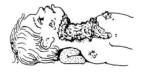

To keep the chin from scarring to the chest, it is very important to keep the head tilted up as the burns heal.

TO HELP BURNS HEAL: When possible, **leave the burns open to the air.**

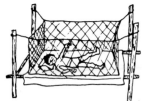

Protect against flies and dust with mosquito netting or by covering the burns with light gauze.

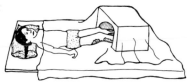

To keep the blanket or mosquito netting off a burned part of the body, cut a cardboard box or make a frame to hold it up.

If burns need to be covered, you can put petroleum jelly *(Vaseline)* on sterile gauze or sterilized cloth and gently cover the burn.

To help healing, and to prevent or control infection of deep or open burns, you can put **bees' honey or sugar** directly on the burn. Or make a paste of bees' honey mixed with sugar. **It is important to wash the burn with water that has been boiled and cooled, and to put on fresh honey 2 or 3 times each day.** (If the honey gets too diluted with oozing from the burn, it will breed germs rather than kill them.)

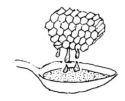

BEES' HONEY IS EXCELLENT FOR HEALING BURNS AND OPEN SORES

Ways to help burns heal faster and better

Skin grafts

Large deep burns heal very slowly and form ugly, stiff scars. Healing can be faster and scarring reduced by using 'skin grafts'. A very thin layer of skin from another part of the body is stretched over the burn. Usually this is only done by a surgeon (although some village health workers have been taught how to do it).

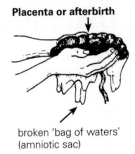

Placenta or afterbirth

broken 'bag of waters' (amniotic sac)

Also, to speed healthy healing, you can use the fresh 'bag of waters' or transparent membrane that comes out with the placenta after childbirth. But only use it if you are certain the mother does not have HIV/AIDS.

This sac must be kept clean Wash it in boiled and cooled, slightly salted water, and put it on the burn as soon as you take it out of the water.

RANGE-OF-MOTION EXERCISES

As soon as burns are covered with new skin or by a scar, gently begin range-of-motion exercises. Slowly straighten and bend the affected joint—a little more each day.

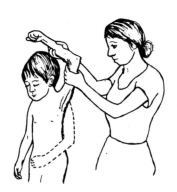

For exercise details, see Chapter 42. If scarring is severe, you may need to continue range-of-motion exercises for years after burns are healed. Scar tissue does not grow and stretch like normal skin. **Skin contractures** often form and may slowly get worse—sometimes even with exercises.

Before beginning exercises, it helps to rub body oil or cooking oil into the healed burn (but never into a fresh burn). Reports from several parts of the world claim that fish oil on healed burns helps prevent thick scarring and skin contractures.

SURGERY

When joints are scarred down or severe contractures form after burns, '**plastic surgery**' may be needed. Sometimes skin is taken from another part of the body and used to add more skin over the joint area (a skin transplant).

In case of severe burns that have destroyed fingers or thumbs, special 'reconstructive' surgery may help to return use of the hand. (This surgery is very costly and usually can only be done by special surgeons in larger hospitals.)

For example, if the thumb has been destroyed, sometimes a finger (or toe) can be attached to the end of the stump so that the child can grasp things better.

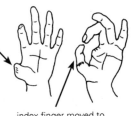

index finger moved to form thumb

PREVENTION of burns is important:

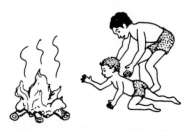

Keep small children away from fires. Where there are open fires, be sure an older child or someone else watches the young children carefully.

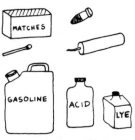

Keep matches and explosives out of reach of children.

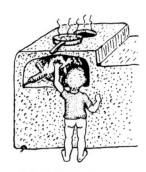

Turn handles of pans on stove so that the small child does not pull them.

Fits

CHAPTER 29

Epilepsy

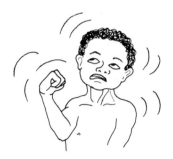

What are they? Fits (also called seizures or convulsions) are sudden, usually brief, periods of unconsciousness or changes in mental state, often with strange jerking movements.

One out of every 10 or 20 children has at least 1 fit by age 15. But only 1 in 50 of these children goes on to have chronic fits (repeated fits over a long period of time)—a condition known as **epilepsy.**

CAUSES OF CHRONIC FITS (EPILEPSY)

Fits come from damage to, or an abnormal condition of, the brain.   Common causes include:

- **Injury to the brain.** This causes at least 1/3 of epilepsies. Injuries may be before birth, during birth, or at any time after. The same causes of brain damage that result in cerebral palsy can cause epilepsy (see p. 91). In fact, **cerebral palsy and epilepsy often occur together. Meningitis** is a common cause of this combination. In small children common causes of fits are **high fever** or **severe dehydration** (loss of liquids). In very ill persons, the cause may be **meningitis, malaria of the brain,** or **poisoning** (see *Where There Is No Doctor,* p. 178). Epilepsy that steadily gets worse, especially if other signs of brain damage begin to appear, may be a sign of a **brain tumor** (or of **hydrocephalus** in a baby—see p. 169). Fits caused by a tumor usually affect one side of the body more than the other. Sometimes, fits may be caused by pork tapeworms that form cysts in the brain (see *WTND,* p. 143).

- **Hereditary.** There is a family history of fits in about 1/3 of persons with fits.

- **Unknown causes.** In about 1/3 of epilepsies, no family history or history of brain damage can be found.

Fever fits. Children who have once had a fit with a high fever often will have fits again when they have a fever—especially if other persons in the family have had fits with fever. Be sure to check for *infections* of the ears and throat, as well as bacterial dysentery (diarrhea with blood and fever), and **treat the cause.**

Fits that come only with fever usually stop occurring by the time the child is 7 years old. Sometimes they may develop into 'non-fever-related epilepsy' especially if the child has signs of brain damage (see "Cerebral Palsy," p. 87 and 88).

WARNING: Fits in a very ill child may be a sign of **meningitis**—for which immediate medical treatment is necessary to save his life. Learn how to check for signs of meningitis (see *Where There Is No Doctor,* p. 185).

MENINGITIS

The spasms of **tetanus** can be mistaken for fits. The jaw shuts tightly (lockjaw) and the body suddenly bends back. Learn to spot early signs of tetanus (see *WTND,* p. 182).

TETANUS

MORE ABOUT FITS (EPILEPSY)

Mental ability. Some children with epilepsy are intelligent. Others are mentally slow. Occasionally, fits that are very frequent and severe can injure the brain and cause or increase *retardation.* Treatment to control fits is important.

Types of fits. Fits may appear very differently in different children. Some may have severe, 'big' or 'major' fits with strong, uncontrollable movements and loss of consciousness. Others may have smaller or 'minor' fits. These can be 'brief spells' with strange movements of some part of the body. They can be sudden unusual behavior such as lip-sucking or pulling at clothes. Or they can be brief 'absences' in which the child suddenly stops and stares—perhaps with blinking or fast movement of the eyelids.

Some children will have both minor and 'big' fits or they may first have minor ones and later develop big ones.

Warning signs or 'aura'. Depending on the kind of fits, the child (and parents) may be able to sense when a fit is about to begin. Some children experience a 'warning' in which they may see flashes of light or colors. Or they may suddenly cry out. In one kind of fit, the 'warning' may be fear or imagined sights, sounds, smells, or tastes. In some kinds of fits there is no 'warning'. The child's body may suddenly jerk or be thrown violently. These children may need to continuously wear some kind of safety hat or other head protection.

Timing of fits. Fits may happen weeks or months apart, or very often. Minor fits or 'absences' may come in groups—often in the early morning and late afternoon.

Fits are usually short. Minor fits may last only a few seconds. Big fits seldom last more than 10 or 15 minutes. Rarely, however, a child may enter into a long 'epileptic state' which may last hours. This is a medical emergency.

Some kinds of fits may appear at any age. Others begin in early childhood and usually disappear or change to other patterns as the child grows older.

Many persons have epilepsy all their life. However, some children stop having fits after a few months or years.

Usually there is no need to know the exact kind of fits a child has. However, some kinds of fits require different medicines. **The chart on p. 240 and 241** describes the main types of fits, when they begin, and their treatment.

WHEN ARE SPECIAL MEDICAL STUDIES NEEDED?

In some poor countries, doctors sometimes prescribe medication for fits without properly checking for signs of causes that may need attention. However, more and more doctors regularly order expensive testing such as an 'EEG' (electroencephalogram). Even if these services are 'free', they are often only available in a distant city, which causes the family much time and expense. Such tests do not usually help much in deciding treatment—unless a brain tumor is suspected. And even if it is a tumor, the possibilities of surgery or successful treatment may be very small, and the costs are often much too high.

> **Usually EEG's and other costly testing are not helpful.**

WHAT TO DO WHEN A CHILD HAS A FIT

- Learn to recognize any 'warning signs' that a fit is about to begin, such as sudden fear or a cry. Quickly protect the child by lying her down on a soft mat or other place where she cannot hurt herself.

- When a 'big' fit starts, do not try to move the child unless she is in a dangerous place.

- **Protect the child as best you can against injury, but do not try to forcefully control her movements.** Remove any sharp or hard objects near her.

- **Put nothing in the child's mouth while she is having a fit**—no food, drink, medicine, nor any object to prevent biting the tongue.

- Between spasms, gently turn the child's head to one side, so that spit drains out of her mouth and she does not breathe it into her lungs.

- After the fit is over, the child may be very sleepy and confused. **Let her sleep.** For **headache,** which is common after a fit, give acetaminophen (paracetamol) or aspirin.

HEAD PROTECTION

To protect the head of a child who falls hard when she has a fit, it may be wise for her to wear some kind of head protection most of the time.

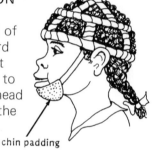

chin padding

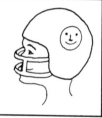
A child who often injures his face with fits may need a 'hard hat' helmet with a face mask.

You can make a 'cage' of stiff wire and wrap it with strips of inner tube, soft cloth, or sponge rubber.

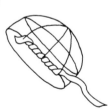

Or cut a piece of old car tire something like this.

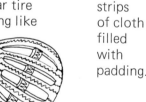

Or sew strips of cloth filled with padding.

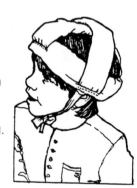

MEDICINES TO PREVENT FITS

There are no medicines that 'cure' epilepsy. However, there are medicines that can prevent the fits of most children—as long as they keep taking the medicine regularly. **As long as a child has epilepsy—which may be for years or all his life—he must continue to take anti-fit medicines.**

Sometimes preventing fits for a long time seems to help stop epilepsy permanently. For this reason, if the child has had many fits in the past, it is usually wise for him to keep taking anti-fit medicines regularly for at least one year after the last fit. Only then should you gradually lower and stop the medication to see if he still needs it.

CAUTION: Great care is needed to select the medicines that help the individual child most, and which do her the least harm. Try to avoid giving so much medicine that she always seems sleepy, dizzy, slow-moving, or loses interest in things. A few fits may be better than too much medicine–which can poison the child.

Choosing medicines

The best medicine (or medicines) for a child with epilepsy is one that is:

WARNING: When child is having a fit **do not put his feet into a fire**, it will not 'frighten him back to life' but will severely burn him.

- effective (prevents the fits).
- safe (has few side effects).
- cheap (because it must be taken for years).
- easy to take (long-acting, few doses a day).
- easy to get.

Many different medicines are used for epilepsy. Some types of fits are controlled better by one medicine and some by another medicine, or by a combination of medicines. Some children's fits are easy to control. Others are very difficult. It may be necessary to try different medicines and combinations to find the most effective treatment. In a few children, no medicines will control the fits completely.

The best medicine to try first for almost all types of fits is usually phenobarbital. Often it is very effective, and is relatively safe, cheap, and easy to take. Usually it is taken 2 times a day, but with some people only once a day at bedtime is enough.

The next best medicine for 'big' fits is usually phenytoin. It is also fairly safe, cheap, and usually needs to be taken only once each night. (For some kinds of epilepsy, however, phenytoin may make fits worse.)

For most epilepsies, phenobarbital and phenytoin are often the best drugs. First try each alone, and if that does not work, try both together. Most other drugs are less likely to be effective, are often less safe, and are much more expensive.

Unfortunately, many doctors prescribe more expensive, less safe, and often less effective medicines before trying phenobarbital or phenytoin. Partly this is due to drug companies that falsely advertise their more expensive products. In some countries, phenobarbital is difficult to get–especially in pill form. The result is that many children's fits are poorly controlled, using drugs that cause severe side effects and that are very costly. *Rehabilitation* workers need to realize this and do what they can to **help provide the safest, cheapest medicines that will effectively control each child's fits.**

CAUTION: To prevent choking, do not give medicines to a child while she is lying on her back, or if her head is pressed back. Always make sure her head is lifted forward. Never give medicines by mouth to a child while she is having a fit, or while she is asleep or unconscious.

It is usually best to **start with only one anti-fit medicine—usually phenobarbital,** if available. Start with a low to medium dose, **and after a week, if fits are not controlled and if there are no serious side effects, increase to a higher dose.** After a few days, if the fits are still not controlled, add a second medication—usually phenytoin, for 'big fits'. Again, start with a low to medium dose and gradually increase as needed.

> *CAUTION:* When you stop or change a child's medicine, do so gradually. Sudden stopping or changing the medicine may make fits worse. Also, it may take several days for a new medicine to have its full effect.

 WARNING: **All anti-fit medicines are poisonous if a child takes too much. Be careful to give the right dose and to keep medicines out of reach of children.**

INFORMATION ON DOSAGE AND PRECAUTIONS FOR ANTI-FIT MEDICINES

Phenobarbital (phenobarbitione, *Luminal*)

For all types of fits. Usually comes in:

tablets of 15 mg.	tablets of 30 mg.
tablets of 60 mg.	tablets of 100 mg.

(It costs less to buy 100 mg. tablets and cut them into pieces.)

Dosage: Because tablet sizes differ, we give the dosage in milligrams (mg.).

The usual dose is 3 to 8 mg. for each kg. of body weight every day (3 to 8 mg./kg./day)—usually given in **2 doses** (morning and evening):

Give 2 doses a day. In each dose give:

children over 12 . . . . 50 to 150mg.
children 7 to 12 years . . . . 25 to 50 mg.
children under 7 years . . . . 10 to 25 mg.

Some children do better with **1 dose** a day instead of 2 doses. Give twice the amount listed here at bedtime. But if the fits return or the child has problems going to sleep or waking up, go back to **2 doses** a day of the regular amount.

SIDE EFFECTS AND COMPLICATIONS

- Too much can cause sleepiness or slow breathing
- Some very active children become over-active or behave badly.
- Rare side effects include mild dizziness, eye–jerking, and skin rash.
- Bone growth problems may occur—especially in retarded chidlren. Extra vitamin D may help.
- Bitter taste. It may help to grind up the tablet and give it with honey or jam.
- Habit forming.

CAUTION: If tablets of 100 mg. are used, be very sure the family understands that they must be cut into pieces. Show them first and then have them do it.

  Giving a whole tablet instead of a small piece can poison the child.

Phenytoin (diphenylhydantoin, *Dilantin*)

For all types of fits except brief fits that suddenly throw the child out of balance ('jolt fits') or 'minor fits' with staring, blinking, or fast movement of eyes. (Phenytoin may make these kinds of fits worse.)

Usually comes in: capsules or tablets of 25 mg., 50 mg., and 100mg.
syrup with 30 mg. in each 5 ml. (1 teaspoon)

Dosage: Give 5 to 10 mg./kg./day in 2 divided doses, but do not exceed 300 mg./day.

Start with the following dose once a day:

children over 12 years ....100 to 300 mg.
children 7 to 12 years ....100 mg.
children 6 or under ....50 mg.

After 2 weeks, if the fits are not completely prevented, the dose can be increased, but not to more than twice the amount.

If child has no fits during several weeks, try lowering the dose little by little until you find the lowest dose that prevent the fits.

SIDE EFFECTS AND COMPLICATIONS

> *WARNING:* Watch for **dizziness, eye-jerking, seeing double,** and **severe sleepiness.** Lower the dose if any of these occur. They are early signs of poisoning, which could cause permanent brain damage.

- **Swelling and abnormal growth of the gums** often occurs with long-time use. It can be partly prevented by good mouth care. **Be sure the child brushes or cleans his teeth and gums well after eating**. If he cannot do it by himself, help him, or better, teach him. If the gum problem is severe, consider changing medicines (See *Where There Is No Dentist*, p. 109.)

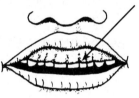

very swollen, sore gums almost covering teeth—caused by not keeping teeth clean while taking phenytoin

- Occasional side effects: increased body hair, rash, loss of appetite, vomiting.
- High dosage may cause liver damage.
- Bone growth problems sometimes occur—especially in retarded children. Extra vitamin D may help.

> *WARNING*: Sudden stopping of phenytoin may cause the child to have a **long-lasting fit.** Therefore, when stopping or changing the medicine, **lower the dosage gradually.**

Carbamazepine (*Tegretol*)

Useful for almost all types of fits as a second choice, or in combination. Especially useful for 'psychomotor' fits (see p. 241). High cost is a disadvantage. (Unfortunately, many doctors prescribe it as first choice when cheaper drugs such as phenobarbital are likely to work as well or better.)

Usually comes in: tablets of 100 mg. or 200 mg.

Dosage: 10 to 25 mg./kg./day divided into 2 to 4 doses. Or you can start with these doses 4 times a day:

children 10 to 15 years ....200 mg.
children 5 to 10 years ....150 mg.
children 1 to 5 years ....100 mg.
children under 1 year old ....50 mg.

It is best to **take it with meals.**

The dose of carbamazepine should be adjusted to the individual. Depending on how well it controls the fits, it can be raised to 30 mg./kg./day (but no higher) or dropped to 10 mg./kg./ day. Try to give the lowest amount of medicine that stops the fits.

SIDE EFFECTS AND COMPLICATIONS

- Rarely causes liver damage or reduces ability of blood to clot.

OTHER DRUGS SOMETIMES USED FOR EPILEPSY

- **Primidone** *(Mysoline)* For all fits. Start with low doses and gradually increase to 10 to 25 mg./kg./day in 2 to 4 divided doses. May cause sleepiness, dizziness, vomiting, or rash.
- **Ethosuximide** *(Zarontin)* First choice for 'minor fits' with blank staring, eye-fluttering, and perhaps strange motions--especially if the fits occur in groups in the morning and evening. Give 10 to 25 mg./kg./day in 1 or 2 doses, with food to avoid stomach ache. Rarely causes liver damage.
- **Valproic acid** *(Depakene)* Used alone or in combination with other anti-fit drugs, except carbamazepine, for 'minor fits' with blank staring or 'absences,' especially when the fits occur in groups. For children between 1 and 12 years. The dosage for a child who weighs up to 20 kg. is initially 20 mg./kg./day in 2 to 3 divided doses. (For example, a child weighing 10 kg. would take 200 mg. a day, and a child weighing 20 kg. would take 400 mg. a day.) Children over 20 kg can start with 400 mg. a day in divided doses, and the dose can be increased until the fits are controlled (usually up to 30 mg./kg./day). Never give more than 60 mg./kg./day. Few side effects. May cause liver damage, so monitor liver function for the first 6 months, especially for children younger than 3 years old.
- **Corticosteroids** *(or corticotropin)* These are sometimes tried for 'baby spasms' and 'jolt fits' (see p. 240) that are not controlled by other medicines. But long-term use of these medicines always causes serious and possibly dangerous side effects (see p. 137). They should be used only with highly skilled medical advice when all other possible medicines have failed.
- **Diazepam** *(Valium)* Sometimes used for 'newborn fits' or 'baby spasms' (see p. 240), but other medicines should be tried first. May cause sleepiness or dizziness. Mildly habit forming. Give about 0.2 mg./kg./day in divided doses.

CAUTION DURING PREGNANCY: Many of the anti-fit drugs, especially phenytoin, **may increase the risk of birth defects when taken by pregnant women.** Also, some of the drug goes into breast milk. Therefore, pregnant women should use these drugs only when fits are common or severe without them. Women taking fit medicine should not breast feed if they are able to feed their babies well without breast milk. Phenobarbital is probably the safest anti-fit medicine during pregnancy.

TREATMENT FOR A LONG-LASTING FIT

When a fit has lasted more than 15 minutes:

- if someone knows how, inject IV diazepam *(Valium)* or phenobarbital **into the vein.**

CAUTION: Diazepam and phenobarbital must both be injected very slowly. For diazepam, take at least 3 minutes to inject the dose for children. For phenobarbital, inject children at the rate of 30 mg./minute or slower, and in adults, not more than 100 mg./minute.

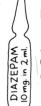 Doses for injectable diazepam:	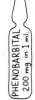 Doses for injectable phenobarbital:
Adults . . 5 to 10 mg. Children 7-12 years . . . 3 to 5 mg. Children under 7 . . . 1 mg. for every 5 kg. of body weight.	Adults . . . . 200 mg. Children 7-12 years . . . . 150 mg. Children 2-6 years . . . . 100 mg. Children under 2 years . . . 50 mg.

- or put a 'suppository' of diazepam, paraldehyde, or phenobarbital up the rectum (asshole).

NOTE: These medicines do not work as fast or well when they are injected into a muscle. If you only have injectable or liquid medicine, put it up the rectum with a *plastic* syringe without a needle. Or grind up a pill of diazepam or phenobarbital, mix with water, and put it up the rectum.

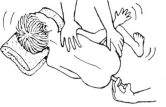

Putting diazepam up the rectum works faster than injecting it into a muscle.

If the fit does not stop in 15 minutes after giving the medicine, repeat the dose.

Types of epileptic fits

Note: This information is for rehabilitation workers and parents because many doctors and health workers do not treat fits correctly. With care, perhaps you can do better. However, correct diagnosis and treatment can be very difficult. If possible, get advice from a well-informed medical worker. Ask her help in using this chart. It is adapted from *Current Pediatric Diagnosis and Treatment* by Kempe, Silver, and O'Brien (Lange Medical Publishing), in which more complete information is provided.

TYPE	AGE FITS BEGIN	APPEARANCE	TREATMENT
Newborn fits	birth to 2 weeks	Often not typical of later fits. May show sudden limpness or stiffness; brief periods of not breathing and turning blue; strange cry; or eyes roll back; blinking or eye-jerking; sucking or chewing movements; jerks or strange movement of part or all of body. *WARNING:* Make sure spasms are not from tetanus or meningitis (see p. 233). With cerebral palsy in the newborn, the baby is usually limp. Stiffness and/or uncontrolled movements usually appear months later, but the baby does not lose consciousness.	Phenobarbital or phenytoin. Add diazepam if not controlled. (Fits due to brain damage at birth are often very hard to control.)
Baby spasms (West's syndrome)	3–18 months (sometimes up to 4 years)	Sudden opening of arms and legs and then bending them— or repeat patterns of a strange movement. Spasms often repeated **in groups** when waking or falling to sleep, or when very tired, sick, or upset. Most children with these spasms are retarded.	Corticosteroids may be tried—but are dangerous. Try to get help from an experienced doctor or health worker. Valproic acid or diazepam may help.
Fever fits (fits that only occur when child has a fever)	6 months to 4 years	Usually 'big' fits (see next page) that happen only when child has a fever from another cause (sore throat, ear infection, bad cold). May last up to 15 minutes or longer. Often a history of fever fits in the family. *WARNING:* Look for signs of meningitis.	A child who has had fever fits on several occasions should be treated with phenobarbital continuously until age 4 or until one year after the last fit. Fits usually do not continue in later childhood.
Jolt or 'lightening bolt' fits (Lennox-Gastaut syndrome)	any age but usually 4–7 years	Sudden violent spasms of some muscles, without warning, may throw child to one side, forward, or backward. Usually no loss of consciousness, or only brief. Many children also have 'big' or generalized fits. May be a history of 'baby spasms' (see above) in earlier childhood.	Try phenobarbital, with valproic acid. If no improvement, consider trying corticosteroids as in baby spasms, or other medicines with medical advice. Protect child's head with headgear and chin padding.

Types of epileptic fits (continued)

TYPE	AGE FITS BEGIN	APPEARANCE	TREATMENT
Blank spells or 'absences' (petit mal). (This type of fit alone is rare.)	3–15 years	Child suddenly stops what she is doing and briefly has a strange, empty or 'blank' look. She usually does not fall, but does not seem to see or hear during the fit. These 'absences' usually happen in groups. She may make unconscious movements, or her eyes may move rapidly or blink. These fits can be brought on by breathing rapidly and deeply. (Use this as a test.) Often confused with 'psychomotor' fits, which are much more common.	Valproic acid or ethosuximide. Since many children also have 'big' fits, add phenobarbital if necessary (or try it first if you think the fits might be 'psychomotor' —see below).
'Marching' fits (Focal fits)	any age	Movement begins in one part of the body. May spread in a certain pattern (Jacksonian march) and become generalized. *Note:* If fits that occur in one part of the body get worse and worse, or other signs of brain damage begin to appear, the cause might be a brain tumor.	Phenobarbital or phenytoin (or both). If poor results, try carbamazepine or primidone.
Mind-and-body fits (psycho-motor fits)	any age	Starts with 'warning' signs: sense of fear, stomach trouble, odd smell or taste, 'hears' or 'sees' imaginary things. Fit may consist of an empty stare, strange movements of face, tongue or mouth, strange sounds, or odd movements such as picking at clothes. Unlike 'blank spells', these fits usually do not occur in groups but alone and they last longer. Most children with psychomotor fits later develop 'big' fits.	Try phenobarbital first —then phenytoin, or both together, then carbamazepine, or all 3 together. Valproic acid may also be useful. Or primidone instead of phenobarbital. Psychological counseling sometimes also helps.
Generalized or 'big' fits (grand mal)	any age	Loss of consciousness—often after a vague warning feeling or cry. Uncontrolled twisting or violent movements. Eyes roll back. May have tongue biting, or loss of urine and bowel control. Followed by confusion and sleep. Often mixed with other types of fits. Often family history of fits.	Try phenobarbital first. Then phenytoin. Then carbamazepine —or combinations. Or combine primidone with one or more of the others.
Temper tantrum fits (not really epilepsy)	under 7 years	Some children in 'fits of anger' stop breathing and turn blue. Lack of air may cause loss of consciousness briefly and even convulsions (body spasms, eyes rolling back). These brief fits, in which the child turns blue **before** losing consciousness, are not dangerous.	No medical treatment is needed. Use methods to help the child improve behavior (see Chapter 40).

HELPING THE COMMUNITY UNDERSTAND EPILEPSY

Fits can be frightening to those who see someone having them. For this reason, epileptic children (and adults) sometimes have a hard time gaining acceptance in the community.

Rehabilitation workers need to help everyone in the community realize that **epilepsy is not the result of witchcraft** or the work of evil spirits. It is **not a sign of madness**, is **not the result of bad actions** by the child or parents or ancestors, is **not an infectious disease,** and **cannot be 'caught' or spread to other people.**

It is important that epileptic children go to school and take part in day-to-day work, play, and adventures in family and village life. This is true even if fits are not completely under control. The schoolteachers and other children should learn about epilepsy and how to protect a child when she has a fit. If they learn more about epilepsy it will help them to be supportive rather than afraid or cruel. (See CHILD-to-child activities, p. 429.)

Although children with epilepsy should be encouraged to lead active, normal lives, certain precautions are needed—especially for children who have sudden fits without warning. Village children can learn to help in the safety of such a child—especially at times when danger is greatest.

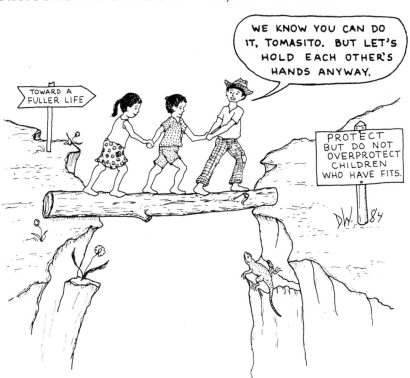

TOWARD A FULLER LIFE

WE KNOW YOU CAN DO IT, TOMASITO. BUT LET'S HOLD EACH OTHER'S HANDS ANYWAY.

PROTECT BUT DO NOT OVERPROTECT CHILDREN WHO HAVE FITS.

PREVENTION of epilepsy

1. Try to avoid causes of brain damage—during pregnancy, at birth, and in childhood. This is discussed under prevention of cerebral palsy, p. 107.

2. Avoid marriage between close relatives, especially in families with a history of epilepsy.

3. When children with epilepsy take their medicine regularly to prevent fits, sometimes the fits do not come back after the medicine is stopped. To make it more likely that fits will not come back, be sure that the child takes her anti-fit medicine for at least a year after her last fit. (Often, however, fits will still return when medicine is stopped. If this happens, the medicines should be taken for at least another year before you try stopping again.)

Blindness and Difficulty Seeing

Difficulty with seeing can be mild, moderate, or severe. When a person sees very little or nothing, we say he is blind. Some children are **completely blind;** they cannot see anything. However, **most blind children can see a little.** Some can only see the difference between light and dark or day and night, but cannot see any shapes of things. Others can see shapes of large objects, but none of the details.

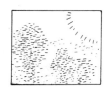

what a child with normal sight can see

Many more children are not blind but do have some **problem seeing things clearly.** For example, they may see fairly well for most daily activities, but have trouble seeing details. The family may not realize that the child has a seeing problem until they notice she has difficulty threading a needle, finding head lice, or reading letters on the blackboard at school. Often these children can see much better with eyeglasses or a magnifying glass. (Children who are completely blind cannot see at all, even with eyeglasses.)

Some children are born blind. Others become blind during early childhood, or later.

> *CAUTION:* Not all children who are blind have eyes that look different. Their eyes may look clear and normal. The damage may be behind the eyes or in part of the brain. So be sure to watch for other signs that can tell you if a child has difficulty seeing.

what a partly blind child may see (large forms but no details)

SIGNS THAT COULD MEAN A CHILD HAS A SEEING PROBLEM

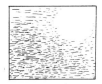

what a child sees who can only tell the direction a bright light is coming from

- Eyes or eyelids are red, have pus, or continually form tears.
- Eyes look dull, wrinkled, or cloudy, or have sores or other obvious problems.
- One or both pupils (the black center of the eye) looks gray or white.
- By 3 months of age, the child's eyes still do not follow an object or light that is moved in front of them.
- By 3 months the child does not reach for things held in front of him, unless the things make a sound or touch him.
- Eyes 'cross', or one eye turns in or out, or moves differently from the other. (Some eye-crossing is normal up to 6 months.)
- Child squints (half shuts his eyes) or tips head to look at things.
- Child is slower to begin using his hands, move about, or walk than other children, and he often bumps into things or seems clumsy.
- Child takes little interest in brightly colored objects or pictures and books, or she puts them very close to her face.
- Has difficulty seeing after the sun sets (night blindness).
- In school, the child cannot read letters on the blackboard. Or he cannot read small print in books, or gets tired or often gets headaches when he reads.

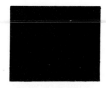

what a completely blind child sees

If the child shows any of these signs, test her vision, and if possible, see a health worker or eye doctor. Sometimes eyesight can be saved by preventive steps or early treatment (see p. 245).

Methods for **testing if a baby sees** and for **measuring the vision of children** are discussed with CHILD-to-child activities on p. 452 and 453, and in *Helping Children Who Are Blind.* For more about that book, see p. 639.

Blindness with other disabilities

Some children with cerebral palsy or other *disabilities* are also partly or completely blind. Parents may not realize this and think that the child's slow development or lack of interest in things is because he is mentally and physically handicapped. In fact, blindness may be a large part of the cause.

Even if a child has no other disability, **blindness can make development of early skills slower and more difficult. If the child does not look at, reach for, or take interest in things around him, check if he can see (and hear).**

Note: Some children with very severe brain damage or mental retardation may seem blind. They may look at things without really seeing them, because their brains are at the developmental level of a newborn baby. With lots of stimulation, little by little some of these children begin to become more aware of things, to follow them with their eyes, and finally to reach for them.

Causes of blindness

Different people have different beliefs about what causes blindness. In some parts of the world, people think a child is born blind as punishment for something the parents have done. In parts of Latin America, villagers believe that a bat's urine fell in the baby's eyes, or that a 'black witch moth' flew by the baby's face. These things do not really cause blindness, and as people get new information, many are leaving these older beliefs behind.

We now know that **child blindness is usually caused by poor nutrition or infection,** and that **most blindness in children can be prevented.**

COMMON CAUSES OF BLINDNESS IN CHILDREN ARE:

1. **'Dry eyes'** (xerophthalmia, or nutritional blindness) is the most common cause of child blindness. It is especially common in parts of Africa and Asia. It results when a child does not get enough vitamin A, which occurs naturally in many fruits and vegetables (and also in milk, meats, and eggs). 'Dry eyes' develops in children who are not regularly fed any of these foods. It often appears or quickly gets worse when these children get **diarrhea** or have **measles, whooping cough,** or **tuberculosis.** It is much more common in children who are not breast-fed.

Dry eyes can be prevented by feeding children foods with vitamin A. Encourage families to grow and eat things like papaya, squash, carrots, and leafy green vegetables in a family garden. **Be sure the child eats these foods regularly, beginning at 6 months old.**

Vitamin A capsules or liquid can also prevent dry eyes, but should not take the place of a well-balanced diet. Give 200,000 units (60 mg. retinol) once every 4 to 6 months (or 100,000 units to babies less than 1 year old). Do not give this large dose more often than 4 to 6 months, because **too much vitamin A can poison the child.** For **treatment,** give 200,000 units (I.U.) of vitamin A at once, 200,000 I.U. the next day, and 200,000 I.U. 2 weeks later. Give half the dose to children under age 1. See a health worker.

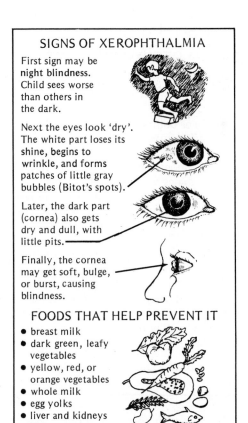

SIGNS OF XEROPHTHALMIA

First sign may be **night blindness.** Child sees worse than others in the dark.

Next the eyes look 'dry'. The white part loses its shine, begins to wrinkle, and forms patches of little gray bubbles (Bitot's spots).

Later, the dark part (cornea) also gets dry and dull, with little pits.

Finally, the cornea may get soft, bulge, or burst, causing blindness.

FOODS THAT HELP PREVENT IT
- breast milk
- dark green, leafy vegetables
- yellow, red, or orange vegetables
- whole milk
- egg yolks
- liver and kidneys
- fish

2. Trachoma is the commonest cause of preventable blindness in the world. It often begins in children and may last for months or years. If not treated early, it can cause blindness. It is spread by touch or flies and is most common in poor, crowded living conditions.

Trachoma can often be prevented by keeping the child's eyes clean and keeping flies away. To prevent blindness from trachoma, treat early with erythromycin or tetracycline eye ointment (see a health worker, or *Where There Is No Doctor,* p. 220).

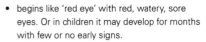
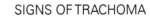

SIGNS OF TRACHOMA

- begins like 'red eye' with red, watery, sore eyes. Or in children it may develop for months with few or no early signs.
- After a month or more, small lumps form inside the upper eyelids.
- White of the eye becomes inflamed or swollen.
- Top edge of the cornea may look cloudy.
- After years the lumps inside eyelids begin to go away, leaving whitish scars.
- The scars may pull the eyelashes down into the eye, scratching the cornea and leading to blindness.

3. Gonorrhea or **chlamydia** in the eyes of newborn babies causes blindness if not treated immediately. The eyes get red, swell, and have a lot of pus. Blindness can be prevented by putting erythromycin or tetracycline eye ointment, or 1 drop of povidone-iodine solution, in the eyes of *all* babies at birth. (A drop of silver nitrate solution will stop blindness from gonorrhea, but not from chlamydia.) The mother can pass these infections to her baby at birth even if she has no signs of infection.

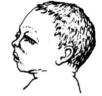

If the baby's eyes get red, swell, and have a lot of pus in them within the first month, he may have one or both of these infections. If you cannot test to find out which disease is causing the infection, give the baby medicines for both.

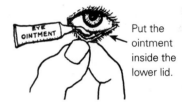
Put the ointment inside the lower lid.

Treatment for gonorrhea: inject 125 mg. of ceftriaxone in the thigh muscle, 1 time only.

Treatment for chlamydia: give 30 mg. erthromycin syrup by mouth, 4 times a day, for 14 days.

If a baby develops gonorrhea or chlamydia of the eyes, both parents must be treated for these infections too. See *Where There is No Doctor* (pages 236, 237 and 360) or *Where Women Have No Doctor* (Chapter 16).

4. River blindness (onchocerciasis) is a very common cause of blindness in parts of Africa and Latin America. (See *Where There Is No Doctor,* p. 227.) It is spread by a kind of black fly that breeds in rivers and streams. There is no cure.

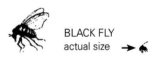
BLACK FLY actual size ➤ 🦟

5. Measles, which can injure the surface of the eyes, is a common cause of blindness, especially in Africa and in children who are poorly nourished.

6. Brain damage causes blindness in many children, usually in combination with cerebral palsy or other disabilities. Brain damage can happen before, during, or after birth. Causes include German measles during pregnancy, delayed breathing at birth, and meningitis. See p. 91.

7. Eye injuries often cause blindness in children. Pointed tools, fireworks, acid, lye, and homemade bombs to dynamite fish are common causes.

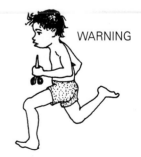
WARNING

8. Also, blindness in children is sometimes caused by other problems such as hydrocephalus (see p. 169), arthritis (see p. 136), leprosy (see p. 219), brain tumors, or certain medicines (see p. 246). Cataracts (clouding of the lens inside the eye) gradually develop in about half of older children with Down Syndrome.

Running with a pointed object is DANGEROUS TO THE EYES.

WARNING ON USE OF EYE MEDICINES

Only use modern medicines or 'home cures' that you are *sure* cannot damage the eyes.

One modern medicine that should not be used often, and only with great caution, is **corticosteroid eye ointment.** Some doctors and health workers prescribe it for almost any eye irritation. **This is a dangerous mistake.** If the irritation is caused by a *virus* (tiny germ), this ointment could make the infection worse and lead to eye damage or blindness!*

Some 'home cures' for eye problems are safe and effective. For example, in Mexico when villagers get a small piece of dirt or sand in the eye, to remove it they put a wet **chia seed** under the eyelid. The smooth seed has a layer of sticky mucus on it, to which the dirt sticks. Then they remove the seed. This is a safe, good home cure.

chia seeds—a helpful home cure

Some home cures are dangerous. Some villagers try to treat 'blurred vision' by putting human feces (shit) around the eye. This is unsafe and does not help. It could lead to dangerous infection. It is also dangerous to put lemon juice, urine, pieces of abalone shell, or *Vicks* ointment in the eye.

*Note: Corticosteroid drops or ointment are important medicine for preventing blindness from iritis (see "Arthritis" and "Leprosy"). But tests with 'fluorescein' should be done first to be sure there is not a virus infection. Get medical advice.

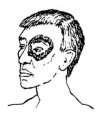

putting feces around the eye—a dangerous home cure

What is the future for a blind child?

With help and encouragement from family and community, a child who is blind can usually develop early skills as quickly and as well as other children. *Helping Children Who Are Blind* (see p. 639) shows ways he can learn to feed, bathe, dress, and care for himself, and to find his way around the home and village without help. Although he cannot see well, he develops an outstanding ability to use his sense of hearing, touch, and even smell. If he can see at all, he can be helped to make the best use of whatever vision he has. He can and should go to school. Although he may not be able to read ordinary writing, he can develop his memory.

As he grows up, he can become a farmer, or a craftsperson. And if he has the opportunity for training, he can learn any of a wide variety of skills. Where blind persons are given a fair chance, they often take active part in their communities and can live full, happy lives. In many countries, blind people have been leaders in organizing disabled persons to become more self-reliant and to work toward their rightful place in society.

Unfortunately, blind children often are not given a chance to develop as quickly or as fully as they could. In some countries more than half of the children who are born blind die of hunger or neglect before they are 5 years old. On the next page are 2 stories of blind children that will help you realize the difference that understanding and help from family and community can make.

SHANTI*

Shanti is a little blind girl, who was born in a small village in India. When they found that she was blind, her parents and grandparents tried to hide the fact from the other villagers. They thought all blindness was sent to a family as a punishment for sin, and that people would look down on them.

Secretly her parents took Shanti to an orphanage and left her there.

Nobody in the orphanage had ever cared for a blind child, and they did not know what to do. There were so many other children who needed care, that there was no time left for her.

Shanti was kept alive, but that was all. Nobody talked to her or held her lovingly or tried to stimulate her. Her blind eyes made the nurses think she could not understand or recognize anything around her. So when other babies began to reach out for objects they saw, and then to crawl toward things they wanted, Shanti was left lying silently on her cot.

People got used to the blind child. She was picked up when necessary, and cleaned and fed. They fed her with a bottle, or pushed food into her mouth. But nobody tried to teach her how to feed herself or how to walk and talk.

As she grew older, Shanti spent most of her time sitting on the doorstep, rocking herself and poking her eyes (see p. 364). She never said a word and only cried when she was hungry. Other children stayed away from her; they were afraid of her dead eyes. Everyone thought she was mentally retarded and that nothing could be done about it.

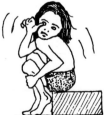

In time, Shanti did begin to talk and walk. But the sad, stony look on her face never disappeared. Now, at age 7 she is in some ways still like a 2-year-old. And in other ways she is no longer a child. We can only guess at her future.

---

*Story adapted from *How To Raise a Blind Child.*

RANI

Rani is also a little blind girl, born in another village in India. Like Shanti's family, when her parents learned she was blind, they were worried about what the villagers would say. But the baby's grandmother, who had slowly lost her sight 5 years ago, said, "I think we should do everything we can for the baby. Look at me. I, too, am now blind, and yet I still have all the same feelings and needs as I did when I could see. And I can still do most of the things I used to do. I still bring water from the well, grind the rice, milk the goats, . . ."

"But you could already do all those things before you went blind," said the father. "How could a blind baby learn?"

"We must help her learn," said Grandma. "Just as I've learned to do things by sound and touch, so Rani must learn. I can help teach her, since I know what it's like. But we can also get advice from the health worker."

The village health worker came the next day. She did not know much about blindness, but she knew a little about early child development. She suggested they give the baby a lot of stimulation in hearing and feeling and smelling things, to make up for what she could not see. "And talk to her a lot," she said.

The family took the advice. They put all kinds of things in Rani's hands and told her what they were. They gave her bells and squeakers, and cans and bottles to bang on. Grandma, especially, took Rani with her everywhere, and had her feel and listen to everything. She played games with her and sang to her. At age 2, Grandma taught her to feel her way along the walls and fence, just as she did. By age 3, Rani could find her own way to the latrine and the well. When she was 4, the health worker talked with the neighbors, and did some CHILD-to-child activities on blindness with their children. After, a few children came to make friends and play with Rani. Sometimes they would all blindfold their faces and try to find something or tell different things apart. At these games, Rani usually won.

When she was 6, Rani started school. The neighbor children came for her every day. When the villagers saw them all walking down the road together, it was hard to guess which one was blind.

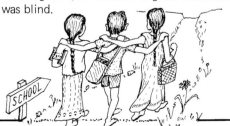

Early stimulation

As Rani's grandmother realized, a child who is blind has all the same needs as other children. She needs to be loved, not pitied. She needs to get to know the members of the family, and other things, by touch, sound, smell, and taste. The whole family can help her to become more aware of her home, and the things that are going on around her.

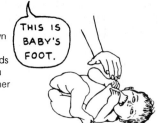

A baby's first plaything is her own body. Since she cannot see her hands and feet move, you may need to help her to feel, taste, smell, and explore them.

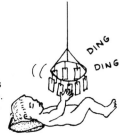

Have him compare by touch and sound his own and other people's faces so that he begins to recognize different people.

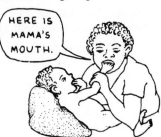

Activities to help a child develop early skills more quickly are discussed in Chapter 35, p. 301 to 318. Most of these activities can help a blind child. But **because he cannot see, he will need more stimulation in other areas, especially sound and touch, and in beginning to reach toward things and move about.** Use toys and playthings that have many different shapes, feel different to touch, and make different sounds (see p. 468 to 476 and *Helping Children Who Are Blind*, described on p. 639).

At first you may need to place the toy in the child's hand, or guide his hand to it. Or hang different things near him so that when he moves his hands they touch them.

At each stage of the child's development, attract her attention with a noisy plaything. Have her reach for it and then try to move toward it.

FIND YOUR RATTLE!

GOOD GIRL!

Praise her when she does well or tries.

In addition to special activities, **be sure the child spends most of each day in a situation where she can keep learning about people and things.** In everything you do, **talk to her,** tell her the names of things, and explain what you and she are doing. At first she will not understand, but your voice will let her know you are near. Listening to words and names of things will also prepare her for learning language skills.

Talk to the child as you do housework. Tell her what makes the sound she hears.

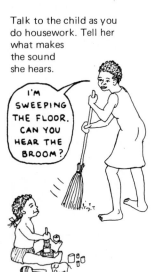

Sing to the child and encourage him to move to music.

Also encourage blind children to make their own music.

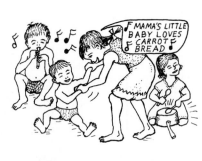

For ideas on homemade musical instruments, see p. 469.

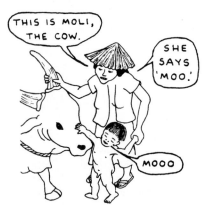

Take the child outside often: to the market, the river, the cowshed, the village square. Show and explain different things to him, and tell him what makes different sounds.

For a blind child, it is important that special help and stimulation start early—in the first months of life. Without this the child will fall far behind in her development. She may become quiet, not do much, and be afraid to move about. So her family does not expect much of her, or provide many learning opportunities. As a result, she falls still farther behind.

However, **if a blind child has the stimulation and help she needs from an early age, she will develop many skills as quickly, or nearly as quickly, as a child who sees.** So her family expects more of her and includes her more in their activities. As a result, she may develop almost as quickly as other children her age. She can probably enter school when they do.

Helping the blind child learn to move about

The child who is blind often is slow at learning to move about and will need extra help and encouragement. Some of the activities in Chapter 35 for creeping, crawling, standing, and walking will help. Here are some other suggestions.

When the child is beginning to scoot or crawl, you can leave toys and other interesting things in different places where he will find them. This will encourage him to explore and discover.

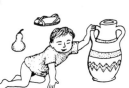

But when the child begins to walk, try to keep everything in its place, so that she does not bump into things unexpectedly and can gain more confidence moving about. If you change the position of something, show her where it is.

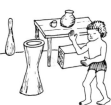

Play games and do exercises that will help the child gain confidence in moving and using his body.

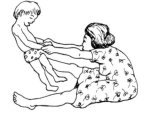

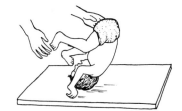

Encourage the child to make adventure, explore, and do all the things a child normally does. Protect her from hurting herself—but do not protect her too much. Remember, all children learning to walk sometimes fall. A blind child is no different.

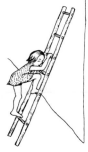

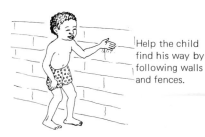

Help the child find his way by following walls and fences.

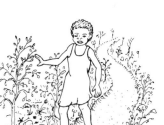

The child can learn to feel the edge of the path with her feet, and to feel plants or other objects with her hands.

If the child does not start walking without help, let him start by pushing a simple walker, chair, or cart.

Do not force the blind child to walk alone before he is ready. One day he will start walking alone, first a few steps only, but finally with confidence.

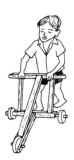

Helping the blind child find her way without holding on

Outside the home, often a blind child will let you lead her by the hand, but may be afraid to take steps or try to find her way alone.

To help her begin to walk alone, first lead her over the area where you want her to walk. Show her and let her feel the different landmarks (posts, trees, bushes, houses) along the way.

A good way to guide a child by the hand is to let her hold one finger and walk a step behind you.

Now walk over the same path, but this time walk backward in front of her, and talk to her while you are walking.

When she feels comfortable with your walking in front of her, start walking behind her. Have her tell you the landmarks.

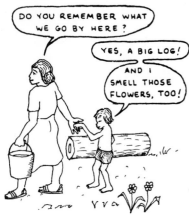
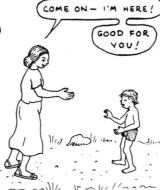
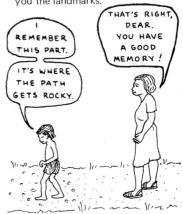

Little by little make yourself less and less needed. Speak less and let her go farther away from you.

Finally let her go the whole way alone. Start by having her walk short distances. Then gradually go farther, with more turns and other things to remember.

When she has progressed this far, the child will have the joy of knowing she can solve some problems alone. She will be ready to learn new things, meet other difficulties, and explore new areas.

Sometimes the child will fall. Have her practice this by falling on soft ground. Teach her to put out her hands and bend her knees as she falls. She will be less likely to hurt herself.

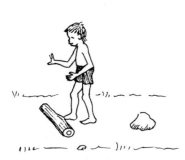

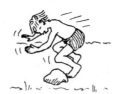

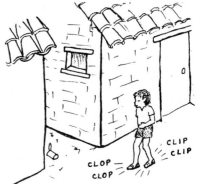

The child needs to learn to 'see' with her feet, and to be prepared for unexpected things in her way. Play games with her. Tell her you have put some things in her path. See if she can get past them without slipping or falling.

Help the child to recognize how the sound of her footsteps (or her stick) changes when she is near a house or wall, and when there is open space. With practice, she can learn to tell the distance from things by the sounds.

Learning to use a stick

Using a long stick can help a child find his way and give him more confidence, especially for walking in places he is not familiar with. With practice, it can also help him to walk in a faster, more normal way, with long, sure steps. This is because he can feel farther ahead of him with his stick than with his feet. The best age to start teaching a child to use a stick is probably about 6 or 7.

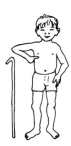

The stick should be thin and light, and tall enough so that it reaches half way between the child's waist and shoulders. The top of the cane can be curved or straight.

At first just give the child the stick and have him lightly touch the ground in front of him as he walks. His arm should be straight.

Play games letting him feel his way. But do not hurry him. Stop before he gets tired of it. At first, 5 or 10 minutes is enough.

After he gets used to the stick, walk beside him and encourage him to take smooth, even steps.

Have him swing the stick from side to side, and see if he can find things in his path.

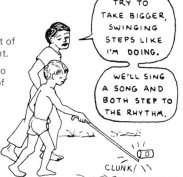

TRY TO TAKE BIGGER, SWINGING STEPS LIKE I'M DOING.

WE'LL SING A SONG AND BOTH STEP TO THE RHYTHM.

CLUNK/

After a time he can learn to use the stick better:

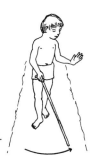

Move the stick from side to side, lightly touching the ground.

The width of the swing should be a little more than the width of his shoulders.

As the stick touches to one side, move the foot on the other side forward.

On a narrow path or rough ground, someone can lead the child by the stick.

Or the child can hold the person's elbow or wrist.

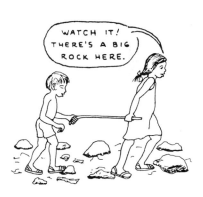

WATCH IT! THERE'S A BIG ROCK HERE.

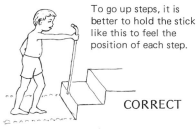

The child can learn to feel the height of steps and curbs, and then to climb them.

To go up steps, it is better to hold the stick like this to feel the position of each step.

CORRECT

Do not hold it like this. This can cause the cane to stop suddenly and hit the child in the stomach.

WRONG

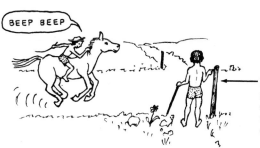

BEEP BEEP

Teach the child to listen carefully before he crosses a path or road where cars or other traffic pass.

Putting posts or other markings where roads or paths cross can help the child find his way or know where to turn.

But whenever possible, **teach him to find his way using 'landmarks' that are already there.**

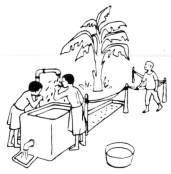

Sometimes putting a guide rope or rail can help the child find his way.

Helping the blind child to use his hands and to learn skills

Help the child who cannot see well to do all kinds of things with her hands, including daily care of herself: eating, dressing, bathing, and toileting. Ideas for learning these skills are in Chapters 36 to 39.

At first you may need to help the child feel things by guiding his hands.

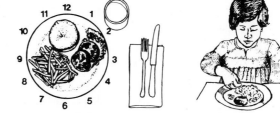

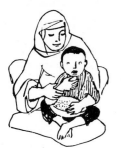

To help the child know where to look for the different foods on her plate, try to always put them in the same place. As the child gets older and learns to tell time, have her think of the plate or bowl as a clock. Tell her at what time each type of food is put on her plate. Here the glass of water is at 2 o'clock. Always put it at 2 o'clock.

Help the child learn to **put in the same place** glasses, cups, bottles, and other things that can be easily spilled or broken. Teach her to remember where she puts things, and learn how to reach out for something and find it without knocking it over. **Reaching out with the back of the hand causes less spilling.** (This will take practice and there will be accidents, but that is the way she learns. Do not hand her everything or do everything for her, just to avoid a mess. Making a mess is part of learning.)

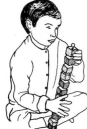

Help the child learn to recognize different shapes, sizes, and the 'feel of things' with her fingers. Let her play with toys and puzzles so that she learns to put different pieces together in a certain pattern or order. Ideas for toys and puzzles are on pages 468 to 476.

Teach the child about things he must be careful with or keep a distance from, to not get hurt: things such as fire, hot pans and dishes, sharp knives, dogs and mules that might bite or kick, deep holes, wells, cliffs, deep ponds or rivers. Do not just tell him "No!" Help him to understand the danger.

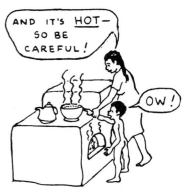

> *CAUTION:* **Whenever possible, keep dangerous things out of reach or put fences around them, and take other precautions to protect the child—especially until he is old enough to be careful.**

Give the child **opportunities to begin to help** in different ways around the house. This will both increase her skills and give her a sense of being part of the life and action of the family.

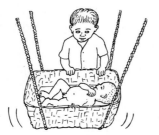

Abdul helps rock his baby brother.

Rani's mother teaches her how to cook by guiding her hand and explaining each step.

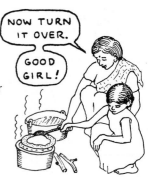

When the child has learned to handle bigger things fairly well, help her learn to feel and handle smaller things. For example:

She can help sister pick the little stones and bits of dirt out of the rice.

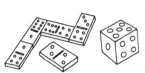

GOOD! YOU CLEAN IT AS WELL AS I DO!

If someone takes the time to teach him, a child can begin to help in a lot of things around the home, and also in village crafts. Weaving of mats, rugs, clothing, and baskets are things many blind children can learn to do well, and it helps them learn to use their hands skillfully.

Also, look for games and toys that help the child develop her ability to feel fine details and small shapes with her fingers.

For example, you can make dominos and dice out of wood. For the dots, hammer round-headed nails into the wood, so she can feel them. Or drill holes.

The child can learn to feel the dots with her fingertips. At the same time, she will begin to learn to count and use numbers.

You can start with 'giant' dominos and dice, and when her fingers learn to feel more skillfully, change to small ones. This will be good preparation for doing many kinds of fine work and perhaps for learning to read braille.

SCHOOL

Blind children should have the same opportunity as other children to go to school. Ideas for how children in the community can help a blind child get to school, and help her in the classroom and with her studies are discussed in the CHILD-to-child activity on blindness (see p. 449).

In most countries there are special schools that teach blind children to read and write **'braille'**. Braille is a system of raised dots that represent letters and can be read with the fingertips. It was invented many years ago by a blind boy from France named Louis Braille.

Most village children do not learn braille in school. However, there are **many other ways** that they can learn in school.

For the blind village schoolchild, one of the best aids for taking notes and reviewing lessons is a small **tape recorder.** The family should try to save money to buy one. Or perhaps the schoolchildren can hold a raffle or collect money to buy one. Other children can help record lessons from school books, and stories and information from other books.

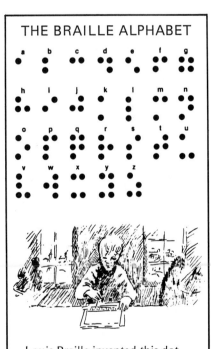

THE BRAILLE ALPHABET

Louis Braille invented this dot alphabet at age 14. The dots are pressed into a thick paper from the opposite side with a pointed tool called a 'stylus'.

IMPORTANT: In order to keep up with her studies a blind child will need help. In school another child can read to her from her books. The child may also need extra help after school. An older brother or sister, or another schoolchild, can perhaps spend time teaching her at home.

Remember, **most 'blind' children have some useful vision. Encourage the child to use whatever sight she has.** If she can see big letters on the blackboard, write big and clear, and be sure she sits in the front. **Be sure the light is good, and that dark letters and things stand out against a light background.**

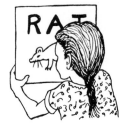

If she can see at all, to help her learn the letters, make them very **BIG**. Use white paper and dark ink.

To help the child learn the shape of letters by feel, you could make them in one of these ways.

rope glued or pinned to wood or cardboard

grooves cut into wood

letter cut out of cardboard and glued to thick paper

letter in plaster or clay

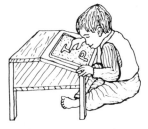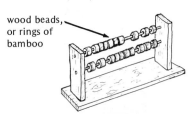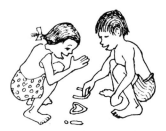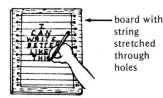

In the schoolroom, a **pan with soft clay or mud** is helpful for learning to write and feel letters.

Children can practice writing outside in **sand, mud,** or **clay.**

→ board with string stretched through holes

When the child begins to write, you can stretch string lines across the paper to help her write in straight lines. Or draw extra dark lines.

To help the child begin to count you can make a simple **'counting frame'.** The child can slide the beads or rings from one side to the other to count, add, and subtract.

wood beads, or rings of bamboo

A pegboard like this can help a child learn numbers through touch—and help him learn to feel small differences in things.

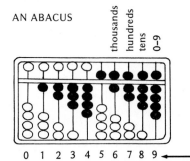

When the child becomes more skilled with numbers, she can learn to use a special counting frame called an **'abacus'** which has beads on wires. The beads slide up and down to form numbers. With practice, a blind child can learn to add and subtract on the abacus as fast or faster than other children can do it on paper.

AN ABACUS

thousands hundreds tens 0–9

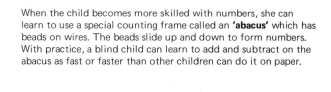

0 1 2 3 4 5 6 7 8 9 ← give these numbers.

(All the beads are really the same color. Here we have made some black to make it clearer how to count.)

The beads in the positions shown give these numbers.

These 4 wires now read 6789.
Notice that each bead above the center bar equals 5 times each bead directly below it.

Work

As a blind child grows up, he or she can learn to do many different kinds of work. On page 509 in Chapter 54 we list many of the different kinds of work that disabled persons can do. Those types of work marked with a * have often been done by blind persons.

The village child who is blind should be given many opportunities to help with work around the home and with farm work. **The blind child should be invited and expected to help in a wide range of daily activities, just like the child who can see.** What starts out as play and imitation ends up as learning of useful skills.

A family that farms the land can begin to include a blind child in gardening and farming activities from an early age.

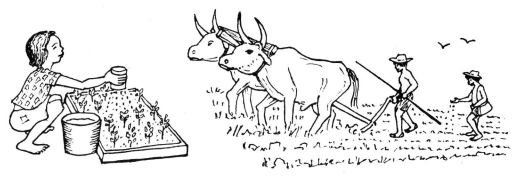

To get an understanding of the whole process of growing the family food, the child can start by planting seeds, watering them, caring for them as they grow, and finally harvesting, cooking, and eating the product.

Later, the child can go with his father or mother to the fields and help with the planting. With his feet he can follow the furrows, or grooves made by the plow.

Try to involve the child with each aspect of housework and farm work. At first show her and guide her as much as is necessary. Then help less and less until finally the child can do the whole job alone.

Social life

The blind child should have all the same opportunities in the community as other children do. Take her with you, and then send her, to the market, well, river, school, and temple. Introduce her to the people you meet. Explain to them that she is an active little girl like any other, except that she cannot see. Ask them, when they see her, to make a point of speaking to her (since she cannot see them), of answering her questions, of helping her to find what she is looking for. Ask them *not* to do everything for her, but instead to help her figure out how to do more for herself. Little by little people will begin to realize that a blind child can do a lot more than they would ever have dreamed possible. And they will begin to respect and appreciate her. For the next blind child in the village, it will be easier.

Take the child to meetings, movies, puppet shows, and town events. Explain to her what she cannot see.

When children who are blind grow up, they can marry and have children. They can be as good parents as persons who see.

PREVENTION of blindness

The best way to prevent blindness is to **try to keep children well fed, clean, and healthy.** During pregnancy, mothers also need to eat enough nutritious foods and to avoid medicines that might damage the baby. For more information, see a book like *Helping Children Who Are Blind* or contact the groups on page 639.

In brief, **steps to prevent child blindness include:**

- When pregnant, keep away from persons with German measles and other infectious diseases, avoid unsafe medicines, and try to get enough to eat.

- Protect the eyes of all newborn babies with erythromycin or tetracycline eye ointment at birth (see p. 245).

- *Vaccinate* children against all the infectious diseases you can.

- Breast feed the baby, and continue to breast feed as long as possible.

- Good nutrition for mother and child—especially foods rich in vitamin A. Children often get diarrhea and then 'dry eyes' after they are taken off the breast. So, when the baby starts to eat other foods, give him mashed papaya, mashed cassava leaves, or other foods with vitamin A, every day.

- Keep the home and child clean. Build and use latrines, and keep them covered. Try to protect against flies. Wash hands with soap and water, especially before eating and after using the latrine (toilet).

- Keep the child's eyes clean. When they get infected or have pus, clean them often with a clean cloth that is wet with clean water, and see a health worker.

- Give children with measles vitamin A rich foods (or vitamin A capsules, see p. 244) because danger of 'dry eyes' increases with measles.

- Treat all persons with signs of trachoma early. For treatment of different eye problems, see a health worker or get information from a book like *Where There is No Doctor.*

- Keep sharp and pointed objects, bullets, explosives, acids, and lye away from children and teach them about their dangers. Warn them about the danger of throwing closed bottles, cans, or bullets into the fire. Also warn them about local plants that can injure the eyes. (For example, the juice of 'hiza', a poisonous fig tree in Mexico, can burn the eyes like lye.) Get good early treatment for any eye injury.

- Warn children about throwing rocks and sticks, or shooting slingshots toward other persons.

- Check babies and children for early signs of eye problems or difficulty seeing. Test how well they can see at 2 months of age and before they begin school.

- Organize children to test the sight of their younger brothers and sisters (see CHILD-to-child, p. 452).

- Help everybody understand that **most blindness in children can be prevented.** Teach people what they can do.

- For special precautions to protect the eyes of persons who have a loss of feeling in their eyes, see Chapter 26 on Leprosy, p. 223.

Deafness and Communication

CHAPTER 31

Different children have different amounts of hearing loss

A few children are **completely deaf**; they do not hear at all. Parents often notice early that their child cannot hear, because she does not turn her head or respond, even to loud sounds.

Much more often, children are **partly deaf**. A child may show surprise or turn her head to a loud noise, but not to softer noises. She may respond to a low-pitched sound like thunder, a drum, or a cow's 'moo', but not to high-pitched sounds like a whistle or a rooster crowing. Or (less commonly) a child may respond to high-pitched sounds but not low ones.

Some children who are partly deaf hear a little when people speak to them. They may slowly learn to recognize and respond to some words. But many words they do not hear clearly enough to understand. They are slow to begin to speak. Often they do not speak clearly, mix up certain sounds, or seem to 'talk through their nose'. Unfortunately, sometimes parents, other children, and teachers do not realize that the child has difficulty hearing. They may treat her as if she is *mentally* slow, or 'dumb'. This only increases the child's problems.

For more information about children with hearing problems, see *Helping Children Who Are Deaf* or the other books listed on page 639.

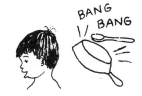

The child who is completely deaf does not respond even to very loud noises. (But he may notice movements or vibrations caused by sudden loud noises. For example, clapping behind the child's head may move the air at his neck and cause the child to turn.)

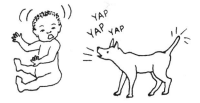

The child who is only partly deaf hears some sounds, but may not hear clearly enough to tell the difference between certain sounds or words. Families are often slow to recognize that these children have difficulty hearing.

Problems that may result

For most growing children, hearing and language are very important for getting to know, understand, and relate to the people and things around them.

> COMMUNICATION is the way in which we **understand** what is said to us and the way we say or **express** to other people our thoughts, needs, and feelings. People who can hear communicate mostly through **speech**.

For a child with a hearing loss, the biggest problem is **learning to communicate.** Because she cannot hear words clearly, it is much more difficult for her to learn to speak. So she has trouble both understanding what people want, and telling them what she wants. This can lead to frequent disappointments and misunderstandings, both for the child and others. It is no surprise, then, that children with hearing loss sometimes are **slow in learning to relate to other people, feel lonely or forgotten, or develop 'behavior problems'.**

The exchange of ideas and information through some form of communication is important for the development of any child's mind. Most deaf children are just as intelligent as other children. But for their mental ability to develop fully, they need to learn to communicate well from an early age.

How deafness affects a child depends on:

1. **when the child became deaf.** For a child who is born deaf or becomes deaf before he begins to speak, learning to speak or 'read lips' will be far more difficult than for a child who loses his hearing after he has begun to speak.

2. **how much the child still hears.** The better the child hears, the more chance he has of learning to speak, understand speech, and 'read lips'.

3. **other disabilities.** Some deaf children also have other problems. A child who is *mentally retarded,* blind, or *'multiply disabled'* will have a harder time learning to communicate than a child who is deaf only. (See "Causes of Deafness.") ⟶

4. **how soon the problem is recognized.**

5. **how well the child is accepted, and how early he is helped to learn other ways to communicate.**

6. **the system of communication that is taught** to the child ('oral' or 'total', see p. 263).

CAUSES OF DEAFNESS

Deafness is *not* caused because the child did something wrong or because someone is being punished.

Common causes before a baby is born:
- **hereditary** (occurs in certain families, although the parents themselves may not be deaf). Usually a child has no other disability, and learns quickly.
- **German measles** during early pregnancy. Often child also has brain damage and learning problems.
- **Rh factor** (see p. 91). Child often has other disabilities also (see p. 283).
- **Prematurity** (born early and small). Two out of 3 have other disabilities also.
- **lack of iodine** in mother's diet (common in areas where many people have goiters). May show signs of mental retardation or cretinism (see p. 282).
- certain **medicines** taken by the mother while pregnant, such as corticosteroids and phenytoin.
- difficult birth, baby slow to breathe.
- dwarfism and brittle bone disease (see p. 125).

Common causes after birth:
- **ear infections**—especially long-lasting repeated *infections* with pus.　pus→
- **meningitis** (often child has other disabilities and *behavioral* problems).
- **certain medicines** (streptomycin, and related antibiotics).
- **frequent very loud noise.**

Other causes. There are many other less common causes of deafness. In 1 out of 3 children the cause is not known.

Importance of early recognition of deafness

During the first years of life, a child's mind is like a sponge; it learns language very quickly. If a child's hearing problem is not recognized early and effective help is not provided, the best years for learning communication skills may be lost (age 0 to 7). **The earlier special training begins, the more a child can learn to communicate.**

Parents should watch carefully for **signs that show if a baby hears or not.** Does the baby show surprise or blink when you make a sudden loud noise? As the baby grows, does he turn his head or smile when he hears familiar voices? Has he begun to say a few words by 18 months of age? Does he say a lot of words fairly clearly by age 3 or 4? If not, he may have a hearing problem. As soon as you suspect a problem, test the child's hearing.

Simple tests for hearing are on p. 450 and 451. If it seems the child does not hear well, when possible, take him to a specialist for testing.

Unless a child is given a lot of understanding and help learning to communicate from an early age, **deafness can be one of the most difficult, lonely, and misunderstood disabilities.** The following 2 stories will help show the difference that it can make to recognize a hearing problem early and provide the extra help that the child needs.

TONIO

Although Tonio was born with a severe hearing loss, his parents did not realize this until he was 4 years old. For a long time, they thought he was just slow. Or stubborn.

Until he was one year old, Tonio seemed to be doing fairly well. He began to walk and play with things. Then his sister, Lota, was born. Lota smiled and laughed more than Tonio when their mother talked or sang to her. So their mother talked and sang to Lota more.

By the time Lota was 1, she was already beginning to say a few words. Tonio had not yet begun to speak. "Are you sure he can hear?" a neighbor asked one day. "Oh yes," said his mother. She called his name loudly, and Tonio turned his head.

When he was 3, Tonio could only say 2 or 3 words. Lota, at age 2, now spoke more than 200 words. She asked for things, sang simple songs, and played happily with other children. Tonio was more moody. Mostly he played by himself. When he played with other children it often ended in fighting—or crying.

Lota behaved better than Tonio. Usually, when her mother told her not to do something and why, she understood and obeyed. Often, to make Tonio obey, his mother would slap him.

One time in the village market Lota asked for a banana and her mother bought her one. A moment later, Tonio quietly picked up a mango and began to eat it. His mother slapped him. Tonio threw himself on the ground and began to kick and scream.

When Tonio's father heard what had happened in the market, he looked angrily at Tonio and said, "When will you learn to ask for things? You're 4 years old and still don't even try to talk. Are you stupid, or just lazy?"

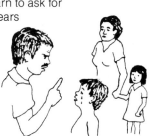

Tonio just looked at his father. Tears rolled down his cheeks. He could not understand what his father said. But he understood the angry look. His father softened and took him in his arms.

Tonio's behavior got worse and worse. At age 4 his mother took him to a health worker, who tested Tonio and found that he was deaf.

Now Tonio's parents are trying to make up for lost time. They try to speak to him clearly and slowly, in good light, and to use some signs and gestures with their hands to help him understand. Tonio seems a little happier and speaks a few more words. But he still has a lot of trouble saying what he wants.

SANDRA

When Sandra was 10 months old, her 7-year-old brother, Lino, learned about testing for deafness as part of the CHILD-to-child program at school (see p. 450). So he tested his baby sister. When he stood behind her and called her name or rang a bell, she did not turn or even blink. Only when he hit a pan hard did she show surprise. He told his parents he thought Sandra did not hear well. They took Sandra to a small rehabilitation center. A worker there tested Sandra and agreed she had a severe hearing loss.

The village worker explained what the family could do to help Sandra develop and learn to communicate. He gave them many drawings of hands held to make 'signs' for common words.

"Every time you speak, make 'signs' with your hands to show what you mean. Include all the signs and gestures that people already use in your village. Teach all the children to use them too. Make a game out of it. At first Sandra won't understand. But she'll watch and learn. In time she'll begin to use signs herself."

"If she gets used to signs, won't that keep her from learning to speak?" asked her father.

"No," said the worker. "Not if you always speak the words at the same time. The signs will help her understand the words, and she may even learn to speak earlier. But it takes years to learn to speak with 'lip reading'. First, she needs to learn to use signs to say what she wants and to develop her mind."

Sandra's family began using signs as they spoke to each other. Months passed, and still Sandra did not begin to speak or to make signs. But now she was watching more closely.

By age 3, Sandra began to make signs. By age 4 she could say and understand many things with signs—even lip read a few words, like 'Yes', 'No', and 'Lino'. By age 5 she had only learned to 'lip read' a few words. But with signs she could say over 1000 words and many simple sentences.

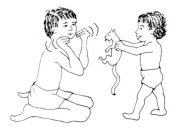

Sandra was happy and active. She liked to color pictures and play guessing games. Lino began to teach her how to draw letters. One day she asked Lino when she could go to school.

WHERE CAN YOU GO FOR HELP?

A child who does not hear well needs extra help. Where you can look for help depends on where you live and on what resources are in your community and in your country. Here are some possibilities:

• **Local deaf persons as teachers.** Even a small village usually has some persons who have been deaf a long time. Probably they will have learned to communicate through signs and gestures. If you ask some of them to become the friends and teachers of a deaf child, and advisers to the family, often they will be glad to do so. They may remember the difficulties and loneliness of their own childhood and want to help provide the understanding and learning opportunities that the deaf child needs.

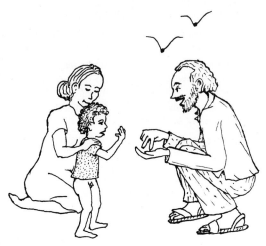

Deaf persons can be especially helpful if they have learned the 'national sign language' and can communicate fully with other deaf persons. If there is no such person in your village, but there is in a neighboring town, perhaps the child can visit that person, or a group of deaf persons.

Deaf persons who have learned to communicate well are often the best teachers of a deaf child and his family.

• **Other families with deaf children.** If several families with a deaf child can come together, share experiences, and learn as a group, this can be a big help. The younger deaf children can learn from older ones, or from deaf adults. Together they can develop a form of communication so that all the children and their families can understand each other.

• **The National Association of the Deaf** (or other group **run by the deaf**). Most countries have associations of deaf persons. These can give you information about the national sign language in your country, and perhaps send books for learning it. They can tell you about training programs for the deaf (government, private, and religious) and can advise which are the best. They may even provide brief training in basic communication skills to a local health worker, teacher, family member, or disabled child—with the understanding that he or she then teach others.

• **'Special education' programs or schools for the deaf.** Many countries have schools where deaf children can live and receive special training. Some of these are good and some are not. Good programs try different methods of communication with each child and then focus on what will probably work best for that child in his community. Bad programs try to make all deaf children communicate only by lip reading or speech. For many children this can lead to failure, anger, and emotional harm (see p. 264). Try to get advice from educated deaf persons.

The Hesperian Foundation book *Helping Children Who Are Deaf* (see p. 640) has many ideas to help deaf children learn a language and communicate to the fullest of their ability. It will also help parents make good decisions about the development of a child who is deaf.

Deciding what to do for a deaf child

Not all children with hearing loss are the same. All need love, understanding, and help learning to communicate. But **different children need different kinds of help, to communicate in whatever way works best for them. We must adapt our methods to the needs of the particular child and to the realities of the community where he lives.**

- If a child is only **partly deaf,** sometimes we can help her to hear more clearly (see p. 262), to understand more speech, and perhaps learn to speak.

- A child who has **no hearing at all** usually cannot be helped to hear. But if he **became deaf after he began to speak,** perhaps he can be helped to 'read' people's lips and to improve his speech.

- If the child was **born deaf and has never heard speech,** learning to lip read and speak is always very slow and difficult, and is usually not very successful. It is better to help the child learn to communicate in whatever ways work best for her: first with her face, body, arms and hands, then possibly adding pictures, reading and writing, finger spelling, and as much lip reading and speech as she is able to learn.

- If the child comes from an **area where there are many deaf people** who communicate with each other in a national sign language, it is probably best to have people in the deaf community help teach the child and her family their language. That way, she can learn to communicate with deaf people as fully and well as hearing people communicate with each other.

- But if the child lives in a **small village where there are few deaf people,** none of whom know the national sign language, learning that language may not help the child much. Probably it makes more sense for her to learn ways to communicate as best she can with those who can hear. Again, this probably means a combination of methods, based on the signs and gestures people already use in the village. With these, the child can also use pictures, and later perhaps, reading and writing.

- Remember, most children with hearing loss can learn quickly. But some may have brain damage or disabilities that affect their ability to learn or to control their hands, lips, or voices. You will need to figure out ways to help these children communicate in whatever way they can: with sets of pictures, head movements, or eye movements.

Note: Some children who hear perfectly well do not develop the ability to speak. Some children with cerebral palsy do not control their mouth or tongue movement well enough to speak. Other children are mentally retarded and may be very late in learning to speak, or never learn. Other children are intelligent in many ways, but for some reason cannot speak. For all of these children, we need to look for ways to help them communicate as best they can.

Helping a child to hear better

Children who are not completely deaf can sometimes be helped to hear better:

- When possible, have the child's hearing and ears examined by a specialist. A few children are born with a closed ear tube or other **defect in the structure of the ear.** Rarely these problems can be corrected by **surgery,** and the children can hear better. (*Note:* For children whose hearing loss comes from brain damage, surgery will not help.)
- Children who have hearing loss because of **ear infections** may begin to hear better if the ear infections are **treated early** and steps are taken to **prevent more infections.** (See p. 276.)
- Some children can hear better with **aids** that make sounds louder. A 'hearing aid' allows some children to understand words fairly well, and can make a big difference in learning to listen and speak. For other children, an aid makes them more aware of sounds (which helps) but does not help them to tell the difference between words. If it appears the child will benefit a lot from a hearing aid, it helps to begin as early as age 1 or 2.

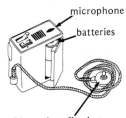

microphone

batteries

The simplest aid is a **hand cupped behind the ear.**

Better is an **'ear trumpet'.** You can make one out of a cow horn, cardboard, or tin.

Better still (for some children) is a **'hearing aid' with batteries. But** usually these are very expensive.
For best results, it should be fitted by a specially-trained worker after the child's hearing has been carefully tested.

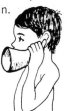

Piece that fits into ear (best if molded to fit the specific child). In a growing child it will need to be changed often.

CAUTION: If you get a child a hearing aid, be sure to ask for instructions on keeping it clean, dry, and working well. Be sure you have a supply of extra batteries and know how to get more.

- Young children who do not hear well can sometimes be helped to **listen more carefully,** and to learn the difference between sounds:

Make different sounds and encourage the child to take notice. When a donkey brays or a baby cries, say clearly and loudly, "Listen to the donkey," or "What was it?" If the child answers or points in the right direction, praise him.

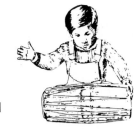

Have the child make different sounds—hitting pans, drumming, ringing bells, and so on. See if he can move or dance to the beat of music or drums.

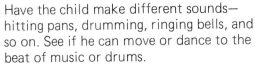

I GIVE YOU SOUP.

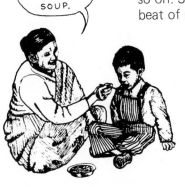

Talk a lot to the child. And sing to her. Tell her the name of different parts of her body, and other things. Ask her to touch or point to them. Praise her when she does.

Experiment to find out how near the child's ear you need to be, and how loud you have to speak, to get the child's attention, or for him to repeat the sounds you make. Then try to speak near and loud enough. Speak clearly, but **do not shout.**

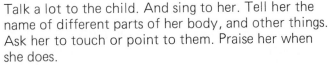

DIFFERENT WAYS TO HELP A CHILD COMMUNICATE

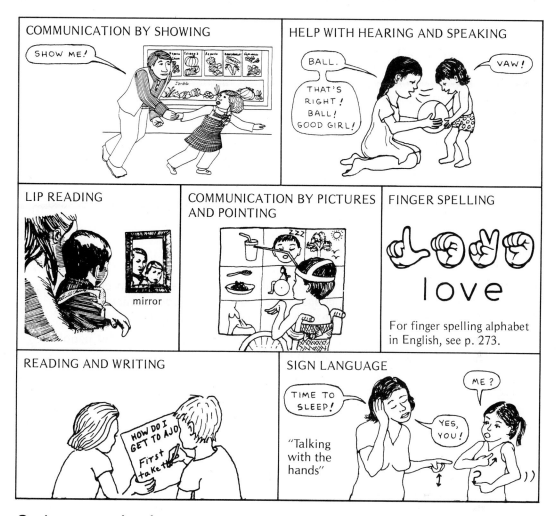

Oral communication

Oral communication (communication by mouth) combines helping a child use her **limited hearing** as much as possible, with **lip reading,** and with learning **to speak.** In many countries, schools for deaf children teach only oral communication. Unfortunately, oral communication usually **only works well for children who can hear the differences between many words, or for children who became deaf after they learned to speak.**

Total communication

Total communication is an approach that encourages a child to learn and use **all the different methods that work well for that child in her particular community.** This might include any (or all) of these:

- the child's own gestures
- sign language
- drawing, reading, and writing
- finger spelling
- whatever hearing the child has, to develop lip reading and speech

IMPORTANT: 'Total communication' as we use the term, does not mean that all the above methods are used for every child. It means that we **try all the methods** that might work for a child. Then we **work with whatever methods will help the child communicate as easily, quickly, and fully** as possible with her family and community. It is an approach that is friendly, flexible, and adaptable to individual and local needs.

WARNING: Beware of programs that teach only oral communication

In many countries, schools for the deaf still try to make all children learn only 'oral communication' (lip reading and spoken words). The results are often disappointing, or even harmful, especially for the child who was born deaf. Lip reading at best gives a lot of problems. A skilled lip reader can only understand about 40 to 50 percent of English words, and has to guess at the rest. (For example, "Mama" and "Papa" look exactly the same on the lips.) Even if the child does learn to lip read and speak some, often his words are unclear or sound strange. As a result, when he grows older, often he prefers not to speak.

The biggest problem with teaching only oral communication is that it slows down a child's language development at the age when children learn language fastest (age 1 to 7 years). A deaf child usually learns to lip read and speak only 5 or 10 words by age 5 or 6. By that age, the same child can easily learn over 2,000 signs—as many words as a hearing child speaks.

Studies have shown that deaf **children who learn to use gestures and signs can communicate easier, earlier, and more fully than those who are taught only oral communication. Learning sign language and other forms of communication first actually makes it easier for a child to learn to speak and read lips.**

For all these reasons, **more and more experts and organizations of deaf people recommend teaching most deaf children a combination of communication methods, including some form of sign language.**

'Total communication' is not new. In villages in many parts of the world, deaf and hearing persons find imaginative and effective ways to talk with each other. They figure out a system of hand signs, objects, face movements, pictures, and certain sounds or words. As a result, deaf persons often manage fairly well in the community. They can "say" and understand a lot. (See p. 276.)

We know families from villages like these who took their deaf child to *'speech therapists'* in the city. Often the parents and child had already begun to communicate with each other by using the local signs and inventing more of their own. The child was happy and learning fairly well. But the therapists told the parents that they were wrong. They told them that they must not let the child use signs, because if he got used to signs he would never learn to speak. They said the child should be put in a 'special education program' and taught 'oral communication'. But since the only programs of this kind are in the cities (and often have a 3-year waiting list) the parents took their child back to the village. Trying to follow the therapist's orders, they tried not to use signs with their child, and punished him when he used them. As a result, both the parents and child felt frustrated, guilty, angry, and hurt. The child's learning and social development were held back. His chances of learning to speak became less than they were when everyone happily used the village system.

Fortunately, most of these families in time realized that they simply could not manage without using signs, and gradually went back to accepting 'total communication'.

In the richer countries more and more special educators and speech therapists are beginning to favor total communication. They have changed to this approach partly because deaf persons have organized and demanded it. **Disabled persons in poor countries, including deaf persons and their families, also need to organize. They need to help professionals listen to them, and to respond to their needs in more realistic ways.**

Helping a child learn 'total communication'

- The learning place should be well lighted, so that the child can see your hands, face, and lips.
- Face the child when you speak to her, and be sure she is watching you.
- Talk to her a lot, even if she does not understand. Talk with your hands, face, and lips, and encourage her to watch them all.
- Speak clear and loud, but **do not shout** and **do not exaggerate the movement of your mouth and lips.** This will help her learn to recognize normal speech.
- Be patient and repeat things often.
- Be sure to let her know that you are pleased when she says something or does something well.
- Encourage her to make whatever sounds she can. This will help her strengthen her voice for possible speech.
- Have a lot of toys, pictures, and other things ready to use in helping her learn the signs and words for them.
- Make learning to communicate fun. Include other children in games like 'Simon says' that help children use their eyes, ears, and bodies, and copy each other (see p. 316).
- Play games that exercise the child's lips, tongue, and mouth *muscles.* In a deaf child, these muscles can get weak. This not only makes speech more difficult, but can make the child's face look dull, or without expression. For activities to strengthen and control the mouth and lips, see p. 314 and 315.
- Make a list of the words that other children her age use, and that you most want the child to learn. Include:

• useful words for learning and games:	• common and interesting things:	• action words:	• people:	• description words:
yes, no, thank you, please, what, do, don't, like, want	body parts, animals, clothing, foods	come, go, eat, drink, sleep, give, put, see, hear, wash, walk, run, play, pee	you, I, he, she, it, we, they, Mama, Papa, Juan, María, and other family members	small, big, up, down, fat, thin, good, bad, hot, cold, day, night

Start with a short list and gradually make it longer. Use the words often, in daily activities (feeding, bathing, dressing), and in play. Have the whole family learn the words on the list and how to make the signs for them. Encourage everyone to use the words and signs together, not only when they talk with the child, but when they talk with each other, and for all the things they do in the home. This way the child will learn about language by playing, watching, listening (as much as he can), and finally by copying—the way most children learn language.

- As the child gets a little older, help her become familiar with letters and written words. You can write the first letter or name of things on different objects around the home. Or make pictures of things with their names in big, clear letters. Or make pairs of 'flash cards' so the child can match pictures with words. This will help the child understand hand signs that are based on letters. It will prepare him for learning the alphabet in writing and signs, and for learning to read and write.

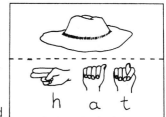

SIGN LANGUAGE

In most villages and communities people use and understand many gestures or signs made with their hands. Most of these signs are 'common sense', or look something like the things they represent. Some children's games use hand signs. For example:

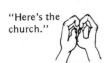 "Here's the church." "And here's the steeple." 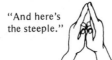 "Open the doors." "And see all the people."

When a family has a deaf child, they begin to use the local signs and also to invent new ones of their own. For example, at a village rehabilitation center in Mexico, a family arrived on muleback with their 6 year old deaf son. The boy got nervous and wanted to go home. So he pulled on his father's shirt sleeve and made these sounds and signs:

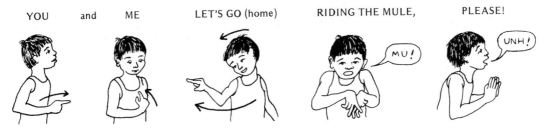

YOU and ME   LET'S GO (home)   RIDING THE MULE,   PLEASE!

MU!   UNH!

The family had begun to figure out its own sign language, without having been taught it. The boy himself had made up the sign for 'RIDING the MULE'.

The sign language that families develop with their deaf children is usually not very complete. Communicating is often still difficult. However, people have joined together to create sign languages which are much more complete. There are hundreds of different sign languages, but there are 3 main types:

- **National and regional sign languages.** In nearly all countries, deaf people have created their own sign languages, in which they can learn to communicate as well and nearly as fast as hearing people. Different hand signs represent different things, actions, and ideas. The structure (grammar) of these languages is different from the spoken language, and therefore is difficult for hearing people to learn. These languages are preferred by people who were born deaf. Examples are American Sign Language (ASL), which is used in the USA and Canada, and Mexican Sign Language.

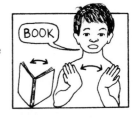
BOOK

- **Sign languages based on spoken languages.** These languages have the same organization and grammar as the local spoken language. They are easier for hearing persons to learn and for persons who became deaf after they learned to speak. Sometimes they use the first letter (finger spelling) of a word as part of the sign. This is harder for children to learn who cannot read, but can make learning to read easier and more fun. Examples are English Sign Language and Spanish Sign Language.

- **Finger spelling.** Each word is spelled out with hand signs that represent the letters of the local alphabet. This method of 'writing in the air' is slow but exact. It is easier for persons to learn who can already read and write. For English, the British use a 2-handed system and the Americans use a one-handed system. Try to learn the system that is most used in your country.

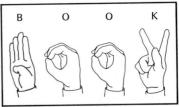
B   O   O   K

Many deaf persons combine these 3 systems. With other deaf persons they use mostly the first, with hearing persons or a 'translator' they use mostly the second, and finger spell difficult words. When 'talking' to someone who does not know sign language, they can write down what they need to say—or use a letterboard.———————➤

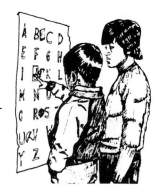

Learning to sign

If possible, contact the Association of the Deaf in your country, and see if you can get a guidebook to sign language adapted to your local area or spoken language. If this is not possible, you can use the local signs and gestures, and invent more signs of your own.

On the next few pages we give ideas for making up signs, and examples for common words. Most are signs used in American Sign Language. You will want to **change them to fit the gestures, customs, and language of your area.** Here are some ideas:

- **Choose signs that will not offend the local people.** (Deaf people already have a difficult time being accepted.) Here are some examples:

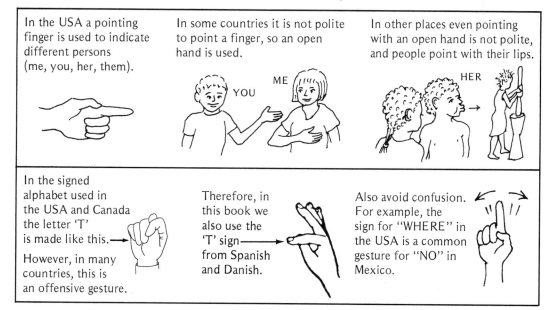

In the USA a pointing finger is used to indicate different persons (me, you, her, them).

In some countries it is not polite to point a finger, so an open hand is used.

In other places even pointing with an open hand is not polite, and people point with their lips.

In the signed alphabet used in the USA and Canada the letter 'T' is made like this.➤ However, in many countries, this is an offensive gesture.

Therefore, in this book we also use the 'T' sign➤ from Spanish and Danish.

Also avoid confusion. For example, the sign for "WHERE" in the USA is a common gesture for "NO" in Mexico.

- **Use local signs.** If people in your area already have a gesture or sign for something, use that instead of a new or foreign one. For example:

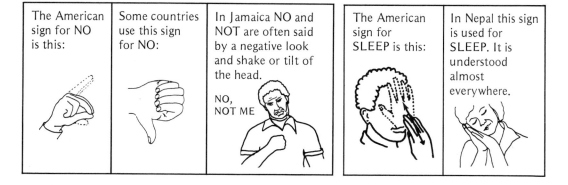

The American sign for NO is this:

Some countries use this sign for NO:

In Jamaica NO and NOT are often said by a negative look and shake or tilt of the head.

NO, NOT ME

The American sign for SLEEP is this:

In Nepal this sign is used for SLEEP. It is understood almost everywhere.

- **Use hand shape, position, movement, and direction to make different signs.** The expression on the face also adds to meaning. For example, here are signs for MOTHER:

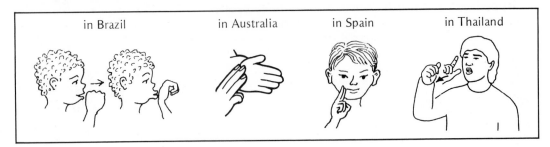

| in Brazil | in Australia | in Spain | in Thailand |

- Try to **make signs look like the things or actions they represent.** To do this you can use a combination of **hand shapes** and **movements.**

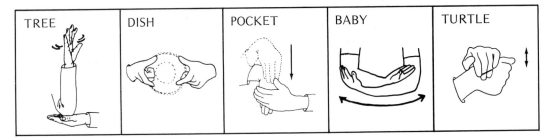

| TREE | DISH | POCKET | BABY | TURTLE |

- Figure out patterns and series of similar signs for related things and actions, and for opposites. For example:

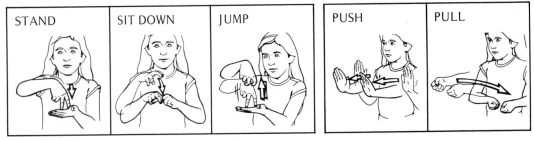

| STAND | SIT DOWN | JUMP | PUSH | PULL |

See other signs with fingers as legs on p. 272.

- Learn new signs by pointing to things.

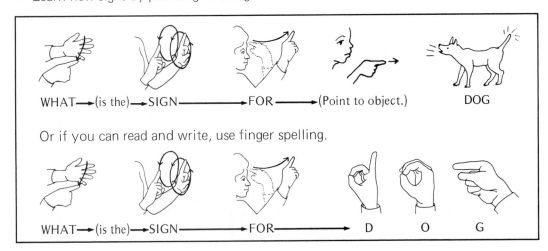

WHAT ➔ (is the) ➔ SIGN ➔ FOR ➔ (Point to object.)   DOG

Or if you can read and write, use finger spelling.

WHAT ➔ (is the) ➔ SIGN ➔ FOR ➔   D   O   G

- **Combine signs for things and actions to communicate ideas or sentences.** The arrangement of words does not need to be the same as in the spoken language—and you can leave out 'extra' words like "the" and "a." Also, words like "to" or "from" can often be left out or can be indicated by the direction of a motion.

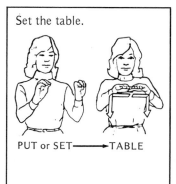

Set the table.

PUT or SET——————➤TABLE

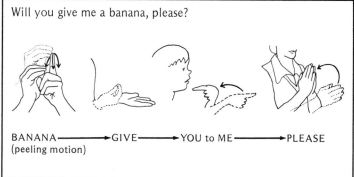

Will you give me a banana, please?

BANANA——————➤GIVE———➤YOU to ME——————➤PLEASE
(peeling motion)

- **Decide whether or not to use letters of the alphabet to make some signs.** In some sign languages the first letter of a spoken (written) word is used as the sign for that word. At first this will mean nothing to a child who cannot read, and will be harder. But it can help prepare the child for learning to read and to finger spell. Again, be systematic:

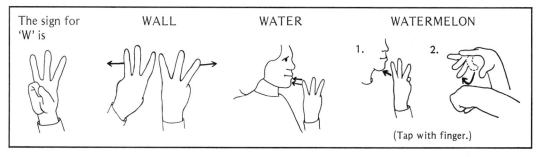

The sign for 'W' is   WALL   WATER   WATERMELON

1.   2.

(Tap with finger.)

Be sure that letter-based signs agree with the word in *your* language. In Spanish, "watermelon" is "sandía," so the English sign makes no sense. The Spanish sign is:

SANDÍA

(Tap with fist.)

- You can make up signs for people's names by **using the first letter of their name,** by showing something that stands for that person, or both.

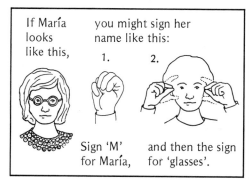

If María looks like this,   you might sign her name like this:

1.   2.

Sign 'M' for María,   and then the sign for 'glasses'.

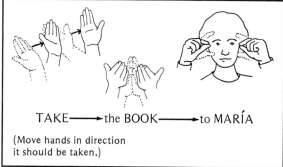

TAKE——————➤the BOOK——————➤to MARÍA

(Move hands in direction it should be taken.)

HOW TO ASK QUESTIONS

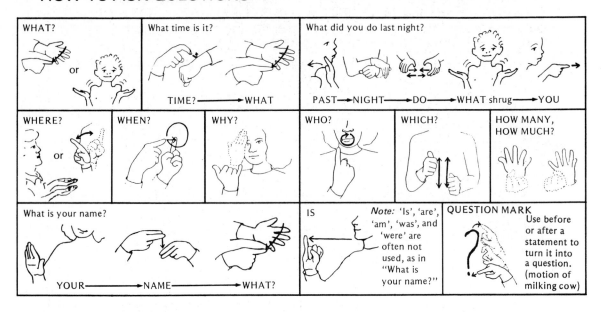

EXAMPLES OF SIGNS

The signs shown here are mostly used in the United States (American Sign Language). A few are from Nepal, Jamaica, and Mexico, because these seem easier to understand. We have chosen signs for things and actions that should be useful for early learning and group games with children. We include them mainly to give you ideas. Change and adapt them to better fit your area.

- **Arrows** (⟶) in the drawings show the direction of hand movement to make the sign.
- **Wavy lines** (〰) used with a sign mean a shake of the hand or fingers.
- **Dotted lines** (------) show how the sign looks when it begins.
- The **darker sign** is how it looks when it ends.

Note: A few signs shown here are based on letters of the alphabet (for example, 'it' uses the letter 'i', and 'we' the letter 'W'). Change these signs if you speak a different language, or if you want to avoid signs based on letters.

I, ME	YOU	THEY, THEM	MALE (MAN)	FEMALE (WOMAN)	*Note:* The male and female signs are used as the base to make signs for boy, girl, father, mother, etc.
		or			
FATHER	MOTHER	BROTHER	SISTER	BOY	GIRL
GRANDFATHER	GRANDMOTHER	FRIEND	BABY	MY	YOUR
HE, HIM	SHE, HER	HIS, HER, THEIR, YOUR — Direct sign toward person.	IT — Or point to object.	WE	OUR

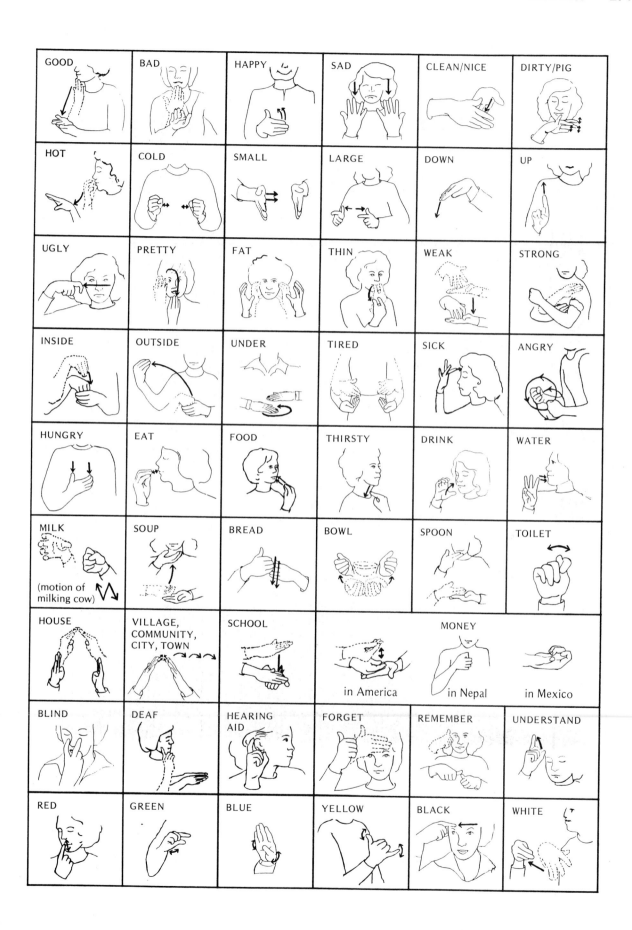

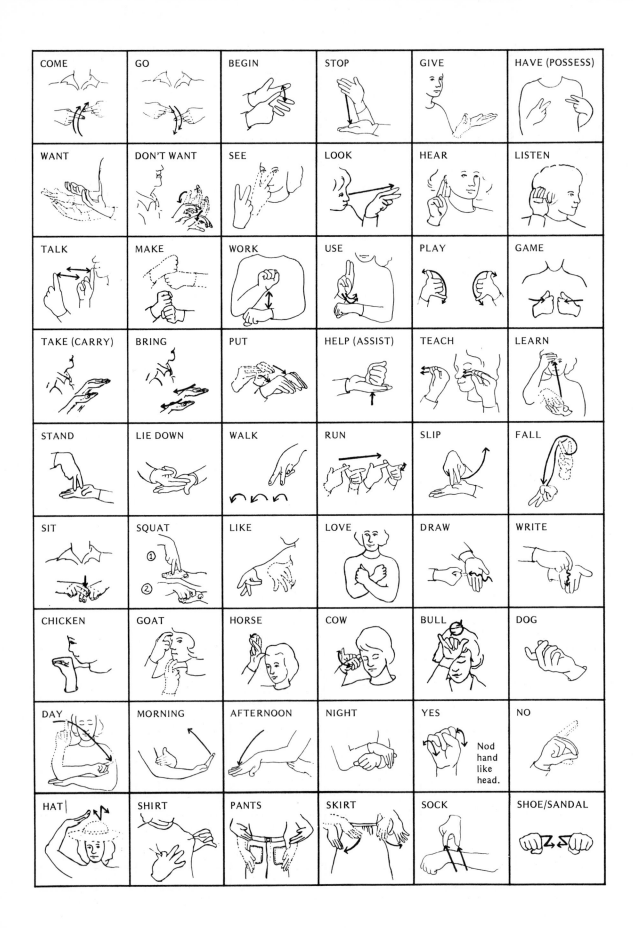

COME	GO	BEGIN	STOP	GIVE	HAVE (POSSESS)
WANT	DON'T WANT	SEE	LOOK	HEAR	LISTEN
TALK	MAKE	WORK	USE	PLAY	GAME
TAKE (CARRY)	BRING	PUT	HELP (ASSIST)	TEACH	LEARN
STAND	LIE DOWN	WALK	RUN	SLIP	FALL
SIT	SQUAT	LIKE	LOVE	DRAW	WRITE
CHICKEN	GOAT	HORSE	COW	BULL	DOG
DAY	MORNING	AFTERNOON	NIGHT	YES (Nod hand like head.)	NO
HAT	SHIRT	PANTS	SKIRT	SOCK	SHOE/SANDAL

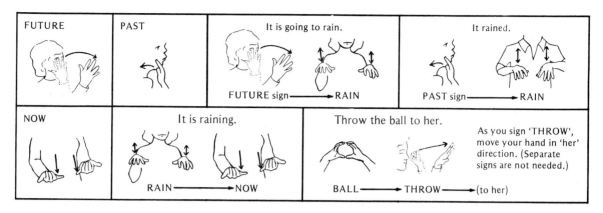

NUMBERS (one of many systems)

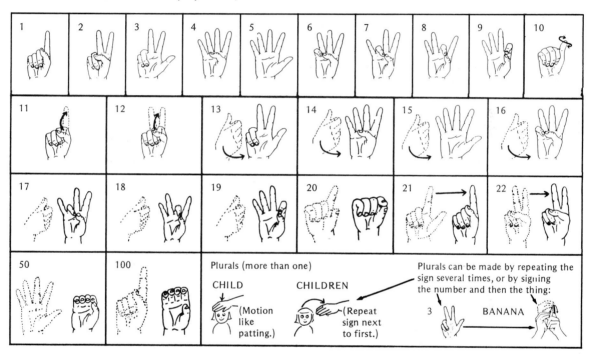

ONE-HANDED SIGN ALPHABET (American)

A	B	C	D	E	F	G	H	I

J	K	L	M	N	O	P	Q	R

S	T American	T Danish	U	V	W	X	Y	Z

Helping the child learn to make sounds and speak

1. If the child hears at all, encourage her to **notice and listen to different sounds,** as discussed on p. 262.

2. Play games and do exercises to help her learn to **use her mouth, tongue, and lips** (see p. 314 and p. 315). Have her press her lips together as if saying

   "mmm," ⟨⟩, make a circle like 'O' ⟨⟩, and stretch her mouth and smile

   as if saying "eee" ⟨⟩ .

   See if she can touch her nose, her chin, and her cheeks with her tongue. Have her blow soap bubbles, or blow out candles. Give her foods to chew and suck.

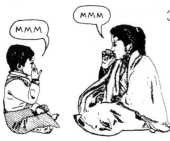

3. Encourage the child to **begin to make sounds.** 'Mmm' is good to start with because it is easy to make. If necessary, show the child how he can hold his lips together to make it. Sit close to him so he can see (and hear?) and copy you. Other sounds that are usually easy to learn are 'ah', 'ay', 'ee', 'aw', 'o', 'p', 'b', 't', and 'd'. (Keep more difficult sounds like 'v', 'w', 'j', 's', 'n', 'r', and 'z' for later.)

4. If the child uses his mouth and lips, but not his voice, have him feel the 'buzz' or vibration in your throat when you make different sounds. To get the 'feel' of different words, you can place his hands on your cheeks, lips, throat, and chest. Then have the child feel his own throat, as he tries to copy you.

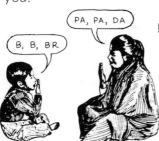

5. Also have the child feel and compare the movement of the air in front of your mouth and his mouth with sounds like 'ha', 'he', 'ho', 'm', 'p', 'b', and 'f'.

   In the same way, have him feel the air move when he 'blows his nose' with his mouth closed. Using this, try to teach sounds like 'n' and 'l'.

6. Begin to teach the child words using the sounds he is learning. First separate the word into different sounds. To say "Ma," first get the child to say "m" with the lips closed. Then "ah" with the mouth open. Then say the word "mah" and have him try to copy you.

7. As the child learns words, teach him what they mean, and have him use them. For example, to teach the child 'nose', have him make the sounds 'n', 'o', and 's'. Then have him put them together. Ask the child to touch his nose as he says the word. Have him copy you. Praise him, and make it a game.

8. Little by little, help the child learn more words and practice using them through games and daily activities. Have her learn her own name and the names of family and friends. Build up a word list as explained on p. 265. But do not try to go too fast. Take time to help her say a few words fairly clearly before going on to the next.

Lip reading

Children with a lot of hearing loss often depend partly on lip reading to understand what people are saying. But lip reading is not easy to learn. Do not try to hurry the child or she (and you) can easily get discouraged. **Do not start teaching lip reading until the child is at least 3 years old.**

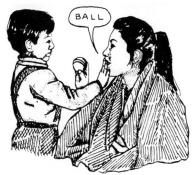

Sit in front of the child in good light, and show him something, for example, a ball. Say "ball," moving your lips clearly and speaking slowly. Let the child see your lips move, and watch your face. Repeat the same word many times.

Then have the child try to imitate you, and feel his own lips as he does.

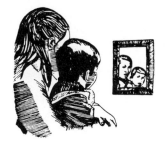

Next, sit with the child in front of a mirror, so that he can see both of your faces. Say the word 'ball' and then have him copy you, watching both of your lips and faces in the mirror.

In this way teach him different words. Start with words where the lips move a lot, and that are easy to tell apart. Pick words that you can use often with him in games and daily activities. When you speak to him, make sure he is watching your face and mouth. Use hand signs when he cannot understand a word. But use the sign *after* speaking the word, not at the same time. He cannot watch both at once.

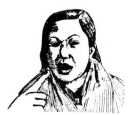

Be sure the child is watching your lips.

You can play games with the child together with children who hear, using 'mime'— that is, acting things out and saying words with the mouth, without making sounds.

Unfortunately, some sounds and words look exactly the same on the lips—the sounds 'k', 'g', and 'h', look the same. 'P', 'b', and 'm' look almost the same. 'T', 'd', 's', and 'z' look the same. And so do 'ch' and 'j'. To help the child tell similar words apart, use hand signs or give him small 'clues', like touching parts of the body, clothes, or food. For example:

If mama wears a dot on her forehead,

and papa has a scar on one cheek,

when anyone at home speaks of them they can also give the 'magic sign'.

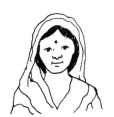

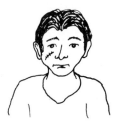

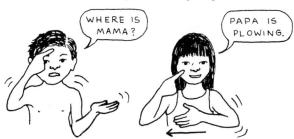

WHERE IS MAMA?

PAPA IS PLOWING.

PREVENTION of deafness

- Take steps to **prevent ear infection** (teach the child not to blow her nose hard when she has a cold). **Treat ear infections at once** when a child gets them. If the child has frequent ear infections, see a health worker or 'ear doctor'. Do not put leaves or plugs of cotton in an infected ear. Let the pus run out. See p. 309 in *Where There Is No Doctor.*
- **During pregnancy, do not take medicines that might harm the baby.** Tell the health worker or doctor you are pregnant, and ask him to check if the medicine he prescribes is recommended during pregnancy.
- **Vaccinate** girls and women against **German measles** (rubella) before they get pregnant (but never when pregnant). Or let young girls catch German measles by letting them play or sleep with a child who has them. This will give them a 'natural' vaccination. Pregnant women should avoid getting near anyone with German measles.
- Have regular medical **check-ups during pregnancy.**
- **Eat as well as possible before and during pregnancy,** use **iodized salt,** and include **foods rich in iron** and other **vitamins** and **minerals.**
- Look for signs of **cretinism** in the baby, and **treat it early** (see p. 282).
- **Vaccinate** the baby against **measles** (and, if possible, **mumps**).
- **Take precautions to prevent brain damage and cerebral palsy** (see p. 107 and 108).
- **Never put,** or let the child put, **pointed objects in the ears.**
- **Avoid** being near very **loud noises.** When a child cannot avoid them, teach him to cover his ears, or use ear plugs.

BANG!

Words to the family of a deaf child

Deaf children can grow up to be loving and helpful sons and daughters, like other children. Try to let your child grow up. Give him the same rights and responsibilities as other children his age.

If there is a chance for your child to go away to a school for the deaf, if it seems right, try to let him go. Deaf children learn in different ways than other children. The special school may provide more opportunities. However, if your child is doing well at the village school, has a teacher who understands and helps him, and has many friends, he might do better there. Help him understand the choices and see what he thinks would be best. Be sure he knows he has a loving family to come home to.

After they finish school, deaf children can do many different kinds of work. Deaf people have become accountants, teachers, lawyers, farmers, health workers, clerks, skilled craftsworkers, and doctors. It is worth the effort to see that deaf children and adults get training and find work.

Be careful that after he has grown up, you do not treat him as a child. He might seem younger than his age. But the best way to help him grow up is to expect him to grow up.

When deaf children grow old enough to marry, they often choose to marry someone else who is deaf, for they can understand each other better. They can have children, and raise them well. Usually a deaf mother and father have children with good hearing.

It is difficult to be deaf. You can help persons who are deaf by letting them communicate in ways they find easy, and by trying to learn to communicate with them yourself.

Mental Retardation

CHAPTER **32**

Down Syndrome, Cretinism, and Other Causes

Mental retardation is a delay, or slowness, in a child's mental development. **The child learns things more slowly than other children his age.** He may be late at beginning to move, smile, show interest in things, use his hands, sit, walk, speak, and understand. Or he may develop some of these skills more quickly, but be slower in others.

Mental retardation ranges from mild to severe. The child who is *mildly retarded* takes longer to learn certain skills. But with help he can grow up to care for himself and take an active, responsible part in the community. The child who is *severely retarded,* as he grows older, may stay at the mental age of a baby or young child. He will always need to be cared for in some ways.

Mental retardation cannot be cured. However, **all mentally retarded children can be helped to progress more quickly. The earlier special help or 'stimulation' begins, the more ability the child is likely to gain.**

IMPORTANT: In this chapter we look at some of the **causes of mental retardation** and briefly describe 2 common forms (Down syndrome and cretinism). However, **mental retardation is only one of the reasons for slow development in children.** A child who is blind will be slow in learning to reach and move about *unless* he has extra help and encouragement. A child who is deaf will be delayed in learning to communicate unless he is helped to learn to 'talk' in other ways than speech. A child who has a severe physical *disability* is often slow in developing use of both his body and mind. Because 'developmental delay' is common with so many disabilities, we include discussion of it in several separate chapters.

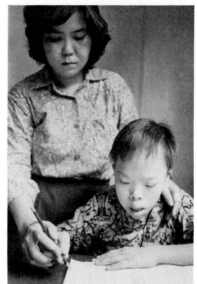

With help, some retarded children can learn to read and write, and do many of the things that normal children do. (Photo of a child with Down syndrome in Indonesia, by Carolyn Watson, Christian Children's Fund.)

Information on helping a child who is mentally retarded or developmentally delayed is in Chapters 34 to 40. Chapters 34 and 35 discuss **early child development** and ways to help or 'stimulate' a child to learn early skills (use of the senses, movement, and communication). Chapters 36 to 39 discuss **learning for self-care** (feeding, dressing, toileting, and bathing). Chapter 40 discusses **child behavior,** and ways to encourage *behavior* that helps learning.

Other ideas for helping retarded children are in the CHILD-to-child activity on pages 442 to 445. The needs and problems of mentally retarded children as they become sexually grown up are discussed in Chapter 52, p. 495.

One important need that we do not include in detail in this book is **education for retarded children.** Some possibilities are discussed in Chapter 53, on education. But often special teaching methods and materials are needed. An excellent book is *Special Education for Mentally Handicapped Pupils.* (See p. 640.) For toys that help a child learn, see Chapter 49.

CAUSES OF MENTAL RETARDATION

There are many causes.

- Often the cause is **not known**.
- Some children are born with a very **small brain,** or the brain does not grow or work normally.
- Sometimes there is a **'mistake' in the 'chromosomes'** or the tiny chemical messages that determine what a child will be like *(inheritance).* This is what happens in Down syndrome.
- Sometimes a mother did not **get enough of a certain food or mineral during pregnancy.** (See "Cretinism," p. 282.)
- **Brain damage** can happen either before, during, or after birth. In addition to being retarded,

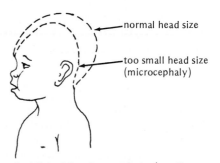

A child with **microcephaly** (small brain) is mentally slow and often also develops certain physical problems. For measurements of head size, see p. 41.

these children may also have cerebral palsy, blindness, deafness, or fits. Common causes of retardation from brain damage are discussed in Chapter 9, and include:

- **German measles** during early pregnancy
- **meningitis** (brain *infection*) from bacteria, tuberculosis, or malaria, most often during early childhood
- **hydrocephalus,** often with spina bifida (see p. 169)
- **head injuries**
- **other causes** include **brain tumor, poisoning** from lead, pesticides (see p. 15), certain medicines and food, and some forms of **muscular dystrophy** or atrophy (see p. 110)

In many parts of the world, the most common causes of mental retardation are brain damage and Down syndrome. But in some mountainous areas, it is very often caused by **lack of iodine** in food and water (see p. 282).

Usually there is no treatment for mental retardation. Therefore, we often do not need to know the exact cause. Instead, we need to help the child develop the best he can. However, in some cases, certain medicines, changes in diet, or prevention of further poisoning can make a big difference. If a child has any signs of cretinism or seems to be gradually losing mental ability, try to get expert medical advice.

Prevention of mental retardation is discussed with its different causes. See especially cerebral palsy (p. 107), Down syndrome (p. 281), and cretinism (p. 282).

MENTAL ILLNESS is different

Some people confuse 'mental retardation' with 'mental illness'. But they are very different. A person who is mentally ill may have normal or high intelligence, and may be highly educated. But because of stressful experiences, or some illness affecting the brain, his behavior becomes strange. When a retarded person behaves in an abnormal way, it is usually because he has not learned the correct way to behave; he needs to be taught. The mentally ill person needs special help—perhaps from a spiritual healer or 'psychiatrist' (soul doctor). **Persons with mental illness are like persons with any other illness. Often they cannot control their strange behavior. We should not blame or punish them, but give them love, protection, and understanding.**

DOWN SYNDROME

In many areas, Down syndrome—or 'mongolism'—is the most common form of mental slowness, or retardation. These children are slower than others in learning to use their bodies and their minds. There are also certain physical signs or problems. (This combination of various signs is called a 'syndrome'.) The baby does not develop normally in the womb because of an error in the 'chromosomes' (material in each cell of the body that determines what a baby will be and look like).

These are the typical **signs of Down** (but *not all* the children have *all* these signs):

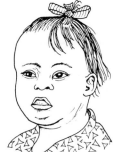

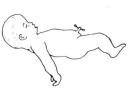

- At birth, baby seems floppy and weak.
- Baby does not cry much.
- The baby is slower than other babies her age to: turn over, grasp things, sit up, talk, walk.
- When suddenly lowered, the baby does not react by spreading her arms, as a normal baby does.

- eyes slant upward; sometimes cross-eyed or poor sight
- ears low
- small mouth, hangs open; roof of mouth is high and narrow; tongue hangs out

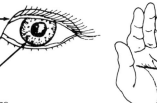

- A fold of skin covers the inner corner of the eyelid.
- Eyelids may be swollen and red.
- The iris of the eye has many little white specks; like sand. These usually go away by 12 months of age.

- short wide hands with short fingers. The little finger may be curved, or have only one fold.
- one deep crease across the palm (sometimes in normal children, too)

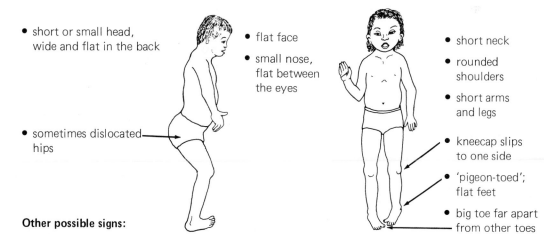

- short or small head, wide and flat in the back
- flat face
- small nose, flat between the eyes
- short neck
- rounded shoulders
- short arms and legs
- sometimes dislocated hips
- kneecap slips to one side
- 'pigeon-toed'; flat feet
- big toe far apart from other toes

Other possible signs:

- Elbow, hip, and ankle joints may be very loose and flexible.
- One out of 3 has heart problems.
- May develop leukemia (blood cancer).
- Check older children for hearing and seeing problems.
- One out of 10 has deformed neck bones which can slip and pinch the nerve cord in the spine. This may cause sudden or slowly increasing *paralysis*—or sudden death.

Care of children with Down and other forms of mental retardation

Mental retardation in children with Down syndrome can be mild, moderate, or severe. Some children never learn to speak. Others talk (and often love to talk). Many can learn to read and write. Most of these boys and girls are very friendly and affectionate, and behave well with people who treat them well. Even those who are more severely retarded, with help and good teaching usually learn to take care of their basic needs, and to help out with simple work. They can live fairly normally with their families and communities.

In rural areas particularly, they can learn to do many important jobs. Sometimes they do repetitive jobs as well or better than other people.

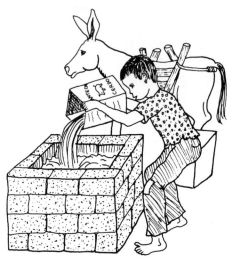

But their physical and mental development is slower than normal. So parents and all those who take care of these children must be very patient with them and from a very early age do all they can to help them develop their mental and physical capabilities. To avoid or solve behavior problems, parents need to be very consistent in how they treat their children and in what they expect of them. The child needs a lot of praise and encouragement for things he does well (see Chapter 40).

In one village, a young man with Down works hauling water from the river, a job he is happy and proud to do.

Some children with Down syndrome can go to school, but they will need extra help. It is important that teachers understand their problem and help other children to treat the retarded child with respect. Unless the child is given understanding and extra help at school, in rural areas it may sometimes be better for the child with Down syndrome to be educated at home through helping his family around the house and in the fields.

There are 3 main concerns in caring for a child with Down syndrome:

1. Help the child to develop her or his mental and physical abilities.

2. Protect the child from infectious diseases.

3. Prevent or correct deformities.

Here we will discuss the last 2 concerns. The first we will cover in other chapters.

IMPORTANT: For a child who has Down syndrome, or is mentally slow, be sure to **read all the chapters on early child development and learning basic skills, Chapters 33 to 41.**

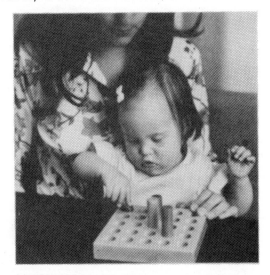

A child with Down syndrome learns to remove pegs from a pegboard. Later she will learn to place the pegs.
Photo from *Teaching Your Down's Syndrome Infant* by Marci J. Hanson.

Protection from infections

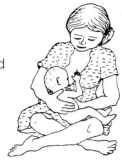

Children with Down syndrome get sick more often than other children. They can easily catch colds, bronchitis, pneumonia, and other infections. So it is very important to protect their health.

- **Breast feed** the child as long as possible. Breast milk has 'antibodies' that help the child to fight infections. (If he cannot nurse well, milk your breasts and feed him the milk, using a spoon or any way that works.)

- Like any baby, at 6 months start giving her other foods such as fruit, beans, eggs, and rice, but also continue to breast feed her. (Like any baby, weigh her each month at the health center to be sure she is growing well.)

- **Vaccinations** can protect her from many childhood diseases. A child with Down syndrome who catches measles or whooping cough can easily get pneumonia.

- **Early medical attention**   When she gets a sore throat, earache, or bad cough, take her to a health worker as soon as possible.

PREVENTION of foot deformities and other problems

- Check all newborns for possible *dislocated* hip, so that it can be corrected as soon as possible (see p. 155).

- For the child whose big toe sticks out,

do not use hard shoes that bend the big toe inward like this.

It is better to wear tennis shoes, or other soft shoes, or sandals.

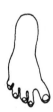

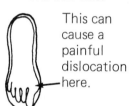

This can cause a painful dislocation here.

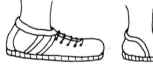

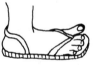

When the big toe sticks out a lot, its position can sometimes be corrected with surgery, so that shoes will fit without problems.

- If the child has **severe** flat feet, a special insole may help. (See p. 118.)

- If any sign of paralysis or lack of feeling develops in the hands, feet, or body, get advice from an orthopedist or a neurosurgeon.

PREVENTION of Down syndrome

One out of every 800 children is born with Down syndrome. Down syndrome is more likely to occur in babies of mothers older than 35 years of age. It is wise for older women to plan their families so as to have no more children after age 35 (see *Where There Is No Doctor*, Chapter 20). Also, if a couple already has one child with Down, the chance of having another is higher than normal (about one in 50).

In some countries a test (amniocentesis) can be done at about 4 months of pregnancy to see if the child will have Down syndrome. If so, the family can consider abortion (in societies where this is permitted).

CRETINISM (Hypo-Thyroidism)

Cretinism is a delay in both mental and physical growth that comes when a child's body does not produce enough 'thyroid'. Thyroid is a substance, or 'hormone', that controls a child's growth and body functions. Without it, everything goes slower.

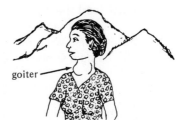

Thyroid is produced by a gland in the front of the neck. To produce thyroid, the gland needs iodine. Most people get enough iodine from water and food. But in some areas, especially in the mountains, the soil, water, and food have very little iodine. In an attempt to obtain more iodine, the thyroid gland sometimes grows very large, forming a swelling called a goiter.

goiter

In areas where there is little iodine and a lot of people have goiters, cretinism is common. In these same areas, often many children have **difficulty hearing** or are somewhat **retarded mentally.** Although they do not show all the typical signs of cretinism, the cause is probably the same. Occasionally, in areas where goiter is not common, cretinism occurs for other reasons than lack of iodine.

SIGNS   Below we show some of the typical signs of cretinism and compare them with Down syndrome, which cretinism resembles in some ways. It is often difficult to tell if a newborn baby has cretinism. She is often born large and then fails to grow normally. The baby may have feeding difficulties, or breathing difficulties or make noises because of the large tongue. She moves and cries little. By 3 to 6 months the mother often becomes worried because the baby looks dull, takes so little interest in things, sleeps so much, and is slow in all areas of development.

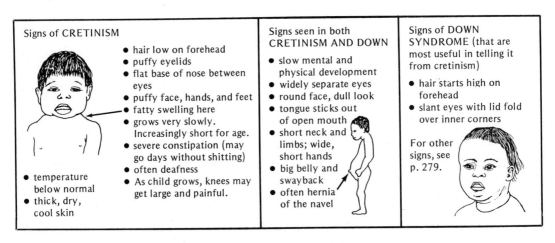

Signs of CRETINISM

- hair low on forehead
- puffy eyelids
- flat base of nose between eyes
- puffy face, hands, and feet
- fatty swelling here
- grows very slowly. Increasingly short for age.
- severe constipation (may go days without shitting)
- often deafness
- As child grows, knees may get large and painful.
- temperature below normal
- thick, dry, cool skin

Signs seen in both CRETINISM AND DOWN

- slow mental and physical development
- widely separate eyes
- round face, dull look
- tongue sticks out of open mouth
- short neck and limbs; wide, short hands
- big belly and swayback
- often hernia of the navel

Signs of DOWN SYNDROME (that are most useful in telling it from cretinism)

- hair starts high on forehead
- slant eyes with lid fold over inner corners

For other signs, see p. 279.

WHAT TO DO   Early and continued treatment with **thyroid medicine** helps improve growth, physical appearance, and sometimes can reduce or prevent mental retardation. For best results, treatment should begin during the first month of life. For this reason, **as soon as you suspect that a baby might have cretinism, get skilled medical advice.**

To help the child develop mentally and physically, and learn basic skills, read Chapters 34 to 41 and use the ideas that can help meet the child's needs. With early treatment and guided learning, many children with cretinism can learn to care for themselves and do simple but important work in the community. For ideas on managing constipation, see p. 212.

PREVENTION   In areas where goiter is common, cretinism (and deafness) can be greatly reduced by encouraging everyone to **use iodized salt.**

The Child with Several Severe Disabilities

Some children have a combination of *severe disabilities.* We say they are 'multiply disabled'. For example, a child may be severely mentally *retarded,* and have little or no physical control of his body. He may also be blind or deaf, have fits, or have difficulty swallowing. Or he may have any combination of these disabilities—and perhaps develop severe *behavior* problems.

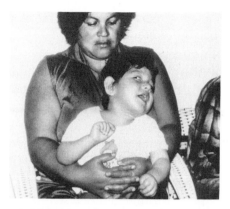

A child with severe cerebral palsy, who is also blind, has fits, and is mentally retarded.

Caring for multiply and severely disabled children is never easy; they need an enormous amount of time, patience, and love. In most communities, parents and close family members will be the main care providers. But **parents will need a lot of support from the community in order to care adequately for the child.** Unless parents have help, they are likely to find that the continual demands of caring for their child are too much. Even the most loving parents, after months and years of continuously caring for a severely disabled child, can easily become frustrated and angry. This is especially true when the child shows little progress or response, and grows up to be a physical adult with the needs of a young child.

It is not uncommon for a parent who for years has poured love and attention into a severely disabled, retarded child, to suddenly hit the child or in other ways begin to neglect or mistreat him.

Before we blame the parent for this, we should try to put ourselves in her position. She has given the child her total love and attention for years. She has waited for a change, for a smile, for some return of warmth and love. But the child remains like a newborn baby, becoming stiffer, more fussy, and more difficult to lift and care for as he grows. Any human being can only give so much without receiving something in return, some sign of recognition or appreciation. In time, the parent is overcome by the unfairness of the situation: the lack of appreciation, the constant demands, the lack of help, the hurt. She reaches her limit and hurts the child in return. Rather than blame her, we should try to understand her. Above all, **we should look for ways to help both the family and child—if possible, long before the mother or other family members reach their limit.**

COMMUNITY SUPPORT

There are several ways in which the community can give assistance to the family of a severely disabled child. In some countries (usually wealthier ones), the most severely retarded, multiply disabled children may be taken care of in special care centers, or **'institutions'.** Although in many cases it is better for the disabled child to stay at home with his own family, there are times when institutional care is needed. This may be because of difficulties in the home situation. Or it may be because the multiply disabled child requires more time and skill than the family can handle.

Institutional care, however, is very costly, and is usually possible only if government pays for it. Few governments of developing countries are willing or able to do that. This means that in poor countries—and especially in the rural areas—most support and assistance for these families must come from the communities themselves.

In areas where a **community rehabilitation program** exists, the program can play an important role. It will usually be neither desirable nor possible for the program to take complete or continual care of the severely disabled child. Yet, the program may be able to help in several ways:

* The community rehabilitation workers can regularly visit the home of the severely disabled child and give **suggestions, assistance,** and **friendship.**

* They can help make or provide **special seating** or **equipment** that can help the family to manage the child more easily.

* They can **teach the family** ways to help stimulate the child's development and can plan with the family a step-by-step approach toward reaching realistic goals.

* Perhaps they can start something like a **'day care center'** where the rehabilitation workers, different parents of disabled children, other concerned parents in the community, or unemployed young persons take turns caring for the disabled children for part of the day. This could be done on a volunteer basis. Or money to pay for caretakers could be raised by the community, either through donations, raffles, bake sales, musical events or other fund-raising activities.

It is very important that the mother and family have rest periods from caring for their severely disabled child.
Such rest periods can often make the difference between whether or not they can handle difficulties and keep treating the child in a loving, supportive way.

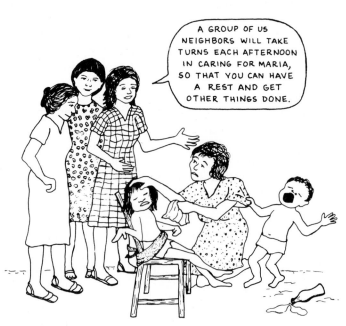

A GROUP OF US NEIGHBORS WILL TAKE TURNS EACH AFTERNOON IN CARING FOR MARIA, SO THAT YOU CAN HAVE A REST AND GET OTHER THINGS DONE.

In some cases it may be better to provide 'day care' in the child's own home. Again, the community may be able to provide either volunteers or paid care-providers.

Whatever the case, often **it is too much to expect the family of a severely, multiply disabled child to care adequately for the child, unless the community offers generous help and support.**

CARING FOR THE SEVERELY DISABLED CHILD

In deciding how to care for and work with the child who has a combination of severe disabilities, it is important to evaluate as best you can both her **disabilities** and **possibilities.** Especially in the very young child, this may not be easy. You must be ready to see new signs and change your *evaluation.* This, in turn, may change your plan for working with the child, so as to best help her to develop whatever skills and responses are possible.

In evaluating and planning activities with the child, try to be realistic. Do not expect too much, because this can lead to disappointment. But at the same time, do not expect too little.

For example, a child with a serious physical disability who is also deaf and/or blind may appear to be mentally retarded simply because her ability to experience and respond to things around her is very limited. The child may, in fact, have a lot more *mental* capacity (or possibility) than she appears to have. It would be wrong not to look for ways of reaching, developing, and appreciating her mind. However, this may take great patience and creativeness by those caring for her.

SOME GOALS IN CARING FOR A SEVERELY AND MULTIPLY DISABLED CHILD:

1. To help her to be physically comfortable, clean, safe, and well-fed.
2. To help her with *positioning* and exercise to prevent further deformity, and to make caring for her easier.
3. To help her learn whatever basic skills she can—in developing head and hand control, and in some form of communication. Also, help her learn to interact with others in a way that her needs are met and her behavior is acceptable.
4. To make caring for the child easier and more enjoyable for those who are responsible for her.

Much of the information and suggestions in Chapters 34 and 35 on early stimulation and development may be helpful for the multiply disabled child. **Look for areas of development where the child seems to be most ready or to have possibilities. Then work out a plan of activity, stimulation, and rewards that will take the child forward one small step at a time.** Some of the suggestions included in Chapter 40, "Ways To Improve Learning and Behavior," may also help. However, you will need to apply them with much patience and repetition.

To help meet the needs of the multiply disabled child, you will also find useful information in the chapters on the different disabilities that affect the child.

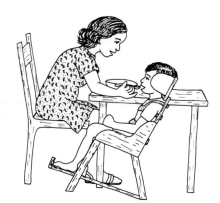

Special seating and positioning, discussed in Chapter 65, may help the child to have more control of her body. This can make feeding, basic communication, and other activities easier.

Special seating can help the severely disabled child by supporting him in a position where he has better control.

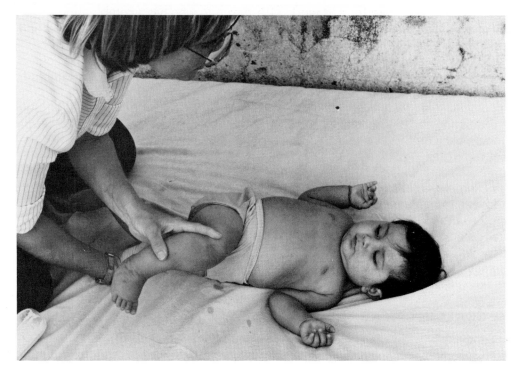

A child who is slower than most in learning to use her mind and body needs extra help. Learning to twist and to roll, and to lift up on her arms and turn, are important early developmental steps. Here a rehab worker first helps 'loosen up' a child by slowly swinging her hips from side to side.

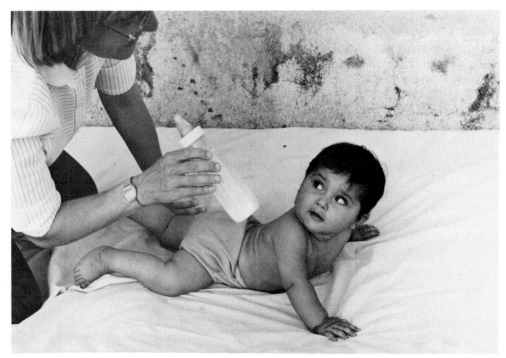

Then she encourages the child to lift up and turn to follow an object she wants.

CAUTION: **Breast feeding is healthier than bottle feeding.** It is usually better to use a toy or rattle to draw the child's attention rather than a bottle.

Child Development and Developmental Delay

CHAPTER **34**

(CP)

In Chapter 32 we discussed some of the primary causes of *'mental retardation'*. Mostly we looked at disabilities that come from **inside a child's head**—conditions where the brain has been damaged, is too small, or for other reasons is not able to work as quickly as other children's brains.

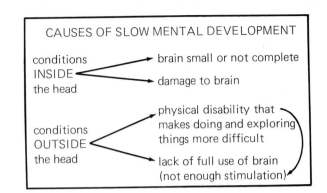

CAUSES OF SLOW MENTAL DEVELOPMENT

conditions INSIDE the head
→ brain small or not complete
→ damage to brain

conditions OUTSIDE the head
→ physical disability that makes doing and exploring things more difficult
→ lack of full use of brain (not enough stimulation)

In this chapter we see how a child's early development also depends on factors **outside the child's head**—on the opportunities a child has to use his senses, mind, and body to learn about the things and people around him. We look at the stages or steps of normal child development, and at ways we can help or 'stimulate' a child to learn and do things more quickly. Our concern is not only to help children who are 'mentally retarded', but those whose development is slow, or 'delayed', for whatever reason.

Usually children whose minds are slow to develop are also slow in learning to use their bodies. They begin later than other children to lift their heads, roll, sit, use their hands, stand, walk, and do other things. **They are physically delayed because of their delayed mental development.**

In other children the opposite is true. Their minds are basically complete and undamaged, but **certain physical disabilities make it harder and slower for them to develop the use of their minds.**

For example, a child who is born deaf but whose brain is normal will have difficulty understanding what people say, and in learning to speak. As a result, she is often left out of exchange of ideas and information. Because language is so important for the full development of the mind, in some ways she may seem 'mentally slow' for her age. However, if the child is taught to communicate her wishes and thoughts through 'sign language' at the age when other children learn to speak, her thinking power (intelligence) will often develop normally (see Chapter 31).

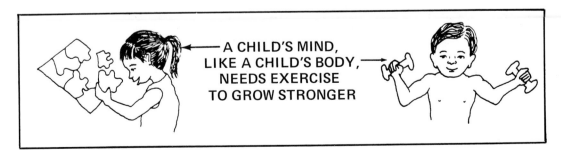

A CHILD'S MIND, LIKE A CHILD'S BODY, NEEDS EXERCISE TO GROW STRONGER

On the next page is a true story that shows how a severe physical disability can lead to slow mental development, and how a family found ways to help their child develop more fully.

(CP)

ENRIQUE'S STORY

Enrique had a difficult birth. He was born blue and limp. He did not start breathing for about 3 minutes. As a result, he developed severe cerebral palsy. His body became stiff and made strange movements that he could not control. His head often twisted to one side and he had trouble swallowing.

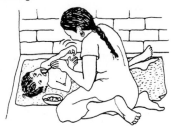

To protect him, his mother kept him on the floor in a corner.

Enrique's mother loved him and cared for him as best she could. But as the years went by, he did not gain any control of his body. His mother kept him on the floor in a corner so that he would not hurt himself. He spent most of his young life lying on his back, legs stiffly crossed like scissors, head pressed back, looking up at the roof and the mud brick walls. By age 3 he had learned to speak a few words, but with great difficulty. By age 6 he spoke only a little more. He cried a lot, had temper tantrums, and did not control his *bowels* or *bladder.* In many ways he remained like a baby. A visiting nurse called him 'retarded'. Still lying alone in the corner, Enrique grew increasingly withdrawn. At age seven—if his mother understood him correctly—he asked her for a gun to kill himself.

Soon after this, Enrique's mother and his older sister took him to a team of village *rehabilitation* workers in a neighboring village. The workers realized that he would probably never have much control of his hands and legs. But he desperately needed to communicate more with other people and see what was going on around him, to be included in the life of his family and village. But how could he do this lying on his back? His mother had tried many times to sit him in a chair, but his body would stiffen and he would fall off or cry.

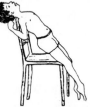

The village workers helped Enrique's family make a special chair for him, with a cushion and hip strap to help him sit in a good position. They taught his mother and sister how to help him sit in a way that would keep his body from stiffening so much.

special cushion (See p. 609.)

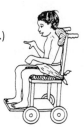

Later, they added wheels to the chair.

With his new chair, Enrique was able to sit and watch everything that was going on around him. He was excited and began to take more interest in things. He could also sit at the table and eat with the family (although his mother still had to feed him). Everyone talked to him and soon he began to talk more. Although his words were difficult to understand, he tried very hard. In time, he spoke a little more clearly. He also began to tell people when he had to use his toilet. He discovered he was no longer a baby, and did not want to be treated as one.

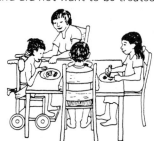

Every day Enrique's sister and brother went to school. One day Enrique begged to go too, and they pushed him there in his chair. Soon he went every day, and began to learn to read. Enrique had begun to develop more control of his head. The village workers helped the teacher make a book holder attached to Enrique's chair, and a head band with a wire arm so that he could turn the pages.

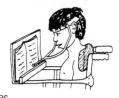

A happier and fuller life had begun for Enrique.

Enrique's story shows how development of the body, mind, and senses all influence each other. Enrique was slow to develop mentally because he did nothing but lie on his back in a corner. His mind did not have the 'stimulation' (activity, exercise, and excitement) it needed to grow strong. He had almost no control of his body movements. However, his eyes and ears were good. When at last his body was placed so he could see and experience more of the world around him, and relate more to other people, his mind developed quickly. With a little help and imagination, he learned to do many things that he and his family never dreamed he could.

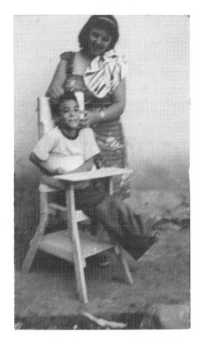

Enrique's sister helps position him in his new chair.

We saw how Enrique's physical disability slowed down his mental development. Similarly, a child who is mentally slow is often delayed in physical development. Development of body and mind are closely joined. After all, the mind directs the body, yet depends on the body's 5 senses (sight, hearing, touch, taste, and smell) for its knowledge of people and things. Therefore:

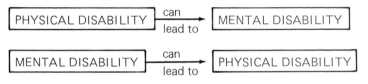

PHYSICAL DISABILITY —can lead to→ MENTAL DISABILITY

MENTAL DISABILITY —can lead to→ PHYSICAL DISABILITY

} **UNLESS** special care is taken to help the child develop BOTH BODY AND MIND as fully as possible.

Each child, of course, has his or her own **special needs.** Parents and rehabilitation workers can try to figure out and meet these needs. (An example is Enrique's need for special *positioning* so that he can see and do things better.)

But **all children** have the same **basic needs.** They need love, good food, and shelter. And they need the chance to explore their own bodies and the world about them as fully as they can.

Early Stimulation

'Stimulation' means giving a child a variety of opportunities to experience, explore, and play with things around her. It involves body movement and the use of all the senses—especially seeing, hearing, and touching.

Early stimulation is necessary for the healthy growth of every child's body and mind. For the non-disabled child, stimulation often comes naturally and easily, through interaction with other people and things. But it is often more difficult for the disabled child to experience and explore the world around him. For his mind and body to develop as early and fully as possible, he will need extra care and special activities that provide easy and enjoyable ways to learn.

> **The younger the child is when a 'stimulation program' begins, the less retarded or delayed he will be when he is older.**

NORMAL CHILD DEVELOPMENT

In order to know how well a child is developing and in which areas she may need special help, we can compare her development with that of other children.

> **An understanding of** *normal child development* **can guide us in planning activities that will help the disabled child progress.**

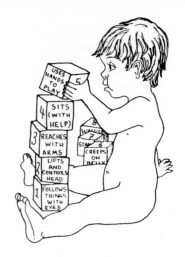

Every child develops in 3 main areas: **physical** (body), **mental** (mind), and **social** (communication and relating to other people). In each area, she develops skills step by step in a certain order. During the first year of life, normally a baby gains more and more control of her body.

A child's abilities develop in a particular order, one upon the other, like building blocks.

Body control develops progressively from the head down:

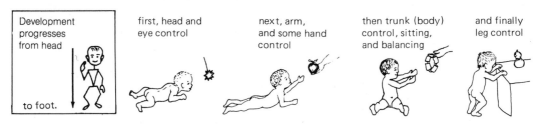

| Development progresses from head to foot. | first, head and eye control | next, arm, and some hand control | then trunk (body) control, sitting, and balancing | and finally leg control |

Before she can begin to walk, a baby needs to go through a series of developmental stages, or 'levels'. First, she has to be able to hold up her head and see what is around her. This encourages her to use her arms and hands so that she can then learn to lift herself to sit. While sitting, she begins to reach, lean, and twist. All this helps her to develop balance and to shift her weight from side to side—skills she will soon need for standing and walking. Normally, the stimulation that a child needs to advance through these stages comes from ordinary day-to-day interaction with people and things.

However, a child who has a disability may need special help to keep progressing. Notice that in the above example, the child's ability to *see* makes her **see things and want to reach for things and explore.** Seeing stimulates her to try to learn and do more. If a child cannot see, this basic part of early stimulation is lacking. To prevent her from falling behind, we must look for other ways to encourage her to learn and do things. We can do this through **touch** and **sound,** adapting the type of stimulation we use to the child's particular stage of development. For example, **if a baby cannot see:**

From the first we should hold her and speak to her a lot. Help her to reach out to touch and feel different things.

Later, we can encourage her to lift and turn her head, and then reach out, toward different sounds.

When she begins to sit, again we can help her to recognize different sounds and reach toward them.

When she begins to walk we can help her find her way with guide poles, and in other ways.

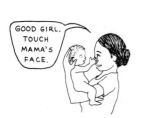
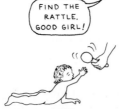
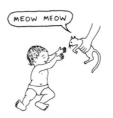
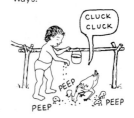

For more ways to help a child who cannot see well, see Chapter 30.

It is important for parents to realize that a child develops control and use of her body in a certain order:

HEAD CONTROL→*TRUNK* CONTROL (SITTING AND BALANCE) →STANDING AND WALKING

This is true even for an older child. Often parents of an older child who is delayed will try to help her learn more advanced skills (which other children her age are learning) before she is ready. This often leads to disappointment and frustration both for parents and child.

For example, Nina is a 3-year-old girl with cerebral palsy. She still has trouble holding up her head or sitting without falling over.

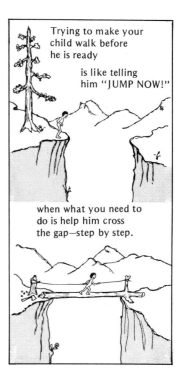

Trying to make your child walk before he is ready

is like telling him "JUMP NOW!"

when what you need to do is help him cross the gap—step by step.

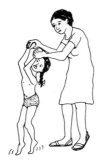

However, her mother is sure she is 'almost ready to walk'. Several times each day she holds Nina in a standing position and moves her forward, so that her feet take stiff, jerky steps on tiptoe. Her mother does not know that this stepping is an 'early reflex' normally only seen in young babies (see p. 311). It means that in some ways Nina's development is still at the level of a 1- to 3-month-old baby. She is not yet ready to walk. Making her 'take steps' will only keep active the early reflex which she needs to lose in order to learn to really walk.

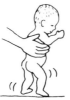

'stepping reflex' in a 1-month-old baby

We must help Nina's mother realize that Nina first needs help with other important developmental steps before she will be ready to learn to walk. To help her develop further, her mother will need to:

1. Figure out what developmental age or stage the child is at.
2. Decide what are the next steps forward, so that the child can build new skills on the ones she has now, **in the same order in which a normal child develops.**

To do these things, Nina's mother should first observe the child carefully. In each area of development, she notes the different things Nina **can do,** the things she **cannot do yet,** and the things she is **just beginning or trying to do,** but still has trouble with. Next, her mother compares what Nina can and cannot do with what other children Nina's age can do. She can then decide at what level her child is at in each area of development, and what are the next steps to work toward.

THE CHART ON NORMAL CHILD DEVELOPMENT

The chart on the next 2 pages shows some of the steps or 'milestones' of normal child development. You can use it to figure out where a child is in her development, and to plan the next steps that she needs help with.

CAUTION: The development chart shows the average ages when children begin to do things. But **the ages at which normal children develop different skills vary greatly.** Just because a child has not developed certain skills by the ages shown does not mean he is backward or has a problem. Be sure to **look at the whole child.**

RECORD
SHEET
6
(page 1)

EVALUATION OF A CHILD'S LEVEL OF *PHYSICAL* DEVELOPMENT

Note: Although on these guides physical and mental skills are separated, the two are often closely interrelated.

These charts show roughly the average age that a normal child develops different skills. But there is great variation within what is normal.

Name: _____
Birth date: _____
Date: _____

PHYSICAL DEVELOPMENT	Average age skills begin	3 months	6 months	9 months	1 year	2 years	3 years	5 years	What to do if a child is behind
Head and trunk control	lifts head part way up	holds head up briefly / holds head up high and well	holds up head and shoulders / turns head and shifts weight						Activities to improve head and trunk control (see p. 302).
Rolling		rolls belly to back	rolls back to belly	rolls over and over easily in play	moves and holds head easily in all directions				Activities to develop rolling and twisting (see p. 304).
Sitting		sits only with full support / sits with some support	sits with hand support	begins to sit without support / sits well without support		twists and moves easily while sitting			Work on sitting. Special seating if needed (p. 308).
Crawling and walking		begins to creep	scoots or crawls	pulls to standing	takes steps	walks / runs	walks easily backward / can walk on tiptoe and on heels	hops on one foot	Activities to improve balance (see p. 306).
Arm and hand control	grips finger put into hand	begins to reach towards objects	reaches and grasps with whole hand	passes object from one hand to other	grasps with thumb and forefinger	looks at small things/pictures	easily moves fingers back and forth from nose to moving object	throws and catches ball	Eye-hand activities. Use toys and games to develop hand and finger control (see p. 305).
Seeing	follows close object with eyes	enjoys bright colors/shapes		recognizes different faces / eyes focus on far object	understands simple words	Sees small shapes clearly at 6 meters (see p. 453 for test).			Have eyes checked (see p. 452). If poor, see Chapter 30.
Hearing	moves or cries at a loud noise	turns head to sounds	responds to mother's voice	enjoys rhythmic music	understands simple words	hears clearly and understands most simple language			Have hearing checked. If poor, see Chapter 31.

Name: _____

Birth date: _____

Date: _____

EVALUATION OF A CHILD'S LEVEL OF *MENTAL AND SOCIAL DEVELOPMENT*

RECORD
SHEET
6
(page 2)

MENTAL DEVELOPMENT	Average age skills begin	3 months	6 months	9 months	1 year	2 years	3 years	5 years	What to do if a child is behind
Communication and language	cries when wet or hungry	coos when comfortable	makes simple sounds	uses certain sounds for different things (WA WA)	begins to use single words (MAMA)	begins to use words together (COW, DADDY.)		uses simple sentences (DADDY GO WORK.)	Speak and sing often to child. If needed, develop alternatives to speech (p. 313).
Social Behavior		smiles when smiled at		begins to understand and respond to "NO!" (COME HERE!)	begins to do simple things when asked	likes to be praised after completing simple tasks (GOOD GIRL!)	interacts with both adults and children	helps with simple work	Consider trying behavioral approach to social behavior (see p. 349).
Self-care	sucks breast	takes everything to mouth		chews solid food; begins to feed self	drinks alone from glass	takes off simple clothes	toilet trained	bathes and dresses	Encourage child to help self if possible. Use behavioral approach to learning (see p. 350).
Attention and interest	grasps things placed in hand	plays with own body; brief interest in toys and sounds	plays with simple objects	develops strong attachments to caretakers	takes longer interest in toys and activities	sorts different objects	builds playthings with several pieces		Early stimulation activities (see Chapter 35). Provide toys and 'fun' objects.
Play				begins to enjoy first social games (peek-a-boo)	imitates and copies people	begins to play with other children	plays independently with children and toys		Guided play, lots of stimulation and interaction with other children.
Intelligence and learning	cries when hungry or uncomfortable	recognizes mother	recognizes several people	looks for toys that fall out of sight	copies simple actions	points to things when asked (WHERE IS YOUR EYE?)	follows simple instructions	follows multiple instructions	Early stimulation (p. 316). Lots of toys, talk, and step-by-step training.

Put a ⬭ circle around the level of development that the child is now at in each area.

Put a ☐ square around the skill to the right of the one you circled, and focus training on that skill.

If the child has reached an age and has not mastered the corresponding level of skill, special training may be needed.

How to use the Child Development Chart

The chart on pages 292 and 293 can be used to:

1. find and record a child's developmental level.
2. plan the next developmental steps or activities with which we can help the child, and
3. and record in which areas the child is progressing, and how much.

Let us suppose that a village health worker wants to help Nina's mother figure out what she needs to do next to help her 3-year-old daughter develop early abilities. Together they look at the chart.

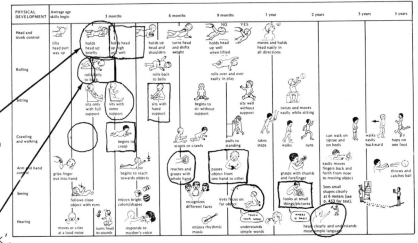

First they put a circle around each of the things that Nina can do. Since she still has trouble holding her head up, they put a circle here.

Nina needs help to roll from her belly to her back, so they put a circle that goes part way around 'rolls belly to back'.

After they circle Nina's level in each area of development, they can see that in her general body movements and control, Nina is still at the level of a 2- to 4-month-old baby. Her hand control is at about 6 months. Her seeing and hearing seem about normal, and her mental development is at about 2 years.

Then they put a square around the next developmental step after each circle. **The squares show which developmental steps Nina now needs help with.** Because Nina's poor head control is holding her back in other areas, they decide to work mostly with this (see p. 302), and also to help her with rolling and twisting her body (see p. 304). Perhaps they can begin to work with sitting and creeping, but probably she will not progress much with these until she gets better head control. The use of her hands is still

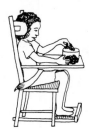

somewhat behind for her age, but this may partly be because of her poor head control. So they decide to have her sit for short periods each day in a special seat. With her head supported in a good position, they can give her games and things to do to help her develop better use of her hands. But, they are careful *not* to keep her head supported for long, because that will not help her to learn to support it herself. Also, they are careful to provide only the least amount of support needed to give her better control of other parts of her body. They will reduce the support as her control improves.

Because Nina's eyes, ears, mind, and speech seem to be developing fairly well, these will probably be what she learns to use best as she grows older. Therefore, her parents decide to do all they can to help her improve these skills. They use pictures, songs, stories, play, and a lot of stimulation to help her develop her mind. But they try to remember that she is still only 3 years old. They must not push her too much. Sometimes it is better to help her gain skill and confidence in only 1 or 2 areas at a time.

To use the Child Development Chart for recording a child's progress, every month or two you can add new circles to the chart. Use a different colored ink each time, and mark the date in the same color. Then add new squares to determine the developmental steps that are next in line. (See p. 49.)

THE NEED FOR EARLY STIMULATION

The parents and family are the key to the development and early learning of any child. Children who are developmentally slow need the same stimulation (talking to them, music, games, adventure, and love) that any child needs. But they need more. They need more help and repeated activities to use their minds and their bodies.

> When a child is delayed, he needs stimulation and activities to help develop all areas of his body and mind.

AREAS OF A CHILD'S DEVELOPMENT THAT CAN BE HELPED THROUGH EARLY STIMULATION AND LEARNING ACTIVITIES

1. **Movement, body control, strength, and balance:** these will help the child move about, do things, play, and work.

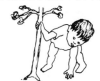

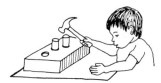

2. **Use of the hands:** increased hand control, and coordination of the hands with what the child sees, allows the child to develop many skills.

3. **The senses:** especially seeing, hearing and feeling. These will help the child recognize and respond to her world.

4. **Communication:** listening, understanding what is said, and learning to speak, or to communicate in whatever way is possible.

5. **Interaction with other people:** smiling, playing, behaving appropriately, and learning to 'get along' with others.

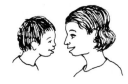

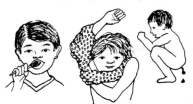

6. **Basic activities for daily living:** eating, drinking, dressing, and control of bowel and bladder (peeing and shitting). These 'self-care' skills help the child become more independent.

7. **Observing, thinking, and doing:** to learn how to make thoughtful, intelligent decisions.

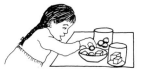

> The goals of an early stimulation program are to help the child become as able, self-sufficient, happy, and kind as possible.

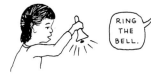

STEPS IN DESIGNING A PROGRAM OF SPECIAL LEARNING AND EARLY STIMULATION

First: Observe the child closely to evaluate what he can and cannot do in each developmental area.

Second: Notice what things he is just beginning to do or still has difficulty with.

Third: Decide what new skill to teach or action to encourage that will help the child build on the skills he already has.

Fourth: Divide each new skill into small steps: activities the child can learn in a day or two, and then go on to the next step.

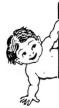

CAUTION: Do not expect too much at once. Be realistic. **Start with what the child can do well** and then encourage him to do a little more. By giving the right help at the right time, both the helpers and the child will feel successful and happy.

SUGGESTIONS FOR DOING LEARNING ACTIVITIES WITH ANY CHILD (DELAYED OR NOT)

Be patient and observant. Children do not learn all the time; sometimes they need to rest. When they are rested, they will begin to progress again. Observe the child closely. Try to understand how she thinks, what she knows, and how she uses her new skills. You will then learn how to help her practice and improve those skills. When talking with the child, give her time to answer your questions. Take turns speaking. Remember that practice and repetition are important.

Be orderly and consistent. Plan special activities to progress naturally from one skill to the next. Try to play with the child at about the same time each day, and to put his toys, tools, clothes, and so on, in the same place. Stay with one style of teaching, loving, and behavior development (if it works!). Respond in a similar way each time to the child's actions and needs. This will help him to understand and to feel more confident and secure.

Use variety. While repetition is important, so is variety! Change the activities a little every day, so that the child and her helpers do not get bored. Do things in different ways, and in various places inside and outside of the house. Take the child to the market, fields, and the river. Give her a lot of things to do.

Be expressive. Use your face and your tone of voice to show your feelings and thoughts. Speak clearly and simply (but do not use 'baby talk'). Praise and encourage the child often.

Have a good time! Look for ways to turn all activities into **games** that both the child and you enjoy.

Be practical. Whenever possible choose skills and activities that will help the child become more independent and be able to do more, for himself and for others. To help prepare the child for greater independence, do not overprotect him.

Be confident. All children will respond in some way to care, attention, and love. With your help, a child who is delayed can become more able and independent.

A special learning program, if well-planned and carefully done, can help a delayed child progress much more than she would without help.

GENERAL GUIDELINES FOR HELPING A CHILD'S DEVELOPMENT

How a family member or rehabilitation worker relates to a child when trying to teach her new skills can make a big difference in her whole development. It can affect how fast or well she learns the new skill. More importantly, it can influence the child's confidence, behavior, and readiness to learn.

There are a few simple methods that you can use to help a child gain a better **understanding of her own body, prepare her for learning language,** and **help her relate to other persons in a friendly, cooperative way.**

These guidelines are especially helpful when doing early learning activities with children who are developmentally delayed:

1. **Praise the child a lot.** Praise him, hug him lovingly, or give him a little prize when he does something well (or when he makes a good effort).

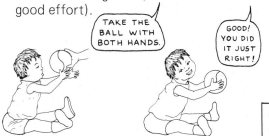

Explanation

Praising success works much better (and is much kinder) than scolding or punishing failure. When the child tries to do something and fails, it is best to ignore it or simply say something like: "Too bad, better luck next time."

> *CAUTION:* **Avoid giving sweets or food as prizes —especially if the child is fat (see box on p. 340).**

2. **Talk a lot to the child.** Using clear, simple words, say everything that you do with him.

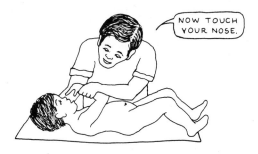

Explanation

A child listens to and begins to learn language long before he begins to speak. Although it may seem as though he does not understand or respond, still talk to him a lot. If you think he does not hear, talk to him but also use 'sign language'. Make sure he looks at you as you speak. (See p. 313 to 314.)

3. When you are helping a child learn a new skill, **guide her movements with your hands.**

For example, to teach a child to bring her hands to her mouth (or to eat by herself) you can,

help her put her finger in a food she enjoys,   and then to put her finger in her mouth.   After the child has learned to do this, let her do it by herself.

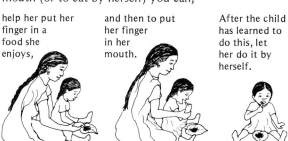

Explanation

It usually works better to gently guide the child than to tell her how to do something. If she tries to do something but has difficulty, guiding her hands so that she is successful will make her a lot more eager to learn the skill than if you say "NO—do it like this!"

4. **Use a mirror** to help the child learn about his body and to use his hands.

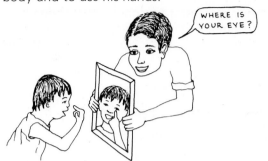

Explanation

The mirror helps the child see and recognize parts of his body. It is especially useful for children who have difficulty relating to different parts of their body or knowing where they are. (This can happen in some forms of mental retardation, cerebral palsy, spinal cord injury, and spina bifida.)

5. **Use imitation (copying).** To teach a new action or skill, do something first and encourage the child to copy you. Turn it into a game.

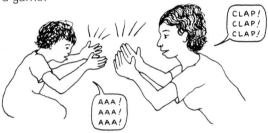

Explanation

Many retarded children (especially those with Down syndrome) love to copy or imitate the actions of others. This is a good way to teach many things, from physical activities to sounds and words.

6. **Encourage the child to reach out or go for what he wants.**

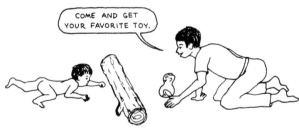

When it gets too easy, put obstacles in the way—but do not make them too difficult.

Explanation

Even at early stages of development, it is a mistake to always place in his hands what a child wants. Instead, use the child's desire as a chance to have him use his developing body skills and language skills to get what he wants—by reaching, twisting, rising, creeping, or whatever he is learning to do.

7. **Make learning fun.** Always look for ways to turn learning activities into play.

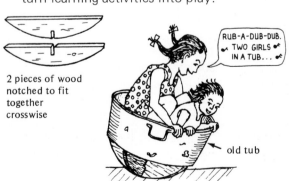

2 pieces of wood notched to fit together crosswise

old tub

Explanation

Children learn best and cooperate more when they enjoy and are excited by what they are doing. **Keep doing an activity as long as it is fun for the child. As soon as it stops being fun, stop the activity for a while, or change it in some way, to put new adventure and excitement into it.**

8. **Let the child do as much as she can for herself. Help her only as much as is needed.**

For example, if the child has trouble putting on clothes because of *spasticity,* help by bending her shoulders and back forward, but let her pull on her clothes herself.

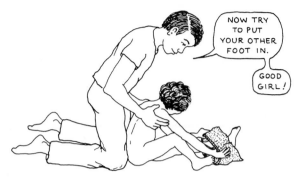

Explanation

This is the "Golden Rule of Rehabilitation." When a child has trouble doing something or seems slow or clumsy at it, parents often want to 'help' by doing it for her. However, for the child's development, it will help her more to let her do it herself—providing encouragement but assisting only in ways that let her do more for herself.

9. **The child often learns best when no teacher is present.**

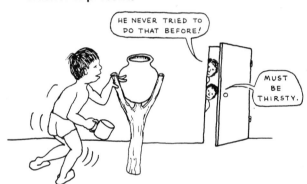

Explanation

Children often try hardest when they want something a lot, and no one is there to help. Teaching is important, but so is giving the child a chance to explore, test his own limits, and do things for and by himself.

10. **Get older brothers and sisters to demonstrate new equipment.**

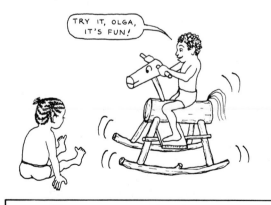

Explanation

Some children may refuse to try, or will be afraid of new playthings, aids, or special seating. If another child tries it first, and shows he likes it, the child will often want to try it also.

REMEMBER: **Good teaching** *will* **make a difference.** *How well* **you teach, play, and express affection is more important than** *how much* **time you spend at it.**

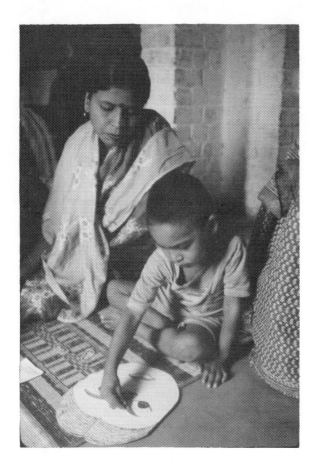

A mentally retarded child learns the parts of a face by placing cut-out cardboard parts on a paper face. (Samadhan, Delhi, India)

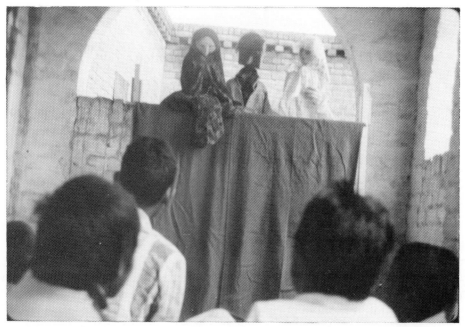

Puppets are used to teach mentally retarded children in Samadhan (India). Each puppet wears clothes of one color and has the name of that color. The children learn the puppets' names—and so begin to learn the colors.

Early Stimulation and Development Activities

On the next pages are activities to help young children's development. They are especially valuable for children who are mentally and physically delayed. They are also useful for children who are mentally normal but whose physical *disabilities* make both *physical* and *mental* development slow or difficult.

In this chapter we describe activities for early skills in the order in which they usually develop. So we start with head control, then progress to more advanced levels: reaching, grasping, sitting and balance, scooting or crawling, standing and walking, and language. (Self-care activities including eating, dressing, and toilet training are discussed in later chapters.)

In any area of development, such as head control or use of the hands, a child also advances through different stages of ability. For example, in developing grip, first a child can grasp only with the whole hand, later with thumb and finger.

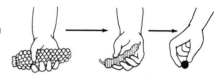

To decide which activities to begin with, start by using the charts on pages 292 and 293 to **determine the developmental level** of your child. Then look through pages 302 to 316 and **pick those activities that are next in line for your child.** After she learns these activities, go on to the next.

A child advances in many areas of development at once. Try to help her in several areas at the same time. **In each area, pick activities that help her do better what she already does, and then to take the next step.**

Often an activity that helps a child to develop in one area also helps in others.

For example, we put the activity with this picture under ──→ **"head control."** But the activity also helps to develop use of **the senses** (eyes, touch, sound), **hand control, eye-hand coordination, balance while sitting,** and **flexibility of the body** (twisting to one side). If done in a friendly way, with praise, it can **develop confidence** and **ability to relate** to other people. And if father talks to the child as they play, naming each object and action, it also prepares the child for learning language.

When helping your child with these learning activities, remember to **introduce new skills in small steps** that the child can easily learn. **Praise her each time she succeeds, or tries hard.** Follow the suggestions on pages 296 to 299 for helping the child develop these new skills.

CAUTION: Many activities in this chapter are useful for children with cerebral palsy or other physical disabilities. However, some must be changed or adapted. Read the chapters that apply to your child's disability. *Above all:* USE YOUR HEAD. OBSERVE HOW YOUR CHILD RESPONDS. NOTICE HOW AN ACTIVITY HELPS—OR HINDERS—THE CHILD'S WHOLE DEVELOPMENT. **DO NOT SIMPLY FOLLOW THE INSTRUCTIONS. ADAPT OR INVENT ACTIVITIES TO MEET YOUR CHILD'S NEEDS.**

1. Activities to help the child lift and control her head (and use her eyes and ears)

(CP)   One of the first skills a normal baby develops is the ability to lift the head and control its movement. Head control is needed before a child can learn to roll, sit, or crawl. Normally, a newborn child can lift or hold her head up for a moment, and she develops fairly good head control in the first months of life. **Children with developmental delay are often slow to develop head control. We need to help them to develop reasonable head control before trying to help them to roll, sit, crawl, or walk.**

To encourage the child to raise her head **when lying face down,** attract her attention with brightly colored objects that make strange or pretty sounds.

TIC
TIC
TIC

If she does not lift her head, to help her, put her like this. Press firmly on the *muscles* on each side of the backbone and slowly bring your hand from her neck toward her hips.

If the baby has trouble raising her head because of a weak back or shoulders, try placing a blanket under her chest and shoulders. Get down in front of her and talk to her. Or put a toy within reach to stimulate interest and movement.

Some children can do more if they lie on a 'wedge' (see p. 571).

If the child has trouble lifting her head when lying face down, lay her against your body so that she is almost upright. This way she needs less strength to lift her head.

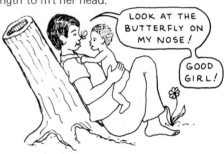

LOOK AT THE BUTTERFLY ON MY NOSE!

GOOD GIRL!

(CP)   To help her develop head control when **lying face up,** take her upper arms and pull her up gently until her head hangs back a little, then lay her down again.

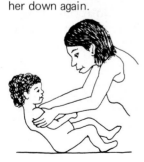

CAUTION: **Do not pull the child up like this if her head hangs back.** As you begin to lift her, watch to see if her neck muscles tighten. If not, do not pull her up. Also, do not pull the child up like this if it causes her legs to straighten stiffly (see "Cerebral Palsy," p. 102).

NOT LIKE THIS

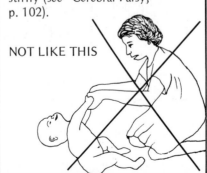

If a child with cerebral palsy stiffens as you pull his arms, try pulling the shoulder blades forward as you lift him up.

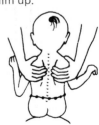

If the child cannot lift his head as you pull him up, then do not pull him up. Instead, sit the child up and gently tilt him back a little, encouraging him to hold his head up. Repeat often, and as he gains strength and control, gradually tilt him farther back—but do not let his head fall backward.

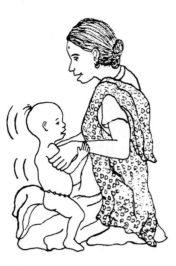

If the baby makes almost no effort to lift or hold her head when you feed her, instead of putting the nipple or food into her mouth, barely touch her lips with it, and make her come forward to get it.

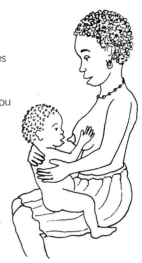

GOOD CARRYING POSITIONS

(CP)

Carrying the child like this helps develop good head control, when he is face down.

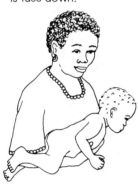

Positions that keep the hips and knees bent and the knees separate help relax and give better control to the child with cerebral palsy whose body straightens stiffly and whose knees press together.

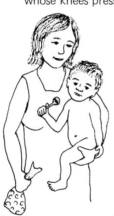

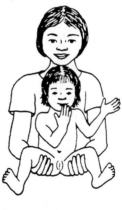

Carrying baby like this frees his head and arms to move and look around.

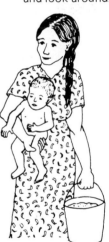

As your child develops better head control, play with him, supporting his body firmly, but with his head and arms free. Attract his attention with interesting objects and sounds, so that he turns his head first to one side and then to the other.

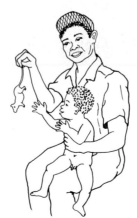

2. Activities to encourage rolling and twisting

After a baby has fairly good head control, usually the next step in development is to roll over. Rolling involves sideways twisting of the head and body. Twisting, or **rotation of the upper body on the lower body, must be learned before a child can learn to crawl and later to walk.**

Babies normally learn by themselves to roll over. But children who are developmentally delayed will learn faster with special help and encouragement. Help the child learn first to lift and turn her head to the side, then her shoulders and body.

Attract the child's attention by holding a rattle or toy in front of her,

Encourage her to reach sideways for the toy,

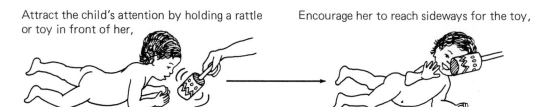

then move the toy to one side, so the child turns her head and shoulders to follow it.

then move the toy upward, so that she twists onto her side and back.

If she does not roll over after various tries, help her by lifting her leg.

Also, help the child learn to roll from her back onto her side. Again, have her reach for a toy held to one side.

(CP)

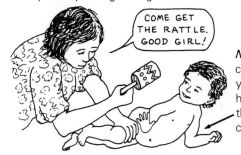

COME GET THE RATTLE. GOOD GIRL!

Note: If the child has *spasticity,* you may need to help position this arm before she can roll over.

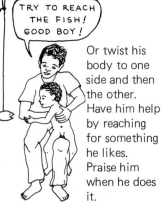

Note: If the child is very stiff, before doing other exercises or activities,

first help to relax him by swinging his legs back and forth,

or curl up the child in a 'ball' and slowly roll his hips and legs from side

to side.

(CP)

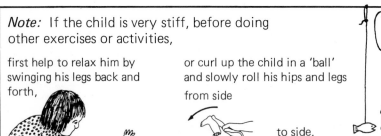

TRY TO REACH THE FISH! GOOD BOY!

Or twist his body to one side and then the other. Have him help by reaching for something he likes. Praise him when he does it.

Remember: THE FIRST RULE OF *THERAPY:* HELP ONLY AS MUCH AS NEEDED, ENCOURAGING THE CHILD TO DO MORE AND MORE FOR HERSELF.

3. Activities to help develop gripping, reaching, and hand-eye coordination

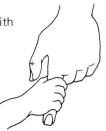

Most babies are born with a 'grasping reflex'. If you put your finger in their hand, the hand automatically grips it—so tightly you can lift up the child.

Usually this reflex goes away, and gradually the baby learns to hold things and let go as she chooses.

Babies who are slow to develop sometimes have little or no 'grasping reflex' and are slow to learn to hold things. For such children, these activities may help.

If she keeps her hand closed, stroke the outer edge of the hand from little finger to wrist.

This often causes the baby to lift and open her hand, and to grip your finger.

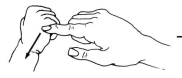 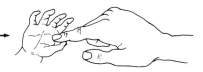 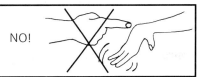

CAUTION: In a child with *spasticity,* stroking the back of the hand may cause her to grip or open the hand stiffly without control. If so, do not do it, but look for ways that give her more control.   NO!

(CP)

When the child opens her hands well, but has trouble holding on,

place an object in her hand, and bend her fingers around it. Be sure the thumb is opposite the fingers.

Gradually let go of her hand and pull the object up against her fingers or twist it from side to side.

When you think she has a firm grip, let go.   GOOD GIRL!

Repeat several times in each of the child's hands.

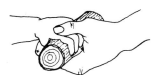 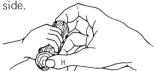

After the child can hold an object placed in her hand, encourage her to reach and grasp an object that just touches her fingertips.
First touch the top of her hand—then place it below her fingertips.

Encourage the baby to grasp by offering her rattles, bells, colorful toys, or something to eat on a stick.

Hang interesting toys, bells, and rattles where the child can see and reach for them.

If the child shows no awareness of her hand, hang little bells from her wrist.

This way the child learns to move her hand forward to take hold of a toy.

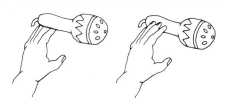 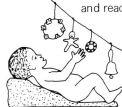

Also, see page 327 for ways to help a child discover her hands by putting a sweet food on her finger and helping her take it to her mouth.

At first a child can only grasp large objects with her whole hand. As she grows she will be able to pick up and hold smaller things with thumb and fingers. Help her do this by playing with objects of different sizes.

To help strengthen grip, play 'tug-of-war' with the child—making it a fun game.

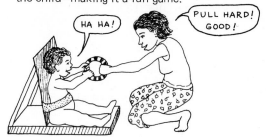

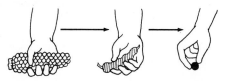

As the child gains more and more control, introduce toys and games that help develop **hand-eye coordination.** For ideas, see p. 318.

Make games of putting things in and out of boxes and jars.

Playing with toys and imitating the work and play of others helps the child gain more skillful use of his hands.

4. Activities for body control, balance, and sitting

After a child gains good head control, he normally starts sitting through these stages.

sits when placed in a sitting position and held

sits, keeping balance with arms

balances with body while sitting, freeing hands for play

sits up alone from a lying position

In order to sit well a child needs to be able to hold her body up, to use her hands to catch and support herself, and finally to balance with her body so that she can turn and reach.

If the child simply falls over when you sit him up, help him develop a protective reaction with his arms. Put him on a log, hold his hips, and slowly roll him sideways. Encourage him to 'catch' himself with a hand.

Or do the same thing with the child on your belly.

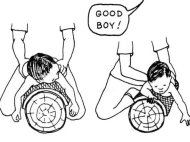

After the child learns to 'catch' herself when lying, sit her up, hold her above the hips, and gently push her from side to side,

and forward and backward so that she learns to catch and support herself with her arms.

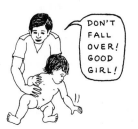

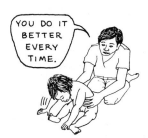

CAUTION: The child must be able to raise and turn her head before she can raise her body.

To help your child gain balance sitting, first sit her on your knees facing you.

Later, you can sit her facing out so that she can see what is going on around her.

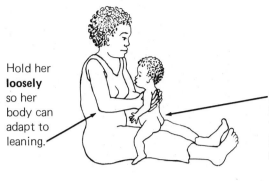

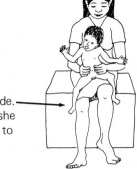

Hold her **loosely** so her body can adapt to leaning.

Slowly lift one knee to lean her gently to one side. Then the other, so that she learns to bend her body to stay seated.

You can do the same thing with the child sitting on a log.

As he gets better balance, move your hands down to his hips and then thighs, so that he depends less on your support.

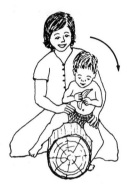

Give him something to hold so that he learns to use his body and not his arms to keep his balance.

With an older child who has difficulty with balance, you can do the same thing on a 'tilt board'.

Or you can do the same on a large ball.

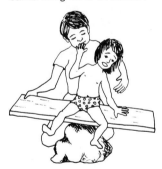

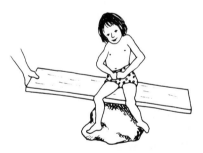

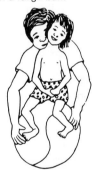

At first let her catch herself with her arms.

Later, see how long she can do it holding her hands together. Make it a game.

Tilt it to **one side and the other** and also **forward** and **back**.

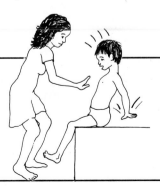

Note: You can also do these exercises by sitting the child on a table and gently pushing him backward, sideways, and forward. But **it is better to tip what he is sitting on.**

Pushing him causes him to 'catch himself' from falling with his arms.

Tilting him causes him to use his body to keep his balance, which is a more advanced skill.

Help the child learn to keep her balance while using her hands and twisting her body,

sitting on
the ground,

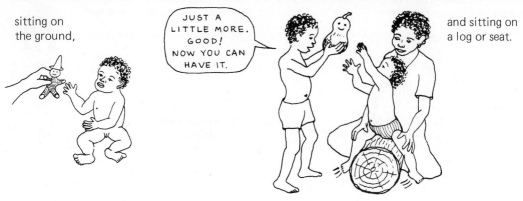

and sitting on
a log or seat.

When the child can sit by herself, help her learn to sit up,

from lying on her back,

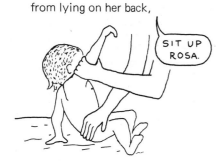

As the child starts to rise,
push on the higher hip.

and from lying on her
belly.

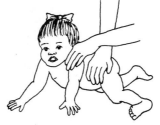

First help her lift her
shoulders.

Press down and
back on hip.

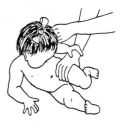

Help her roll to one
side, rise onto one
elbow, and sit.

Help her to sit up herself. **Do not pull her up. Praise her each time she does well, or tries hard.** Help her less and less until she can sit up alone.

Some children will need seating aids to sit well. To help improve balance, the aid should be **as low as possible** and still let the child sit straight. Often, firmly supporting the hips is enough. Here are 2 examples:

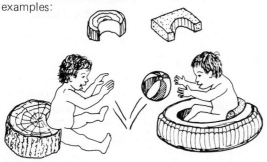

For the child who needs higher back support, simple 'corner seats' can be made of cardboard, wood, or poles in the ground.

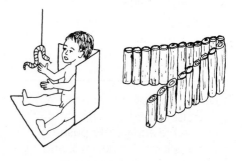

For more ideas on special seating and *positioning,* see Chapters 64 and 65. For sitting aids, see p. 573.

5. Activities for creeping and crawling

To move about, many babies first begin to **creep***, 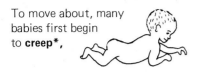 and then to **crawl***, 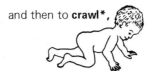 or to **scoot** on their butt.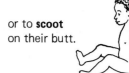

> *Note:* **Some babies never crawl** but go directly from sitting to standing and walking. Whether or not they crawl often depends on cultural patterns and whether the family encourages it.

If the child can lift her head well when lying on her stomach, encourage her to begin creeping in these ways:

Put a toy or food the child likes just out of reach.

At first it may help to support his feet.

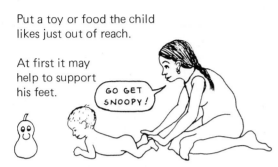

GO GET SNOOPY!

> *CAUTION:* If the child has cerebral palsy, supporting the feet may cause legs to straighten stiffly. If this happens do not support her feet.

If the child cannot bring her leg forward to creep, help her by lifting the hip.

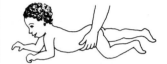

If the child has difficulty beginning to creep or crawl:

Let her 'ride' your knee. Play 'horsey'. Slowly move your knee up and down and sideways so that she shifts her weight from side to side.

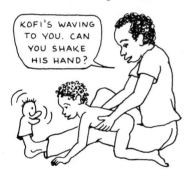

KOFI'S WAVING TO YOU. CAN YOU SHAKE HIS HAND?

Encourage her to lift one hand off the ground and shift her weight to the other. Then help her to move forward.

Or put the child over a bucket or log. To help him bear weight with his elbows straight, firmly push down on his shoulders and release. Repeat several times.

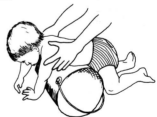

If the baby has trouble beginning to crawl, hold him up with a towel like this. As he gains strength, gradually support him less.

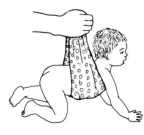

Move him from side to side so he shifts weight from one arm and leg to the other.

Older brothers and sisters can help.

Encourage the child to first reach—and later crawl—for something he wants.

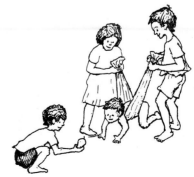

---

*North American therapists use these terms in the reverse way (creep for crawl and crawl for creep).

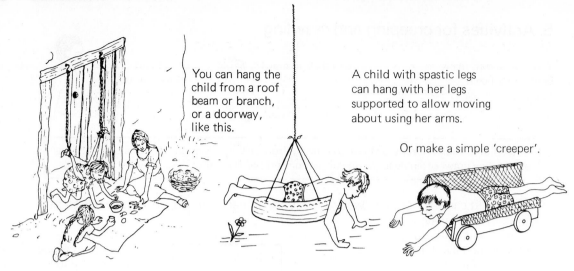

You can hang the child from a roof beam or branch, or a doorway, like this.

A child with spastic legs can hang with her legs supported to allow moving about using her arms.

Or make a simple 'creeper'.

When the child has learned to crawl fairly well, have him play crawling games.

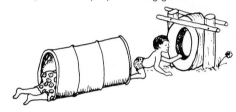

She can crawl up and down a small hill or pile of straw. This will help improve her strength and balance.

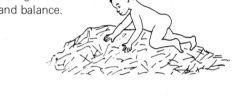

To help an older child with balance problems to prepare for walking, encourage him to **crawl sideways and backward.**

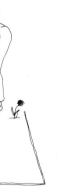

Also, have him hold one leg or arm off the ground and shift his weight back and forth.

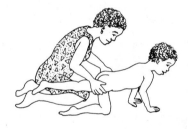

At first, you may need to hold up one limb while you slowly rock him from side to side.

Later, have him practice holding one arm and the opposite leg off the ground at the same time.

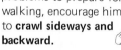

LET'S SEE HOW LONG YOU CAN HOLD IT! 1, 2, 3, 4...

A 'rocker board' is fun and helps balance.

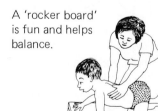

After a child gets her balance on hands and knees, you can help her begin to stand—and walk—on her knees. She can walk sideways along the rope.

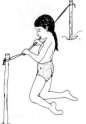

CP

CAUTION: Do not do this in a child with spasticity whose knees bend a lot when she stands.

There are many ways the child can practice standing on her knees and shifting her weight—ways that are fun and include her in family activities.

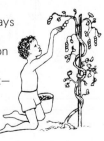

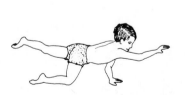

6. Activities for standing, walking, and balance

Normally a child progresses through these stages:

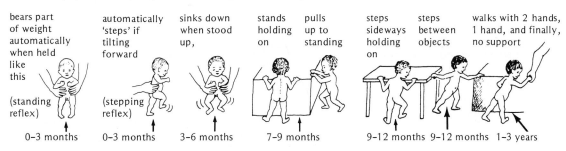

bears part of weight automatically when held like this (standing reflex)	automatically 'steps' if tilting forward (stepping reflex)	sinks down when stood up,	stands holding on	pulls up to standing	steps sideways holding on	steps between objects	walks with 2 hands, 1 hand, and finally, no support
0–3 months	0–3 months	3–6 months	7–9 months		9–12 months	9–12 months	1–3 years

You can prepare a child for walking by encouraging each of the above stages as the child develops.

> *CAUTION:* **If the child cannot balance when sitting, do not work on walking yet. Help her develop sitting balance first.**

Hold the baby so that she uses the **early stepping reflex** to strengthen her legs. You can even bounce the baby gently.

> *CAUTION:* **In children with spasticity, this activity may increase muscle stiffness. DO NOT DO IT. (See p. 93 and 291.)**

When the child begins to stand, support her hips with your hands. Spread her feet apart to form a wide base. First do this from in front, later from behind.

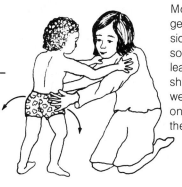

Move her gently from side to side, so that she learns to shift her weight from one leg to the other.

As she gains better balance, you can provide a light support at the shoulders.

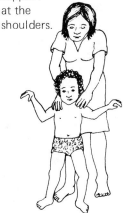

Or have the child hold a hose or rope. Because it is flexible, he needs to balance more.

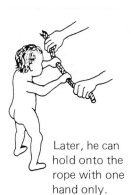

Later, he can hold onto the rope with one hand only.

To encourage a child to pull up to standing, put a toy he likes on the edge of a table.

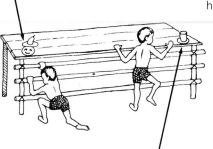

To encourage him to take steps, put something he likes at the other end of the table.

When a child can almost walk alone but is afraid of falling, tie a cloth around his chest.

Hold the cloth, but let it **hang completely loose.** Be ready to catch him if he falls.

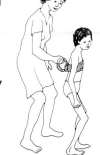

> *CAUTION:* Do not let the child hang by the cloth. Have him bear his own weight. The cloth is only to catch him if he falls.

Other activities for **improving balance:**

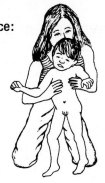

Hold the child **loosely** under the arms and gently tip him from side to side and forward and backward. Allow him to return to a straight position. Turn it into a game.

At first support the child while you do this. When his balance improves, do it without supporting him—but be ready to catch him if he falls.

Practice walking sideways and backward.

Note: Walking backward helps children who tend to walk tiptoe to bring their heels down.

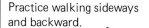

It is better to hold a child:

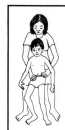

LIKE THIS

His balance is centered in his body.

NOT LIKE THIS

His balance is off center.

Support your child only as much as he needs, until he can walk by himself.

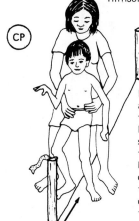

Draw a square on the ground and help him to take steps forward, sideways, and backward. Follow the 4 sides of the square, always facing the same direction. Make it fun by having him collect a different colored tag or piece of puzzle at each corner—or however you can.

For the **older child** with poor balance, a homemade **balance board** will turn developing better balance into a game. Move slowly at first—especially with a child with cerebral palsy.

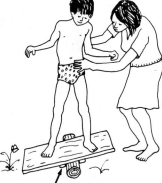

A balance board with a wide rocker is better because it rocks more smoothly. (See p. 576.)

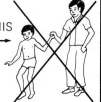

Some children will need a pole to hold onto.

Blocks to prevent rolling sideways.

Simple homemade **parallel bars** can help a child with weak legs or a balance problem get started walking.

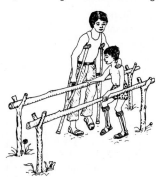

Homemade **pushcarts** or **walkers** can provide both support and independence for the child who is learning to walk or who has balance problems.

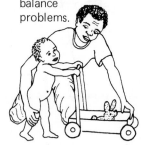

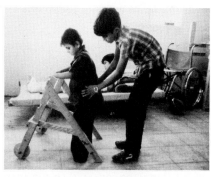

A simple **wooden walker** with plywood wheels helps this developmentally delayed child begin to walk. (For designs of walkers, see p. 581.)

7. Activities for communication and speech

A normal child's ability to communicate develops through these stages:

expresses needs through body movements, looks on the face, and crying	makes 'happy sounds'—coos and gurgles	babbles—listens to sounds and tries to imitate	says a few words	begins to put words (and ideas) together
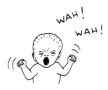				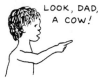
0–1 month	1–2 months	4–8 months	8–12 months	12 months–3 years

> **Learning that prepares a baby for speech begins early, long before she says her first word. Speech develops out of body movement, use of the mouth and tongue in eating, and use of the senses—through interaction with people and things.**

One of the early stages in a baby's development of speech is noticing and responding to different sounds. A delayed child may need extra help and stimulation:

Make noises with bells, rattles, clickers, and drums, first directly in front of the baby, then to one side, so that she turns her head.

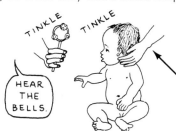

If she does not turn her head, bring the toy back so she can see it, and move it away again.

Or, gently turn her head so that she sees what makes the sound. Help her less and less—until she turns her head alone.

Repeat the babble of the child: have conversations with him in his language. But when he begins to say words, repeat and pronounce them clearly and correctly—**do not use 'baby talk'.**

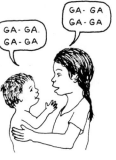

To get the child used to language, **explain everything you do with him.** Use clear, simple words—the same ones each time. Name toys, objects, body parts. Repeat often.

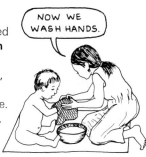

Understanding language depends not only on hearing, but also on watching lips and looks. So **speak to the child on her level.**

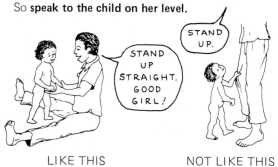

LIKE THIS   NOT LIKE THIS

A child understands words before he can speak them. Play **question games** to help him listen and learn; he can answer your questions by pointing, nodding, or shaking his head.

Repeat words. Make small requests. Reward successes.

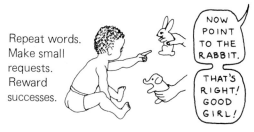

Rhythm is important to language development. **Sing songs, play music,** and **have the child imitate body movements:** clap your hands, touch your toes, or beat a drum.

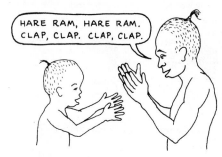

HARE RAM, HARE RAM. CLAP, CLAP. CLAP, CLAP.

Imitate the sounds that baby makes and have him copy the same sounds when you make them. Then say words similar to those sounds.

Also, imitate use of the mouth: open wide, close tight, stick out tongue, blow air, push lips in and out.

CAUTION: Encourage use of gestures, but not so much that the child does not feel the need to try to use words.

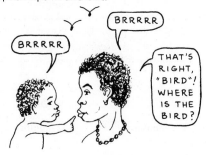

BRRRRR

BRRRRR

THAT'S RIGHT, "BIRD"! WHERE IS THE BIRD?

SPECIAL PROBLEMS IN SPEECH DEVELOPMENT

A mouth that hangs open or drools is a passive (inactive) mouth. It makes development of language more difficult. Often children with Down syndrome or the floppy type of cerebral palsy have this problem.

Here are some suggestions to help correct the problem of drooling and to help strengthen the mouth, lips, and tongue for eating and speaking ability.

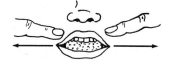

CAUTION: If the child's mouth hangs open and she drools, do not keep telling her to close it! This will not help and will only frustrate the child.

Stroke or tap the upper lip, or gently press the lower lip several times.

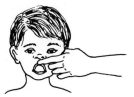

Or, gently stretch the lip muscles. This may help the child to close his mouth.

To strengthen the tongue and lips, put honey or a sweet, sticky food on the upper and lower lips. Have the child lick it off.

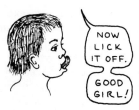

NOW LICK IT OFF.

GOOD GIRL!

You can also put sticky food on the inside of the front teeth and roof of the mouth. Licking this food helps prepare the tongue for saying the letters T, D, N, G, H, J, and L.

JAM

Also have the child lick sticky food from a spoon and lick or suck 'suckers' and other foods or candies.

Put food into the side of the mouth and behind the teeth so that the child exercises the tongue. Also, have the child try to take food off a spoon with his lips.

Begin to give the child solid foods, and foods she needs to chew, as early as she can take them (after 4 months). This helps develop the jaw and mouth.

CAUTIONS: 1. Do not do licking exercises in a child with cerebral palsy whose tongue pushes forward without control. This can make the 'tongue thrusting' worse.
2. After giving the child sweet or sticky food, take extra care to clean teeth well.

Play games in which you have the child:

suck and blow bubbles through a straw	blow soap bubbles	blow air	blow whistles

 CP

> *CAUTION:* For children with cerebral palsy, these blowing exercises may increase the uncontrolled tightening of muscles or twisting of the mouth. If so, DO NOT USE THEM.

Encourage mouthing and chewing on clean toys (but not thumb sucking).

Help the child discover how to make different sounds by flapping her lips up and down with your finger, BRRR 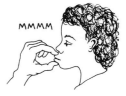 or by squeezing them together as she makes sounds. MMMM

CP

For a child with cerebral palsy, you can help him control his mouth for eating or speaking by stabilizing his body in a firm position. Choose the position in which he is most relaxed (least spastic). This usually means bending the head, shoulders, and hips forward. For this reason it is sometimes said:

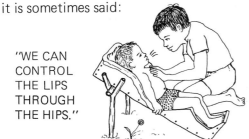

"WE CAN CONTROL THE LIPS THROUGH THE HIPS."

You can help the child make different sounds by pushing on and jiggling his chest.

Imitate the sounds he makes and encourage him to make them by himself.

If the child has trouble with controlling his jaw when he tries to speak, try using **'jaw control'** with your fingers, like this. (See p. 323.)

Have him repeat sounds that require jaw movement.

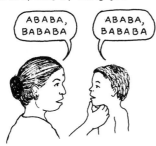

ABABA, BABABA

ABABA, BABABA

When the child has difficulty pronouncing words, **do not correct her.** Instead, repeat the words correctly and clearly, showing that you understand.

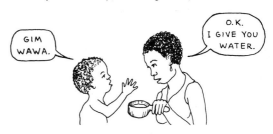

GIM WAWA.

O.K. I GIVE YOU WATER.

REMEMBER—The child needs a lot of stimulation of all her senses to develop language. Play with her, speak to her, and sing to her often. Ask her questions and give her time to answer. **Do not try to 'make her learn', but give her many learning opportunities.** Ask questions that need words for answers, not just 'yes' or 'no'.

———————●———————

Is your child deaf? If your child is slow to speak, check his hearing (see p. 447). Even if he hears some noises, he may not hear well enough to understand speech.

Also, some children who hear well may never be able to speak. For example, certain children with cerebral palsy cannot control their mouth, tongue, or voice muscles. For these children, as for young deaf children, we must look for other ways to communicate. (See Chapter 31.)

8. Early play activities and toys

Play is the way children learn best. **So try to turn every activity you do with a child into some kind of play or game.**

It is not what you do, but **how you do it** that makes something play. As long as it is fun and the child wants to do it, it is play. But if it stops being fun, or the child does it only because 'he has to', it stops being play. Small children (and big children who learn slowly) only stay interested in the same thing for a short time. The child soon gets bored and stops learning. Therefore, for activities to be play and stay play,
1. continue with the same activity for a short time only, and
2. look for ways to keep changing the activity a little so that it is always new and interesting.

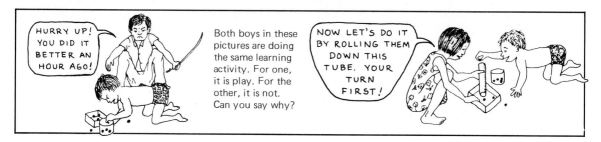

Not all play has to be organized or planned; often the child learns most when it is not. Play needs some aspect of **adventure, surprise,** and **freedom.** It is important that a child learn to **play with other children.** But it is also important that she be given the chance and encouraged to **play alone.** She needs to learn to enjoy and live with other people—and with herself.

We do not talk much about play separately, because mostly it is not a separate activity. It is the best way to do almost any activity. For this reason, in this whole chapter—and book—we often give ideas for turning exercise, therapy, and learning into play.

Play activities, like other activities, should be picked so that they 'fit' a child's level of development and help him move one step farther. They should be HARD ENOUGH TO BE INTERESTING, but EASY ENOUGH TO BE DONE WELL. For example:

If the child is at the level of a very young baby, play games that help him use his eyes and hold up his head.

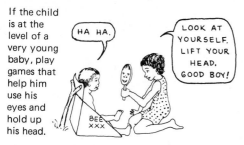

If the child is at the level where she sits, but finds it hard to keep her balance or open her knees, look for play that helps her with these.

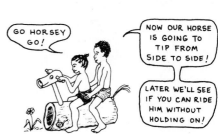

If in preparation for standing and walking the child needs practice shifting weight from one knee to the other, you might try imitation games. Here are 2 ideas:

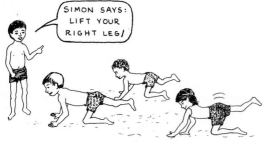

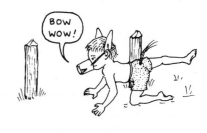

TOYS AND PLAYTHINGS TO STIMULATE A CHILD'S SENSES

Play is more important than toys. Almost anything—pots, flowers, sandals, fruit, keys, an old horseshoe—can be used as a toy, if it is used in play.

Toys—or 'playthings'—offer stimulation for a child, both when she plays by herself and when she plays with others. Many simple things in the home can be used as toys, or can be turned into them.

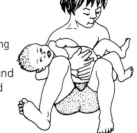

Hanging toys for baby to admire, touch, and handle can be made of many things.

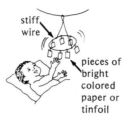

thread spools

slices of plastic bottle

metal bottle caps

top half of plastic bottle

stiff wire

pieces of bright colored paper or tinfoil

Caring for babies provides a learning experience that combines work and play for the child who is gentle.

CAUTION: **Take care that toys are clean and safe for the child.**

Here are a few examples of interesting toys. Use your imagination and the resources of your family to make toys.

Toys for touching

soft clothes or blanket
baby animals
corn on the cob
finger paints
inner tubes for
  swimming, bathing
nuts and bolts
toes and fingers
seed pods
mushy food
cloth doll
gourds
sand

clay
string
chain
pulley
gears
rocks
beads
fruits
mud

flowers
dough

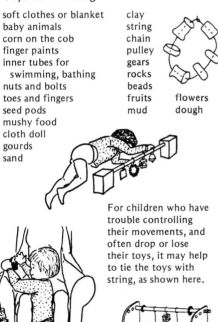

For children who have trouble controlling their movements, and often drop or lose their toys, it may help to tie the toys with string, as shown here.

Toys for seeing

mirrors
colors
colored paper or tinfoil
daily family activity
puppets
old magazines with pictures
crystal glass pieces (rainbow maker)
flashlight (touch)

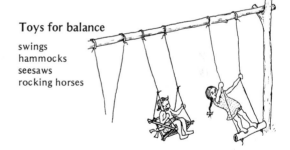

finger puppets

Toys for balance

swings
hammocks
seesaws
rocking horses

Toys for hearing

rattles
guitar
flutes
drum
bells
bracelets on
  baby's wrist
  and ankles
  that tinkle
  when baby
  moves

marimba or
  xylophone
wind chimes
whistles
pet birds
animal sounds
seashells or
  other echo toys
talking
laughing
singing

a pan as
a drum

Toys to taste or smell

foods
flowers
fruits
animals
spices
perfumes

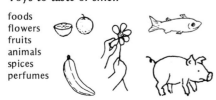

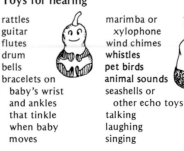

HELLO, LUPE.

HI, MARIA.

tin can telephone

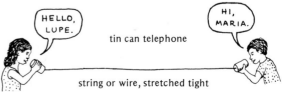

string or wire, stretched tight

TOYS TO DEVELOP A CHILD'S MIND AND HAND-EYE COORDINATION

Learning to fit things into things

Start simple—dropping objects into a jar, then taking them out again.

As the child develops, make things more complex.

rings of wood, woven string, baked clay, old bones, or buckles

wood or corncob

base of wood or several layers of cardboard →

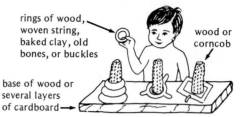

Note: Rings can be of different sizes, colors or shapes so that the child can also learn to match these.

To help develop controlled movement of the hands and arms, the child can move beads or blocks along a rod or wire.

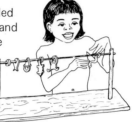

Using animals or funny figures makes the exercise more fun. Other children will be more likely to join in the game.

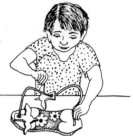

Matching games

The child can match objects of similar shape, size, and color.

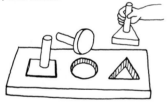

Small pegs glued onto cut-out pieces help develop fine hand control.

peg

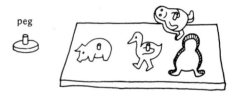

Start with simpler games with square or round figures.

ball, round fruit, or pill bottle

cardboard box →

blocks or match boxes

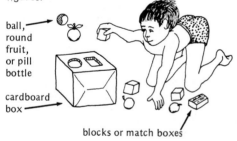

Then progress to more complicated games with different shaped figures.

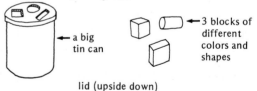

← a big tin can

3 blocks of different colors and shapes

lid (upside down)

lid of wood, or layers of cardboard →

Inside ring tightly fits into can.

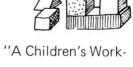

Puzzles

Jigsaw and block puzzles and building blocks also help a child learn how shapes and colors fit together. Suggestions for making different puzzles are on p. 476.

Many more ideas for simple toys are included in Chapter 49, "A Children's Workshop For Making Toys," p. 463 to 476.

CHAPTER **36**

Feeding

Feeding is one of the first abilities that a child develops to meet her needs. Even a newborn baby has reflexes that cause her to:

(CP)

turn her head to seek the breast when her cheek is touched,

suck and swallow,

and cry when hungry.

By a few months of age, the child learns to take solid food in her mouth and eat it.

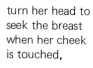
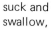
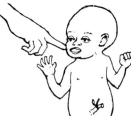
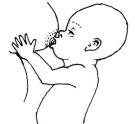
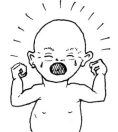
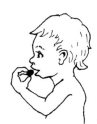

Normally a child's feeding skills gradually increase without any special training. She learns first to use her lips and tongue to suck and swallow liquids. Later she learns to bite and chew solid foods, and to take food to her mouth with her hands. The early head-turning and sucking reflexes gradually go away as she learns to control her feeding movements.

Some children, however, do not develop feeding skills easily or naturally. This may be because the child's whole **development is slow** *(retarded)*. Or, because the child has a particular **physical difficulty** (such as a hole in the roof of her mouth—see "Cleft Palate," p. 120).

Children with **cerebral palsy** often have feeding difficulties, which are sometimes severe. Difficulty with sucking (or being unable to suck) may be the first sign in a child who later develops other signs of cerebral palsy. Or the child may have trouble swallowing, and easily choke on food. Uncontrolled movements of the body, pushing out the tongue, or floppy, inactive lips may also be a problem.

(CP)

One reason that some disabled children are slow to develop self-feeding skills is that their families continue to do everything for them. Because of a child's other difficulties, her family may continue to treat her as a baby. They may give her only liquids, and put everything into her mouth, rather than encouraging her to do more for herself.

REMEMBER: Helping the child develop feeding skills as early as possible is of special importance because **good nutrition is essential for health and life. The food needs of a disabled child are the same as for any child.**

Good use of the lips and tongue when feeding is also important for future speech.

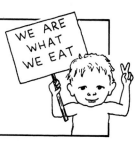

POOR NUTRITION IN DISABLED CHILDREN

Poor nutrition or 'malnutrition' usually results from not getting enough to eat and is one of the most common causes of health problems. With its signs of weakness, thinness, failure to grow, and reduced ability to fight off illness, poor nutrition might be considered a *'disability'* itself. It affects at least 1 out of every 6 of the world's children, mainly those who live in poor countries.

In this book, we do not discuss the problems of malnutrition in detail, because they are covered in most primary care handbooks (see *Where There Is No Doctor,* Chapter 11). However, a special warning is called for.

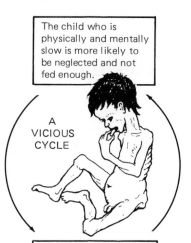

The child who is physically and mentally slow is more likely to be neglected and not fed enough.

A VICIOUS CYCLE

Not eating enough slows down both physical and mental development.

> *WARNING:* **Disabled children are often in greater danger of malnutrition than are other children.**

Sometimes this is because the child has difficulty sucking, swallowing, or holding food. Sometimes it is because the family gives more food to the children who are stronger and more able to help with daily work. Sometimes, however, it is because parents, although they treat their disabled child with extra love and care, keep bottle feeding him (with milk, rice water, or sugared drinks) until he is 3 or 4 years old or older. They keep treating—and feeding—their child like a baby, even though he is growing bigger and needs the same variety and quantity of foods that other children need.

To give a child only—or mainly—milk and sweet drinks after 6 months of age may keep the child fat. But he will slowly become malnourished. Milk and sweet drinks lack iron, so that the child may become more and more pale, or anemic (weak blood).

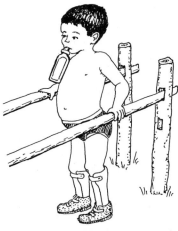

This 4-year-old with spina bifida has no difficulty eating any foods. Yet his family still treats him like a baby —complete with a baby bottle filled with a sweet drink—just because he is 'disabled'.

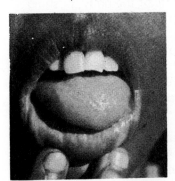

Normal: Lips, tongue and finger-nails have a reddish, healthy color.

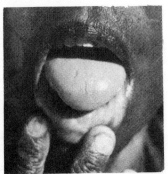

Anemic: Lips, tongue and finger-nails, pale. Lack of energy. Tires quickly.

> *CAUTION:* It is important that disabled children get enough to eat. It is also **important that they do not eat too much and get fat.** Extra weight makes it more difficult for a weak child to move about. If the child is getting fat, give him less fatty foods and sweets.
>
> DO NOT LET A DISABLED CHILD GET FAT!

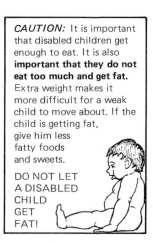

> *REMEMBER:* **A disabled child needs the same foods that other children of the same age need.**

THE BEST FOOD FOR YOUR YOUNG CHILD

The first 6 months

Give **breast milk** and **nothing else**.

BREAST IS BEST because breast milk contains the ideal combination of foods that the child needs, is clean, and is always the right temperature. Also, **breast milk contains 'antibodies'** from the mother that protect the baby against infections.

Therefore, breast milk is especially important for children more likely to get infections, such as a child with Down syndrome (see p. 279) or a child who often chokes on her food and might get pneumonia.

Breast milk is healthier for babies than other milks or 'formula'.

If the baby cannot suck, a mother can milk her breasts:

and then give the baby her milk with a cup and spoon.

WARNING:

Avoid baby bottles whenever possible. They often spread infections.

Cup and spoon feeding is safer.

After 6 months

Continue breast feeding and also begin to give the baby other foods—juices and fruits rich in vitamins, mash of green leafy vegetables, beans (boiled, skinned, and mashed), peanuts (skinned and mashed), egg yolks, and other local staples such as rice, corn, plantains, or cassava.

Small stomachs need food often. Feed children under 1 year old at least 5 times a day— and give them snacks between meals.

If the child has trouble eating solid foods, do not keep giving only milk or formula or 'rice water'. Even mother's milk alone is not enough after 6 months. Mash or grind up other foods to form a drink or mush.

By 8 months to 1 year of age the child should be eating the same food as the rest of the family—even if it has to be mashed or turned into liquids.

HIV/AIDS and breast feeding

If a woman has HIV/AIDS, sometimes this disease can pass to the baby through her breast milk. But if she does not have access to clean water, her baby is more likely to die from diarrhea, dehydration, and malnutrition than from AIDS. Only the mother can evaluate the conditions in her home and community and decide what to do.

Babies older than 6 months have less danger of dying from diarrhea because they are bigger and stronger. A woman with HIV/AIDS who has breast fed her baby should stop at 6 months, and feed him with other milks and foods. This way the baby will have less risk of getting HIV/AIDS.

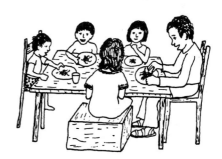

Successful feeding involves the whole child

The more difficult it is for a child to control his body movements, the more difficult it will be for him to feed himself. A child with Down syndrome may have trouble feeding because of weak mouth and lips and poor head control. But the feeding problems of a child with cerebral palsy are more complex. They may include: lack of mouth, head, and body control; poor sitting balance; difficulty bending hips enough to reach forward; poor hand-eye coordination; and difficulty holding things and taking them to his mouth. We must consider all these things when trying to help the child feed more effectively.

It is not enough simply to put food or pour drink into the mouth of a child who has difficulty sucking, eating, and drinking. First, we must look for ways to help the child learn to suck, swallow, eat, and drink more normally and effectively. Here are some suggestions.

POSITIONS FOR FEEDING

Be sure the child is in a good position *before* you begin feeding her. The position will make feeding either easier and safer, or more difficult and unsafe.

Do not feed the baby while she is lying on her back because this increases the chance of choking.

In a child with cerebral palsy, it often causes backward stiffening, and makes sucking and swallowing more difficult.

WRONG

Feed the baby in a half sitting position with her **head bent slightly forward.**

In a child with cerebral palsy, to keep the head from pushing back, hold the shoulders forward, **keep the hips bent, and push firmly on the chest.**

RIGHT

Do not let the head tilt backward. It makes swallowing harder and may cause choking.

In a child with cerebral palsy, **avoid pushing the head forward** like this. It will cause the baby to push her head back more forcefully.

WRONG

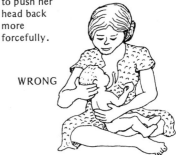

Positions for feeding with a bottle, spoon, or finger are like those for breast feeding.

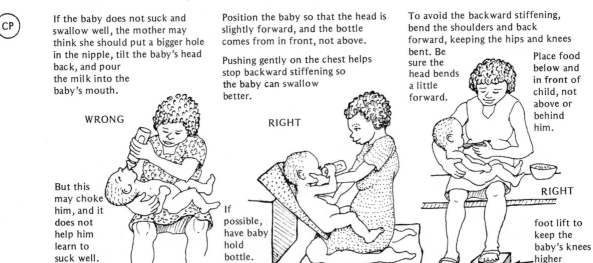

If the baby does not suck and swallow well, the mother may think she should put a bigger hole in the nipple, tilt the baby's head back, and pour the milk into the baby's mouth.

WRONG

But this may choke him, and it does not help him learn to suck well.

Position the baby so that the head is slightly forward, and the bottle comes from in front, not above.

Pushing gently on the chest helps stop backward stiffening so the baby can swallow better.

RIGHT

If possible, have baby hold bottle.

To avoid the backward stiffening, bend the shoulders and back forward, keeping the hips and knees bent. Be sure the head bends a little forward.

Place food below and in front of child, not above or behind him.

RIGHT

foot lift to keep the baby's knees higher

A simple **'baby seat'** can help the baby hold a good position while eating. Here is one idea using an old plastic bucket.

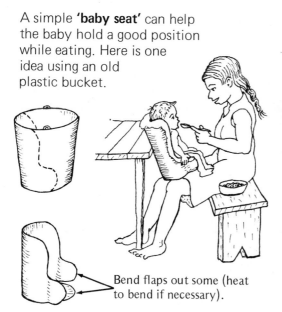

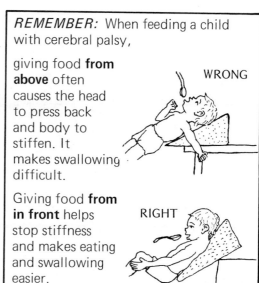

REMEMBER: When feeding a child with cerebral palsy,

giving food **from above** often causes the head to press back and body to stiffen. It makes swallowing difficult.

WRONG

Giving food **from in front** helps stop stiffness and makes eating and swallowing easier.

RIGHT

Bend flaps out some (heat to bend if necessary).

For other seating ideas, see p. 326.

HELPING CONTROL MOUTH FUNCTION

The child may also need help in improving the **sucking-swallowing reflex,** and her ability to eat from a **hand or spoon** and to **drink from a cup.** Sometimes these can be improved by using what is called 'jaw control'.

Jaw control. Before giving the breast, bottle, spoon or cup, place your hand over the child's jaw, like this:

if you sit beside the child   if the child is facing you

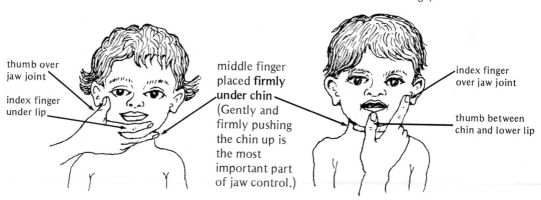

thumb over jaw joint

index finger under lip

middle finger placed **firmly under chin** (Gently and firmly pushing the chin up is the most important part of jaw control.)

index finger over jaw joint

thumb between chin and lower lip

At first the child may push against your hand, but after she gets used to it, it should help her control the movement of her mouth and tongue. Be sure not to push her head back, but keep it bent forward slightly.

While you feed the child, **apply gentle, firm steady pressure**—not off and on.

Good positioning together with jaw control will help with several problems common in cerebral palsy, such as pushing the tongue forward, choking, and drooling (dribbling). **As mouth control improves, gradually lessen and finally stop jaw control.**

For more suggestions for controlling drooling and improving use of the lips and tongue, see the section on developing speech, p. 314.

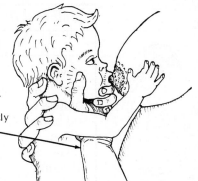

For the child who has difficulty breast feeding (or bottle feeding), as you apply jaw control try bringing her cheeks forward with your fingers.

At the same time, push gently against the child's chest with your wrist. (This may help the child who tends to stiffen backward.)

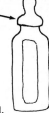

If you bottle-feed the baby, an 'old-fashioned' large round nipple usually works best.

If the child still has trouble sucking, try making the hole in the nipple bigger and thickening the milk with corn meal, gelatin, or mashed food.

CAUTION: Jaw control helps in many children with developmental delay and cerebral palsy—but not all. After trying it for 2 or 3 weeks, if the child still resists it or shows increased problems, stop using jaw control.

Spoon feeding

The child who has no sucking-swallowing reflex needs to be fed with a spoon.

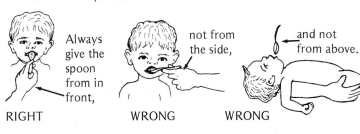

Always give the spoon from in front,

RIGHT

not from the side,

WRONG

and not from above.

WRONG

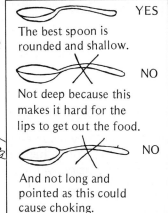

YES
The best spoon is rounded and shallow.

NO
Not deep because this makes it hard for the lips to get out the food.

NO
And not long and pointed as this could cause choking.

'Tongue thrusting'

A baby sucks by moving her tongue forward and backward. For this reason, when the child begins to eat from a spoon, her tongue will at first push part of the food out of her mouth. She has to learn to use her tongue differently—pushing the food between the gums to chew, and to the back of her mouth to swallow. Children with developmental delay or cerebral palsy may have trouble learning to do this, and continue to push or 'thrust' the tongue forward for some time. **Do not mistake this for meaning she does not like the food.**

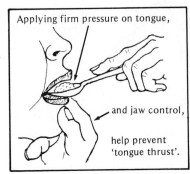

Applying firm pressure on tongue,

and jaw control,

help prevent 'tongue thrust'.

Jaw control, although helpful, may not be enough to prevent this tongue thrusting. It also helps to **apply firm pressure with the back of the spoon on the tongue** as you feed the child. This helps keep the tongue from pushing forward and lets the child use his lips and tongue better.

CAUTION: Better to use a strong (metal) spoon and **NOT** a thin plastic one that might break when you push down the tongue.

Do **NOT** scrape the food onto the upper lip or teeth as you take the spoon out. Instead, let the child try to get the food off the spoon onto her tongue. To make it easier for her, start by putting only a little food on the end of the spoon. As you take the spoon out, make sure the mouth is closed so that the tongue can move the food inside the mouth and cannot push it out.

WRONG

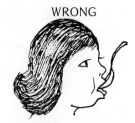

If eating with fingers is the custom, or if spoon feeding is too difficult, use your fingers.

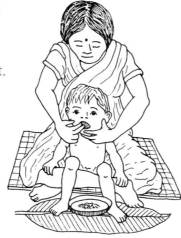

Here a mother holds her child in a good position on her lap, using her legs and body to give support.

With one hand she gives jaw control while she feeds him with the fingers of the other hand. Place a little food on the side or middle of the tongue—not on the front of it.

For spoon or finger feeding, it is best to start off with soft, mushy foods rather than liquids. Milk (even breast milk) or egg yolk can be mixed with rice paste, boiled corn, or mashed beans. You can also give small pieces of fruit, mashed greens and vegetables, and yogurt or soft cheese.

Hardest for the child to eat are combinations of liquids and solids—such as vegetable soup.

> *CAUTION:* Remember to wash your hands before feeding child with your fingers.

Chewing

To help the child learn to chew, **put a bit of firm food in the side of her mouth between her teeth.** Use very small pieces of bread crust, tortilla, or chapati. Help her close her mouth using jaw control.

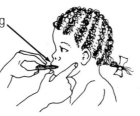

Biting off can be encouraged by pulling slightly on a long thin piece of food.

Or rub the piece of food against the teeth before putting it between them.

> *CAUTION:* Do *NOT* open and close the child's jaw or help her chew. After she bites the food, **her jaw must stay closed or almost closed to chew.** To help her do this, apply steady firm pressure with jaw control. This should lead the child to make chewing motions. Let the jaw move some on its own. But **do NOT make chewing motions for the child!** This will only encourage abnormal movements.

If the child has difficulty chewing and chokes on pieces of food, try this:

Cut a piece of clean, soft cotton cord, or braid thin strips of cotton cloth. Soak or cook the cord in a tasty good food and hold the end while she bites and chews on it, squeezing out the nutritious juices. Help with jaw control.

This method is completely safe. Because you hold on to the cord, the child cannot bite off pieces and choke on them. It is best to practice this at the beginning of a meal while the child is still hungry.

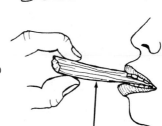

> *CAUTION:* If a piece of food slips back into the child's throat and gets stuck, bend the child far forward, and keep calm. The food should drop out. Do NOT pat the child on the back as this could cause the child to breathe in the food.
>
> If the food does not fall out and the child cannot breathe, suddenly and forcefully squeeze the child's lower chest (see *Where There Is No Doctor*, p. 79).

A finger-shaped piece of tough cooked or dried meat or very tough chicken (old rooster) can be used instead of the cord. Be sure it is too tough for the child to chew pieces off of it, but juicy or tasty enough to give her pleasure.

Drinking

Successful drinking, like eating, involves the whole child. Body position is important. For example, in a child with cerebral palsy, to drink from a regular cup or glass, his head must be tilted back. But this can cause uncontrolled backward stiffening and possible choking.

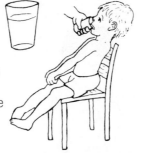

You can make a special cup from a plastic bottle.

Cut it like this.

However, if he uses a **plastic cup with a piece cut out,** he can drink without bending his head back.

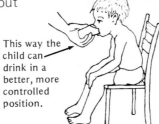

Gently heat the rim and gradually bend it out with a round smooth rod or stick.

The cup should have a projecting rim.

Cut out a space to fit around the child's nose.

This way the child can drink in a better, more controlled position.

At first you may need to apply jaw control to help the child close her lips on the rim of the cup. Tilt the cup so that the liquid touches the upper lip and let the child do the rest. Do **NOT** take away the cup after each swallow as this may trigger pushing the head back or tongue out. It helps to start with thick liquids—like cooked cereals, maize mush, or yogurt.

Self-feeding

To be able to feed herself, a child needs more than control of her mouth, lips, and tongue. She also needs to be able to **sit with her head up,** to **pick things up,** and to **take them to her mouth.**

To prepare for self-feeding, encourage the child to play, taking his hands and toys to his mouth. Also, encourage him, when sitting, to balance while he uses both hands (see p. 105 and 307).

A child with poor balance or uncontrolled movements will at first need special seating adapted to her needs.

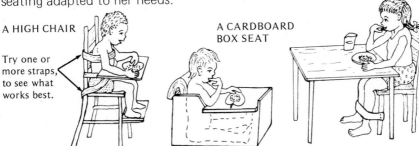

A HIGH CHAIR

Try one or more straps, to see what works best.

A CARDBOARD BOX SEAT

Some children with cerebral palsy may only need a **foot strap** to stay in a good position (to keep the body from straightening stiffly as shown above).

CAUTION: Seats or straps that limit movement should be used only until the child learns to control her position without being tied or held. **Special seating should help the child to do more and to move more freely. It should not become a prison!** For more seating ideas, see p. 323, 573, and Chapter 65.

When a child is slow in using her hands to grasp things, or to take things to her mouth, you can help her discover how to use her hands and feed herself, like this:

Put the child's finger in a food she especially likes.

Then lift her finger to her mouth.

Help her to do more and more, step by step, until she does it alone.

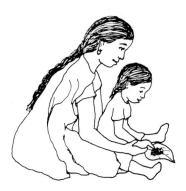 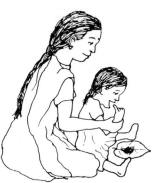 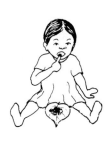

Little by little help her less and less. Lift her hand to her mouth and touch her lips with the food. See if she will then put it into her mouth. When she has learned this, lift her hand near her mouth and see if she will do the rest. Next just put her finger in the food and encourage her to lift it to her mouth. **Each time she does more for herself, praise her warmly.**

This method is part of a 'behavioral approach' to teaching new skills. The same approach can be used for teaching the child many skills related to eating, such as using a spoon or drinking from a glass. To learn more about this approach, see Chapter 40, "Ways to Improve Learning and Behavior."

IMPORTANT: Try to **make mealtime a happy time.** Remember that it takes time for any child to learn new skills, and that a child learns best when he plays. When any child first learns to eat for himself, he makes a mess. Be patient, help the child to become more skillful at eating, praise him when he does well, but at the same time let him enjoy himself and his food. Remember, even normal children often do not learn to eat cleanly and politely until they are 5 or 6 years old—or even older.

A cover or 'bib' like this, of plastic or waterproof cloth, is a big help. The pocket at the bottom catches spilled food.

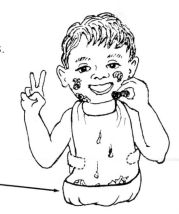

While it is important not to push or hurry children too much in developing feeding skills, the opposite is also true. Often parents wait too long and do not expect enough from their disabled child. On the next page is a 'trick' that a rehabilitation worker uses to help parents awaken to the ability of their retarded child to learn new skills.

THE 6 MINUTE BISCUIT TRICK
FOR DEVELOPMENTALLY DELAYED CHILDREN

by Christine Miles of Peshawar, Pakistan, and Birmingham, United Kingdom

The 'trick' gets parents to open their eyes to what their child actually can do and learn to do. I see many parents with developmentally delayed children between 15 and 30 months. They have realized that the child is not functioning at a level appropriate for his age. But often they cannot describe what the child actually can do, and do not seem to realize that children gain new skills by **learning.** Parents complain that "He doesn't speak. He can't do this, he can't do that," as though there is something wrong with the machinery or someone has failed to push the correct button.

I ask them whether the child can eat a biscuit (cookie). "No, he only has milk and mush. He can't feed himself." I get a biscuit and put it into the child's hand. I guide the hand up to the mouth. Sometimes the child will bite on the biscuit; sometimes it needs to be tapped gently against his teeth and wetted with his lips and tongue until a piece breaks off and is eaten. I move the child's hand away from the mouth, then repeat the process. Usually by the time half the biscuit has gone, the child has learned how to do it, and finishes the biscuit happily without help. The parents usually say "Oooh!"

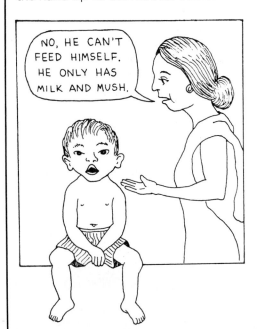

In 6 minutes the parents have watched their child **learn** an important skill, by our using a simple directed action and a strong reward (tasty food). Whether their child is temporarily delayed in development or will be permanently retarded, the parents gain some vital information about the child's ability to learn. Whether or not they remember anything else that I say to them, they go away with a whole new experience to think about. Almost always they have consulted several doctors before coming here, without gaining any useful advice.

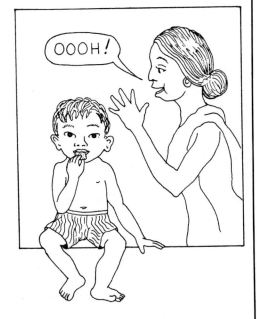

Of course, it is not guaranteed to work. But it does work surprisingly often. The 6 minute biscuit trick is a powerful stimulant to parents to actually observe their child and to help the child learn.

SELF-FEEDING SUGGESTIONS FOR THE CHILD WITH CEREBRAL PALSY

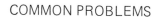

CP

COMMON PROBLEMS

The less-used arm pulls up and back or moves about.

Head twists to side and back.

Child has a weak, awkward grip, and poor control of arm movement.

Whole body stiffens backward.

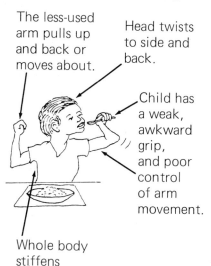

SUGGESTIONS

Help the child to control arm at shoulder.

Help him learn to hold the spoon firmly.

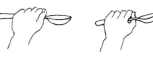

WRONG   BETTER

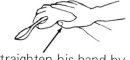

Straighten his hand by turning it out gently from the base of the thumb.

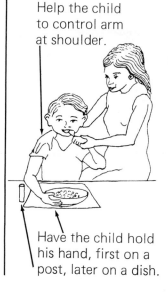

Have the child hold his hand, first on a post, later on a dish.

Sometimes you can help her with head control by gently pressing one hand flat against her chest.

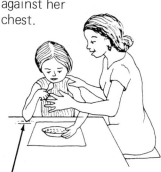

A child who has difficulty controlling her hand for eating may gain better control by resting her elbow on the table.

Raising the table may make it easier for some children.

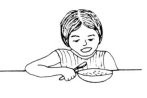

Where the custom is to eat sitting on the floor, a child may be helped by making a low table out of a box.

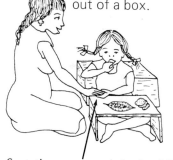

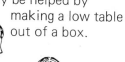

Sometimes you can help the child avoid twisting to one side by bending the less-used arm across the belly, and turning the palm up.

When head and body are difficult to control, it may help to sit on a bench or log in a 'riding' position.

If he sits with a rounded back, it may help to support the lower back.

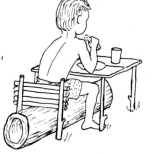

A child who has trouble controlling a cup with one hand can often do better if the cup has two handles.

Ask a local potter to make one.

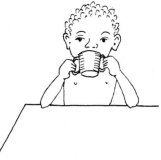

Homemade equipment to help eating

A plate with steep sides makes eating easier for the child who uses only one arm. When that arm is very weak, it helps if the dish is low on one side and high on the other, to push food against.

This boy, whose arms and hands are paralyzed, lifts his spoon by raising and lowering his shoulder. His forearm is on the table edge, so that when he lowers his elbow, his hand lifts.

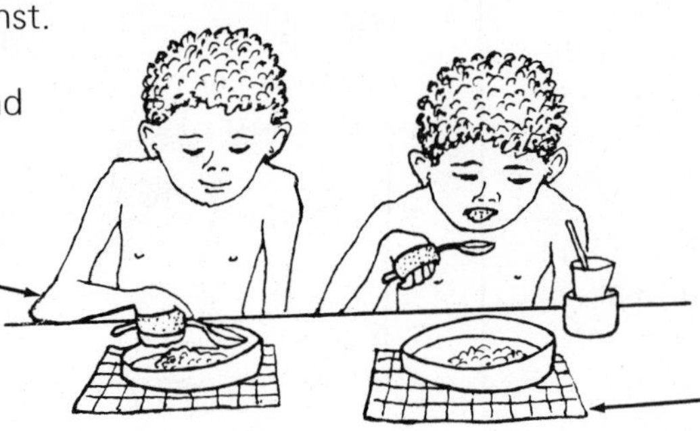

A non-slip mat under the plate can be made from strips of tire tube woven over a stiff wire frame.

The spoon slips into a leather or rubber (tire tube) hand band. (Also, see p. 577.)

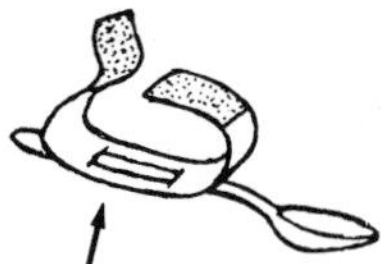

Velcro (or buckle)

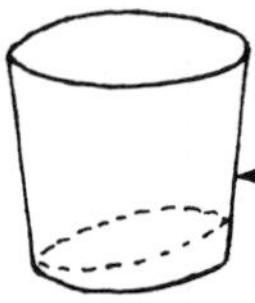

The special plate can be made from a small plastic bucket.

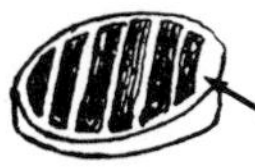

To prevent slipping, you can glue (with a waterproof glue) strips of tire tube on the bottom.

A **non-spill cup holder** can be made using 2 plastic bottles.

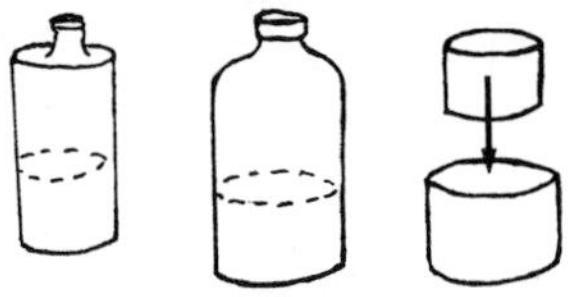

Fill space between containers with fine sand, plaster, or cement.

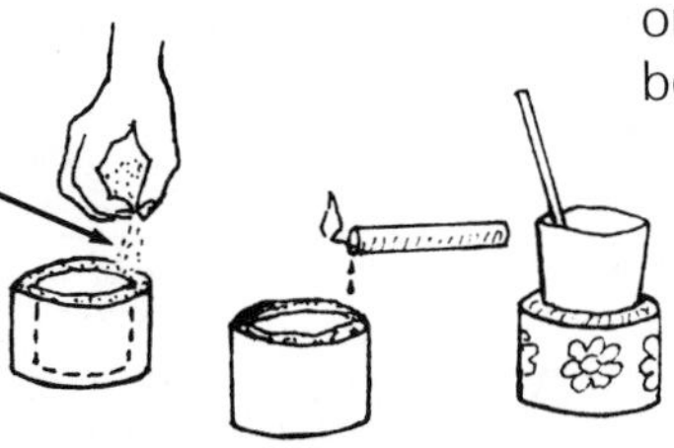

Seal with wax or waterproof glue.

Or, glue a plate or tin to the bottom of the cup.

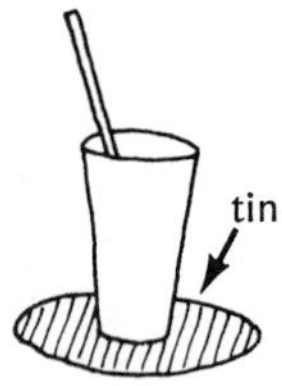

Spoon handles for easy gripping

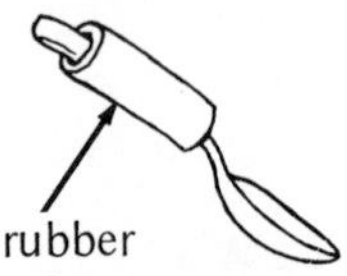

rubber tube

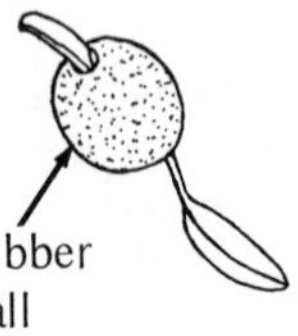

rubber ball

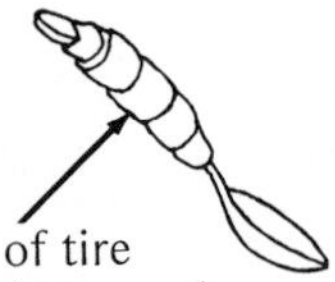

strip of tire tube (wrapped)

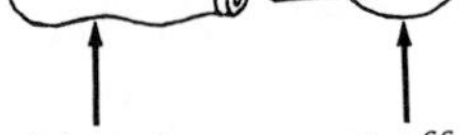

old tool handle

cut off spoon

piece of wood

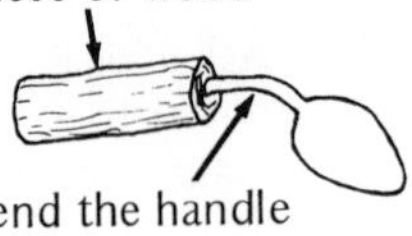

bend the handle to fit the child's grip

Tortilla or chapati holder

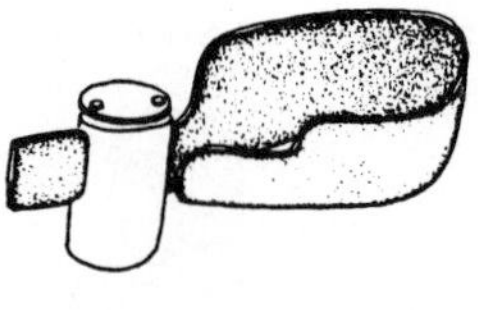

From *UPKARAN Manual.* (See p. 642.)

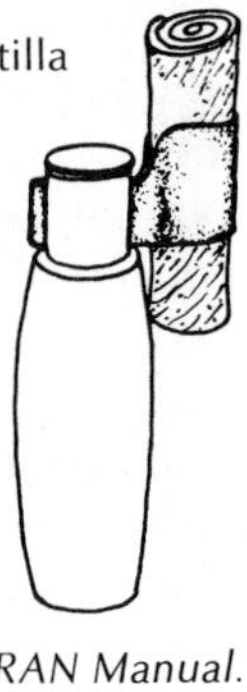

From *UPKARAN Manual.* (See p. 642.)

Swing-a-sling eating aid

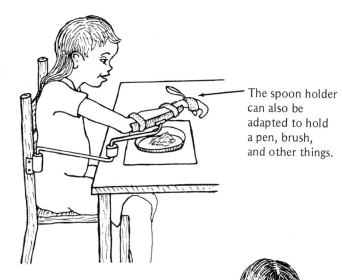

This eating aid lets a child with very little strength in her arm feed herself. However, it must pivot smoothly but firmly at 3 points. It will take a skillful and imaginative craftsperson to make it.

The spoon holder can also be adapted to hold a pen, brush, and other things.

Arm rocker—for a child whose arm is too weak to lift

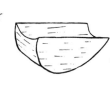

Carve it out of wood—or glue together layers of *'Styrofoam'* (stiff foam plastic) or cardboard.

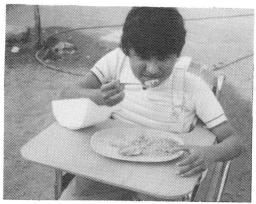

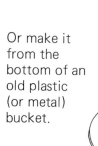

Or make it from the bottom of an old plastic (or metal) bucket.

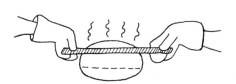

Heat the plastic along the lines with a hot strip of metal.

Straps may or may not be needed.

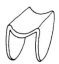

And bend it like this.

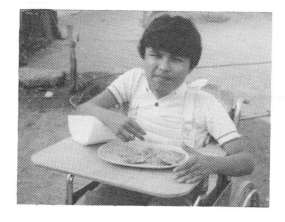

A boy with muscular dystrophy, whose arm is too weak to lift it to his mouth, eats with the aid of an arm rocker. This arm rocker, cut out of *Styrofoam*, took about 5 minutes to make.

Feeding aids for a child with no hand use

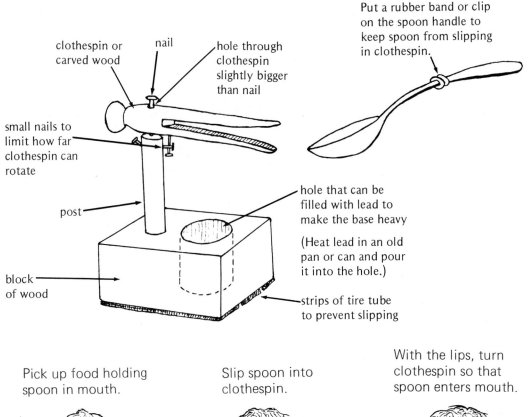

clothespin or carved wood

nail

hole through clothespin slightly bigger than nail

Put a rubber band or clip on the spoon handle to keep spoon from slipping in clothespin.

small nails to limit how far clothespin can rotate

post

hole that can be filled with lead to make the base heavy

(Heat lead in an old pan or can and pour it into the hole.)

block of wood

strips of tire tube to prevent slipping

Pick up food holding spoon in mouth.

Slip spoon into clothespin.

With the lips, turn clothespin so that spoon enters mouth.

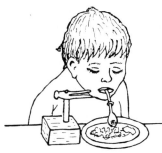
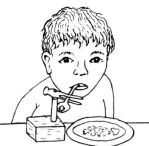
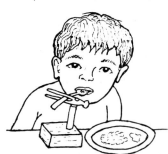

Note: **If other children laugh at the child's awkwardness, let him practice alone until he gains some skill.**

Children with no use of their arms can feed themselves by lowering their mouths to their food. It helps if the plate can be lifted nearer to the face. A pot like this helps to stabilize the plate. If the plate has a rounded bottom, the child can tip it bit by bit as it is emptied.

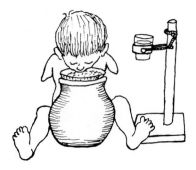

A rack allows the child to drink from a cup that he can tip with his mouth.

Or simply use a straw.

Use your imagination **to think of many other ways to help the disabled child eat and do other things for herself.**

Dressing

Children with *disabilities,* like other children, should be encouraged from an early age to help with their own dressing. It is important, however, not to push a child to learn skills that are still too difficult for her level of development.

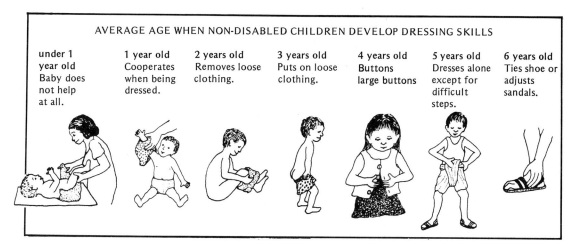

AVERAGE AGE WHEN NON-DISABLED CHILDREN DEVELOP DRESSING SKILLS

under 1 year old	1 year old	2 years old	3 years old	4 years old	5 years old	6 years old
Baby does not help at all.	Cooperates when being dressed.	Removes loose clothing.	Puts on loose clothing.	Buttons large buttons	Dresses alone except for difficult steps.	Ties shoe or adjusts sandals.

Children may learn dressing skills at different ages depending on local customs and on how much importance parents give to learning these skills. Observe what other children in your village can do at different ages. Children may begin to take off their clothes before they are 2 years old, yet may not learn to put on all their clothes correctly until they are 5 or 6 years old. Often a normal 6-year-old may put a shirt on backward, or the left sandal on the right foot.

Children who are slow in their development or who have difficulty with movements may be slower to learn dressing skills. It may seem quicker and easier for mother or sister to simply put the clothes on her, without interacting with the child. However, this will only delay the child's development more.

It is important to **use dressing as an opportunity to help the child develop in many areas at once: awareness, balance, movement, and even language.**

As you dress the child, talk to her. Help her learn her body parts, the names of clothes, and the way these relate: "The arm goes into the sleeve," "The foot goes into the pants," and so on. This will help the child begin to learn language and connect parts of her body to her actions and things around her.

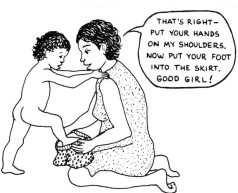

THAT'S RIGHT— PUT YOUR HANDS ON MY SHOULDERS. NOW PUT YOUR FOOT INTO THE SKIRT. GOOD GIRL!

Helping the child gain dressing skills takes time and patience. Let her try to do as much as she can for herself. Be ready to help if it gets too difficult, but only as much as is needed. It is not good to frustrate the child so much that she will not want to try again. Be sure the task is not too advanced for the child's level of development.

(CP) POSITIONS FOR DRESSING

Try dressing the child in different positions, to see what works best.

Body position is especially important when dressing a child with spastic cerebral palsy. Often his body tends to bend stiffly backward if he is dressed lying on his back.

A bad position: (child's body stiffens backward)

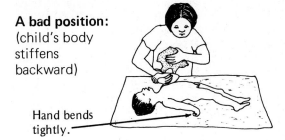

Hand bends tightly.

It often works better to dress a child with *spasticity* with his body and hips bent forward.

A good position:

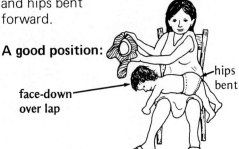

face-down over lap

hips bent

For changing that needs to be done **face-up,** try putting a firm pillow under the head, and keep knees and hips bent. This may help the baby relax and not stiffen up.

knees bent

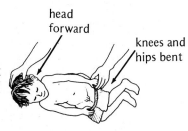

head up

Lying on the side is often a good position for a child with spasticity who is beginning to dress himself. He may need to roll from one side to the other to pull on clothes— but he should keep his knees, hips, and head bent to avoid stiffening.

head forward

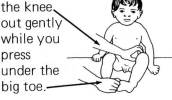

knees and hips bent

To help the child **dress while sitting,** be sure he is in a steady position. You can help him keep his hips bent and body forward like this.

first with help

then alone →

If balance when sitting is still not good, or if the child tends to stiffen backward, try sitting in a corner to dress.

Sitting with the feet forward and knees apart is a good position for play and dressing. If legs press together stiffly, try pushing the knee out gently while you press under the big toe.

When a child with athetoid cerebral palsy tries to raise her arms or to speak, her feet may come off the ground or her legs spread.

Try pressing down over the knees, keeping them together. Or press on top of the feet.

Help the child find the position that allows the best control for dressing.

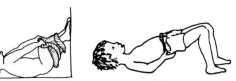

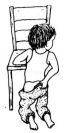

SUGGESTIONS FOR DRESSING

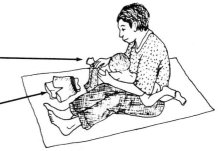

- If one arm or leg is more affected than the other, it is easier if you **put the clothes first on the affected side.**

- Put the clothes where the child can see and reach them easily, so he can help in any way possible.

- If the arm is bent stiffly, first try to **straighten it slowly,** then put the sleeve on. (If you try to straighten it forcefully or quickly, it may become more stiff.)

- If the legs straighten stiffly, bend them gently in order to put on pants or shoes.

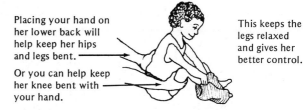

Placing your hand on her lower back will help keep her hips and legs bent.

Or you can help keep her knee bent with your hand.

This keeps the legs relaxed and gives her better control.

- Begin any dressing activity for the child, but let him finish it for himself. Little by little have him do more of the steps. If he can do it all by himself, give him time. Do not hurry to do it for him if he is struggling to do it himself. Praise him when he does well or tries hard.

- Use loose-fitting, easy-to-put-on clothing. Here are some ideas:

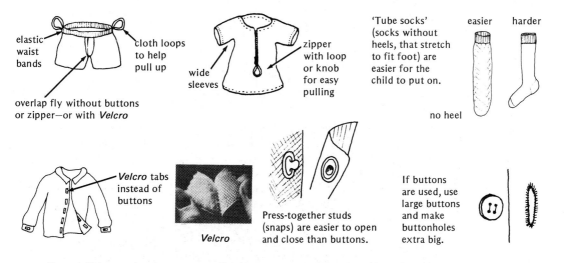

elastic waist bands

cloth loops to help pull up

overlap fly without buttons or zipper—or with *Velcro*

wide sleeves

zipper with loop or knob for easy pulling

'Tube socks' (socks without heels, that stretch to fit foot) are easier for the child to put on.

easier   harder

no heel

Velcro tabs instead of buttons

Velcro

Press-together studs (snaps) are easier to open and close than buttons.

If buttons are used, use large buttons and make buttonholes extra big.

- For children who have poor finger control, make a simple tool to button and unbutton buttons.

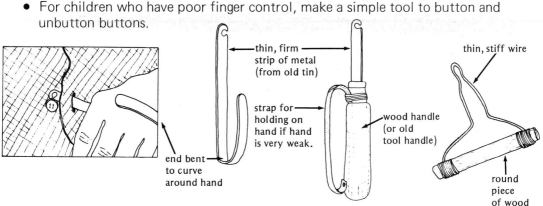

thin, firm strip of metal (from old tin)

strap for holding on hand if hand is very weak.

end bent to curve around hand

wood handle (or old tool handle)

thin, stiff wire

round piece of wood

- For the child who often puts her dress on backward, or her sandals on the wrong foot, try to build in 'reminders' that will help her do it right. For example:

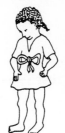

Sew a colorful bow on the front of her dress.

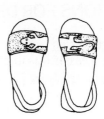

Draw half an an animal on each sandal or shoe so that the 2 halves make the whole animal when she puts them on right.

- For the child who has difficulty reaching his feet, a **stick with a hook** may help.

for pulling

for pushing

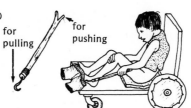

An all-purpose tool

comb

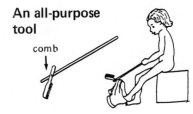

Ideas for shoes

- For toes that claw up, or bend under, you can cut off the top of the shoe, or use a sandal.

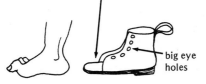

big eye holes

Velcro straps (instead of buckles)

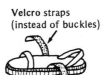

- Tennis shoes or other shoes that open all the way down to the toes are easier to put on.

Velcro straps for easy fastening can make many children more independent in dressing.

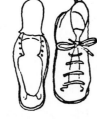

A leather or cloth loop sewed on the heel makes it easier to pull on shoe.

Consider using shoes that fit loosely— about one size too large.

- If the foot stiffens downward so much it is hard to get a shoe on, you can cut the back of the shoe open and put the foot in from the back.

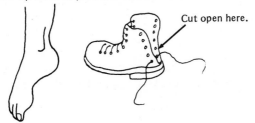

Cut open here.

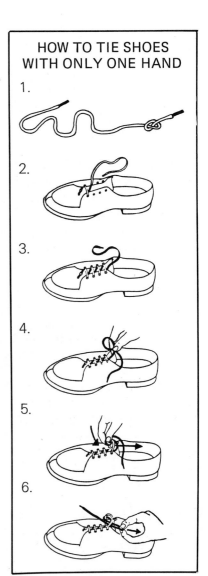

HOW TO TIE SHOES
WITH ONLY ONE HAND

1.

2.

3.

4.

5.

6.

For special footwear designs for feet that do not feel, see p. 224 and 225.
For shoe adaptations for braces, see p. 544.

CHAPTER 38

Toilet Training

By **'toilet training'** we mean **helping a child learn to stay clean and dry.** A child is toilet trained when:

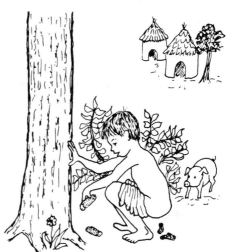

- He knows when he needs to shit or pee (make stool or urinate) and has learned to 'hold on' so he does not go in his clothing or on the floor (*bowel* and *bladder* control).

- He tells people when he needs to do his toilet,

  or (if he is physically able) . . .

- he takes himself to a special place (pot, toilet, latrine, or at least outside the house), removes necessary clothing, 'goes', cleans himself in the customary way, puts his clothing back on, and does whatever may be necessary to get rid of the waste.

'Toilet training' is important for the development of a child's independence and dignity. Yet it is very often neglected in disabled and *retarded* **children.** Often we see children 5, 10, even 15 years old who are still in *diapers (nappies)* and who are still completely dependent on their mothers for being changed and cleaned. This situation is hard on both child and family. With a little instruction and encouragement, we have found that many of these children have become 'toilet trained' in a few days or weeks. Many could have learned years earlier.

The age when normal children become toilet trained varies greatly from child to child. It also varies from place to place, according to local customs, what clothes children wear (if any), and how much the family helps. With training, many children can stay dry and clean by age 2 or 2½. With little or no training, most normal children learn to stay clean and dry by age 4.

Children who are developmentally slow, or physically disabled, are often late in learning to stay clean and dry. This may be partly due to **their disabilities.** But often it is because the **parents have not provided the opportunity, training, and help** that the child needs. For example, one mildly retarded deaf 10-year-old boy in Mexico still depended on his mother to change his diapers. His mother had never seriously tried to teach him and thought he could not learn. Yet with a little help from a village *rehabilitation* worker, he became completely toilet trained in 3 days!

Handicapped children should be helped to become as independent as possible in their toileting. With help, **most retarded or disabled children can become completely toilet trained by ages 3 to 5.**

Of course, children with *severe physical disabilities* may always need help with clothing or getting to the pot. But they can learn to tell you when they have to go, and do their best to 'hold on' until they are on the pot.

Children who lack bladder and bowel control because of **spina bifida** or **spinal cord injury** have special problems. But even these children can often learn some control and become relatively or completely independent. The special problems and training of these children are discussed in Chapter 25.

WAYS TO MAKE TOILET TRAINING EASIER

1. Start when the child is ready

Just as training should not be delayed, it also should not be started too early. If a child's body is not yet able to control her bladder and bowel, trying to train her can lead to failure and frustration—both for the child and her parents. Normally a child is 'ready' by age 2 or 2½. But in some children, training may need to be delayed to age 3 or 4, or sometimes later.

Most children learn to keep clean a long time before they learn to stay dry. However, because a child pees much more often than she shits, if training aims at 'staying dry', 'staying clean' usually follows.

There are **3 simple tests to check if your child is 'ready' for toilet training.** These are: bladder control, readiness to cooperate, and physical readiness.*

- **Bladder control**

  Does your child pee a lot at one time and not dribble every few minutes?

  Does he often stay dry for hours?

  Does he seem to know when he is about to pee? (The look on his face, holding himself between the legs, etc.)

  If the child does these 3 things (or at least the first 2) he probably has enough bladder control and awareness of peeing to make training possible.

- **Readiness to cooperate.** To test whether the child has enough understanding and cooperation, ask her to do a few simple things: lie down, sit up, point to parts of her body, put a toy in a box, hand you an object, and imitate an action like hand clapping. If she does all these things willingly, she is probably mentally ready for toilet training.

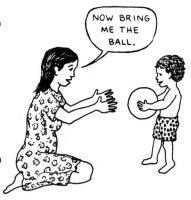

NOW BRING ME THE BALL.

- **Physical readiness.** Can the child pick up small objects easily? Can she walk or move herself fairly well? Can she squat, or sit on a stool, and keep her balance? If so, she is probably physically able to do her toilet by herself. If not, she can probably still be trained but may need physical assistance.

Most children more than 2 years old can pass these 3 tests. If not, it is usually better to wait before trying toilet training, or to help the child become more ready.

---

*These tests and many of these suggestions on toilet training are adapted from *Toilet Training in Less Than a Day.* Azrin and Foxx. Pocket Books, N.Y. 1974.

SPECIAL PROBLEMS

If the child still **does not have enough bladder control or awareness,** it is best to wait until she is older. For example, some children with cerebral palsy are slow in developing bladder control.

If the child **does not hear or understand simple language,** or is mentally retarded, more of the training needs to be done by *showing* and less with words. Special gestures or 'signs' need to be worked out for 'wet', 'dry', 'dirty', 'clean', and 'pot' or 'latrine'. Instead of teaching by using a doll, it is more helpful to have another child demonstrate toilet use.

If the child is **stubborn, refuses to cooperate** when asked to do simple things, or often cries and screams whenever he does not get what he wants, toilet training will be more difficult. Stubbornness and refusal to do what they are told are common in many handicapped children—mainly because they are often overprotected or spoiled. Before trying to toilet train such children, it is wise to work first on improving their attitude and *behavior.* This is discussed in Chapter 40.

If a child's **physical disability** makes it difficult for her to get to the toilet place, to lower her pants, to squat or sit, or to clean her butt, various aids or ways must be looked for to help her become as independent as possible. These will be discussed on the next pages.

2. Put the child on the pot at the times when she is most likely to use it

Before beginning toilet training, for several days notice at **what time of the day** the child shits and pees. Usually there will be certain times when she usually does so—for example, soon after the first meal of the day.

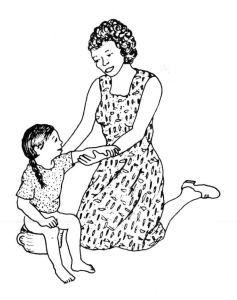

Begin to put her on the pot or latrine at these times, encouraging her to make 'poo' or 'pee' (or whatever she calls it).

Leave her on the pot until she 'goes'—or for no more than 10 minutes.

If the child 'goes', clap your hands, kiss her, show her what she has done, and let her know how pleased you are.

If she does not 'go', just ignore it. Do not scold or make her feel bad, or she may begin to fear or dislike the pot, and refuse to use it.

3. Reward and praise success

In toilet training—as in any form of education—it works better **to reward success than to punish failure.** When the child shits or pees where she should, give her praise, hugs, kisses and other signs of approval. However, **make sure that the child knows you are pleased with her,** not because she shits and pees, but **because she is staying dry or clean.** When training, check the child often to see if she is 'dry' or 'clean'. When she is, praise her. Also, teach her to check herself. ──────────

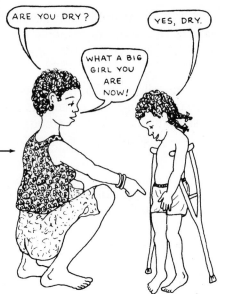

When the child has 'an accident' and wets or dirties herself **do not punish or scold her.** It is better to quietly clean up the mess or change her. At most, say something friendly (but not approving) like, "Too bad!—Better luck next time!"

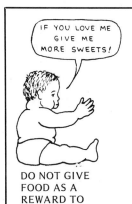

DO NOT GIVE FOOD AS A REWARD TO CHILDREN WHO ARE FAT

CAUTION: As a general rule, do not offer a child candy, sweets or other food as a reward for doing something right. This can lead the child to associate food with love or approval—and therefore to make constant demands for sweets. Avoiding food rewards is especially important for children whose disability makes them less active, so that they easily get fat. Extra weight makes moving around harder for both child and parents. So . . . DO NOT LET DISABLED CHILDREN GET OVERWEIGHT.

For children who are thin and active, it may make sense to sometimes give foods as rewards. But be sure to include healthful foods like nuts and fruits—not just sweets.

4. Guide the child's movements with your hands—not your tongue

When the child has difficulty carrying out a physical task—for example, lowering his pants—do not do it for him (if it is something he can learn to do for himself). And do not tell him his mistakes or how to correct them. Instead, gently guide his hands with yours so that he learns how to do it himself.

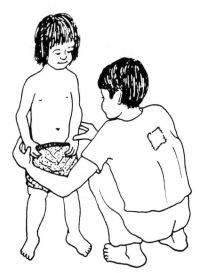

guiding the child's hands

5. Use models, examples, and demonstrations

Setting an example is one of the best ways of teaching—especially if the example is set by persons the child loves, admires, and tries to copy. Even before children are old enough to be toilet trained, help prepare them by letting them watch their brothers and sisters use the pot or latrine. Tell them that when they are big enough they will be able to do it that way too.

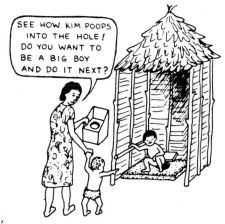

SEE HOW KIM POOPS INTO THE HOLE! DO YOU WANT TO BE A BIG BOY AND DO IT NEXT?

Using a **doll that wets** is another good way to introduce toilet training. Dolls that 'wet' can be bought, or you can make one out of,

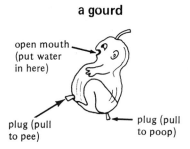

a gourd

open mouth (put water in here)

plug (pull to pee)

plug (pull to poop)

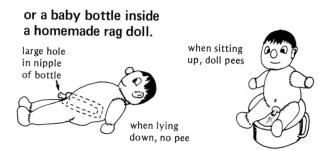

or a baby bottle inside a homemade rag doll.

large hole in nipple of bottle

when sitting up, doll pees

when lying down, no pee

Show the child how the doll pees in the pot. Or better, ask your child to help you toilet train the doll. Be sure to include each step that will be needed for the child to become as self-reliant as possible. For example:

First have the child show the doll how to get to the latrine or pot— and then help the doll lower his pants.

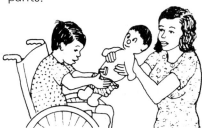

Next have the child teach the doll how to get onto the pot, and sit there until he pees. Try to make the situation as nearly like that of the child as you can—using the same pot in the same place that he will use it.

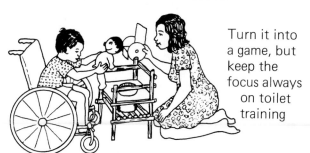

Turn it into a game, but keep the focus always on toilet training

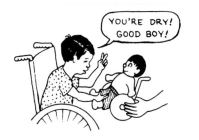

YOU'RE DRY! GOOD BOY!

After the doll has finished peeing, have the child pull up the doll's pants. Ask him to feel the doll's pants and check whether they are dry. If so, have him praise the doll.

To repeatedly see real persons (not just dolls) *enjoy* and be rewarded for using the pot or toilet is especially important for a child who is retarded or who has language difficulty.

6. Adapt toileting to the special needs of the child

Many handicapped children can be helped to become independent in their toileting if special aids or *adaptations* are made. Different children will require different adaptations. However, the following are often helpful:

- If the child has trouble pulling down pants or panties—**use loose fitting clothing with elastic or 'Velcro' waist band.**

Correct position of hands, for lowering pants

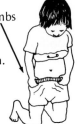

Hook thumbs inside pants and push down.

for raising pants

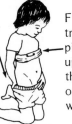

Put hand inside pants to pull over butt.

For training, pin shirt up out of the way— or do not wear one.

- Use short 'training pants' made of towel-like material that will soak up urine.

 CP

- For a child with cerebral palsy or spina bifida, it may be easier lying down—you might provide a clean mat.

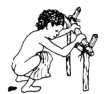

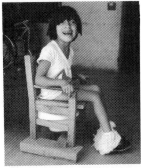

Some children, like this girl with cerebral palsy, need to sit. This potty seat was adapted from a child's wood chair.

- If people by custom squat to shit, and the child has trouble, a simple hand support can help.

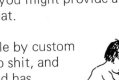 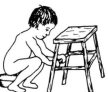

- Latrines can also be adapted

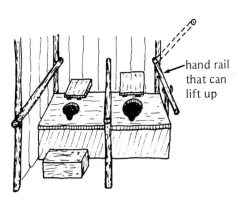

hand rail that can lift up

2-seater latrine with child-sized hole and step

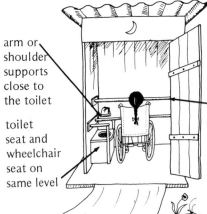

arm or shoulder supports close to the toilet

toilet seat and wheelchair seat on same level

high hand rail to make moving from wheelchair to toilet easier

Make the outhouse (latrine) and its door big enough so that a wheelchair can fit inside. Position the door so that the wheelchair can enter right beside the latrine without having to turn around.

Be sure the path to the latrine is level and easy to get to from the house.

● A simple pot or 'pottie' is one of the best aids for toilet training of young children. It can be adapted in various ways for disabled children.

simple pot

more complex pots sold in some countries

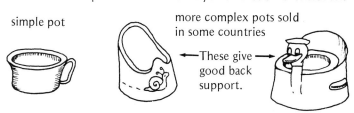

←These give→ good back support.

'Baby Relax Toilette' with removable pot— gives good back and side support.

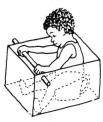

(CP)

For the child severely disabled with cerebral palsy, the pot can be placed between mother's knees. This provides good back support. Mother holds his shoulders forward, his hips bent and his knees separated.

Later it may be possible to put the child on a corner seat like this— which also holds arms and shoulders forward and helps keep hips bent.

A cardboard box can also make a good sitting frame.

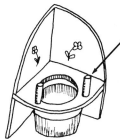

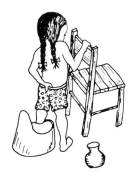

2 posts may be needed to keep knees apart.

bucket

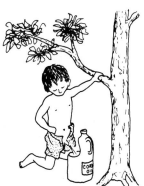

Use your imagination and whatever materials you can get to make it easier for your child to do it by herself.

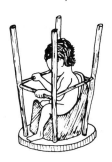

For severely handicapped children, 'toilet seats' can be built into specially designed chairs.

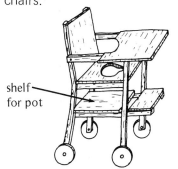

shelf for pot

A cushion can be made to fit over the toilet seat for ordinary sitting.

Put a shelf for the pot.

Or leave the space under the seat open, so that the whole chair can be rolled over a toilet.

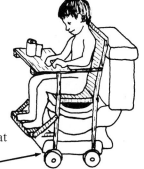

For the child who cannot sit up, you might make a wedge-shaped toilet box like this.

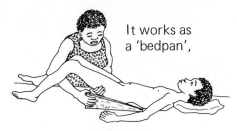

It works as a 'bedpan',

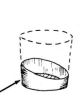

An old plastic bucket can be cut at the same angle as the bedpan so that it fits snugly under the hole.

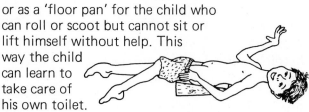

or as a 'floor pan' for the child who can roll or scoot but cannot sit or lift himself without help. This way the child can learn to take care of his own toilet.

(CP) For the child who has *spasticity* or poor balance, you can make a seat like this. The bar can be put in after the child has been seated.

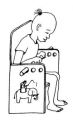

The seat can be made to fit over a bucket, over a floor-hole latrine, or over a standard toilet.

Tire potty seat—soft, safe, washable*

Tire can be used alone,

or over a 'hole-in-the-floor' toilet,

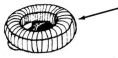

To keep urine from getting inside the tire, you can wrap long strips of inner tube tightly around the tire.

or on a wood or metal frame over a toilet seat.

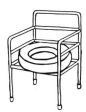

Try to pick size of tires to match the size of the child. For small children, scooter or very small car tires may work well.

Cane or rattan toilet seat with climb up bars*

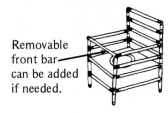

Removable front bar can be added if needed.

Enclosed wood or plywood toilet*

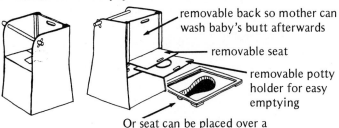

removable back so mother can wash baby's butt afterwards

removable seat

removable potty holder for easy emptying

Or seat can be placed over a hole-in-the-floor toilet.

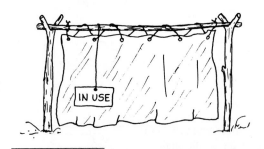
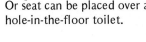

IN USE

REMEMBER: As the disabled child grows, she will feel the same need of privacy as any child would for toileting and other personal acts. **Help the child to obtain the privacy she needs.**

*Ideas from India—UPKARAN manual. See p. 642.

CHAPTER **39**

Bathing

Regular bathing is important for all children. Bathing the severely disabled child, however, is often not easy. Children whose bodies get stiff or whose knees pull together may be very difficult to clean. As the child gets older and heavier, the difficulties often increase. Here are some aids and ideas that may make bathing easier.

(CP)

For the baby or small child, some kind of a tub may be a big help.

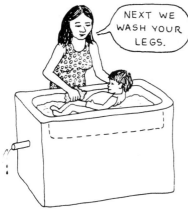

NEXT WE WASH YOUR LEGS.

A rectangular tub of the size you need can be made out of mud or mud bricks (or dried bricks) and covered with a thin layer of cement.

IMPORTANT: Talk or sing to the baby as you bathe her. Tell her each thing you do, and the name of each body part you wash, even if she cannot understand. A child must spend a long time listening before she can say her first words. So **get an early start.**

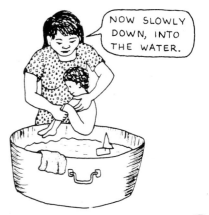

NOW SLOWLY DOWN, INTO THE WATER.

This is a good way to hold the child who stiffens and bends backward, or throws open her arms when you pick her up.

(CP)

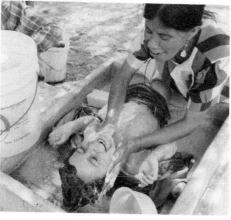

A mother bathes her child in a cement wash tub. (PROJIMO)

A baby that tends to stiffen backward can sometimes be held like this for bathing.

Gently spread the child's legs as wide as possible to clean between them. Also, lift arms high above the head. In this way, **bathing can be combined with range-of-motion exercises** (see Chapter 42).

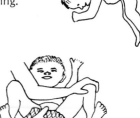

(CP)

As the child grows, make every effort to help her take part in bathing herself. Help her do more and more until she can bathe herself without help, if possible.

> **Our goal in bathing is SELF-CARE, even for the child who is fairly severely disabled or *retarded*.**

For many children **balance is a problem,** even while sitting. Anything that can help the child keep his balance, and stay in a position where he has the most control, will help make bathing easier. **Here are some aids and suggestions for helping the child manage better.**

The child who has trouble sitting because she stiffens backward may need some kind of back support to sit while bathing.

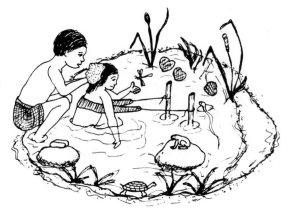

CAUTION:
Be sure water is clean and does not spread disease.

2 old car tires (or inner tubes) tied together

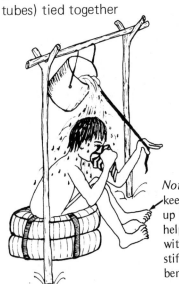

Note: Anything that keeps the hips bent up like this will help keep a child with *spasticity* from stiffening and bending backward.

Especially for the child who does not have good *bowel* or urine control, it is very important to carefully clean her *butt* and between her legs. An inner tube on poles, like this, holds her in a good position for washing.

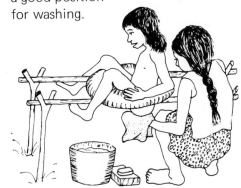

a bath seat made from half a plastic bucket or laundry basket on a tube frame

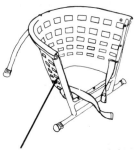

Heat the edges to bend them around the tubing.

a stool with a seat woven from strips of car tire inner tube

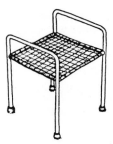

From the UPKARAN Manual. See p. 642.

a washing platform of wooden slats for the child who washes (or is washed) lying down

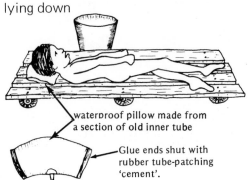

waterproof pillow made from a section of old inner tube

Glue ends shut with rubber tube-patching 'cement'.

Also see the bicycle inner tube mat on p. 200.

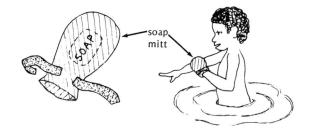

A soap mitt, made of a piece of towel and a tie string (or *Velcro* straps), lets the child who has difficulty grasping use both the washcloth and soap more easily.

Bath time is a good time to help a child develop many different skills. Encourage her to handle and play with toys in the water, repeat words, and imitate actions. Let her feel the difference between a sponge and a cloth, or dry and wet and soapy. To learn to use both hands together, let her squeeze water out of the sponge.

To help the child learn how to bathe herself, let her first wash her toys and dolls. Show her how and encourage her to copy you.

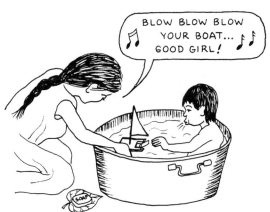

For a child who is afraid of the water, letting her bathe a doll or toy first may calm her fears.

Toys that float in the water make bathing more fun. Use corks, bits of wood, or plastic bottles with lids on them. Making little boats with sails or 'paddle wheels' makes it more fun and helps the child learn to use her hands better. The child with weak lips or who drools can play by blowing the boat across the water.

For the child with limited control or strength, it is often easier to play in the water with toys that float than it is to play with toys out of the water.

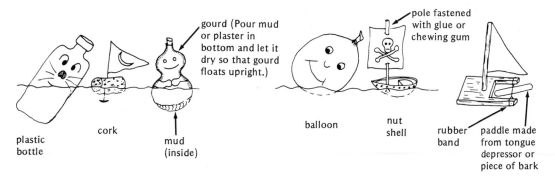

Drying the child can also become a game that aids development. Rub the child, sometimes gently and sometimes briskly, with a rough cloth or towel. Name the different parts of her body as you rub them. Remember, as you bathe and dry the child, talk about each thing you do—or sing a song about it! Move the towel with the music, and encourage the child to move with you. Use your imagination to make it more fun and to help her learn.

Use bath time as an opportunity for learning and play.

CARE OF THE TEETH AND GUMS

Many disabled children develop problems in their teeth and gums. There are many reasons:

- In children who have poor mouth and tongue control, food often sticks to gums and teeth and is not cleaned away by the natural movement of the tongue.
- Many disabled children (even those with no eating problems) are fed soft, sticky 'baby foods' long after they should be eating rougher, more solid 'adult foods'. So, their gums get soft, weak, and unhealthy.
- Sometimes children with *disabilities* are 'spoiled' by giving them extra sweets—which increases tooth decay.
- Some medicines for fits (epilepsy) cause swollen, unhealthy gums. (See p. 238.)
- (CP) Dental care is more difficult in some disabled children—especially those with cerebral palsy. (In some places, dentists refuse to care for these children.)

For these reasons, **we must take care to keep the gums and teeth of the disabled child healthy and clean.**

STEPS IN CARING FOR GUMS AND TEETH:

1. **Avoid foods and drinks with lots of sugar**—especially between meals.

2. **Start child on solid food as early as he can take them.** Toast, crackers, carrots, raw fruit, and other foods that rub the teeth and gums clean are especially helpful.

3. **Clean the child's teeth and gums,** if possible after every meal.

Before the baby has teeth, clean his gums with a soft cloth over your finger. First, dip the cloth in boiled water with a little salt or baking soda in it.

After the child has teeth, clean them with a small, soft toothbrush. Or use a piece of thick cloth or a bit of towel wrapped on a stick.

Toothpaste is not necessary. Instead you can use salt, salt mixed with baking soda, or a burned and powdered piece of bread, chapati, or tortilla, or just water.

Clean all surfaces of the teeth well, and also rub or brush the gums.

RIGHT   WRONG

This is a good position to clean the child's teeth and gums. Be sure the head bends down.

If his head bends up, he will be more likely to choke or gag.

Or use a stick from a Neme tree or other non-poisonous plant.

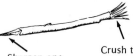

Sharpen one end to form a 'toothpick'.

Crush the other end to form a 'brush'.

4. Help the child learn to do whatever she can to clean her own teeth and gums. At first you can guide her hand, then have her do a little more each time, and praise her when she does it well.

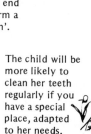

The child will be more likely to clean her teeth regularly if you have a special place, adapted to her needs.

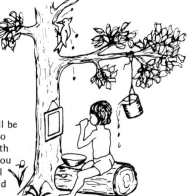

REMEMBER: **Brushing the gums is just as important as brushing the teeth!**

For more information, see *Where There Is No Dentist,* Chapter 5, "Taking Care of Teeth and Gums" (see p. 637).

Ways to Improve Learning and Behavior

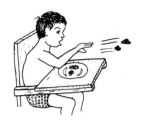

"I still feed Raúl myself because when I let him try to eat by himself he throws his food all over the place. The more I punish him the worse he gets."

"Erica begins to cry and scream every time I put her down for a minute. It's worse when I take her out where there are other people. At the river she has such tantrums that I can't finish washing the clothes."

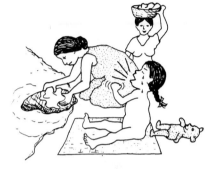

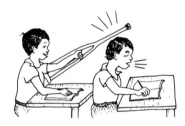

"Jorge is always starting fights with other children or doing other bad things—at home and in school. He seems to enjoy making people mad at him!"

These and other *behavior* problems can occur in both non-disabled and disabled children. But some disabled children have special difficulty learning acceptable and appropriate behavior. Children who are *mentally retarded* may develop poor behavior because they are confused by the unclear or conflicting messages they get from their parents and others. Children who are *physically disabled* sometimes act in 'naughty' or self-centered ways because they have become dependent on others to do things for them. They lack self-confidence, and are afraid of being forgotten. On the other hand, children who are often neglected or ignored when they are quiet and behave well, may learn to behave badly to get attention.

As a rule, **if children repeatedly behave badly, it is because they get something satisfying or rewarding from their bad behavior. Therefore, to help children learn acceptable behavior, we need always to CLEARLY LET THEM SEE THAT 'GOOD' BEHAVIOR IS MORE SATISFYING THAN 'BAD' BEHAVIOR.**

In this chapter we explore ways to do this, using a 'behavioral approach' which you can divide into 5 steps:

1. Carefully observe the circumstances of your child's unacceptable behavior.
2. Try to understand why your child behaves as he does.
3. Set a reasonable goal for improvement based on his immediate needs and his developmental level.
4. Plan to work toward the goal in small steps, always rewarding 'good' behavior and making sure 'bad' behavior brings no pleasure, attention, or reward.
5. After the child's behavior has improved, gradually move toward a more natural (less planned) way of relating to him.

A BEHAVIORAL APPROACH TO LEARNING AND IMPROVED BEHAVIOR

Step 1. Observe the circumstances of your child's behavior.

To help your child to behave more acceptably, start by carefully observing what is happening around and with the child when he begins his acts of disturbing behavior. **Observe carefully for a week or two.** To notice patterns more clearly, it helps to **write down your observations.** Try to **make your records clear, specific, and simple.** Take note of everything that might lead to your child's acts of 'bad' behavior, and **what he seems to gain from it.** For example, Raúl's mother might write these notes:

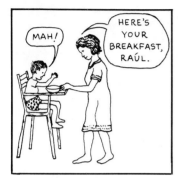

"I put him in his chair, and gave him food."

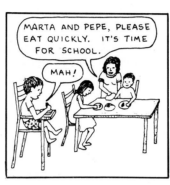

"Then I got the older children ready for school."

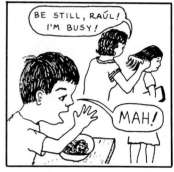

"He kept calling to me, but I was busy and told him to keep quiet."

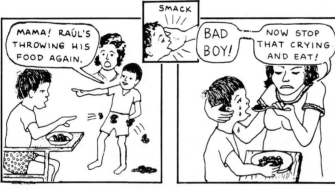

"Raúl began to throw his food!" "I slapped him." "He started crying. To quiet him, I fed him his breakfast."

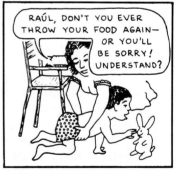

"Then I put him down to play with his toys."

Step 2. Based on your observations, try to figure out why your child behaves as he does. Look for answers to these questions:

- What happens that leads to or 'triggers' his unacceptable behavior?
- Is his behavior partly due to **confused or unclear messages** from you or other persons?
- **What satisfying results does his behavior produce that might make him want to do it again?**
- Is the child's behavior partly from feeling afraid or insecure?

By repeatedly observing what happened before Raúl began to throw food, his mother started to find some answers:

- "Raúl throws food most often when I leave him alone with it—especially when I am busy with the other children."

- "My own messages to Raúl are confusing and contradictory. At the same time that I scold him, I also give him the attention and care that he wants—like feeding him as if he were still a baby.

- By throwing food, Raúl gets a lot of satisfaction.

POSSIBLE EXPLANATION FOR RAÚL'S FOOD THROWING

TRIGGERS	WHAT HE LOSES BY THROWING FOOD	WHAT HE GETS
• Raúl is being ignored. He is left out while his mother is busy with the other children. • He may be afraid that if he feeds himself, he will be left out even more. He is very dependent on his mother's care and attention.	• His mother gets angry, slaps, and scolds him. 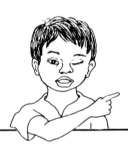	• He gets the whole family's attention. • His mother quickly leaves the other children and goes to him. • If he cries when she slaps or scolds him, she quickly comforts him and cares for him like a baby. • And then he gets to play with his toys. • By being fed like a baby, he calms his fears of growing up and losing his mother's care and attention.

Step 3. Set a goal for improvement of the child's behavior.

If the child has several different behavioral problems, it is usually best to try to improve one at a time. Be positive. Try to **set the goal in terms of the good behavior that you want,** not just the bad behavior that you wisn to end. For Raúl, the goal might be 'to learn to feed himself quietly' (not simply 'to get him to stop throwing his food').

Be sure that **goals are possible for the child at his developmental level.** (See p. 354.)

Step 4. Plan a way to help the child improve his behavior.

Consistently reward 'good behavior'. Each time the child behaves as you want, **immediately show your appreciation.** Rewards can be words of praise, a hug, a special privilege (perhaps the chance to play with a favorite toy). Or give the child a bit of favorite food. However, food rewards should mostly be used only for very thin children or if nothing else works. **Avoid giving food as rewards to fat children** (see p. 340).

As much as possible, **ignore rather than punish 'bad' behavior.** Rewarding 'good' behavior rather than punishing 'bad' behavior brings improvement with much less bad feeling for both parent and child.

Always reward 'good' behavior and never reward 'bad' behavior. This is the key to the behavioral approach.

For example, whenever Raúl eats by himself, without throwing his food, the whole family can applaud and praise him.

Raúl finds that good behavior brings rewards and attention.

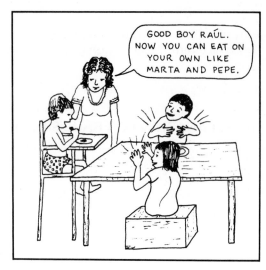

But whenever he throws his food, the family ignores him, except perhaps to say "I'm sorry you did that, Raúl," or, "Once more and I'll have to take your food away because I'm tired of having to clean up the mess." (Make this a result, not a punishment.) **Always do what you say you will do.**

He quickly learns that throwing his food now brings no reward.

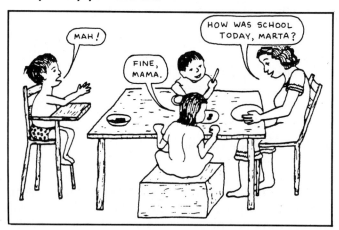

ADDITIONAL GUIDELINES:

- **Be consistent** in how you respond to your child's behavior. If you sometimes reward good behavior and at other times you ignore it, or if you sometimes ignore bad behavior and at other times either scold or do what the child demands, this is confusing. His behavior is not likely to improve.

- *WARNING:* When using this approach, **at first the child may actually behave worse.** When Raúl does not get his mother's attention by throwing his food, he may try throwing his bowl too. It is very important that his mother not give in to his demands, but rather be consistent with her approach. Only if she is consistent will he learn that he gets more of what he wants with 'good' behavior than with 'bad'.

- **Move towards the goal little by little, in small steps.** If steps forward are small and clearly defined, often the child will learn more easily, and a beginning period of worse behavior can sometimes be avoided.

For example, it would be too much to expect Raúl to suddenly eat by himself quietly when mother is busy with the other children. Instead, mother can help him work toward this goal little by little.

A possible first step is for Raúl's mother to give him his food after the other children have left for school. This way she can stay close to him as he eats it.

The next step might be for mother to do her work while Raúl eats, but to keep talking with him and praising him when he does well.

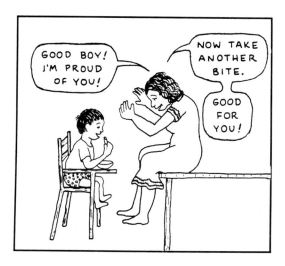
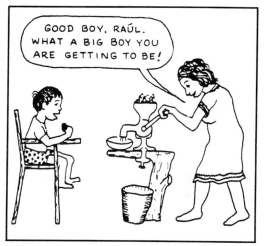

In this way, Raúl will learn that eating by himself does not mean being left alone, but gets more attention from his mother than does throwing food.

Step 5. After the child's improved behavior has become a habit, gradually move toward a more natural way of relating to the child.

To help the child improve his behavior, the 'behavioral approach' just described often works well. Your responses to your child's acts are carefully planned and consistent. However, such a controlled approach to person-to-person relationships is not natural. Parents and children, like other people, need to learn to relate to each other not according to a plan, or because each action earns a reward, but because they enjoy making each other happy.

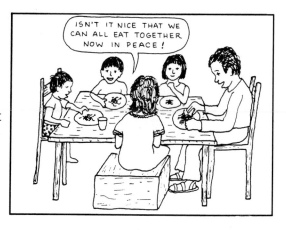

Therefore, the last step, after the child's new behavior has been established, is to **gradually decrease immediate rewards while sharing the pleasure of an improved relationship.**

Setting reasonable goals—based on the child's developmental level

Be realistic when setting a goal for improvement in behavior, or a new skill that you want your child to learn. First try to determine the child's developmental level, and set a goal consistent with that level. (To determine the child's developmental level, see Chapter 34, '' Child Development and Developmental Delay.'')

Consider Erica, the girl on p. 349 who has *tantrums* (crying and screaming fits) whenever her mother puts her down. Erica is retarded, which means she is developmentally slow for her age. Depending on her developmental level (*not* her age), her mother can plan steps to help her avoid tantrums:

Suppose **Erica is at the development level of a very young child.** She has poor hand control and no ability to play by herself, or to imitate (to copy) others. She will need to begin with very basic steps and clear, simple messages. Her mother can put her down briefly, then praise, talk, or sing to her as long as she does not have a tantrum. When she does have a tantrum, her mother should try to give her as little attention as possible, and never give in to her demands. She can pay attention and reward her during those moments when she stops screaming—if only to catch her breath. This way Erica will begin to learn that she gets more of what she wants through good behavior than through tantrums.

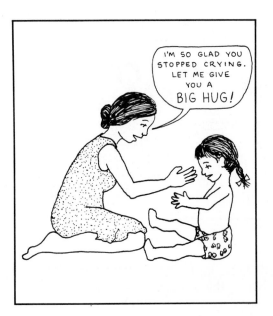

Now suppose that **Erica is at a more advanced level of development.** She likes using her hands and imitating her mother. Steps for improving her behavior can start from this level. Perhaps her mother can have Erica sit at the river's edge and pretend to help her mother wash clothes. This way Erica will feel closer to her mother and will be less afraid of being left alone. Her mother can talk to her and praise her all the time.

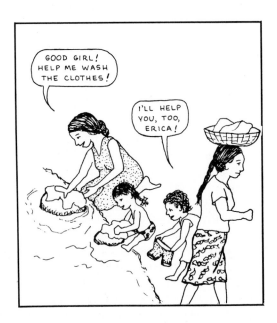

Note: At this level, Erica will not be able to stay with one activity for very long. To avoid tantrums, her mother will need to keep the activities interesting by changing them often, and talking to her a lot. In all of this, other children can be a big help.

Helping the child make sense of his world

The 'behavioral approach' to learning and development that we have discussed is similar to what is called 'behavior therapy' or 'behavior modification'. However, we prefer to put the emphasis on **improving communication** to help the child make sense of the world around him. Instead of our 'changing the child's behavior', we would rather **help the child to understand** things clearly enough so that he chooses to act in a way that will make life more pleasant for everyone.* To achieve this, **parents first learn to understand and change their own behavior in relating to their child. They look for ways to communicate with the child that are consistent and supportive, and that reinforce good behavior.**

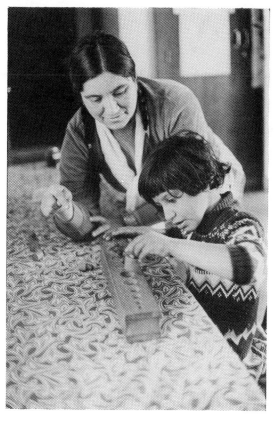

A behavioral approach can often help **children who are mentally retarded or developmentally delayed,** such as Raúl and Erica, to relate to other persons better and to learn basic skills more quickly.

Giving lots of attention, encouragement, and praise when he makes an effort is one of the best ways to help a child learn new skills. Photo by Sonia Iskov from *Special Education for Mentally Handicapped Pupils,* see p. 640.

The approach can be used at almost any age. It is often easier with younger children (developmental age from 1 to 4). Starting at a young age can prevent small behavioral difficulties from becoming big problems later. For the very young or severely retarded child, goals must be kept basic, and progress toward the goals must be divided into small steps. To master each step, **much repetition may be needed** with consistent praise and rewards for each small advance.

Mentally normal children with physical disabilities sometimes also develop unacceptable patterns of behavior. A behavioral approach may help them also. The story on the next page tells how this approach helped Jorge, from p. 349, to behave better.

---

*This is the point of view in Newson and Hipgrave's *Getting Through to Your Handicapped Child,* from which many ideas in this chapter are taken, and which we strongly recommend.

THE STORY OF JORGE

Jorge is an intelligent 10-year-old whose legs are paralyzed by polio. He lives with his grandmother. He is noisy, rude, bad tempered, and whenever he plays with other children, it turns into a fight. Jorge has caused so much trouble in the classroom that his teacher recently told his grandmother he will throw Jorge out of school if he does not change. Both his teacher and grandmother have tried scolding him and whipping him, but it only seems to make Jorge's behavior worse. As his grandmother says, "He loves to make people angry at him."

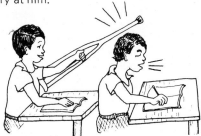

Not long ago, Jorge's grandmother took him to the village rehabilitation center to ask for advice. A village worker helped her to observe both Jorge's and her own behavior more closely to better understand why Jorge acts the way he does. She realized:

- When Jorge is quiet and well-behaved (which is not often), everyone ignores or forgets him.

- As a result, Jorge feels unwanted, unloved, and useless. Starved for emotional human contact, he gets it by making people angry with him.

- Jorge's bad behavior, therefore, brings him a lot of person-to-person contact, even though it is painful. The few times he tries to be good, he is made to feel unwanted and unneeded.

"I really do love him," said his grandmother. "But I guess I don't show it much. He makes me worry so much!"

To begin to behave better, Jorge needed to find out that friendly and helpful behavior can bring him closer to people than bad behavior. For this reason, the village worker—together with the grandmother, the schoolteacher, the schoolchildren, the rehabilitation team, and Jorge himself—helped figure out ways that would let the boy see that 'good' behavior is better than 'bad' behavior.

At home, grandma began to look for things Jorge could do to help her, and to show him how happy she was when he did them. She made a backpack, open at the sides, so that he could help bring firewood. Also, she learned to quietly turn her back when he misbehaved, and to let him know how happy she was when he would sit quietly doing his homework or shelling the maize.

THANK YOU SO MUCH FOR BRINGING THE FIREWOOD. COME EAT A CAKE I BAKED JUST FOR YOU.

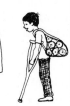

At school, the teacher discussed with the other children ways to include Jorge in their games. When they all played football (soccer), they let him be 'goalie'. To everyone's surprise, Jorge was an excellent goalie. With his crutches he could reach farther and hit the ball farther than anyone else. Soon all the children wanted Jorge to play on 'their team'. At first Jorge started a few fights. But when he did, he was quietly asked to sit on the sideline. Soon he learned to stop hitting other children so that he could keep hitting the ball.

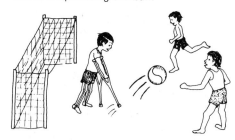

In the village rehabilitation center, the village worker invited Jorge to help make educational toys for young and disabled children. He helped Jorge get started and praised him for each toy Jorge completed. Soon Jorge learned to make the toys by himself and took great pride in his work. When he saw other disabled children playing and learning things with his toys, it made him very happy. He decided he wants to be a rehabilitation worker when he grows up.

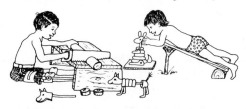

'Time Out' or 'non-reward' instead of punishment

The story of the way family and friends used the 'behavior approach' to help Jorge sounds fairly straightforward and simple. But in real life it is seldom that easy. 'Bad' behavior may sometimes be so bad that it cannot be ignored.

In general, the best way to make 'bad' behavior seem boring to the child and not worth the trouble is to give no rewarding response. At the same time, make sure to reward 'good' behavior. This means everything satisfying stops as a result of 'bad' behavior (instead of the usual situation where everything satisfying starts).

For example, when Raúl throws his food, instead of entertaining him by scolding and feeding him, his mother should remove both the food and herself for 3 or 4 minutes—making the situation as boring as possible.

Removing food may seem like punishment. But it is best to aim at **making the situation less interesting** rather than making it unpleasant. To make things less interesting, sometimes we may remove the child from the situation for a brief time. This is often called **'time out'.**

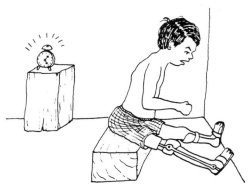

For example, when Jorge's grandmother first began using the behavioral approach, to try to make her angry he would shout and hit the chickens with his crutches. But instead of her usual scolding, grandma now simply told him that if he did not quiet down she would ask him to take 'time out' in the corner. Then, if he continued to make trouble, she would lead him to the corner and tell him that he would have to stay there for 5 minutes from the time he was quiet. She set an old alarm clock to ring in 5 minutes. At first Jorge would continue to shout from the corner, but each time he did, grandma would set the alarm to ring in another 5 minutes from the time he was quiet. Meanwhile she gave him no attention and continued her work.

In this way Jorge learned while he was in the corner that the only way to make life interesting again was to stop making a disturbance. Because he was clever, he learned fast. (Slower children often take longer.)

We should try to use 'time out' as a 'non-reward' and not a punishment. However, because time out is something an adult makes a child do, it can seem like punishment. Try to use it only when less forceful methods of avoiding rewards do not work. It is best to start with a 'time out' period of no more than 5 minutes (less for a very young child). If the child does not behave better in 5 minutes, consider with the child adding another 5 minutes. **Never leave the child in 'time out' for more than half an hour,** even if he has still not become quiet.

CAUTION: **For a child who is younger than 5 years old or severely retarded, do not extend time out to more than 15 minutes, checking frequently with the child to see if he is ready to behave acceptably.**

A BEHAVIORAL APPROACH TO CHILD DEVELOPMENT AND LEARNING NEW SKILLS

In this chapter we have talked mainly about correcting 'bad' behavior. However, the behavioral approach can also be used to help children learn basic skills for their continuing development. The approach is often useful for children who are slow to develop—for either mental or physical reasons.

In Chapter 34 on child development, we introduced the key features of a behavioral approach: (1) make messages clear, (2) consistently reward things learned, and (3) advance toward new skills through small steps. You will also recognize this behavioral approach in the chapters on 'feeding', 'dressing', and 'toilet training'. Here we would like to review ways of applying a behavioral approach to a child's basic development and learning.

Looking at the whole child to decide where to begin

In considering how to help a child's development, start by looking at what the child can and cannot do. In terms of behavior, we can group our observations into 4 sections:

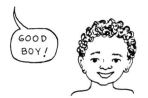

- **Positive behaviors:** Skills and characteristics the child now has—particularly those that may help him in learning something new. (For example, he enjoys being praised.)

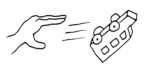

- **Negative behaviors:** Things he does that are dangerous, disturbing, or prevent his progress. (For example, breaking things, hitting people, screaming when bathed, throwing toys rather than playing with them.)

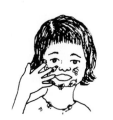

- **In-between behaviors:** These have both positive and negative aspects, and need to be worked with to make them more positive. (For example, for a child who is beginning to feed herself, but who smears food all over: we encourage feeding herself (which is positive), but not smearing (which is negative). Even screaming or crying in order to express a need might be considered positive for a child who has great trouble communicating. We need to help this become more satisfactory communication.)

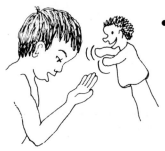

- **Key needs:** These are problems in the child's behavior that need to be solved to make progress with learning. They differ depending on the stage of development. (For example, for a child to learn from his mother, he needs to respond to his own name, to look at her when she speaks to him, and to stay still and give attention for at least a few seconds. These 'key needs' suggest the first steps in learning to speak, play, or develop new skills.)

It may help to write a list of these different behaviors. Here is a list that a little girl's mother made with the help of a village health worker who studied this book.

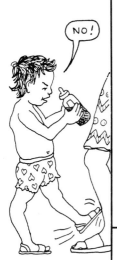

Child: Celia
Age: 4

POSITIVE BEHAVIORS —ones she now has that we can build on	IN-BETWEEN BEHAVIORS—ones that have both good and bad points	NEGATIVE BEHAVIORS—ones that prevent her progress or disturb the family
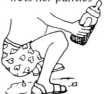• smiles when praised • can feed herself with her fingers • can put 3 rings on a peg • undresses herself • enjoys rough play • enjoys being bathed • says 6 words: mama, dada, bottle, sweets, pee-pee and NO!	• plays only a moment with toys— then throws them • says 'pee-pee', then wets her panties • **will not sit still** for a minute—except for food	• kicks people when she gets upset • carries around a baby bottle all the time, and screams when it is taken away • spits her food at others 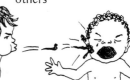

KEY NEEDS (in order that new skills and behavior can develop)
• sitting down and giving attention for a longer time
• getting rid of the baby bottle to free hands for other things

Deciding where to begin

After they listed these behaviors and considered Celia's key needs, the health worker helped her mother plan where to begin. He explained that, since **we cannot change everything at the same time,** we need to **decide what things need to be done first** (choose priorities for action). So we choose the behavior we most want to introduce or change.

- If we are trying **to introduce a new behavior or skill,** we need to think of all the **different parts** that make up the behavior. Next we plan the separate **small steps** that lead to the skill. We encourage the child to advance step by step, making clear what we expect for each step and consistently giving **praise and small rewards.**

- **To improve an 'in-between behavior',** we can help the child by working with a skill she has already developed a little. First we need to think about the various **parts of her behavior** that concern us. Then we decide **which parts seem helpful and which do not.** We then **reward the good behavior and ignore the bad.** As the child gradually improves, we can expect more of her before giving a reward, until the whole improved behavior is achieved.

- If we are trying **to reduce or stop an old behavior** we need to do 2 things. First we note **when** and **where** the behavior happens, and **what happens before, during, and afterward.** We observe carefully **both what the child does and what we ourselves do.** Second, we try to guess what the child gains from her 'bad' behavior. We can then try to **change things so that 'good' behavior is more worthwhile than the 'bad'.** To do this we **reward the new 'good' behavior and refuse to give attention for her 'bad' behavior.**

Thinking about Celia's behavior, her mother realized that she already has the beginnings of **many valuable skills.** She uses her hands well and has begun to develop skills for **feeding** and **dressing** herself. She also **speaks a few words**—although it would be nice if she could say "yes" as well as "no."

It is important that she **likes praise** and hugs, and bathing, and rough play. This means she will probably learn well with a reward-based approach.

However, **certain things seem to be stopping** Celia from developing her skills more. Not being able to sit still and give attention makes it hard for her to learn from other people, or even to learn to enjoy her toys (which she always throws). Also, her **baby bottle is a big problem.** She is much too old for it, but her mother is afraid to take it away because Celia screams. Her mother fills the bottle with sweet drinks (which have already begun to rot Celia's teeth). The biggest problem is that by always holding her bottle, Celia's hands are not free to do other things—such as play with her toys or take down her panties when she has to pee-pee.

For these reasons, Celia's mother decided that the 'key needs', which need to be solved in order to advance in other areas, are:

- **helping Celia learn to sit quietly and give her attention to something**

- **helping Celia grow out of her need to always hold her bottle**

The health worker discussed with Celia's mother what she might do. To help Celia learn to sit quietly and pay more attention to things, her mother decided to start with the times when Celia was already willing to sit fairly quietly—which was mealtime and bathtime. For example:

After giving Celia her food, but before her final 'sweet', her mother or her older brother, Oscar, plays quietly with her for 5 minutes or so, praising her whenever she gives attention.

Her mother also uses bathtime as an opportunity to help her concentrate on toys and to give attention to words and sounds.

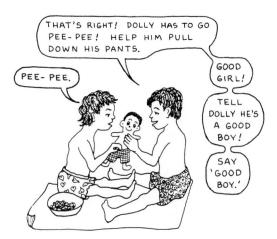

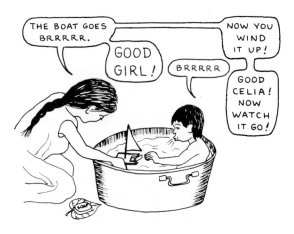

To make a paddle wheel boat, see p. 475.

Celia's mother decided to help her outgrow the bottle little by little. For a start, she filled it with water only. After a few days, she refused to fill it at all.

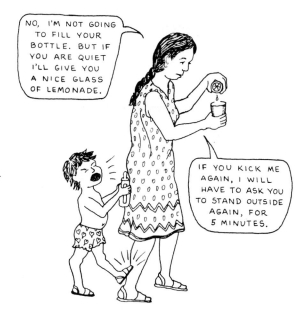

At first Celia screamed and kicked. But her mother did her best not to give Celia any attention when she acted that way. As soon as Celia was quiet, however, she would give her a tasty drink from a glass, or some other reward.

Sometimes Celia would throw her empty bottle in anger. But after a while she began putting it down, more and more often, to pick up other toys or objects. Finally, her mother simply removed the bottle from sight.

After Celia had forgotten her bottle, she started to explore more with her hands. When she needed to go 'pee-pee', she began to lower her panties by herself; in a few weeks she was 'toilet trained'. She also began to play with her toys more, instead of just throwing them. As she learned to give longer attention to things, she discovered lots of things that gave her pleasure. Many of her behavior problems such as screaming, spitting food, and kicking began to disappear. Her mother, father, and brother spent more time playing and talking with her. They praised her when she behaved well, and did their best to ignore her 'bad' behavior.

Where it seemed necessary, her mother began to use a behavioral approach to help Celia develop other skills: dressing, eating, and talking. To increase her language skills, together they looked at picture books and listened to songs.

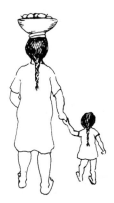

As a result of her family's efforts, Celia has grown up a lot, and is a much happier and more able little girl. Thinking about the changes that took place, her mother said, "I think my behavior has changed as much as Celia's. I was still treating her like a baby—bottle and all! Now that I expect more from her and show her how much I appreciate her effort, she has developed a lot faster, and is a lot easier to live with. She and I have both come a long way!"

Examples or methods for helping children develop basic skills using a behavioral approach are discussed in other chapters: Feeding, Chapter 36; Dressing, Chapter 37; and Toilet Training, Chapter 38. We suggest you also read again the chapter on child development, Chapter 34, and consider how a behavioral approach can be useful for helping a child through many difficult areas of development.

PARTICULAR BEHAVIOR PROBLEMS THAT OCCUR IN SOME DISABLED CHILDREN

Tantrums

'Tantrums' are fits of crying, screaming, and angry or destructive behavior. The child may try to break, throw, kick, bite, or in other ways damage anything or anyone within reach—sometimes including himself.

Tantrums can be frightening, both to the child and the family. After a tantrum begins, it is difficult to 'reason' with the child and calm him. Punishment often makes it worse.

Children—including some retarded and physically disabled children—may learn to use tantrums to get what they want. Erica, on p. 354, is one example. Here is another:

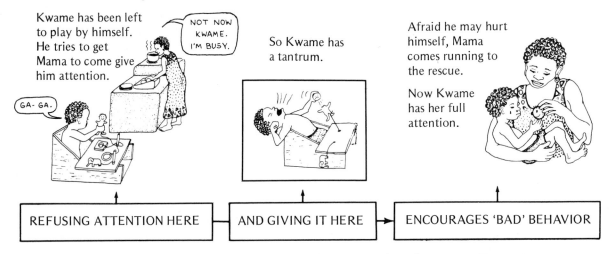

In this way children discover that tantrums get them what they want. To help a child have fewer tantrums, parents need to help the child find other, more acceptable ways of showing his wants and fears. And most important, parents need to **reward the acceptable ways,** and at the same time **refuse to give the child attention** when he is having a tantrum. Let's look at how Kwame's mother learned to do this:

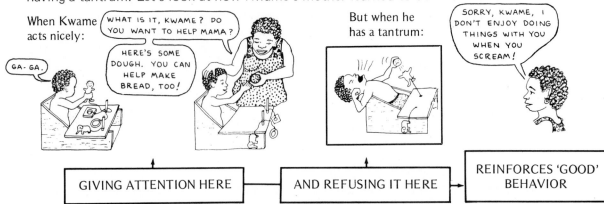

Thus, by rewarding Kwame's good behavior and by refusing to give attention to his demands when he does have tantrums, Kwame's mama helped him learn that **tantrums do not get him what he wants.** At first he had more violent tantrums than ever. But when even these failed to give exciting results, little by little he stopped having tantrums. He found that other forms of communication gave more satisfying results.

Holding breath

"Not giving attention during a tantrum sounds very nice. But my child **gets so angry, he stops breathing and turns blue!** I can't just do nothing!"

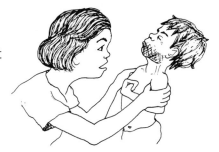

But doing nothing is often the best way to prevent your child from holding his breath more often!

The **child will not hurt himself by holding his breath.** At worst, he will lose consciousness and begin to breathe normally, long before the lack of air causes any damage.

Once a child learns that holding her breath frightens and confuses her parents, she is likely to repeat it every time she gets angry at them. (Many completely normal children do this.) We need to try *not* to show worry or concern when the child holds her breath and turns blue. Instead, we should wait until she gives up trying to frighten us and begins to breathe normally again. Then we can do something to show her how much we love her. But *not* while she is holding her breath!

Head banging, biting, and other self-damage

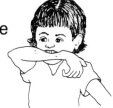

Children may do these things for the same reason they hold their breath—to frighten and punish their parents.

Sometimes, however, children with brain damage, epilepsy or severe mental problems may form habits of biting themselves, banging their heads, pulling out their hair or other self-destructive behavior.

Whatever the cause, acts of self-destruction cannot be ignored. Parents should look for the most simple and calm way possible to gently stop the child from injuring herself. For example, they can hold the child's arms to keep her from biting herself.

However, often a behavioral approach helps solve these problems. Take care **not to get excited or give the child extra attention** when she hurts herself. At the same time, make every effort to reward positive behavior and to help the child gain self-confidence, learn new skills, play with toys and other

To stop a child who is hurting himself, hold him from behind tightly, but quietly, so that he does not see you and gets as little response from you as possible.

children, and have friendly interaction with other people. Of course, some children's mental ability will not allow much learning or play. Showing these children a lot of affection, hugging them, talking and singing to them, and doing things with them that they like, **at times when they are not harming themselves,** may help them to stop such acts. **Rewarding a child when she stops a self-destructive act** may help a child to not act that way so often. But be sure to reward and give the child even more attention at times she has not been harming herself. When possible, get advice from a child psychologist.

STRANGE BEHAVIOR

Children with different disabilities sometimes develop unusual habits or patterns of behavior. This is especially true for retarded or brain-damaged children who may be confused or frightened because they have difficulty understanding what goes on around them.

In helping children through such difficulties, first try to understand what might 'trigger' or be the cause of the behavior. For example:

Rocking

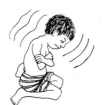

"Joel often starts rocking back and forth, and seems to escape into his own world! He then shows no interest in anything that is happening around him. Sometimes he rocks for almost an hour."

"When does this happen most?"

"Mainly when he is with a group of other children, or when there are guests. But sometimes when he's just alone."

Joel seems to withdraw into his world of rocking when things get too confusing, frightening, or even boring, for him. To stop rocking he may need to be helped, little by little, to discover that interaction and play with other persons and things can be enjoyable. But to avoid confusing and frustrating him, new people, toys, and activities will need to be introduced gently, a little at a time, by the persons he knows and trusts most. You might praise or reward him when he smiles or shows any interest in playing with other children, or with new toys. When he starts to rock, try to interest him in things you know he likes. (But make sure to spend **more time doing things he likes with him when he is not rocking.** Otherwise you will be encouraging him to rock more often to get your attention.)

Eye poking

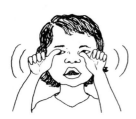

"My 5-year-old daughter, Judy, is blind and somewhat retarded. She has a habit of poking her fingers deep into her eyes. As a result, her eyes often get infected."

For Judy, who lives in the dark, life is not always very interesting. She cannot see things to play with. When she tries to explore, she bumps into things. She has found that poking her eyes causes flashes of light, so she has made a game of this. Also, she has discovered that when she pokes her eyes her mother comes running. Sometimes mother slaps her hands, but at least she gets attention!

For Judy to learn not to poke her eyes, she will need a lot of help to find things to do that are more interesting and rewarding:

- toys that have interesting shapes and surfaces and that make different sounds.
- perhaps her own 'space' or part of the house where everything is always kept in the same place so she can learn her way around and find her toys. (See Chapter 30 on blindness.)
- giving her more attention and praise when she does not rub her eyes than when she does.

———————●———————

Whenever your child develops behavior that you have trouble understanding, it may help to ask: **What does the child gain from the behavior? What are his alternatives and in what way do they offer him less reward?** And, **how can we help provide alternatives that are more rewarding to him?**

'Learning Disabilities' in Children with Normal Intelligence

Some children, whose minds in most ways seem quick and normal, have difficulty learning or remembering certain things.

For example, a child may have great difficulty learning to read, often mixing up certain words, letters or numbers. Or he may have trouble remembering names of persons, things or places. These 'blocks' to learning may happen in a child who is as intelligent, or even more intelligent, than most children the same age.

In developed countries at least one child in 30 is thought to have a learning *disability.* In poor countries nobody knows how many. Any child who in the first years of life seems to develop abilities and understanding

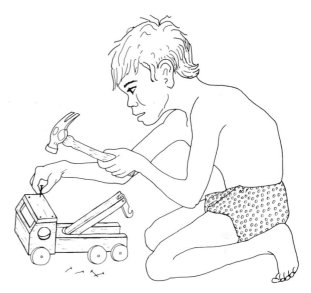

The child who has difficulty learning or remembering certain things may show unusual skills or talents in other ways. In some ways, he may prove to be more intelligent than average.

about as quickly as other young children, yet at a certain age begins to show difficulty learning or remembering certain things, may have this kind of 'special learning disability' (or call it what you like). Often these children are unusually active, have a hard time sitting still, or may develop certain *behavior* problems.

WHAT TO DO

- These children (even more than most) have a great need for love, understanding, and appreciation of the things they do well.

- It is very important not to treat these children as stupid or 'retarded'. **Praise the child and try to help her** develop in areas where she shows interest or ability.

- Often the best way to help a child learn in the area where she has special difficulty is to introduce it, little by little, through activities the child likes and can do well.

For example, a child who has difficulty learning and using numbers, but likes building things, can gradually begin to take measurements for cutting and shaping the pieces for the things he builds.

- Do not blame, scold or punish the child for not learning, or for 'not trying'. This may only make things worse. A child can easily become frustrated with her special learning difficulty. Trying to force or shame her into learning can make her more restless, angry, or rebellious. Some children will not admit to themselves and others that they have trouble learning something. Instead they hide their difficulty by pretending they do not want to learn. Thus a child who has a special learning disability may be mistaken for one who is simply stubborn, lazy or a trouble-maker. The child may become defensive and uncooperative. You will need to show a lot of understanding, patience, and proof of your respect for the child in order to win his trust and cooperation. But after trust and respect are established, he may become as eager and considerate as he was stubborn and troublesome before.

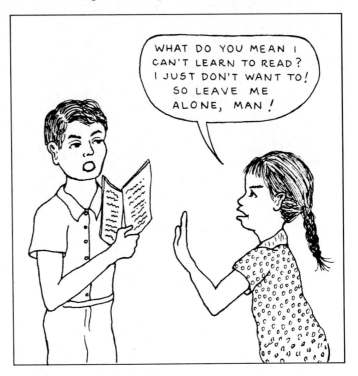

- Special help with learning may be needed. It often works best to move forward in small steps, with much repetition, so that the child finds it easier and gains confidence. (See Chapter 34.) Make study periods short and mix them with activities that the child likes. And of course, try to make learning fun.

- Let the child learn, and use what she learns, at her own speed. Do not hurry her. Help her to relax. It has been found that when children who have difficulty with reading or writing are given all the time they need to take tests, they often do as well as other students.

- Some very intelligent children never learn to read or write. Some of these children, if given a chance to study with the help of tape recorders or other means, have completed university degrees. Others have preferred to leave school and learn other skills. Many have become leaders in their communities or work places. What is important is to help and encourage these children to develop in the areas where they are strongest.

WARNING: Some doctors are quick to treat learning disabilities with medicines—especially when the children are very active. **Use of medicine is often not helpful, and may do more harm than good.** Try to get advice from several experienced persons before giving any medicines.

Range-of-Motion and Other Exercises

All children need exercise to keep their bodies strong, flexible, and healthy. Most village children get all the exercise they need through ordinary daily activity: **crawling, walking, running, climbing, playing games, lifting things, carrying the baby,** and **helping with work** in the house and farm.

As much as is possible, disabled children should get their exercise in these same ways. However, sometimes a child's *disability* does not let him use or move his body, or parts of it, well enough to get the exercise he needs. *Muscles* that are not used regularly grow weak. Joints that are not moved through their full range of motion get stiff and can no longer be completely straightened or bent (see Chapter 8 on *contractures*). So we need to make sure that the disabled child uses and keeps strong whatever muscles he has, and that he moves all the parts of his body through their full range of motion. Sometimes a child may need help with these exercises. But as much as possible, he should be encouraged to do them himself, in ways that are useful and fun.

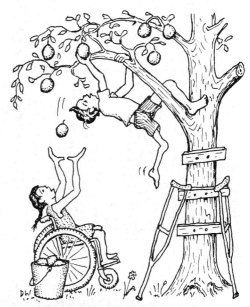

As much as possible, disabled children should get their exercise in ways that are useful and fun!

Different exercises for different needs

Different kinds of exercises are needed to meet the special needs of different children. On the next two pages we give an example of each kind of exercise. Then we look at some of the different exercises in more detail.

Purpose of exercise	Kind of exercise	Pages with good examples
To maintain or increase joint motion	1. range-of-motion exercises (ROM)	224, 368, 378
	2. stretching exercises	83, 368, 383
To maintain or increase strength	3. strengthening exercise **with motion:** exercises that work the muscles and move the joint against resistance	368, 378, 388
	4. strengthening exercises **without motion:** exercises that work the muscles without moving the joint	140, 141, 368
To improve position	5. practice at holding things or doing things in good positions	96, 149, 164
To improve control	6. practice doing certain movements and actions, to improve balance or control	306, 325, 369

DIFFERENT KINDS OF EXERCISES AND WHEN TO USE THEM

1. Range-of-motion exercises (ROM)

Ram is 2 years old. Two weeks ago he became sick with polio and both legs became *paralyzed*.

Ram needs range-of-motion exercises **to keep the full motion of his joints,** so they will not develop contractures (see p. 370).

At least 2 times a day, his mother slowly bends, straightens, and moves all the joints as far as they normally go.

All these are exercises for his knee. For other ROM exercises he needs, see p. 378 to 381.

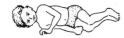
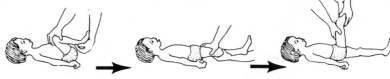

2. Stretching exercises

Lola, who is now 4, had polio at age 2. She did not have any exercises to keep the range of motion in her joints, and now she has severe **contractures** especially of the knees.

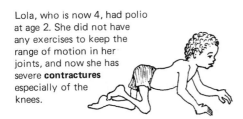

Lola's mother does stretching exercises several times a day, **to straighten the joints a little more each day.** Stretching exercises are like ROM exercises, but the joint is held with firm, steady pressure in a position that slowly stretches it.

3. Strengthening exercises with motion

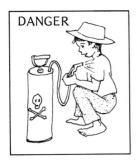

DANGER

Chon was 6 years old when he got his clothes and body wet with a poison his father used to kill weeds. A week later his legs became so weak he could not stand. Now, 2 months have passed, and Chon is a little stronger. But he still falls when he tries to stand.

To help strengthen the weak muscles in his thighs, Chon can raise and lower his leg like this—first without added weight and later with a sandbag on his ankle. As his leg gets stronger the weight can be increased.

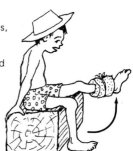

4. Strengthening exercises without motion

Clara, who is 9 years old, has a very painful knee. It hurts her to move it and her thigh muscles have become so weak she cannot stand on the leg. She cannot do exercises like Chon does because it hurts her knee too much.

But Clara can do exercises to strengthen her leg without moving her knee. She holds it straight and tightens the muscles in her thigh.

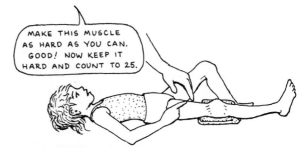

MAKE THIS MUSCLE AS HARD AS YOU CAN. GOOD! NOW KEEP IT HARD AND COUNT TO 25.

For more information on 'exercises without motion', see p. 140.

5. Exercises to improve position

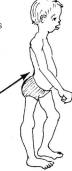

Ernesto is 8 years old and has early signs of muscular dystrophy. Among other problems, he is developing a swayback.

Ask Ernesto to stand against a wall and to pull in his stomach so that his lower back comes as close to the wall as possible. Ask him to try to always stand that way, and praise him when he does.

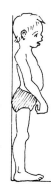

Because swayback is often partly caused by weak stomach muscles, strengthening the stomach muscles by doing 'sit-ups' may also help. See if Ernesto can still do sit-ups—at least part way, and have him do them twice a day.

It is best to do sit-ups with the knees bent. (With legs straight, the hip-bending muscles may do more work than the stomach muscles.)

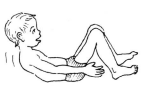

6. Exercises to improve balance and control

Celia is 3 and still cannot walk without being held up. She has poor balance. Many exercises and activities might help her improve her balance and control of her body. Here are 2 ideas for different stages in her development. For other possibilities, see Chapter 35 on Early Stimulation.

Play games with her to see if she can lift one leg, and then the other.

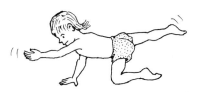

This will help her shift her weight from side to side and keep her balance.

After Celia has learned to walk alone, if she still seems unsteady, walking on a log or narrow board may help her to improve her balance.

COMBINED EXERCISES

Often several kinds of exercises, involving different parts of the body, can be done through one activity—often an ordinary activity that children enjoy.

For example, Kim, who is 8 years old, had polio as a baby. His right leg is weak, his knee does not quite straighten, and the heel *cord* of his right foot is getting tight. He is also developing a swayback.

Many of the exercises Kim needs he can do by riding a bicycle.

The biking position helps **improve the position** of his back.

Learning to ride **improves his balance and his control,** so that all parts of his body work smoothly together.

The movement of pedaling gives **range-of-motion** and **stretching** exercises to his knee.

Pushing the pedal down **strengthens** the thigh muscle.

Pushing down on the pedal **stretches** the tight heel cord.

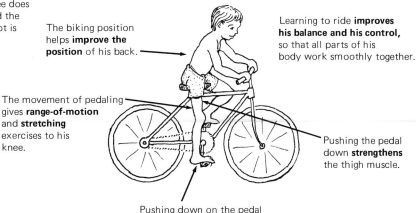

Note: Ordinary activities that exercise the whole body, like riding a bicycle or swimming, can provide many of the exercises that a child needs. But sometimes specific exercises using special methods are needed. Some special exercises are included in this chapter.

RANGE-OF-MOTION (ROM) EXERCISES

What are they?

Range-of-motion exercises are regularly repeated exercises that straighten or bend one or more joints of the body and move them in all the directions that a joint normally moves.

Why?

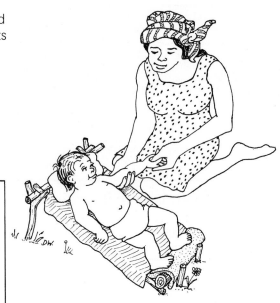

The main purpose of these exercises is to keep the joints flexible. They can help prevent joint stiffness, contractures, and deformities.

> Range-of-motion exercises are especially important for **prevention of joint contractures.** This danger is greatest when paralysis or spasticity causes **'muscle imbalance'**— which means the muscles that pull a joint one way are much stronger than those that should pull it the other way, so that the joint is continuously kept bent or kept straight (see p. 78).

Who should do them?

Range-of-motion exercises are important for:

- babies born with cerebral palsy, spina bifida, club feet, or other conditions that may lead to gradually increasing deformities.

- persons who are so sick, weak, or badly injured that they cannot get out of bed or move their bodies very much.

- persons who have an illness or injury causing damage to the brain or *spinal cord,* including:
  - polio (during and following the original illness)
  - meningitis or encephalitis (*infections* of the brain)
  - spinal cord injury
  - stroke (paralysis from bleeding or blood clot in the brain, mostly in older adults, see *Where There Is No Doctor,* p. 327)

- children with parts of their bodies paralyzed from polio, injury, or other causes, especially when there is muscle imbalance, with risk of contractures.

- children with *progressive* nerve or muscle disease, including muscular dystrophy and leprosy.

- children who have lost part of a *limb* (amputation).

How often?

ROM exercises should usually be done at least 2 times a day. If some joint motion has already been lost and you are trying to get it back, do the exercises more often, and for longer each time.

at least twice a day

When should range-of-motion exercises be started?

Early! Start before any loss in range of motion begins. With gentleness and caution, help a severely ill or recently paralyzed child to do range-of-motion exercises from the first few days. For precautions, see p. 374 to 376. **Starting range-of-motion exercises EARLY can reduce or prevent disability.**

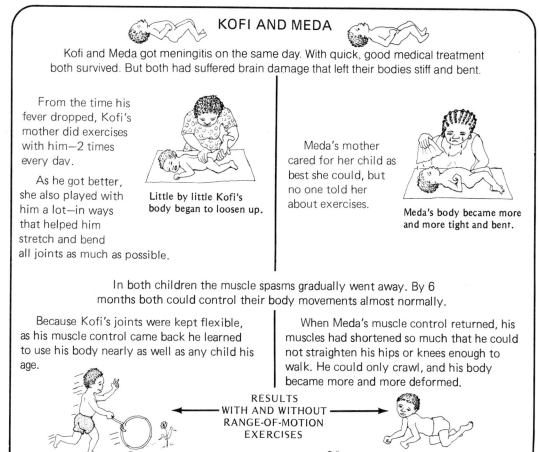

KOFI AND MEDA

Kofi and Meda got meningitis on the same day. With quick, good medical treatment both survived. But both had suffered brain damage that left their bodies stiff and bent.

From the time his fever dropped, Kofi's mother did exercises with him—2 times every day.

As he got better, she also played with him a lot—in ways that helped him stretch and bend all joints as much as possible.

Little by little Kofi's body began to loosen up.

Meda's mother cared for her child as best she could, but no one told her about exercises.

Meda's body became more and more tight and bent.

In both children the muscle spasms gradually went away. By 6 months both could control their body movements almost normally.

Because Kofi's joints were kept flexible, as his muscle control came back he learned to use his body nearly as well as any child his age.

When Meda's muscle control returned, his muscles had shortened so much that he could not straighten his hips or knees enough to walk. He could only crawl, and his body became more and more deformed.

RESULTS WITH AND WITHOUT RANGE-OF-MOTION EXERCISES

It is much easier to prevent these problems than to correct them.

WHY DIDN'T SOMEONE TELL ME SOONER?

For how long should range-of-motion exercises be continued?

To prevent contractures or deformities, **range-of-motion exercises often need to be continued all through life.** Therefore it is important that a child learn to **move the affected parts of his body through their full range of motion as part of work, play, and daily activity.** If the range of motion remains good, and the child seems to be getting enough motion through daily activities, then the exercises can be done less often. Or simply check every few weeks to be sure there is no loss in range of motion.

Which joints?

Exercise all the joints that the child does not move through normal range of motion during her daily activities. For a child who is very ill or newly paralyzed, this may mean **exercising all the joints of the body.** For a child with one paralyzed limb, range-of-motion exercises usually only need to be done with that limb (including the hip or shoulder). Children with arthritis may need range-of-motion exercises in all their joints, including the back, neck, and even jaw and ribs.

GUIDELINES FOR DOING STRETCHING AND RANGE-OF-MOTION EXERCISES

1. When doing these exercises, **consider the position of the whole child,** not just the joint you are moving. For example:

The knee will often straighten more (and you will be stretching different muscles) when the hip is straight,

than when the hip is bent.

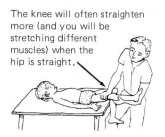
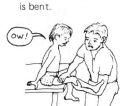
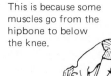

This is because some muscles go from the hipbone to below the knee.

To prove this, try to touch your toes with your knees straight. You will feel the muscles stretch, and the cords tighten here.

In a similar way, movement in the ankle is affected by the position of the knee (see p. 29), and movement of the fingers by the position of the wrist (see p. 375).

2. If the joints are stiff or painful, or cords and muscles are tight, often it helps to **apply heat to the joint and muscles** before beginning to move or stretch them. Heat reduces pain and relaxes tight muscles. Heat can be applied with hot water soaks, a warm bath, or hot wax. For methods, see p. 132 and 133.

For a stiff, painful joint,

apply heat for 10 or 15 minutes

before doing the exercises.
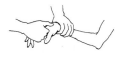

3. **Move the joint SLOWLY through its complete range of motion.**

If the range is not complete, try to stretch it slowly and gently just a little more each time. Do not use force, and stop stretching when it starts to hurt.

Hold the limb in a stretched position while you count to 25.

Then slowly stretch the joint a little more and hold it again for a while.

Continue this way until you have stretched it as far as you can without forcing it or causing much pain.

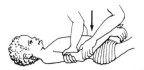
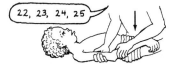
22, 23, 24, 25
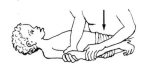

The more often you repeat this, the faster the limb will get straighter.

4. **Have the child herself do as much of the exercise as she can.** Help her only with what she cannot do herself. For example:

Instead of doing the child's range-of-motion exercise for her,

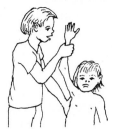

have her do the exercise using her own muscles as much as she can.

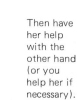

Then have her help with the other hand (or you help her if necessary).

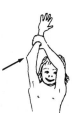

Whenever possible, exercises that help to **maintain or increase joint motion** should also help to **maintain or increase strength.** In other words, **range-of-motion, stretching, and strengthening exercises can often be done together.**

THERE ARE 3 MAIN WAYS OF DOING RANGE-OF-MOTION EXERCISES

1. **Passive exercise.** If the child cannot move the limb at all, either you can do it for him . . .

or he can move the limb through its full range with another part of his body.

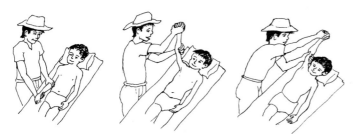

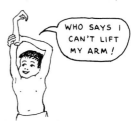

WHO SAYS I CAN'T LIFT MY ARM!

2. **Assisted exercise.** If the child has enough strength to move the affected part of her body a little, have her move it as far as she can. Then help her the rest of the way.

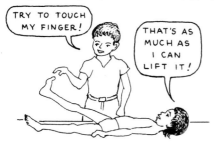

TRY TO TOUCH MY FINGER!

THAT'S AS MUCH AS I CAN LIFT IT!

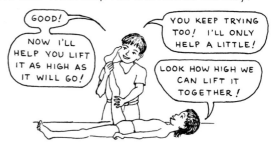

GOOD!

NOW I'LL HELP YOU LIFT IT AS HIGH AS IT WILL GO!

YOU KEEP TRYING TOO! I'LL ONLY HELP A LITTLE!

LOOK HOW HIGH WE CAN LIFT IT TOGETHER!

3. **Active exercise.** If the child has enough strength to move the body part by itself through its full, normal range of motion, then he can do the exercises without assistance, or 'actively'. When the child can do it, **active exercise is usually best, because it also helps maintain or increase strength.**

If muscle strength is poor, have the child move his limb while in a position so that he does not have to lift its weight.

If necessary, support the limb with your hands, in a sling, or on a small roller board.

If he can lift the weight of his limb through its full range of motion, let him exercise in a position to do it. For example, he can lie on his side and lift his leg up sideways.

If he can lift the limb's weight easily, add resistance by pushing against the limb or by tying a sandbag to it. This helps strengthen the muscles for that motion.

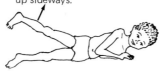

cloth bag filled with sand

As the child gains strength, gradually increase resistance (add more weight).

For many exercises, resistance can be added with **stretch bands.** Cut rubber bands from an old inner tube. The wider the band, the more resistance it will give.

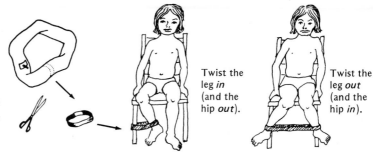

Twist the leg *in* (and the hip *out*).

Twist the leg *out* (and the hip *in*).

This child is doing range-of-motion and strengthening exercises at the same time.

COMMON SENSE *PRECAUTIONS* WHEN DOING EXERCISES

Every child's needs are different. Please do not simply do, or recommend, the same exercises for each child. First THINK about the child's problems and needs, what exercises might help her most, and what could possibly harm her. **Adapt the exercises to the child's needs, and to how she responds.** Here are some important precautions:

1. **Protect the joint.** Weak joints can easily be damaged by stretching exercises, unless care is taken. **Hold the limb both above and below the joint** that you are exercising. And **support as much of the limb as you can.**

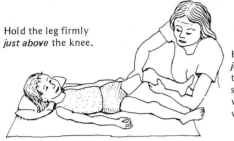

Hold the leg firmly *just above* the knee.

Hold the leg *just below* the knee and support the whole leg with your arm.

Do *not* push directly on the joint.

Do *not* pull far from the knee.

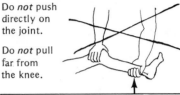

WARNING: Pulling here can dislocate the knee (or break the bone).

(CP) 2. **Be gentle—and move the joints SLOWLY—** especially when a child has spasticity, or when joints are stiff or painful.

WARNING: Moving spastic joints rapidly makes them stiffer. SLOW DOWN!

For example, Teresa has juvenile arthritis and her joints are very painful. She holds them in bent positions that are leading to contractures. Move the joints very slowly and gently, as far as you can without causing too much pain. Straighten them little by little, like this:

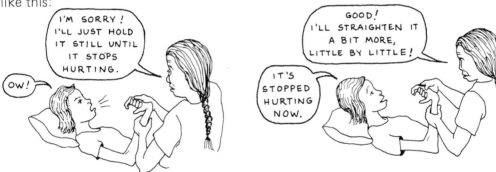

OW!

I'M SORRY! I'LL JUST HOLD IT STILL UNTIL IT STOPS HURTING.

IT'S STOPPED HURTING NOW.

GOOD! I'LL STRAIGHTEN IT A BIT MORE, LITTLE BY LITTLE!

A common mistake is to rapidly move the limb back and forth like the handle of a pump. This does no good and can do harm. **Go slow, with gentle, steady pressure.**

3. **Do no harm.** In children who have recently broken their neck, back, or other bones, or who have serious injuries, exercises should be done with great caution. Be careful not to move the broken or injured part of the body. This may mean that some joints cannot be exercised until the bones have joined or wounds healed. (For broken bones, usually wait 4 to 6 weeks.)

4. **Never force** the motion. Stretching will often cause discomfort, but it should not be very painful. If the child cannot tell you, or does not feel, be extra careful. Feel how tight the cords are to be sure you do not tear them.

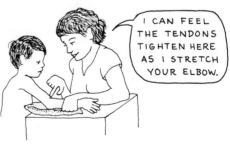

I CAN FEEL THE TENDONS TIGHTEN HERE AS I STRETCH YOUR ELBOW.

5. **Do not do exercises that will increase the range of motion of joints that are 'floppy' or that already bend or straighten more than they should.**

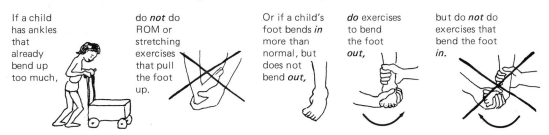

If a child has ankles that already bend up too much, do *not* do ROM or stretching exercises that pull the foot up.

Or if a child's foot bends *in* more than normal, but does not bend *out*, *do* exercises to bend the foot *out*, but do *not* do exercises that bend the foot *in*.

Do exercises in the opposite direction of the deformity or contracture, so that they help to put the joint into a more normal position.

6. Before doing exercises to increase the range of motion in certain joints, **consider whether the increased motion will make it easier for the child to do things.** Sometimes, certain contractures or joint stiffness may actually help a child to do things better.

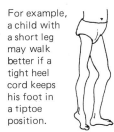

For example, a child with a short leg may walk better if a tight heel cord keeps his foot in a tiptoe position.

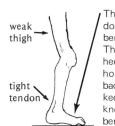

Similarly, a child with paralysis in the thigh muscles may actually walk better if a tight heel cord prevents his foot from bending up. (See p. 530.)

weak thigh

tight tendon

This foot does not bend up. The tight heel cord holds the leg back and keeps the knee from bending.

Stretching exercises to bend the foot up may cause the weak knee to bend when the child tries to walk.

A child with cerebral palsy or arthritis often needs exercises to maintain or improve the movement of the back. However, a child with spinal cord injury or muscular dystrophy may do better if the back is allowed to stay stiff—especially if it is in a fairly good position.

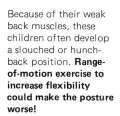

Because of their weak back muscles, these children often develop a slouched or hunch-back position. **Range-of-motion exercise to increase flexibility could make the posture worse!**

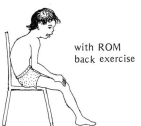

with ROM back exercise

Allowing the child's back to stiffen in a good position may help him to sit straighter.

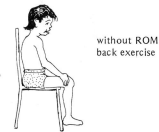

without ROM back exercise

In persons with **quadriplegia** or other paralysis that affects the fingers, **avoid stretching open the fingers with the wrist bent back.**

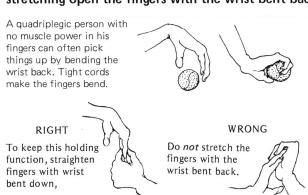

A quadriplegic person with no muscle power in his fingers can often pick things up by bending the wrist back. Tight cords make the fingers bend.

For the same reason, the quadriplegic child should also learn to support herself on her hands with her fingers bent, not straight.

RIGHT

To keep this holding function, straighten fingers with wrist bent down,

WRONG

Do *not* stretch the fingers with the wrist bent back.

RIGHT

WRONG

7. In doing range-of-motion exercises for a stiff neck, caution is needed to make sure the neck bones do not slip and cause damage to the *spinal nerves.* This damage can cause total paralysis or even death. The danger is especially great in persons with arthritis, Down syndrome, or neck injury. **Do not use any force to help the person bend her neck. Let her do it herself, slowly, with many repetitions, and without forcing.**

CP
8. In children with **cerebral palsy,** sometimes the **standard range-of-motion exercises will increase spasticity** and make bending or straightening of a particular joint difficult or impossible. Often the spastic muscles can be relaxed by *positioning* the child in a certain way before trying to exercise the limb. For example:

When a child with spasticity lies straight his back, his head and shoulders may push back. His legs also stiffen and will be hard to bend.

But if we position the child with his back, shoulders, and head bent forward, this helps to relax his stiff legs and will make motion easier.

It may also help to rotate the leg outward before trying to bend the knee.

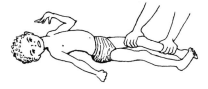

It may be very hard to bend the spastic legs of a child in this position.

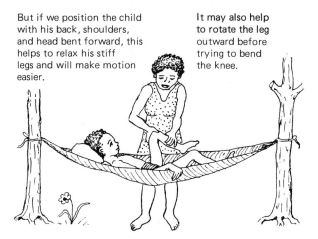

REMEMBER: Fast movements increase spasticity.
Do exercises VERY SLOWLY.

A hammock is good for positioning the child with cerebral palsy who stiffens backward.

CAUTION: **Range-of-motion exercises are very important for many children with spasticity,** but special techniques are needed. More examples of how to relax spasticity are given in Chapter 9 on cerebral palsy. However, you can learn a lot by trying different positions until you find the ones that help relax the spasticity.

9. In joints where there is **muscle imbalance** (see p. 78), **do exercises to strengthen the weaker muscles, not the stronger ones.** This will help to prevent contractures by making the muscle balance more equal.

If the muscles that straighten the knee are weak,

then do exercises that strengthen the weaker side.

Do *not* do exercises that strengthen the stronger side.

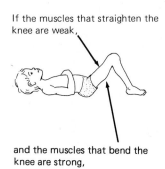

and the muscles that bend the knee are strong,

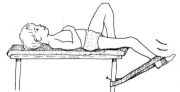

This will make stronger the muscles that straighten the knee. It helps prevent contractures.

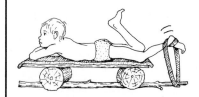

This will make the muscles stronger that bend the knee—and make contractures more likely.

In daily activities, also, look for ways to give weak muscles more exercise than strong ones. This advice is discussed in more detail in Chapter 16 on juvenile arthritis.

IDEAS FOR MAKING EXERCISES FUN

Exercises can quickly become boring, and the child will not want to do them. So turn them into games whenever possible.

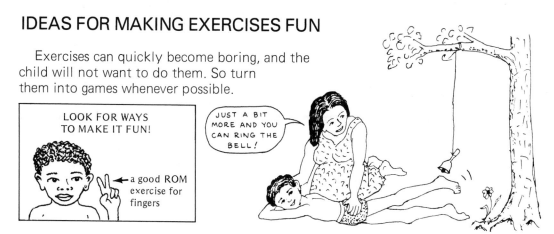

LOOK FOR WAYS TO MAKE IT FUN!

← a good ROM exercise for fingers

JUST A BIT MORE AND YOU CAN RING THE BELL!

One good way is to involve the children in games with other children. Try to think of ways to **adapt games so that they help to stretch the joints and exercise the muscles that most need it.**

A boy with cerebral palsy rolls a ball so that a girl with juvenile arthritis can kick it. This helps her to straighten her knees, and to strengthen the muscles that straighten them.

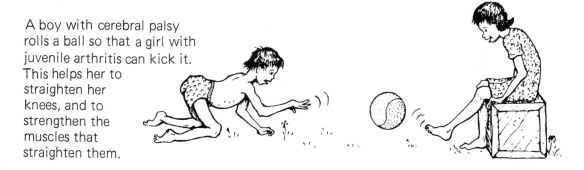

In the picture below, children play ball to help María, a girl with juvenile arthritis, stretch her stiff joints and muscles.

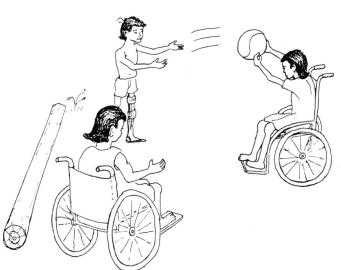

Can you see how the 2 children on the left are helping María with 'range-of-motion' exercises?

Which of María's joints are they exercising?

Answers:

The children form a triangle, so that to catch the ball María has to twist her body to one side, and to throw it she has to twist to the other side. This helps loosen her stiff back and neck. Also, sometimes they throw the ball high so that she has to lift her head and raise her arms high to catch it.

This way María exercises her neck, back, shoulders, elbows, wrists, hands, and fingers. And the play helps her forget the pain of movement—pain that often makes range-of-motion exercises seem like punishment. But this way she has fun.

Complete range-of-motion exercises—upper limbs*

Do these exercises slowly and steadily. Never use force, as this could damage a joint.

Do one joint at a time. Hold the limb steady (stabilize it) with one hand just above the joint, and place your other hand below the joint to move the part through its full range of motion. Here we show the basic exercises only. But remember, try to do them in ways that make it fun!

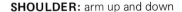

SHOULDER: arm up and down

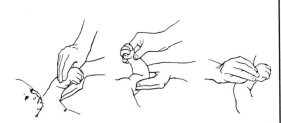

Raise arm straight forward, and up.

Stabilize here.

SHOULDER: arm back and forward

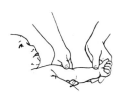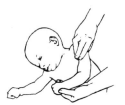

Move arm all the way back,

and then all the way forward over the chest.

SHOULDER: rotation

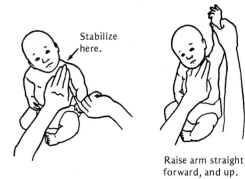

With elbow bent

turn the arm all the way up,

then all the way down.

SHOULDER: out to side

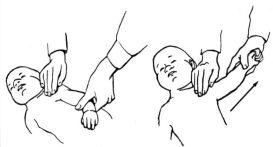

Raise arm straight out to side.

ELBOW: straighten and bend

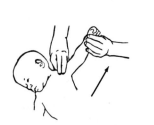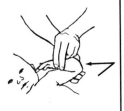

Straighten the arm out from the side,

then bend the elbow to bring hand up to shoulder.

FOREARM: twist

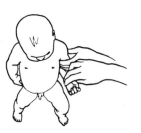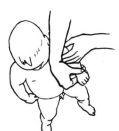

Holding the wrist twist the hand up,

and then twist it down (gently).

*Drawings on pages 378 to 380 are adapted from *Range-of-Motion* by Hewitt/Jaeger. (See p. 640.)

WRIST: up and down

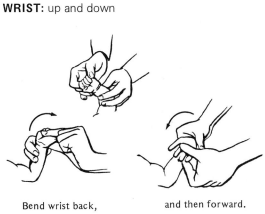

Bend wrist back,   and then forward.

WRIST: side to side

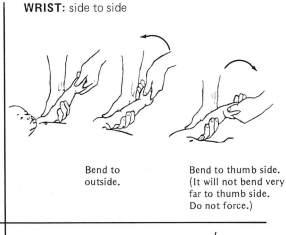

Bend to outside.

Bend to thumb side. (It will not bend very far to thumb side. Do not force.)

FINGERS: close and open

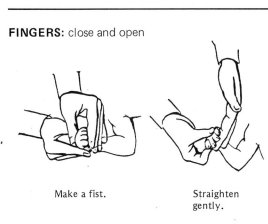

Make a fist.   Straighten gently.

FINGERS: spread

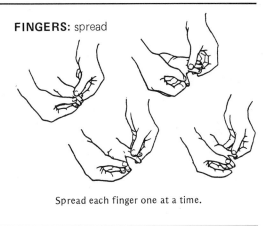

Spread each finger one at a time.

FINGERS: straighten while bent at hand

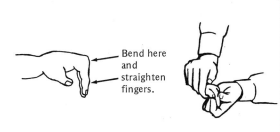

Bend here and straighten fingers.

THUMB: for grasping

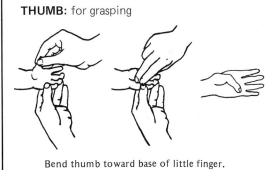

Bend thumb toward base of little finger.

THUMB: shut and open

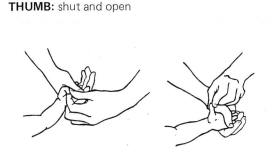

Bend the joints of the thumb in all the way,   then open thumb all the way to the side.

THUMB: up and down

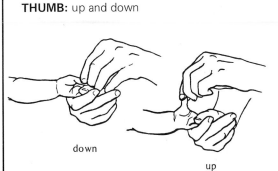

down

up

Move straightened thumb down and then up, with palm flat and fingers open.

Range-of-motion exercises—lower limbs

(Also see the exercise sheets on pages 382 to 386.)

KNEE

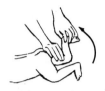

Bring heel back as far as possible,

then straighten leg as much as possible.

HIP: straighten   in an older child
(Also see p. 385.)

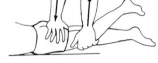

Be sure hip stays flat against a firm surface as you bend leg up.

HIP: bend

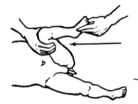

Bend knee to chest.   Straighten all the way.

HIP: spread

leg out   and in

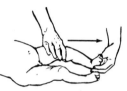

Spread hips open as far as you can by moving leg out to the side.

HIP: twist (rotation) — leg straight

Twist the leg,   not the foot.

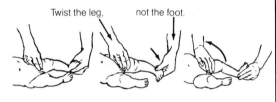

Roll leg and foot to inside,   then to outside.

HIP ROTATION: leg bent

Twist the upper leg,   not the foot.

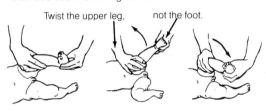

With knee bent,   swing leg out,   then in.

ANKLE AND FOOT: down and up
(Also see p. 83.)

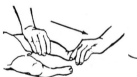
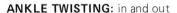

Bend foot down.   Pull heel down and bend foot up.

IMPORTANT: To stretch a tight heel cord, pull heel down as you push foot up.

Pull heel harder than you push on foot—or you may dislocate foot upward instead of stretching the ankle cord and muscles. (See p. 382 and 383.)

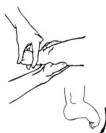

ANKLE TWISTING: in and out

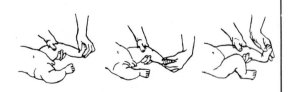

Twist in.   Twist out.

TOES: up and down

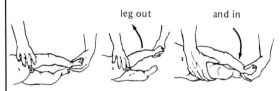
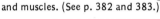
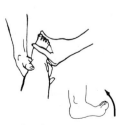

Bend toes up.   Bend toes down.

Range-of-motion exercises — neck and trunk

We show these as active exercises. Usually they should be done by the person himself. If any help is given it should be very gentle, with no force, especially when exercising a stiff neck. (See precaution on p. 376.)

NECK

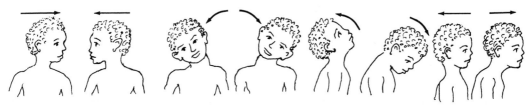

Turn head to left and to right,   side to side,   up and down,   and back and forward.

TRUNK

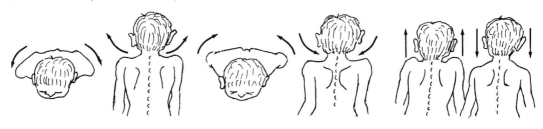

Bend back.   Bend forward.   Bend sideways.   Twist.

UPPER BACK (shoulder blades):

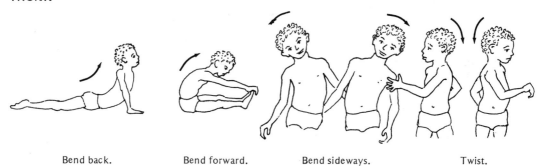

Bringing shoulders forward, pulls the shoulder blades wide apart.   Pulling shoulders back, pushes the shoulder blades close together.   Pull shoulders up toward ears.   Push shoulders down.

RIBS

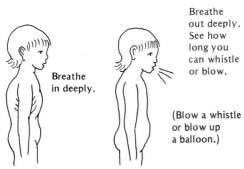

Breathe in deeply.

Breathe out deeply. See how long you can whistle or blow.

(Blow a whistle or blow up a balloon.)

JAW

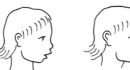

Pull jaw back,   and push forward.   Open mouth wide.

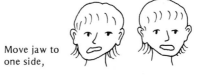

Move jaw to one side,   and then to the other side.

EXERCISE INSTRUCTION SHEETS—For Giving To Parents

If you give the family pictures of the exercises that their child needs, they will be more likely to do them—and do them right.

On the next few pages are samples of **exercise sheets** that you can copy and give to families. They show some of the home exercises that we have found are needed most often.

However, these exercise sheets should not be a substitute for hands-on demonstration and guided practice. Instead, **give them to the family after you teach them how to do the exercises.** In teaching an exercise or activity:

1. First show and explain.

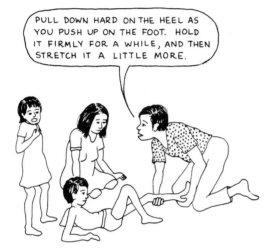

2. Next have the family and child practice until they do it right and understand why.

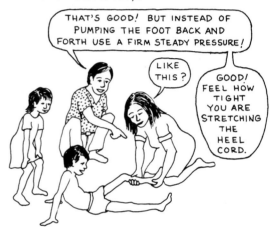

3. Then give her the instruction sheets and explain the main ideas again.

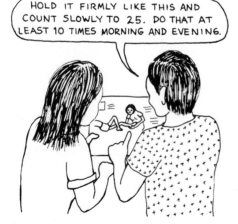

4. For exercises to correct contractures, consider giving the family a 'flexikin'. Show them how to measure and record the child's progress. This lets them 'see' the child's gradual improvement, so they are likely to work harder at the exercises. (See "Flexikins" in Chapter 5.)

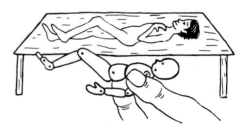

You may want to prepare more sheets showing other exercises, activities, or play ideas that are included in this book. Better still, make sheets showing **exercises and activities in ways that fit your local customs and that help the child to take part in the life of the community.** (See Chapters 1 and 2.)

STRETCHING EXERCISE—TO HELP YOUR CHILD PUT HER FOOT DOWN FLAT (TO CORRECT A 'TIPTOE' CONTRACTURE)

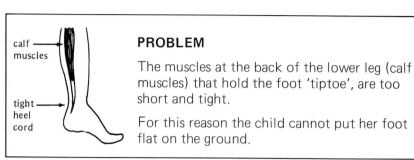

PROBLEM

The muscles at the back of the lower leg (calf muscles) that hold the foot 'tiptoe', are too short and tight.

For this reason the child cannot put her foot flat on the ground.

calf muscles

tight heel cord

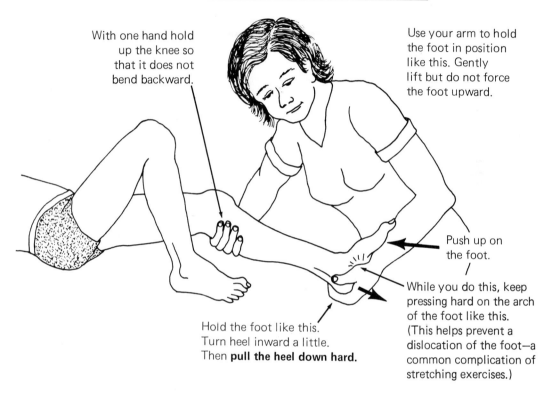

With one hand hold up the knee so that it does not bend backward.

Use your arm to hold the foot in position like this. Gently lift but do not force the foot upward.

Push up on the foot.

While you do this, keep pressing hard on the arch of the foot like this. (This helps prevent a dislocation of the foot—a common complication of stretching exercises.)

Hold the foot like this. Turn heel inward a little. Then **pull the heel down hard.**

Pull down on the heel and push up on the foot, firmly and steadily while counting slowly to 25. Relax, then do it again. Repeat this exercise 10 to 20 times—in the morning, at noon, and in the evening.

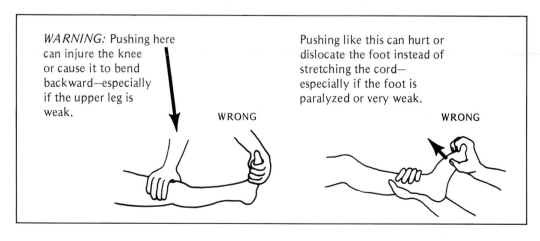

WARNING: Pushing here can injure the knee or cause it to bend backward—especially if the upper leg is weak.

WRONG

Pushing like this can hurt or dislocate the foot instead of stretching the cord—especially if the foot is paralyzed or very weak.

WRONG

STRETCHING EXERCISE—TO STRAIGHTEN A STIFF KNEE (KNEE CONTRACTURE)

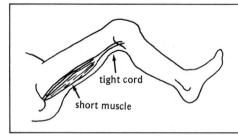

PROBLEM

The muscle and cord here are too short and tight. For this reason the knee will not straighten.

tight cord

short muscle

Ask the child to straighten his knee as much as he can by himself (if he can do it at all). Then help him slowly straighten it as far as it will go.

Both of you keep working to hold the knee as straight as possible while you count slowly to 25. Repeat several times. Do this exercise 3 times a day.

If the foot also has a contracture, try to hold or bend it up while you stretch the cord behind the knee.

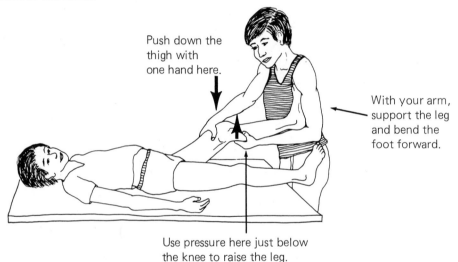

Push down the thigh with one hand here.

With your arm, support the leg and bend the foot forward.

Use pressure here just below the knee to raise the leg.

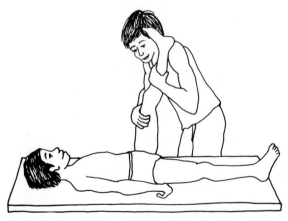

When you get the knee as straight as you can with the hip extended, gradually lift the leg higher, keeping the knee straight.

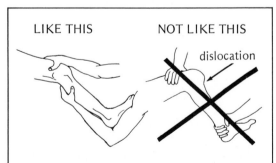

LIKE THIS

NOT LIKE THIS

dislocation

BE CAREFUL. Never try to straighten the leg by pulling the foot. Instead of stretching the cord, this could dislocate the knee or break the leg. The danger is especially great when the leg is very weak or when the child cannot walk.

STRETCHING EXERCISE—FOR A BENT-HIP CONTRACTURE

PROBLEM

The thigh is pulled forward by tight cords and cannot straighten backward.

tight cord →

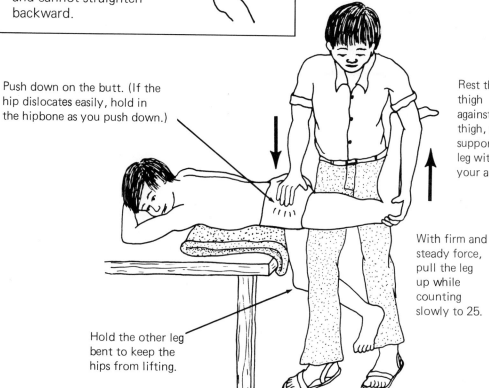

Push down on the butt. (If the hip dislocates easily, hold in the hipbone as you push down.)

Rest the thigh against your thigh, and support the leg with your arm.

With firm and steady force, pull the leg up while counting slowly to 25.

Hold the other leg bent to keep the hips from lifting.

Repeat several times. Do this exercise 3 or more times a day.

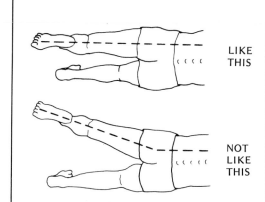

VIEW FROM ABOVE

Do the exercise with the leg in a straight line with the body.

LIKE THIS

NOT LIKE THIS

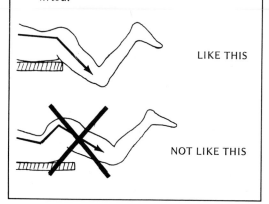

Make sure the hips are against the table and that they do not lift up as the leg is lifted.

LIKE THIS

NOT LIKE THIS

EXERCISES AND POSITIONS TO HELP AVOID PRESSURE SORES AND CONTRACTURES

Children who spend a lot of time lying or sitting, or have lost feeling in their butts, should NOT SPEND ALL DAY SITTING DOWN. This can cause pressure sores, contractures of the hips and knees, and back deformities.

PREVENT THIS   *PREVENT THIS*

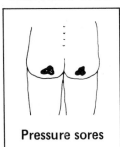

Pressure sores

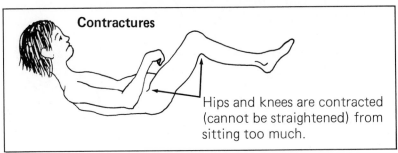

Contractures

Hips and knees are contracted (cannot be straightened) from sitting too much.

When you spend time sitting in a wheelchair (or any chair) lift yourself up with your arms like this and count to 25 every 15 or 20 minutes.

Be sure to use a soft cushion.

Lifting up often is especially important for people who do not have feeling in their butt, so that they do not get sores on their bottom.

Spend a part of the day lying down with your shoulders up like this. (For other designs see p. 199 and 500.)

You can do schoolwork lying down. Try to arrange things with the teacher so that you can spend part of your day lying down.

cushions or foam rubber wedges

BE CAREFUL: To avoid sores, it is important to put foam rubber cushions to protect the body where bones press against skin—especially if you cannot feel in parts of your body.

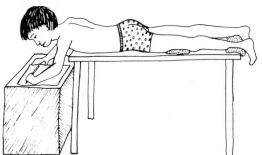

If the child cannot straighten enough to lie on the floor, he can lie on a table, and work or play with his hands at a lower level, as shown here.

EXERCISE FOR A STRAIGHTER BACK

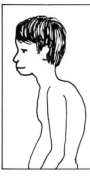

PROBLEM

The upper back bends forward (in older persons this is a common cause of high back pain). Often the shoulders and shoulder blades are also stiff.

Lie face down and move the arms as shown. This helps keep the shoulder blades and upper back flexible.

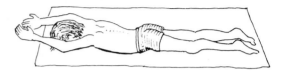

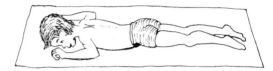

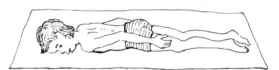

Put a strap around the upper body and bend backward as far as you can.

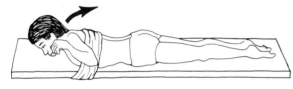

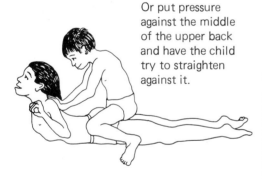

Or put pressure against the middle of the upper back and have the child try to straighten against it.

CAUTION: Bending back like this usually bends the lower back too much and does little or nothing to help straighten the upper back. It may make the problem worse.

NO!

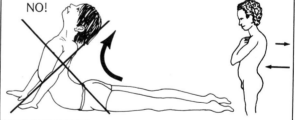

Stay in this position while you count to 25. Do the exercise 2 or 3 times a day.

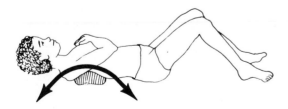

Also, for at least half an hour a day, lie with a rolled up towel or cloth under the middle of the curve in your back. Breathe deeply, and every time you breathe out, try to let your body bend backward over the roll.

Note: Some experts believe that the exercises that bend the back up and back, as shown above, may also help keep a mild sideways curve of the spine (scoliosis) from getting worse. But the exercises will not help much if the curve is severe.

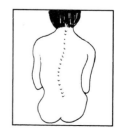

STRENGTHENING EXERCISES—
TO GET ARMS READY TO WALK WITH CRUTCHES

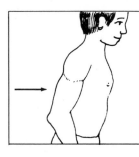

OBJECTIVE

These exercises help make your arms stronger so that you can walk with crutches.

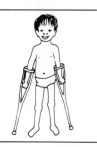

Sit like this and lift yourself up with your arms.

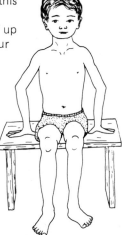

Go up and down until your arms are so tired you cannot lift yourself another time.

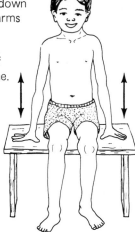

It is better to use bricks or books to lift yourself higher.

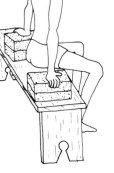

Note: If the child's arms are too short to lift himself up on open hands, he can use his fists.

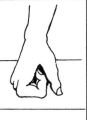

Try to lift yourself with your elbows out, like this,

and not like this.

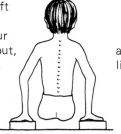

To practice for using crutches, make 'handgrips'.

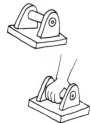

Or use a sawed-off crutch.

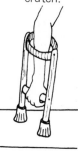

Or you can do these exercises in your wheelchair.

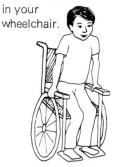

pulley

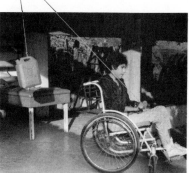

Weight lifting. Increase the weight little by little as the arms get stronger.

Do these exercises 3 or 4 times a day. Every day try to lift yourself more times without resting, until you can do it 50 times.

STRENGTHENING EXERCISES—
TO HELP YOUR CHILD HAVE STRONGER THIGHS

EXERCISE
SHEET
7

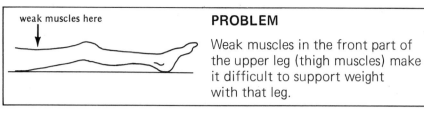

weak muscles here

PROBLEM

Weak muscles in the front part of the upper leg (thigh muscles) make it difficult to support weight with that leg.

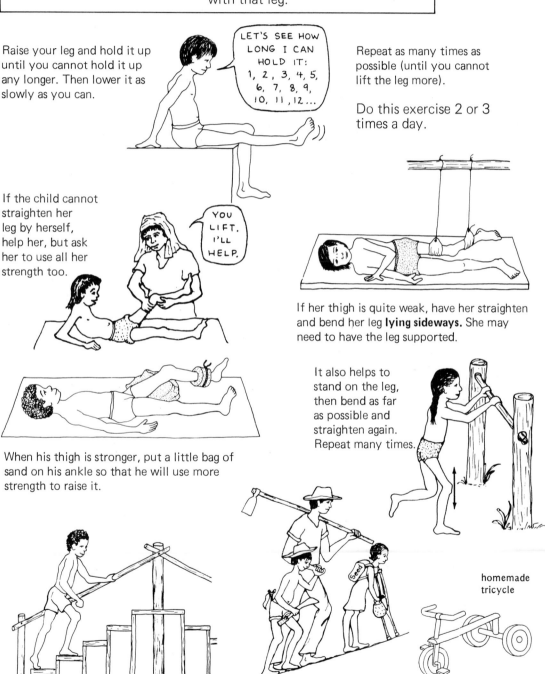

Raise your leg and hold it up until you cannot hold it up any longer. Then lower it as slowly as you can.

LET'S SEE HOW LONG I CAN HOLD IT: 1, 2, 3, 4, 5, 6, 7, 8, 9, 10, 11, 12...

Repeat as many times as possible (until you cannot lift the leg more).

Do this exercise 2 or 3 times a day.

If the child cannot straighten her leg by herself, help her, but ask her to use all her strength too.

YOU LIFT. I'LL HELP.

If her thigh is quite weak, have her straighten and bend her leg **lying sideways.** She may need to have the leg supported.

When his thigh is stronger, put a little bag of sand on his ankle so that he will use more strength to raise it.

It also helps to stand on the leg, then bend as far as possible and straighten again. Repeat many times.

homemade tricycle

If the leg gets strong enough, practice going up and down steps. Start with low steps and slowly progress to higher ones.

Climbing hills or riding a tricycle or bicycle also helps strengthen the thighs.

STRENGTHENING EXERCISE—
FOR THE MUSCLES ON THE SIDE OF THE HIP

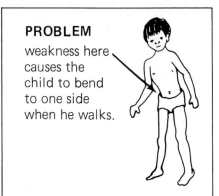

PROBLEM
weakness here
causes the
child to bend
to one side
when he walks.

Lie on your side and raise
your leg as high as you can.

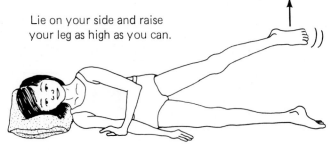

Keep your leg up until you get so tired that
it falls by itself.

If the child cannot raise his leg by
himself, help him a little, but be
sure that he uses as much strength
as he can.

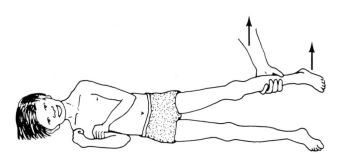

Or have the child
lie on his back and
move his leg to the
side. You can hang
the leg like this
so that he can move
it more easily.

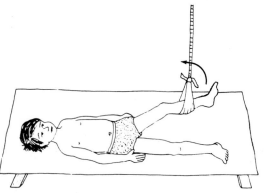

As he gets stronger,
move the rope more to
the other side to
make him work harder.

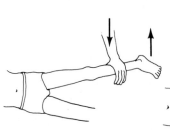

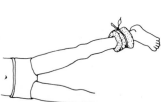

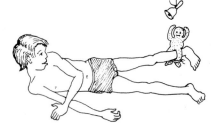

If the child can raise her leg
easily, add weight with your
hand,

or with a little bag of sand.

Think of ways to make the exercises
fun.

Repeat 3 times. Do this 3 times a day.

RANGE-OF-MOTION AND STRENGTHENING EXERCISES— FOR THE HAND AND WRIST

These exercises can help bring back or maintain strength and range of motion of the hand. They are useful after **injuries** (or surgery) to the hand, after **broken arm bones** near the wrist have healed, and for **arthritis,** or partial **paralysis** from any cause (polio, spinal cord injury, stroke).

To do these exercises, the person should move the hand as much as possible without help. Then, if motion is not complete, use another hand to bend and straighten the fingers or wrist as much as possible without **forcing.**

Repeat each exercise 10 to 20 times, at least 2 times every day.

1. Close and spread the fingers as much as possible.

2. Open. Bend like this. Make a fist.

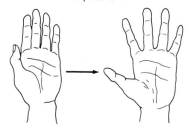

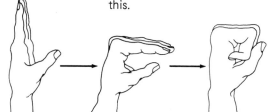

3. Make 'O's with the thumb and each finger.

After you can make the large 'O's, repeat making the 'O' as small as you can.

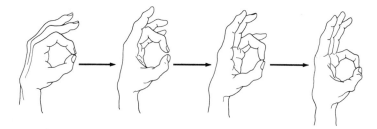

4. Bend wrist forward and backward. (Backward is more difficult but is especially important.)

5. Spread and close the thumb.

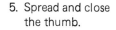

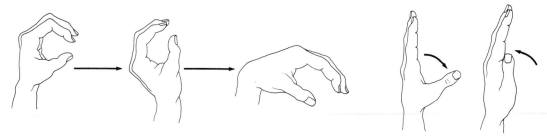

6. Bend the wrist from side to side.

7. Turn hands upward and downward—as far as you can.

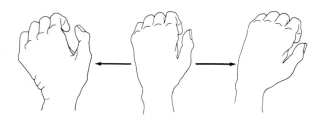

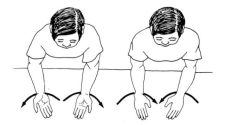

MAKING HAND EXERCISES FUN OR USEFUL

Look for ways to make hand exercises fun.

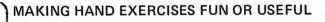

For example, try to learn sign language from a deaf child (see p. 266).

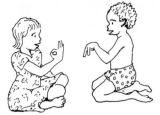

Or play 'shadow puppets' with a light.

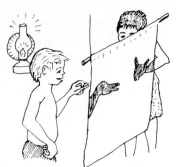

Aids for hand exercise

You can buy a simple hand exerciser like this.

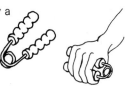

Or make one like this. If the child makes it herself, that will also be good exercise for her hands.

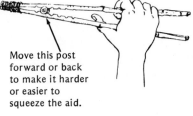

Move this post forward or back to make it harder or easier to squeeze the aid.

This **'acrobatic bear'** is more work to make, but even more fun to exercise and play with.

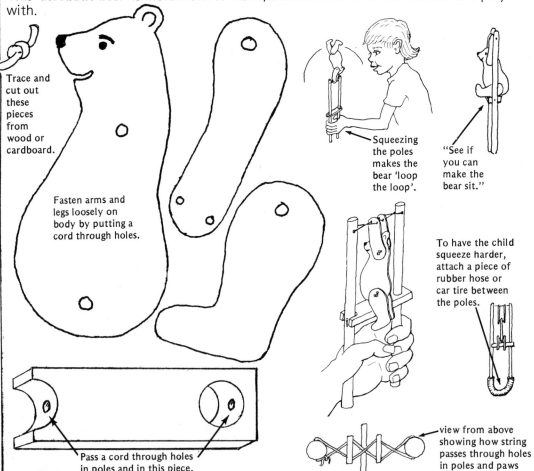

Trace and cut out these pieces from wood or cardboard.

Fasten arms and legs loosely on body by putting a cord through holes.

Squeezing the poles makes the bear 'loop the loop'.

"See if you can make the bear sit."

To have the child squeeze harder, attach a piece of rubber hose or car tire between the poles.

Pass a cord through holes in poles and in this piece.

view from above showing how string passes through holes in poles and paws

A child can also get squeezing exercise with the hands by **milking goats, cutting with scissors or shears, punching holes in leather or paper** with a hand punch (while making things), by **washing and wringing clothes,** and in many other ways.

For examples of how different kinds of exercises are used for different disabilities, look under 'Exercises' in the INDEX.

Crutch Use, Cane Use, and Wheelchair Transfers

CHAPTER 43

USE OF CRUTCHES

MAKING SURE THE CRUTCH FITS THE CHILD

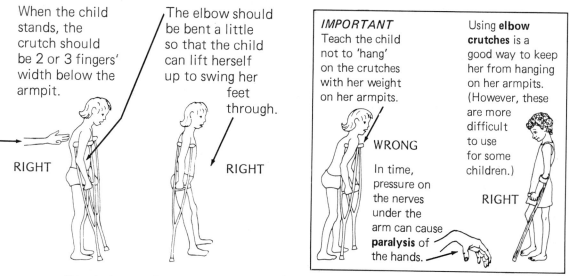

When the child stands, the crutch should be 2 or 3 fingers' width below the armpit.

RIGHT

The elbow should be bent a little so that the child can lift herself up to swing her feet through.

RIGHT

IMPORTANT
Teach the child not to 'hang' on the crutches with her weight on her armpits.

WRONG

In time, pressure on the nerves under the arm can cause **paralysis** of the hands.

Using **elbow crutches** is a good way to keep her from hanging on her armpits. (However, these are more difficult to use for some children.)

RIGHT

For designs and measurements of different crutches, see p. 584 to 586.

Walking with crutches

TAKING STEPS

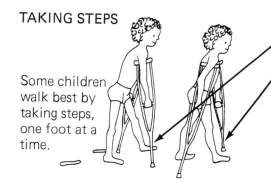

Some children walk best by taking steps, one foot at a time.

For better balance and position, move the right crutch forward together with the left leg, and then the left crutch together with the right leg.

Her 'tracks' should look like this.

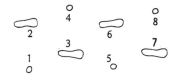

'SWING TO' WALKING

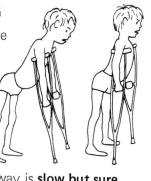

Many children who have difficulty taking steps use crutches by pulling or swinging both feet forward to the level of the crutch tips. Then they advance the crutches and pull themselves forward again. This way is **slow but sure.**

'SWING THROUGH' WALKING

Although at first they may be afraid to try it, many of these children can learn to 'swing through' between their crutches, like this.

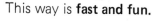

This way is **fast and fun.**

USE OF A CANE

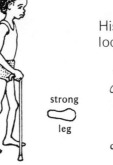

It usually works best to hold the cane on the side opposite the weaker leg.

Move forward and put down the weaker leg and the cane together.

For different crutch and cane designs, see Chapter 63.

His 'tracks' should look like this.

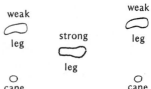

WHEELCHAIR TRANSFERS

Persons who use wheelchairs become much more independent if they can learn to **transfer** (get in and out of their wheelchairs) by themselves, or with limited help. For those who need some help, it is important to find ways to transfer that make it easiest both for the disabled person and the helper.

Too often, as disabled children get bigger and heavier, mothers and fathers hurt their own backs.

Different persons will discover their own 'best way' to transfer with or without help, depending on their own combination of strengths and weaknesses.

Here we give some suggestions of ways to transfer that many people have found to work well.

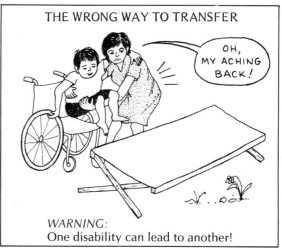

THE WRONG WAY TO TRANSFER

OH, MY ACHING BACK!

WARNING:
One disability can lead to another!

Notice that it is often easier to transfer sideways out of a chair, and also back into it. To transfer sideways, however, a *wheelchair without armrests,* or with at least one **removable armrest,** is needed. Therefore, **for many disabled children, make an effort to get or make wheelchairs without armrests or with removable armrests.** Unfortunately, most wheelchairs in many countries have fixed, often very high, armrests. We therefore will give examples of transfers both with and without armrests.

A good way to transfer the child who needs help is like this.

Put the child's feet on the floor and lean her forward against your body. Have her hold on as best she can.

Lift her like this and swing her onto the bed.

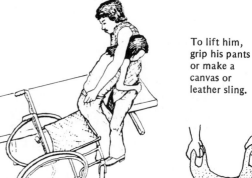

To lift him, grip his pants or make a canvas or leather sling.

Ideas for wheelchair design, adaptation, and use are in Chapters 64, 65, and 66.

Transfer from cot or bed to wheelchair without armrests

CAUTION: Make sure brakes are 'on' and footrests are 'up' out of the way.

To transfer from the wheelchair to the cot, follow the same steps in reverse.

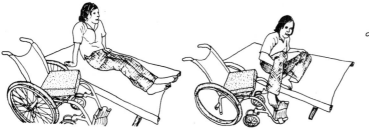

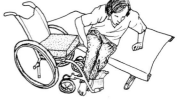

1. Push yourself to a sitting position.

2. Reach under knees one at a time.

3. Move legs so that feet are on the floor.

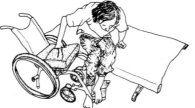

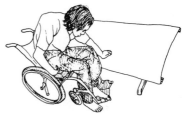

4. Make sure brakes are locked. Then push up on arms while leaning forward with head facing down. Weight should be over knees.

5. Move body into wheelchair.

Transfer from cot or bed to wheelchair with armrests

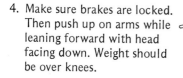

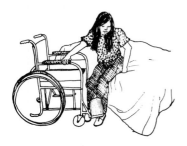

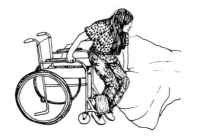

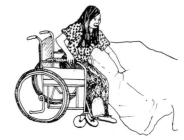

1. Position your wheelchair so that you can swing body past armrests.

2. Place one hand on bed and one on the far armrest. Push yourself up while leaning forward with head down, weight over knees.

3. Swing body into wheelchair.

Transfer forward from wheelchair to cot or bed (often works well for children)

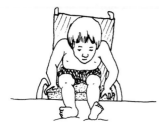

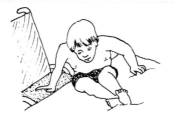

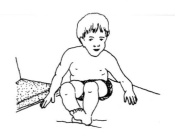

1. Lift feet onto bed and wheel the chair forward against bed. Put on brakes. Then bend forward and lift butt forward on chair.

2. With one hand on the cushion and one on the bed, lift the body sideways onto the bed.

3. Repeated lifts and lifting of legs may be needed.

Transfer with sliding board—without help

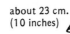 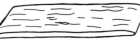

SLIDING BOARD

For getting into
and out of bed,
a car, etc.

about 23 cm.
(10 inches)

round
ends

about 65 cm. (2 feet)

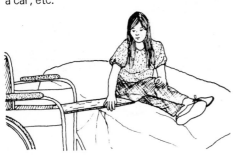 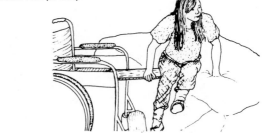

1. Place board under hip by leaning to opposite side or by pulling up leg.

2. Lean forward, with your head and weight over knees.

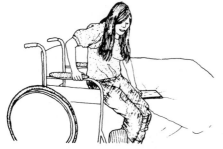 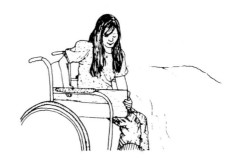

3. Push yourself along the board.

4. When you are in the chair, remove the board and put it where you can easily get it.

Transfer with sliding board—with help

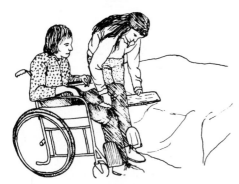 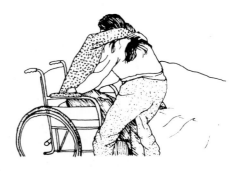

1. Lift leg and put board under hip.

2. Have person put arms around neck (if possible) while you put your hands under his *butt*, or grab his pants.

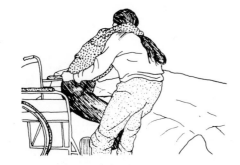 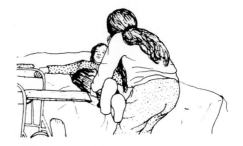

3. Slide the person along board to bed.

4. Lift legs onto bed.

Transfer from floor to wheelchair — with help of a low seat

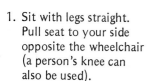
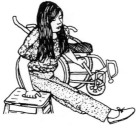
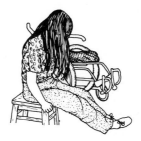
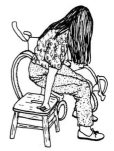

1. Sit with legs straight. Pull seat to your side opposite the wheelchair (a person's knee can also be used).

2. With hands on each chair, push up, with your head forward over knees.

3. Swing onto the seat.

4. Now, with your head forward over your knees, swing body onto the wheelchair.

Transfer from wheelchair to floor — and back again — without help of a stool

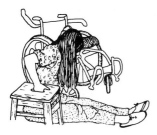

1

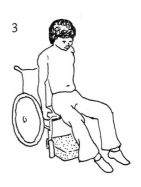

2

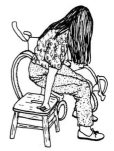

3

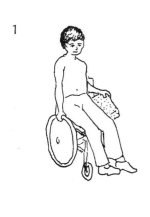

4

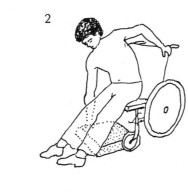

5

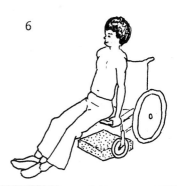

6

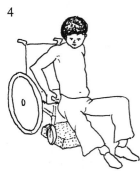

7

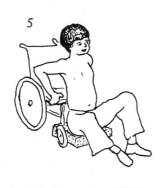

8

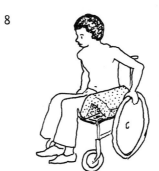

9

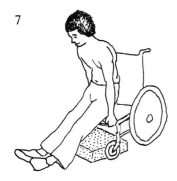

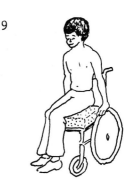

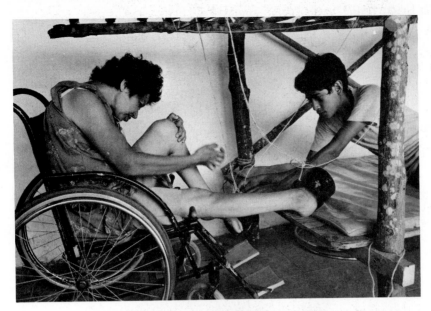

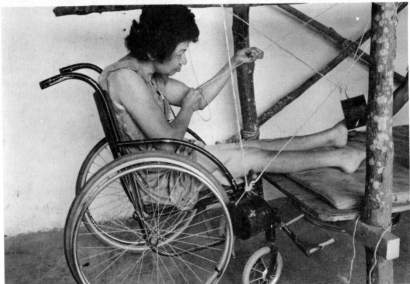

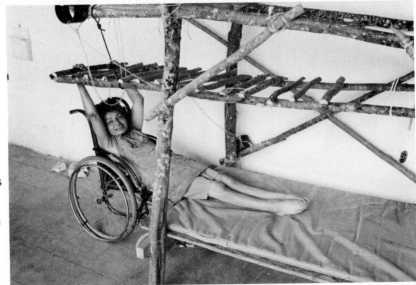

This woman, who has severe spasticity, transfers from wheel-chair to bed using tin cans, ropes, and a wood frame over her bed. (Photo: John Fago, PROJIMO.)

WORKING WITH THE COMMUNITY

Village Involvement in the Rehabilitation, Social Integration, and Rights of Disabled Children

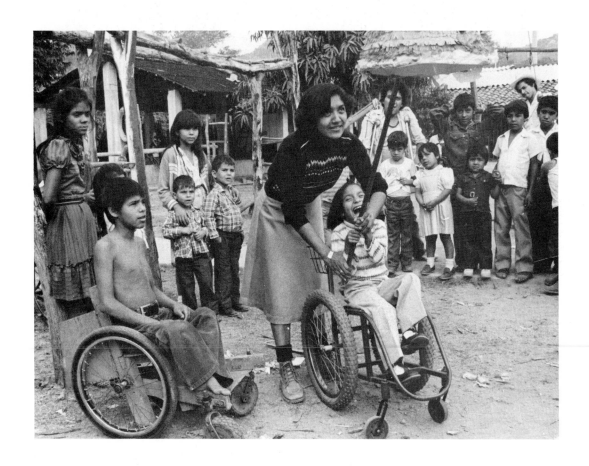

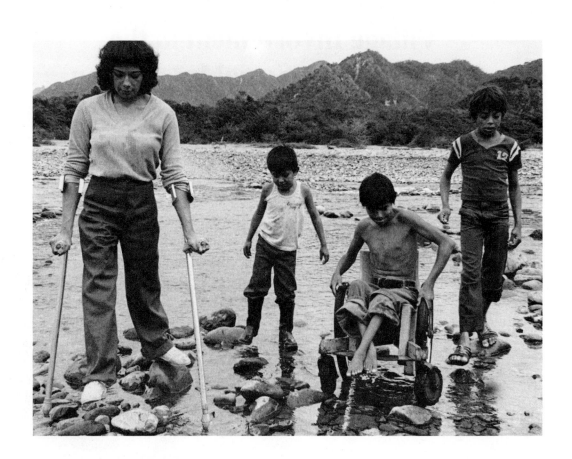

INTRODUCTION TO PART 2

Disabled Children in the Community

In PART 1 of this book, we discussed ways of working with individual children according to their particular disabilities. However, a lot of what can make life better—or more difficult—for a child comes not from the child's disability itself, but from the way that people in the family and community look at and treat the child.

In this part of the book (PART 2) we look at ways to actively involve members of the community—disabled persons, their families, concerned adults, schoolchildren, and others—in meeting the needs of disabled children and in helping them find a meaningful place in the community.

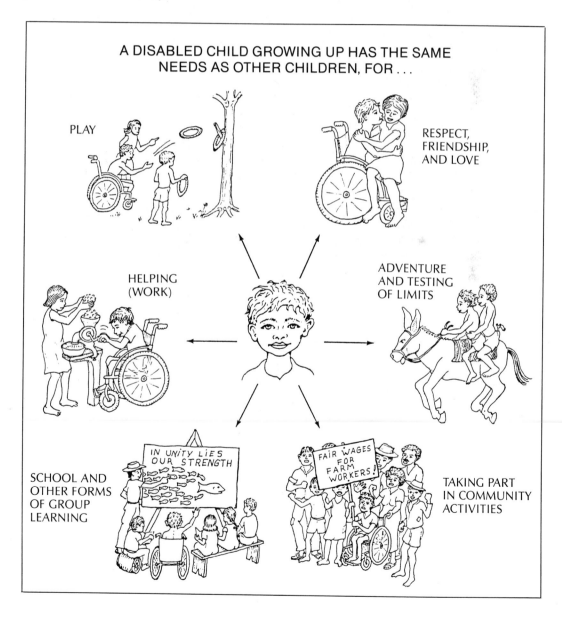

A DISABLED CHILD GROWING UP HAS THE SAME NEEDS AS OTHER CHILDREN, FOR . . .

PLAY

RESPECT, FRIENDSHIP, AND LOVE

HELPING (WORK)

ADVENTURE AND TESTING OF LIMITS

SCHOOL AND OTHER FORMS OF GROUP LEARNING

IN UNITY LIES OUR STRENGTH

FAIR WAGES FOR FARM WORKERS!

TAKING PART IN COMMUNITY ACTIVITIES

In every society, disabled children have the same social needs as other children. They need to be loved and respected. They need to play and explore their world with other children and adults. They need opportunities to develop and use their bodies and minds to their fullest ability, whatever that may be. They need to feel welcome and appreciated by their family and in their community.

Unfortunately, in most villages and neighborhoods, disabled persons—including children—are not given the full chance they deserve. Too often people see in them only **what is wrong** or different without appreciating **what is right.**

DIFFERENT COMMUNITIES REQUIRE DIFFERENT APPROACHES

The way people treat disabled persons differs from family to family, community to community, and country to country.

- **Local beliefs and customs** sometimes cause people to look down on disabled persons. For example, in some places, people believe that children are born disabled or deformed because their parents did something bad, or displeased the gods. Or they may believe that a child was born defective to pay for her sins in an earlier life. In such cases, parents may feel that to correct a deformity or to limit the child's suffering would be to go against the will of the gods.

- **Lack of correct information** often leads to misunderstanding. For example, some people think that *paralysis* caused by polio or cerebral palsy is 'catching' (contagious), so they refuse to let their children go near a paralyzed child.

- In many societies, children who have fits or *mental* illness are said to be possessed by the devil or evil spirits. Such children may be feared, locked up, or beaten.

- **Failure to recognize the value and possibilities of disabled persons** may lead to their being neglected or abandoned. In many countries, parents give their disabled children to their grandparents to bring up. (In return, many of these children when they grow up take devoted care of their aging grandparents.)

- **Fear of what is strange, different, or not understood** explains a lot of people's negative feelings. For example, in communities where polio is common, a child who limps may be well accepted. However, in a community where few children have physical disabilities (or where most who do are kept hidden), the child with a limp may be teased cruelly or avoided by other children.

- **How severe a disability** is often influences whether or not the family or community gives the child a fair chance. In some parts of Africa, children with polio who manage to walk, even with braces or crutches, have a good chance of becoming well accepted into society. The opposite is true for children who never manage to walk. Even though most could learn important skills with their hands and perhaps become self-sufficient, the majority of non-walkers die in childhood, largely from hunger or neglect.

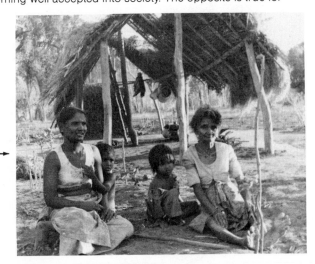

- **Where poverty is extreme,** a child's disability may seem of small importance. When this family in ——→ Sri Lanka was asked about their disabled child, the mother said her biggest worry was that the roof of their hut leaked. The village rehabilitation workers organized neighbors to help build a new roof. Only when the basic needs of food and shelter were met, could the mother give attention to her child's disability.

(Photo: Philip Kgosana, UNICEF, Sri Lanka.)

Overprotection

Certainly not all disabled children are neglected or treated cruelly. In Latin America (where this book was written) a disabled child is often treated by the family with an enormous amount of love and concern. It is common for parents to spend their last peso trying to cure their child, or to buy her vitamins or sweets, even at the cost of hardship for the other children.

Providing too much protection is one of the biggest problems in Latin America and elsewhere. The family does almost everything for the child, and so holds her back from developing skills and learning to care for herself. Even a child with a fairly *mild disability* is often not allowed to play with other children or go to school because her parents fear she will be teased, or unable to do as well as the others.

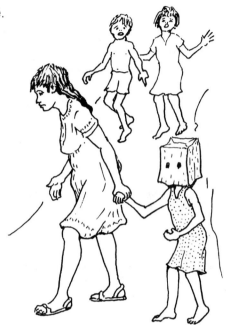

Even in Latin America, where families usually provide loving care for their disabled children, **they often keep them hidden away.** Seldom do you see a disabled child playing in the streets, helping in the marketplace, or working in the fields. Partly because disabled persons are given so little chance to take part in the life of the community, everyone assumes that they cannot—and should not. Disabled children often grow up as outsiders in their own village or neighborhood. They are unable to work, unable to marry and have children, unable even to move about and relate freely to others in the community. This is not because their disabilities prevent them, but because society makes it so difficult.

In one Latin American border town, a mother brought her child to a clinic with her head covered by a paper bag—to hide a deformity of her mouth (cleft lip).

Yet things do not have to be like this. In the village of Ajoya, Mexico, people used to stare at, turn their backs on, or express their sorrow for the occasional disabled child whom they saw. But now things have changed. Ajoya has become the base of a community *rehabilitation* program (PROJIMO) run mainly by disabled young people.

In Ajoya, disabled children and their parents are now comfortable about being seen in public. Non-disabled and disabled children play together in a 'playground for all' built by the village children with their parents' help. The community has helped build special paths and ramps so wheelchair riders can get to the stores, to the village square, in and out of some homes, and to the outdoor movie on Saturday nights.

Mari, a young woman who is paraplegic (paralyzed from the waist down), first came to Ajoya from a neighboring village for rehabilitation. She soon became interested in the village program and decided to stay and become a worker. Today Mari keeps the records, helps interview and advise disabled children and their families, and is learning how to make plastic leg braces. She has become one of the most important members of the PROJIMO team.

But Mari does not want to go back to her own village. "It's depressing there!" she says. "I never go out of the house. I don't want to. The people don't treat me like myself anymore. They don't even treat me like a person. They treat me like a cripple, a nothing. One time I tried to kill myself. But here in Ajoya it's a different world! People treat me just like anybody else. I love it here! And I feel useful."

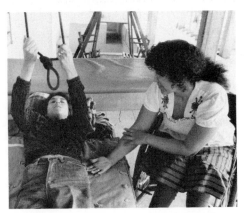

Her fellow team members in the village rehabilitation center are trying to convince Mari to go back sometime to her own village as a rehabilitation worker. They offer to help her change people's attitudes there, too. Mari is still uncertain. But the PROJIMO team has begun to visit Mari's village. Already the families of disabled children there have begun to organize. The village children have helped build a 'playground for all', and adults have built a small 'rehabilitation post' next to it. So, things have begun to change in Mari's village too. The 'different world' has begun to grow and spread.

Mari helps another spinal cord injured girl with her exercises.

In PART 2 of this book we look at ways to help the community respond more favorably to disabled children and their needs. Usually, of course, a village or neighborhood does not decide, on its own account, to offer greater assistance, acceptance, and opportunity to disabled persons and their families. Rather, **disabled persons and their families must begin to work together, to look for resources, and to re-educate both themselves and their community.** Finally—when they gain enough popular understanding and support—they can **insist on their rights.**

The different chapters in PART 2 discuss various approaches and possibilities for bringing about greater understanding of the needs and possibilities of disabled children in their communities. We start by looking at what disabled persons and their families can do for themselves and each other. We look at possibilities for starting a **family-based rehabilitation program,** and the importance of starting **community-directed rehabilitation centers** run by disabled villagers themselves. We explore ways to include village families and school children. Finally, we look at specific needs of the disabled child growing up within the community—needs for group play, schooling, friendships, respect, self-reliance, social activities, ways to earn a living or to serve others; also needs for love, marriage, and family.

EXAMPLES, NOT ADVICE

In this part of the book, which deals with community issues, we will try mostly to give examples rather than advice. When it comes to questions of attitudes, customs, and social processes, advice from any outsider to a particular community or culture can be dangerous. So as you read the experiences and examples given in these pages, do not take them as instructions for action. Use, adapt, or reject them according to the reality of the people, culture, needs, and possibilities within your own village or community.

> **Each community is unique and has its own obstacles and possibilities.**

Starting Village-Based Rehabilitation Activities

CHAPTER 45

TOP-DOWN OR BOTTOM-UP?

Around the world today there are many examples of what have sometimes been called 'community-based rehabilitation programs'. Some of these programs are 'top down'; others are 'bottom up'.

Top-down: Chain of command

Top-down programs or activities are mostly planned, started, organized, and controlled from outside the community: by government, by an international organization, or by distant 'experts'. And the local leaders are usually persons in positions of authority, influence, or power.

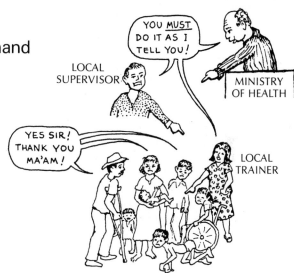

Bottom-up: Equality in decision-making

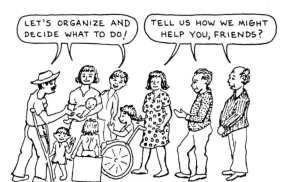

Bottom-up programs or activities are those that are largely started, planned, organized, and controlled locally by members of the community. Much of the leadership and direction comes from those who need and benefit most from the program's activities. In brief, the program is **small, local,** and **'user-organized'**.

Community participation is important to both top-down and bottom-up programs. But it means something different to each:

In top-down programs, people are asked to participate only in ways that have already been decided from above. For example, a decision might be made by a team of foreign specialists that certain persons in each community be selected as 'local supervisors'. The local supervisors are taught several pre-decided 'packages' of cookbook-like information. Each supervisor then instructs a given number of 'local trainers' (family members of the disabled) how they 'must train' each particular disabled person. Thus 'community participation', from the viewpoint of the experts, means 'getting people to do what we decide is good for them'.

In bottom-up programs, 'community participation' means something else. The program develops within a village or neighborhood, according to the needs and wishes of its members. It may take an outsider with some knowledge in rehabilitation and skill in organizing people to help get things started. But it is the people themselves, especially disabled persons and their families, who make the decisions about their own program. They can learn from other programs and from the experts. But they do

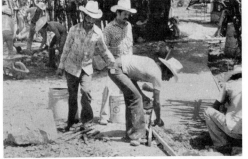

In the village of Ajoya, Mexico, over 60 families participated in building a cement walkway from the rehabilitation center to the main street.

not simply copy or follow others. They pick and choose from whatever advice and information they can get in order to plan activities that fit the needs and possibilities of their particular village, and their particular children.

There are advantages and disadvantages to top-down and bottom-up. For a central government, a standardized, top-down approach is easier to introduce, administer, and *evaluate* in many communities at the same time. But in primary health care, it has become clear that top-down programs frequently fail or have serious weaknesses, mainly because they do not have enough popular leadership, understanding, and personal commitment. These are especially important for rehabilitation. Every disabled child is different and has her unique combination of needs. An imaginative, problem-solving approach is essential. If decisions and plans come pre-packaged from above, rehabilitation measures often do limited good and sometimes even harm.

In a bottom-up approach there is a greater sense of equality, and of arriving at decisions together. People do not just follow instructions. They consider suggestions. They want to know *why.* This greatly increases the chances that exercises, aids, and activities will really fit the individual needs of the child. It also makes rehabilitation more interesting, meaningful, and valuable for all concerned. It helps both parents and children become more independent.

A bottom-up approach to rehabilitation has the advantage of flexibility and adaptability that comes from being organized and controlled locally. **Planning is a continuous learning process** that responds to the changing needs, difficulties, and possibilities within the community. Especially when disabled persons and family members play a leading role, participants at every level are likely to develop a spirit of respect, friendliness, and equality that keeps a program human and worthwhile.

Above all, a bottom-up program organized by those it serves, decentralizes and redistributes power: people who have been powerless begin to find strength through unity. You can never be sure where things may lead, how far people may go in terms of taking charge of their own lives or in demanding their rights.

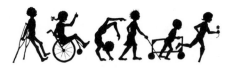

On the following pages we look at community rehabilitation activities and programs from a 'bottom-up' approach in a village situation. This is where our own experience lies. For a different approach with more of the planning from above, we suggest you see the World Health Organization's *Training Disabled Persons In the Community* along with the supplementary materials (see p. 637). For a sharp analysis of different approaches, read Mike Miles' *Where There Is No Rehab Plan* (see p. 641).

STARTING IN A VILLAGE—WHERE TO BEGIN?

Rehabilitation of disabled persons within a village or neighborhood usually has two major goals:

1. To create a situation that allows each disabled person to live as fulfilling, self-reliant, and whole a life as possible, in close relation with other people.

2. To help other people—family, neighbors, school children, members of the community—to accept, respect, feel comfortable with, assist (only where necessary), welcome into their lives, provide equal opportunities for, and appreciate the abilities and possibilities of disabled people.

One of the best ways to bring about better understanding and acceptance of disabled people is to involve both disabled and non-disabled persons in shared activities. The next few chapters discuss selected community activities that can help improve people's understanding and respect for the disabled. These can be introduced either as part of a rehabilitation program, or independently by concerned persons such as parents, school teachers, or religious leaders. Some of these activities, in fact, have proved to be good ways to create interest and open discussion with local people about starting a small community-based program.

There are many possibilities for getting people in a village or neighborhood more actively involved. Often a good way to start is to **call a meeting to bring together disabled persons and family members of the disabled.** Sometimes one or more leaders in the community happen to have a child or close relative who is disabled. These persons, with a little encouragement, may take the lead in organizing other families with disabled children, or in starting a local rehabilitation program.

It makes sense to **start where people express their biggest concern.** For example, in Peshawar, Pakistan, a community program for *retarded* children was started because families of these children expressed a strong need. In Nicaragua, a group of disabled revolutionaries with *spinal cord injuries* started a program to produce low-cost wheelchairs to meet their particular needs. In Mexico, *physically disabled* village health workers started a community program for disabled children and their families. Today, these 3 programs have all expanded their coverage to include a far wider range of disabilities than they started with.

Some children have several disabilities, so it is hard to limit attention only to certain ones. We must try to meet the needs of the whole child, within the family and within the community. However, it often works best to start in a **small and fairly limited way, wherever people are ready.** Let things grow and branch out from there, as new concerns arise and new people become involved.

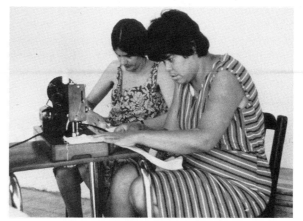

In a community program everyone helps out. Here the mother of a boy with polio sews cloth to form 'stockings' for use under plaster casts.

Who gets things started?

Within a community or neighborhood there will often be persons eager to become involved in starting rehabilitation activities or even a program. All it may take is something to 'spark the idea'. This spark can be in the form of a person, a pamphlet, or even a radio program that triggers people's imaginations with ideas or basic information.

For example, we know of one village medic, herself disabled by polio, who received a WHO magazine with an article on "Rehabilitation for All." As a result, she began to organize the villagers to build a simple rehabilitation playground. In a similar fashion, CHILD-to-child activity sheets have sometimes inspired teachers to conduct activities that help school children to prevent certain disabilities or to behave toward disabled children in a more friendly, welcoming way.

Often, to get things started, it takes a person with some background in rehabilitation and in community work, to stay for a while in a village or neighborhood. Her role is to bring together people with similar needs, helping them to form a plan of action and to obtain the information and special resources they need.

Such a 'resource person' is sometimes called an **'agent of change'**. She need not be a highly-trained professional in rehabilitation or social work. In fact, persons who have professional degrees often have the hardest time accepting that parents and disabled persons can and should be the primary workers and decision makers in a community rehabilitation program.

What is necessary is that the agent of change be someone who respects ordinary people, and is committed to helping them join together to meet their needs and defend their rights.

The agent of change should be a counselor, not a boss; a provider of information and choices, not orders or decisions. Especially when such a person comes from outside the community, her role is to stay in the background, to help the people make their own decisions and run their own program. At all costs she avoids taking charge.

Staying in the background, however, is easier said than done, especially for an agent of change who is deeply committed. To make sure that a program is run by the people, not by outsiders, it is often a good idea that agents of change and any visiting professionals not be present all the time. Instead, they should encourage the program to continue without them. Perhaps the final test of an agent of change's success is to leave the community forever, without her absence being much noticed. These ideas are said beautifully in this old Chinese verse:

> Go in search of Your People:
>   Love Them;
>   Learn from Them;
>   Plan with Them;
>   Serve Them;
>   Begin with what They have;
>   Build on what They know.
>
> But of the best leaders
>   when their task is
>   accomplished,
>   their work is done,
>   The People all remark:
>   "We have done it Ourselves."

To help start a program for the disabled, it often works out better if the agent of change is also disabled. This helps make the *outsider* an *insider.*

Disabled persons as leaders and workers in rehabilitation activities

Some of the most exciting and meaningful community rehabilitation activities in various parts of the world are those that are **led and staffed by disabled persons themselves.** When the leaders and workers in a program are disabled, they can be excellent role models for disabled children and their parents. When they see a team of disabled persons working together productively, doing more to help other people than most able-bodied persons do, and enjoying themselves in the process, it often gives both family and child a new vision and hope for the future. This alone is a big first step toward rehabilitation.

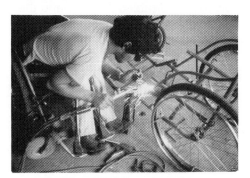

Another reason for recruiting leaders and workers who are mostly disabled persons (or their relatives) is that they are more likely to work with commitment, to give of themselves. From their own experience, they understand the problems, needs, and possibilities of disabled persons. Because they, too, have often suffered rejection, misunderstanding, and unfair treatment by society, they are more likely to become leaders in the struggle for a fairer, more fully human community. Their weakness contributes to their strength.

Disabled workers give an example to disabled children that they can lead a helpful, full life. Polo Leyva, severely disabled by polio, has become a skilled welder and wheelchair maker.

> Examples of community rehabilitation programs run by local disabled persons are in Chapter 55.

Kinds and levels of village-based activities

There is no formula or blueprint for starting a village rehabilitation program. How things get started will depend on various factors: the size of the village, the number and nature of disabled children, the interests and talents of parents and other persons, the resources available, the distance and difficulties for getting specific rehabilitation services elsewhere. Also consider the possibilities for getting assistance (voluntary, if possible) from *physical therapists* and other rehabilitation professionals, craftspersons, health workers, schoolteachers, and others with skills that could be helpful.

If rehabilitation is ever to reach most of the children who need it, **most rehabilitation activities must take place in the home** with the family members as the primary rehabilitation workers. And even where plenty of money and professional services are available, the home and community are still the most appropriate place for most of the rehabilitation of most disabled children.

For home-based rehabilitation to be effective, however, parents need carefully prepared and selected information, friendly encouragement, and assistance. And at times they will need back-up services of rehabilitation and medical workers with different kinds and amounts of skills.

A good arrangement, perhaps, is a **referral chain,** starting with rehabilitation in the home with guidance from a small community center run by local, modestly trained workers. If possible, the center has close links with the nearest low-cost or free *orthopedic* hospital and professionally-run rehabilitation center, to which the relatively few children with disabilities requiring surgery or complex *therapy* can be referred. Outside professionals (*orthotists, therapists,* and others) can help by making periodic teaching visits to village rehabilitation centers. They can also invite village workers to visit and apprentice with them in their city shops and clinics. (*Apprentice* means to learn by helping someone more skilled.)

Some villages will be too small or lack the resources to start their own community rehabilitation center. However, it has been found in several countries that once a modest center in one village opens, the word spreads. Disabled children with family members soon begin arriving from surrounding villages. In time the rehabilitation team may be able to help disabled persons and their families in neighboring villages to organize their own sub-centers. Disabled workers from these sub-centers can learn by 'apprenticing' at the original center.

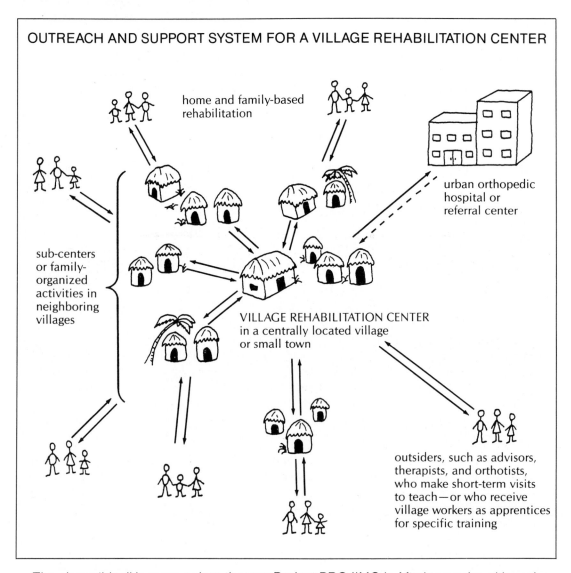

OUTREACH AND SUPPORT SYSTEM FOR A VILLAGE REHABILITATION CENTER

home and family-based rehabilitation

urban orthopedic hospital or referral center

sub-centers or family-organized activities in neighboring villages

VILLAGE REHABILITATION CENTER in a centrally located village or small town

outsiders, such as advisors, therapists, and orthotists, who make short-term visits to teach—or who receive village workers as apprentices for specific training

The above 'ideal' is more or less the way Project PROJIMO in Mexico works, although with certain difficulties and obstacles.

The role of a villager-run rehabilitation center

Some of the most important rehabilitation activities take place with the family in the home. Others take place in the school, the marketplace, the village square, and, when necessary, in the nearest orthopedic hospital. **The key to helping all this happen can be the village rehabilitation center.** (See the next page.)

A village rehabilitation center run by modestly trained disabled workers, together with the families of disabled children, can provide a wide range of services. These may include training and support of families, community activities, non-surgical orthopedic procedures, and making orthopedic and rehabilitation aids. The program need not try to do everything at first, but can start with what seems most important and gradually add new skills and activities as needs and opportunities arise.

Eventually, a community team can gain considerable skill in many areas. For example, the village team of PROJIMO is able to adequately attend the needs of about 90% of the disabled children it sees (except for blind or deaf children for whom its services are still not adequate). Only about 10% need referral to orthopedic hospitals or larger rehabilitation centers. Visiting experts have found that at times the therapy or aids provided by PROJIMO are more helpful than those previously provided to the same children by professionals in the cities.

The chart on the following page gives an idea of possible activities and functions of a village rehabilitation center. It also lists activities of possible 'sub-centers' in neighboring villages, as well as referral and support services needed from urban orthopedic and rehabilitation centers, and outside specialists.

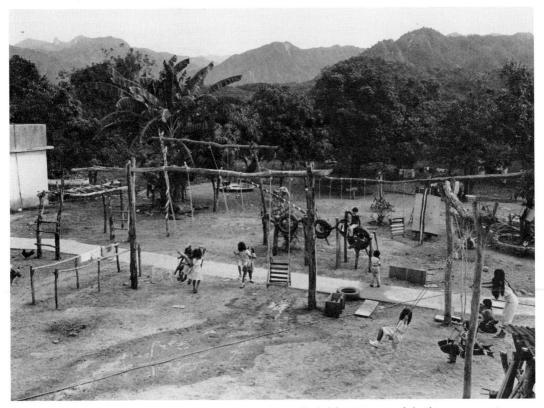

Organizing the community to build a 'playground for all children' is one of the best ways to increase participation and to integrate disabled and non-disabled children in a way that everyone enjoys.

POSSIBLE ACTIVITIES AND FUNCTIONS OF REHABILITATION CENTERS AT DIFFERENT LEVELS

VILLAGE REHABILITATION CENTER
(serving children and their families from a group of villages)

- **all of the activities listed for the sub-centers. And also:**

- family and small group training in basic care, therapy, and development of disabled children (guidelines and advice)

- workshop for making and repairing (and teaching families how to make and repair) orthopedic and rehabilitation aids including:
  - braces
  - crutches
  - walkers
  - special seating
  - wheelchairs
  - artificial limbs
  - special footwear
  - therapy aids

- non-surgical orthopedic procedures (straightening joints with series of casts, etc.)

- arrangements within village to provide room and board for visiting disabled children and family members from neighboring villages

  This may include:
  - village families who are willing to take in visiting families at low cost
  - a 'model home' where visiting families can stay, equipped with low-cost adaptations and equipment for better function and self-care by the disabled
  - coordination, informal training, visits and advice to parent groups or sub-programs in neighboring villages

- workshops and/or agricultural projects where disabled youth can learn income-producing skills to bring in some income to the program or family

- prevention campaigns, for example:
  - *vaccination* against polio and childhood diseases, with special focus on underserved families and communities
  - education campaign against overuse and misuse of injections

- activities to involve and include as much of the community as possible (adults and children) in the program; possibly,
  - help with therapy
  - help with play and entertainment
  - accompany disabled children on outings, help them get to school, etc.
  - village support committee
  - a toy-making workshop where village children make toys for disabled children and also for their little brothers and sisters

- 'outreach' to help start neighboring sub-centers, with provision of training, back-up referral services, and regular visits

Sub-centers in neighboring villages

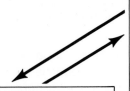

- parent meetings, mutual assistance and shared child care between families of disabled

- playground for all children (disabled and non-disabled)

- group action to get disabled children into school

- special group activities for children who cannot attend normal school

- community awareness raising activities:
  - skits
  - CHILD-to-child
  - involving school-children and villagers in building playground, improving accessibility, making toys and equipment

- organized (group) visits to the village rehabilitation center in the neighboring village

- educational and preventive activities

- perhaps one or more 'village rehabilitation assistants' to help with basic therapy and rehabilitation, under guidance from rehabilitation workers from the village rehabilitation center

Urban orthopedic and rehabilitation referral centers, and **outside specialists**

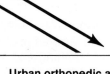
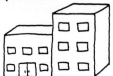

- **referral services for:** orthopedic evaluation, advice and surgery as needed (at low or no cost)

- orthopedic and rehabilitation equipment too complicated to be made at village level

- periodic visits by orthopedic surgeons to village rehabilitation center to evaluate possible surgical needs of selected children

- **short teaching visits** (3 days to 1 month) by visiting specialists (physical therapists, occupational therapists, special teachers, brace makers, limb makers, rehabilitation engineers, etc.) to **teach and advise the village team** (It is important that such visitors play a secondary, background role and not be present all the time, nor take charge or work independently with children.)

- **apprenticeship opportunities:** learning for village workers in the centers of the different specialists

The importance of community-run rehabilitation centers

In an attempt to get the focus of rehabilitation out of big institutions and into the home, some community-based rehabilitation programs have tried to manage without any kind of local rehabilitation centers. 'Local supervisors' make home visits and work directly with the families of the disabled. However, when additional assistance or aids are needed, the local supervisor often has nowhere to turn. She has to send the disabled person to professionals in the city. For reasons of distance, cost, fear, or failure of the support system, these referrals too often do not work out. As a result, rehabilitation is often incomplete, and people get discouraged.

Of course, referral to large city hospitals or centers will still be important for selected individuals. However, there are several **strong arguments in favor of setting up a small village or community-based rehabilitation center run by local concerned persons:**

1. It is a visible, practical, low-cost base for coordinating rehabilitation activities in the home, and for providing back-up services outside the home.

2. It can produce a wide range of rehabilitation equipment and aids quickly and cheaply, using local resources, with participation of families, schoolchildren, and local craftspersons, when possible.

3. It can include a 'playground for all children' and organize activities to encourage understanding and interaction with the disabled.

4. It can provide meaningful work and training experience for local, otherwise often untrained and unemployed disabled persons. It gives the families of disabled children and other villagers the chance to see what a useful, helpful, and rewarding role disabled persons can have in a community.

5. Although the best place for day-to-day rehabilitation is often the home, there are families for whom this may be very difficult. These include families in which one or both parents have left or are dead, or have drinking problems, or where step-parents or other family members are cruel to the child, neglect her, or abuse her sexually (a fairly common problem). In many homes, the family does the best it can. But the extra work of trying to care for a *severely disabled* child may simply be too much for the family that has to work long hours just to survive. Under any of these circumstances, special care at a community center may be of enormous benefit to both the child and the family.

6. If many small community centers join to form a 'network', they can exchange ideas and learn from each other. Or different centers can 'specialize' in producing different supplies or equipment. For example, one village center might make wheelchairs, another toys, and another low-cost plaster bandage for casting. Then different centers or programs can supply each other at low cost.

Home-based rehabilitation often works much better with the help of a local, community-run center.

How small, local programs spread to new villages and areas

Bottom-up programs tend to spread through popular demand. As the news of the program travels from family to family and town to town, even a small program based in a single village can reach far in its impact. For example, Project PROJIMO is based in a village of less than 1000 and has a staff of a dozen disabled villagers. In its first 4 years, PROJIMO has attended to the needs of over 1,000 disabled children from over 100 towns and villages and the slums of several large cities. (Since roughly one child in every 100 people is moderately to severely disabled, PROJIMO is in effect serving a population of over 100,000.)

There are various ways that bottom-up or 'people-centered' programs tend to spread. We speak of their growth as 'organic' because they grow and spread in a living, whole sort of way, like seeds into trees.

In Project PROJIMO, some of the young people from neighboring communities, who first come for rehabilitation, decide to stay and to work for a while in the program. In the process they learn skills which they can use to help in the rehabilitation of other persons when they return to their own communities. In some cases, other villages and village-based health programs have sent young disabled persons to apprentice with PROJIMO for several months, in order to help start similar activities on return to their communities.

Another people-centered program that started small and has spread to many other towns is the Community Rehabilitation Development Program in Peshawar, Pakistan. This is discussed on p. 520.

ACTIVITIES IN THE COMMUNITY TO WIN INTEREST AND UNDERSTANDING

Group activities in a village or neighborhood can help improve understanding of and interaction with the disabled children. Four types of activities that have proved especially useful are discussed in the next 4 chapters:

- **A 'Playground for all children'**
- **CHILD-to-child activities**
- **Popular theater**
- **A children's workshop for making toys**

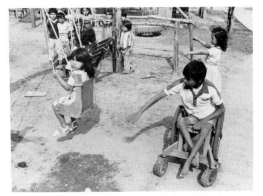

Any of these activities may be used to gain people's interest and involvement when starting a community rehabilitation program. Or they can be used to increase understanding even where no special program is planned. For example, the workers in a village with a rehabilitation center can visit neighboring villages and

Playground for all children—PROJIMO

put on skits or puppet shows about disability prevention. They might also talk with school teachers, local health workers or concerned parents about developing CHILD-to-child activities, or organize local children to build a 'playground for all children'. Project PROJIMO took a truckload of school children to a neighboring village to help the children there build their own playground. Nearly 100 children and adults built the playground in one day.

After these 4 chapters, we will explore other aspects of social integration and opportunities for the disabled.

Playgrounds for All Children

A good way to start a village or neighborhood *rehabilitation* program is to involve the local people in building a low-cost 'rehabilitation playground'. It is important that the playground be built **for use by all children — both *disabled* and non-disabled.**

With a little help from adults, the local children can build most of the playground themselves. To prevent the playground from being destroyed or vandalized, you may wish to invite some of the roughest local children and 'gang leaders' to help lead the project. Or you can appoint them as 'maintenance chiefs'.

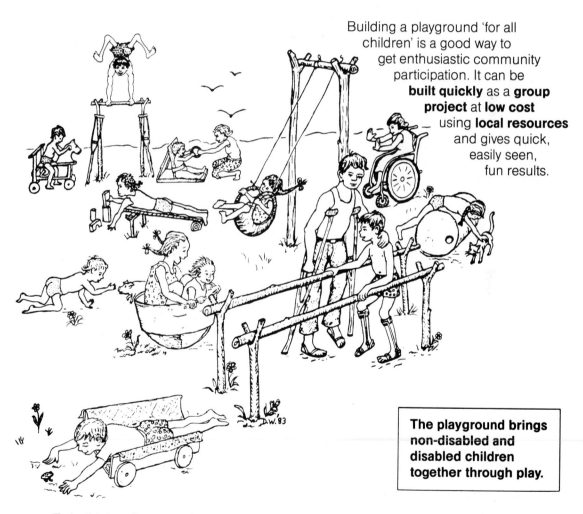

Building a playground 'for all children' is a good way to get enthusiastic community participation. It can be **built quickly** as a **group project** at **low cost** using **local resources** and gives quick, easily seen, fun results.

The playground brings non-disabled and disabled children together through play.

To build the playground, it is best to **use local, low-cost materials,** and **simple construction.** One of the playground's main purposes is to give disabled children and their parents a chance to try different playthings and exercise equipment. Whatever works for their child, a family can easily build at home, at no or low cost. For this reason, a playground made of tree limbs and poles, old tires, and other 'waste' materials is more appropriate than a fancy metal playground built by skilled craftsmen at high cost. (Also, metal gets very hot in hot, sunny climates.)

These pages will give you some ideas for simple playground equipment. Although most of the photos come from PROJIMO in Mexico, many of the ideas shown are based on a playground in Thailand (see p. 425) and on designs by Don Caston (see p. 642).

A 'playground for all' built by children—PROJIMO, Mexico

When disabled village health workers in the small village of Ajoya decided to start a rehabilitation program for disabled children, one of the first activities was to involve the local children in building a playground.

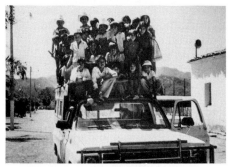

1. First the children went into the forest to cut poles and vines.

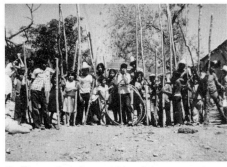

2. These they brought back to an empty lot at the edge of the village.

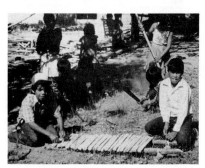

3. While some children cleaned up the lot, others began to build the playground equipment.

4. They built ramps or 'wedges' like this one, which can be used in many ways for play and exercise. Here a child with cerebral palsy walks up the ramp to help improve balance and stretch his feet upwards to prevent **contractures.**

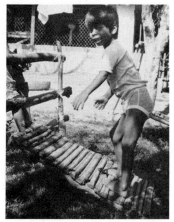

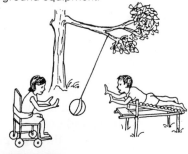

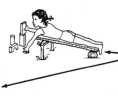

The wedges can also be used for severely disabled children to lie on, so that they can lift their heads and play with their hands.

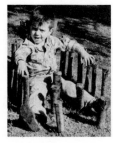

Pole seats like this help a child sit who still lacks balance, or has trouble controlling his position.

These separators will hold apart the legs of a child whose legs pull together (*spasticity*).

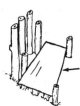

Putting front posts the same height allows a shelf to be placed for play.

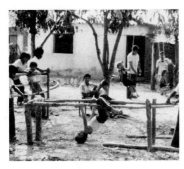

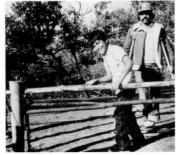

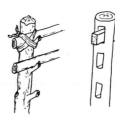

Simple parallel bars can be used as gymnastic bars by the able-bodied children . . .

and as bars for learning to walk by disabled children.

Bars need to adjust to different heights for different children. Here are 2 simple ways.

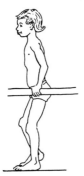

For most children, the bar should be about hip height, so that the elbows are a little bent (the same height as the handles of crutches).

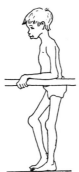

A child with very weak upper arms may find it easier to rest his forearms on the bar. The bar will need to be elbow high.

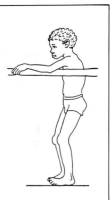

A child who tends to slump forward may be helped to stand straighter if the bar is high, so that he has to stand straighter to rest his arms on it.

SEPARATION OF BARS

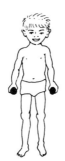

Bars should be close enough to leave only a little room on either side of the child's body. Too close, they get in the way. Too far apart makes weight bearing more difficult.

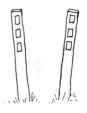

Smaller children require closer bars. Therefore, put uprights so they are wider higher up.

Simple, homemade bars, adjusted to the individual child's needs, often provide more benefit than expensive walkers or other equipment.

TEETER BRIDGE

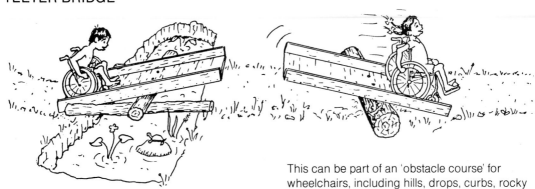

This can be part of an 'obstacle course' for wheelchairs, including hills, drops, curbs, rocky ground, sand pits, and zig-zags between posts.

A simple seesaw or **teeter-totter** like this is fun and helps disabled children gain balance. The one in the photo was made by putting a pole in the crotch of a mango tree.

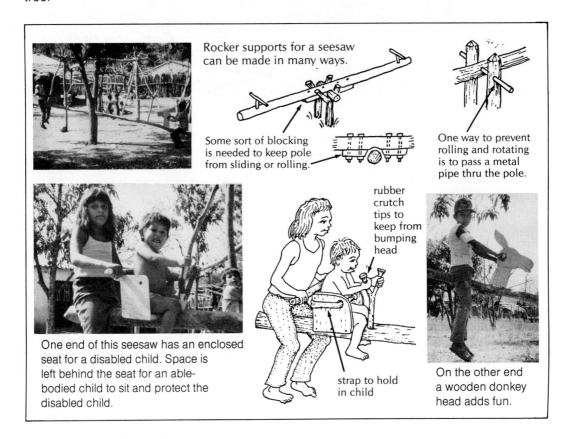

Rocker supports for a seesaw can be made in many ways.

Some sort of blocking is needed to keep pole from sliding or rolling.

One way to prevent rolling and rotating is to pass a metal pipe thru the pole.

rubber crutch tips to keep from bumping head

One end of this seesaw has an enclosed seat for a disabled child. Space is left behind the seat for an able-bodied child to sit and protect the disabled child.

strap to hold in child

On the other end a wooden donkey head adds fun.

Here are some other ideas for seesaws.

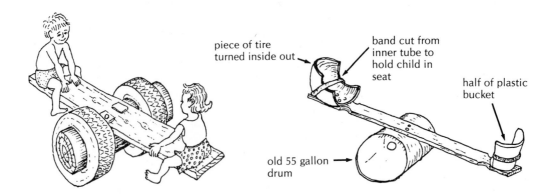

piece of tire turned inside out

band cut from inner tube to hold child in seat

half of plastic bucket

old 55 gallon drum

PRECAUTIONS

1. To avoid accidents, be sure the pole for the seesaw is strong enough. Test it every few weeks by having 2 adults put their full weight on the ends of the pole.

2. To avoid coming down too hard, put old tires under the ends of the seesaw (see p. 425).

3. Make sure the seesaw will not roll lengthwise or sideways (see above).

For another seesaw idea, see p. 425.

CLIMBING FRAME AND HIGH BAR

Children can make a simple climbing frame out of poles, by nailing them or tying them together with string.

The climbing frame can be used for all kinds of play, for helping disabled children pull up to sitting or standing, and for therapy exercise.

High bars (horizontal bars) at different levels for different children can be used for exercise and gymnastics.

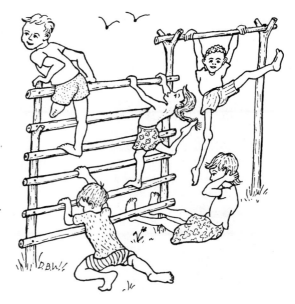

TIRE GYM

Climbing gyms can be made out of many materials, including old tires.

Gym will be more solid if tires are bolted together.

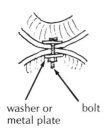

washer or metal plate   bolt

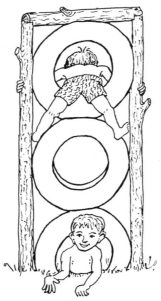

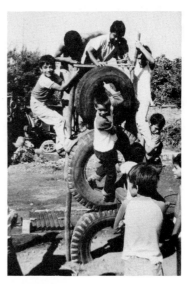

The children in the village of Ajoya, Mexico helped those in a nearby town build their own rehabilitation playground. This tire climbing gym was one of the playthings they created.

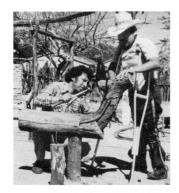

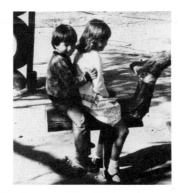

Building and riding a rocking horse made of logs.

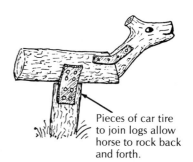

Pieces of car tire to join logs allow horse to rock back and forth.

SWINGS

A wide variety of swings can be built out of different local materials. Swinging is fun; it can help develop balance, head control, coordination, and strength. Swings with special features can be built for the needs of particular children.

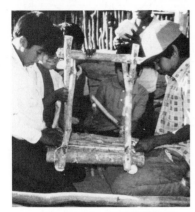

Here children in PROJIMO make an enclosed swing.

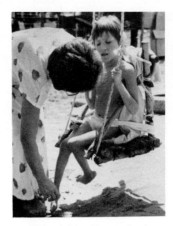

This child with cerebral palsy had never had a chance to swing before. At first he was afraid . . .

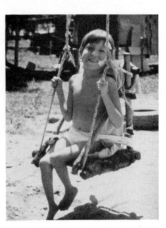

but after a while, he loved it.

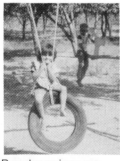

Regular swings are placed next to special and enclosed swings, so that non-disabled and disabled children learn to play side by side.

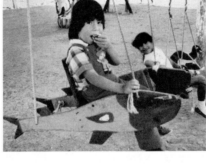

Swings in the form of animals or fish add to the fun.

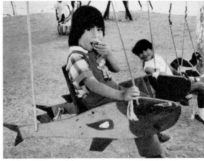

Extra wide swings allow 2 children to swing together— one assisting the other.

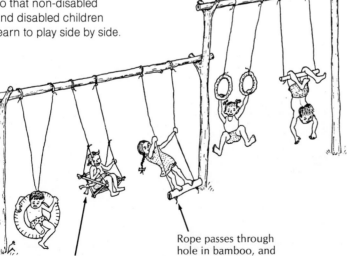

tie to hold child in swing

Rope passes through hole in bamboo, and is knotted.

Rings for swinging and many games can be made by cutting out the inner rims of old car tires.

SWINGS AND PLAYTHINGS USING OLD TIRES AND TUBES

This swing made of an old tire is especially good for children with spasticity because it bends their backs, heads, and shoulders forward.

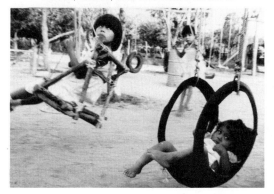

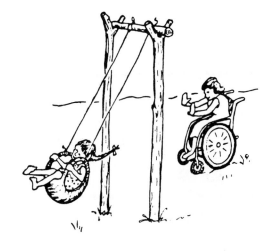

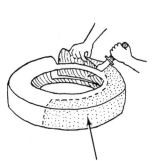

Cut away this part of the tire.

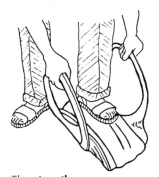

Then **turn the tire inside out.**

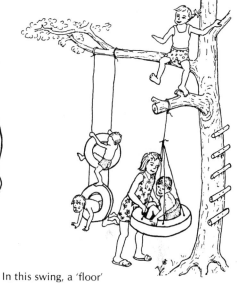

In this swing, a 'floor' of sticks can be put in the tire and covered with straw or a mat.

This **flat-hanging tire** swing is especially useful for the severely disabled or delayed child who is just beginning to learn to move his body. The child can lie across the tire and move this way and that by pushing the ground with his hands.

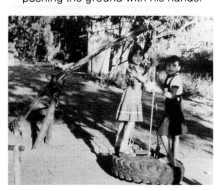

It swings! It spins! It bounces! Fun for the able-bodied! Fun for the disabled! Several children can play on it at once!

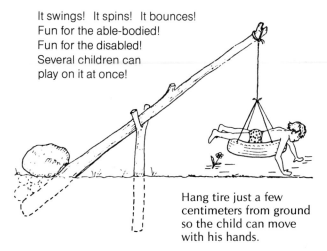

Hang tire just a few centimeters from ground so the child can move with his hands.

WHIRLYGIG CIRCULAR SWING

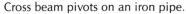

Cross beam pivots on an iron pipe.

Hole in beam is soaked in old motor oil to make it turn around easier.

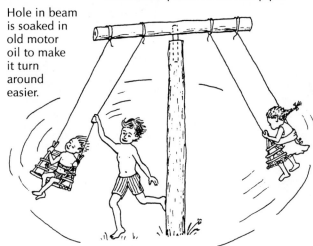

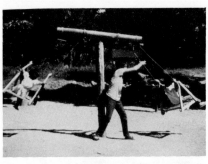

Circular swing in PROJIMO rehabilitation playground. (Here the child pushing the swing has cerebral palsy. The twisting motion he uses is excellent therapy.)

> *CAUTION:* Be sure both the pole and beam are of strong hard wood. Test them occasionally with adults' weight.

BOUNCING TUBE (from *Low Cost Physiotherapy and Low Cost Walking Aids,* see p. 642.)

see p. 642.

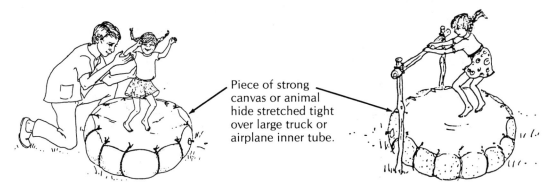

Piece of strong canvas or animal hide stretched tight over large truck or airplane inner tube.

BOUNCING TIRE HOBBY HORSE (OR COW)

loops of car inner tube

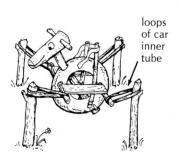

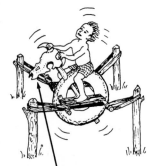

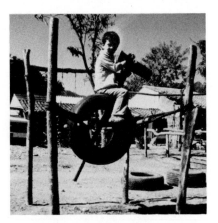

Be sure to notch poles and attach tubes so they do not slip.

A cow's skull makes a good head for many playground toys. The child holds onto the horns. (Cut off the points.)

Note: It is much easier to put holes through tires that do not have steel wire in them.

MAYPOLE

Disabled children who can sit and hang on can play with non-disabled children on the maypole. But to start turning round the circle, they may need another child to help push them.

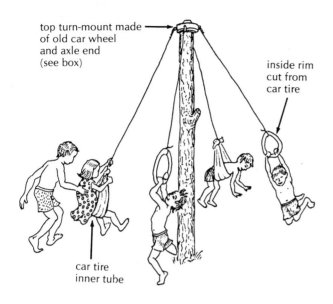

top turn-mount made of old car wheel and axle end (see box)

inside rim cut from car tire

car tire inner tube

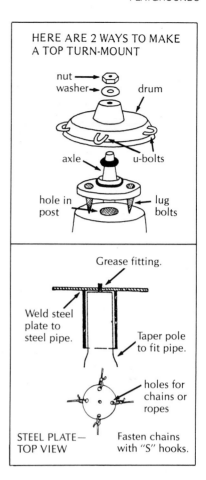

HERE ARE 2 WAYS TO MAKE A TOP TURN-MOUNT

nut
washer
drum
axle
u-bolts
hole in post
lug bolts

Grease fitting.

Weld steel plate to steel pipe.

Taper pole to fit pipe.

holes for chains or ropes

STEEL PLATE— TOP VIEW

Fasten chains with "S" hooks.

HANGING SEESAW SWING

OBSTACLE COURSE

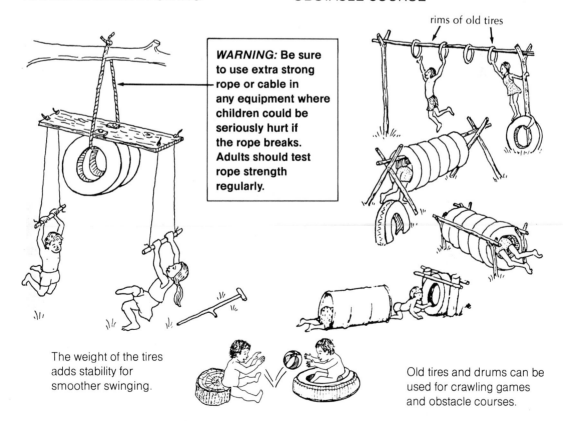

WARNING: Be sure to use extra strong rope or cable in any equipment where children could be seriously hurt if the rope breaks. Adults should test rope strength regularly.

rims of old tires

The weight of the tires adds stability for smoother swinging.

Old tires and drums can be used for crawling games and obstacle courses.

BALANCE BOARDS

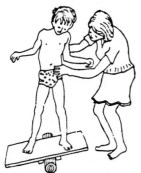

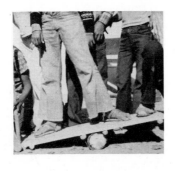

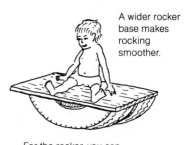

A wider rocker base makes rocking smoother.

For the rocker, you can use 2 pieces of old tire.

For more balance boards and balance beams, see p. 576.

ROLLS

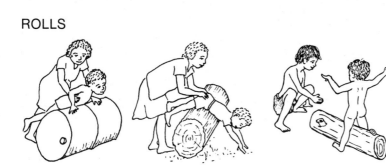

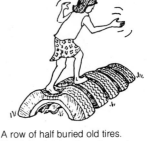

A row of half buried old tires. The tires sink in when stepped on. A test of balance and great fun!

Old barrels, oil drums, paint cans, and logs make good playground equipment—for therapy and fun.

CRAWL-THROUGH DRUMS

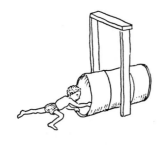

HANGING CRAWL-THROUGH DRUMS

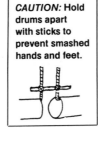

CAUTION: Hold drums apart with sticks to prevent smashed hands and feet.

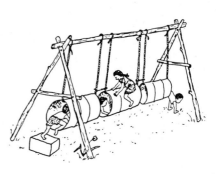

RING-TOSS

rings of tire rims or anything else

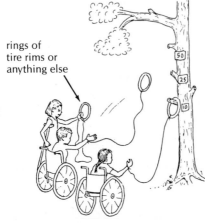

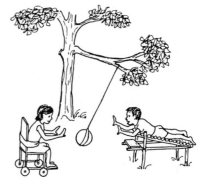

For children who have trouble going after dropped balls or rings, tying a string to the toy allows the children to pull it to them.

Examples from the 'bamboo playground' in the Khao-i-dang refugee camp, Thailand

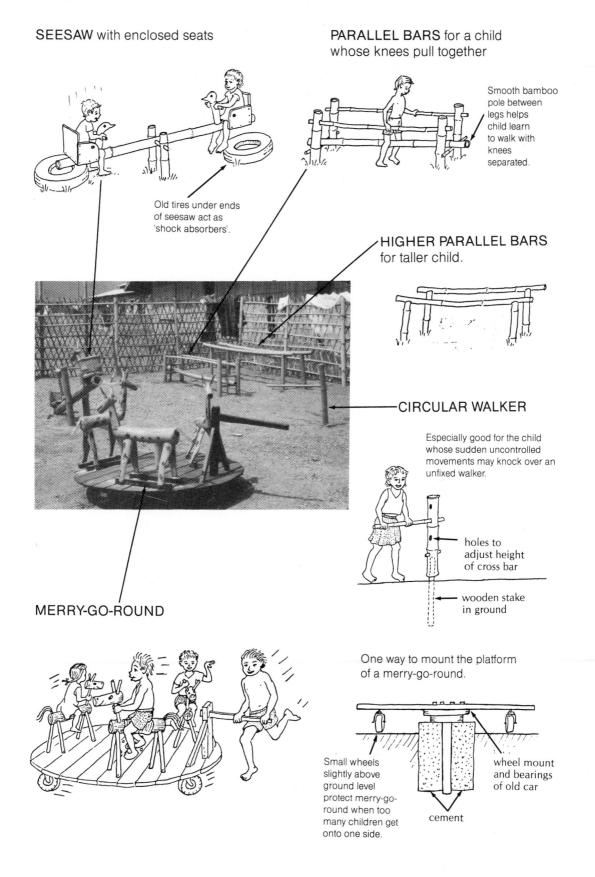

SEESAW with enclosed seats

PARALLEL BARS for a child whose knees pull together

Smooth bamboo pole between legs helps child learn to walk with knees separated.

Old tires under ends of seesaw act as 'shock absorbers'.

HIGHER PARALLEL BARS for taller child.

CIRCULAR WALKER

Especially good for the child whose sudden uncontrolled movements may knock over an unfixed walker.

holes to adjust height of cross bar

wooden stake in ground

MERRY-GO-ROUND

One way to mount the platform of a merry-go-round.

Small wheels slightly above ground level protect merry-go-round when too many children get onto one side.

cement

wheel mount and bearings of old car

PRECAUTIONS AND SUGGESTIONS FOR A SUCCESSFUL ALL-CHILDREN'S PLAYGROUND

1. Involve as much of the community as possible in building and maintaining the playground.

2. Keep the playground simple and build it from local low-cost materials. Only this way can it serve as a model for families of disabled children to build the most useful equipment for their child in their own homes. Resist offers from the local mayor or politicians to build an impressive metal frame playground. This will eliminate community participation and makes the equipment too costly for poor families to build at home.

3. For poles that are put into the ground, use a kind of wood that does not rot quickly. Or paint the posts with old motor oil, creosote, tar, copper sulfate or some other insect and fungus resistant substance.

   If poles are used that will rot quickly, to avoid accidents, **check strength of poles frequently** and replace them at regular intervals—especially during the hot rainy season.

4. Swings can be hung from ropes or chains. Rope or vines are cheaper but may rot or wear through fairly quickly. Plastic or nylon rope will not rot in the rains, but will gradually grow brittle and weak with the sun. As with posts, **to avoid accidents, check the strength of ropes frequently** by having several heavy persons hang on them at one time. **Replace ropes at regular intervals,** before they get weak.

5. Regular maintenance of the playground is essential, and this will require planning and organization. Perhaps once a month the village children can take an expedition to cut new poles to replace rotting ones, to repair old equipment, and to build new. Adult coordination of such activity is usually necessary.

6. To boost enthusiasm, keep lists in a public place of all the children and adults who help with the playground—and put a star for each time they help.

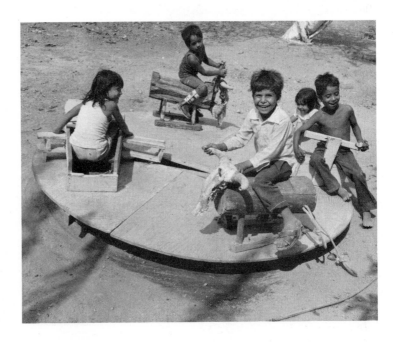

Children play on a 'merry-go-round' in PROJIMO. Enclosed 'cars' protect more severely disabled children. A cow's skull provides handles for a rider.

CHILD-to-child
Helping Teachers and Children Understand Disabled Children

Children can be either very cruel or very kind to a child who is different. They may be cruel by teasing, laughing, imitating, or even doing *physical* harm. But more often they are cruel simply by not including the disabled child in their games or activities, by rejecting the child, or by pretending she does not exist.

Often children act in a cruel way because they fear what they do not understand. **When they gain a little more understanding, children who may have been cruel or felt uncomfortable with the child who is different, can become that child's best friends and helpers.**

It is important that children in every neighborhood or community have a chance to better understand persons who, for whatever reason, are different from themselves — in color, in dress, in beliefs, in language, in movements, or in abilities.

One way to help a group of children gain appreciation of the disabled child and learn ways to be helpful is through **CHILD-to-child activities.**

CHILD-to-child is a non-formal educational program in which school-aged children learn ways to protect the health and well-being of other children — especially younger children and those with special needs. The children learn simple preventive and curative measures appropriate to their own communities. They pass on what they learn to other children and their families.

The CHILD-to-child program began during the International Year of the Child, 1979. David Morley (author of *Paediatric Priorities in the Developing World* and *See How They Grow*) brought together a group of health workers and educators from many countries. They designed a series of 'activity sheets' — or guidelines — to be adapted by teachers and health workers for children in different countries and situations.

Thirty-five activity sheets for children, including 5 activity sheets about disabled children, are available in a book called *Child-to-Child: A Resource Book, Part 2* from Teaching Aids at Low Cost (TALC), PO Box 49, St. Albans, Herts. AL1 5TX, United Kingdom. The activity sheets in the packet include:

* *Children with disabilities*
* *Helping children who do not see or hear well*
* *Mental handicap and children*
* *Polio*
* *Helping children who experience war, disaster or conflict*

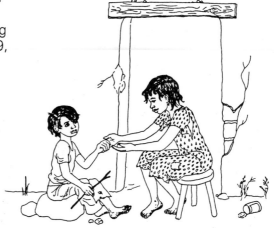

Other activity sheets in *Child-to-Child: A Resource Book, Part 2* that include **disability** prevention are:

- *Feeding young children: feeding children aged 6 months to 2 years*
- *Feeding young children: how do we know if they are eating enough?*
- *Caring for children with diarrhea*
- *Preventing accidents*
- *Our neighborhood*
- *Playing with young children: playing with babies*
- *Playing with young children: play for pre-school children*
- *A place to play*
- *Caring for children who are sick*
- *Safe lifestyles*

CHILD-to-child activities can be introduced:

- by schoolteachers with schoolchildren,
- by schoolchildren (who have practiced the activities in school) with younger schoolchildren, or with children who do not go to school,
- by health workers or community *rehabilitation* workers,
- by parent groups or any concerned persons in the community.

The purpose of CHILD-to-child activities that relate to disability is to help children:

- gain awareness of different disabilities and what it might be like to be disabled,
- learn that although a disabled person may have difficulty doing some things, she may be able to do other things extra well,
- think of ways that they can help disabled children feel welcome, take part in their play, schooling, and other activities, and manage to do things better,
- become the friends and defenders of any child who is different or has special needs.

From the CHILD-to-child activity sheet:

ACCIDENTS

Help children learn how important it is to:

- Make sure that their younger brothers and sisters do not go too close to the cooking fire.

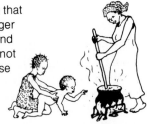

- Keep matches out of the reach of small children. (They can even make a small basket or shelf for matches to be stored high on the wall.)

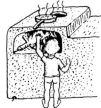

- Be sure that handles of pans are turned so that the child does not pull them.

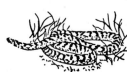

- Warn younger children about where snakes, scorpions, and bees live.

- Clear grass and weeds away from paths.

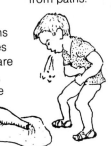

- Make sure poisons such as medicines and insecticides are kept out of reach, and that kerosene is not stored in drink bottles.

Rehabilitation programs in several countries have developed their own, more complete CHILD-to-child activity sheets. Here we combine versions from Kenya (Africa), the Philippines, and Mexico (where some of the original sheets were developed and tested). The 3 activities we include in this chapter are:

"Understanding children with special problems" (p. 429)
"Children who have difficulty understanding" (p. 442)
"Let's find out how well children see and hear" (p. 447)

CHILD-to-child ACTIVITY:
UNDERSTANDING CHILDREN WITH SPECIAL PROBLEMS

Group discussion

Encourage a class or group of children to talk about children who have some special problem or 'handicap'. Ask questions like:

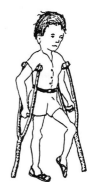

- Do you know any child who cannot walk or run or talk or play like other children?
- Why can't this child do everything the same as you can?
- Is the child to blame?
- How do other children treat this child? Are they kind to him? Are they mean? Do they make fun of him? Do they include him in their games?
- How would you feel if you had a similar problem? How would you want other children to treat you? Would you like them to laugh at you? To pay no attention to you? To feel sorry for you? To do things with you and become your friend?

Games and role playing

Children will better understand the child with a special problem if they can 'put themselves in his shoes'. They can **play a game in which one child pretends to have a handicap.**

For example, tie a stick to a child's leg. Then have him run in a game or play tag.

The other children act out different ways of behaving toward the child. Some are friendly. Some ignore him. Some make fun of him. Some help him. Some include him in their games. Let the children think up their own ideas and act them out.

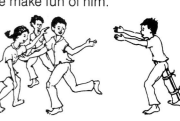

After several minutes, another child can pretend to have a handicap. Let several children have a turn with a handicap. Try to make the pretend handicap seem real.

Also ask the children what they might be able to do to make things better or fairer for the disabled child. Try or 'act out' their different suggestions. For example:

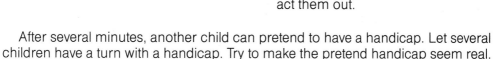

WE COULD ASK HIM TO PLAY GAMES WHERE HIS HANDICAP DOESN'T MATTER.

WE COULD GIVE EACH OF US A "HANDICAP". OR GIVE HIM SOME ADVANTAGE, SO WE COULD ALL BE EQUAL ... LIKE WE COULD ALL TIE OUR FEET TOGETHER!

CAUGHT YOU!

WE SHOULDN'T LAUGH AT HIM IF HE DOES THINGS IN A FUNNY WAY, BUT ENCOURAGE HIM TO DO HIS BEST, WHATEVER WAY HE CAN.

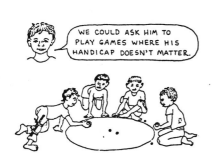

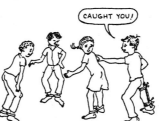

For a more severe physical disability, the group of children can invent ways to 'find out what it is like'. For example, to learn about a child with almost no use of her legs, the children might tie the legs of one of their group together, like this.

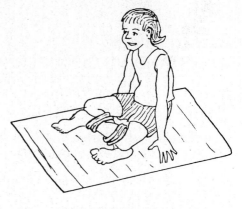

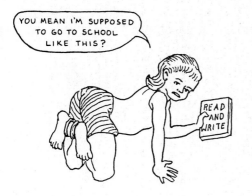

YOU MEAN I'M SUPPOSED TO GO TO SCHOOL LIKE THIS?

READ AND WRITE

Then the children can ask the child to do some of their day-to-day activities—like moving around the house, going to the latrine, and going to school.

After talking with the child about her difficulties, the children can try to think of ways to make it easier for her to move about.

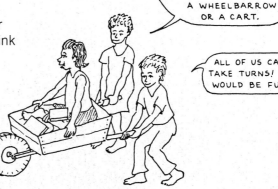

MAYBE WE COULD TAKE HER TO SCHOOL EVERY DAY IN A WHEELBARROW OR A CART.

ALL OF US CAN TAKE TURNS! IT WOULD BE FUN!

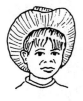

ALL OF US CHILDREN COULD TAKE UP A COLLECTION TO BUY HER A WHEELCHAIR. THEN SHE COULD GO PLACES WITHOUT SO MUCH HELP.

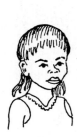

OR WE COULD MAKE HER A WHEELCHAIR OUT OF AN OLD CHAIR AND A COUPLE OF BIKE TIRES. MY FATHER'S A CARPENTER AND COULD HELP US.

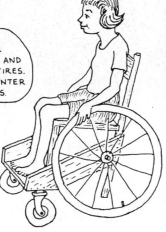

Note: With the help of their teacher or parents, children can, in fact, make simple wheelchairs and other aids for disabled children. For simple designs, see PART 3 of this book.

REMEMBER: Children are usually kind to a child with a very severe disability. They are often more cruel to a child with a less severe problem, such as a limp.

Help the children gain an understanding of the particular difficulties of any disabled child in their village.

For example, if there is a child with spastic legs who has trouble walking because his knees press together, have a child try to walk with her knees tied together with a band of car tire inner tube.

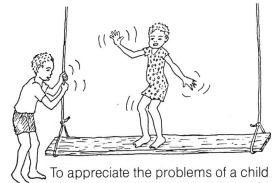

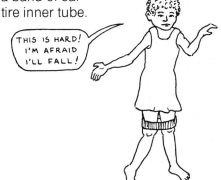

THIS IS HARD! I'M AFRAID I'LL FALL!

To appreciate the problems of a child who has trouble with balance (cerebral palsy), have one of the children try to walk on a hanging board (or other moving surface).

If there is a child with arthritis in the village, some of the children can put small stones in their shoes or tie small stones to the bottoms of their feet. Then the other children can invite them to run and play games. Ask the children why a child with arthritis might not want to play games.

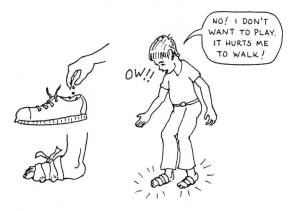

OW!!

NO! I DON'T WANT TO PLAY. IT HURTS ME TO WALK!

Ask the children, "Do you know any children who cannot use their hands like you can?" If they answer yes, help them experience the difficulties of such a child. Have the children work in pairs.

One child can wrap a strip of cloth around the other child's hand and fingers so that he has trouble moving his fingers.

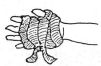

Now have the child try to do things like:

- write
- turn pages of a book
- fill a cup with water
- eat
- get something from a pocket
- button a shirt

Have the children try to figure out ways to make it easier. For example, wrap cloth or a piece of inner tube around a pencil or spoon, to make it easier to hold.

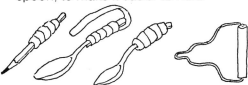

Note: For more ideas and tools for persons with disabled hands, see pages 223 and 330.

buttoning tool (See p. 335.)

Things that a disabled child can do well

A disabled child cannot do **everything** as well as other children. But often there are **some things** she can do as well, or even better. Try to have the children think of examples.

A child with weak legs, who has to walk with crutches, often develops very strong arms and hands.

Or a blind child may learn to hear things extra well.

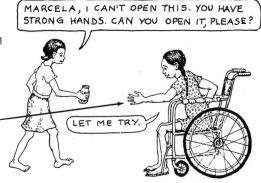

MARCELA, I CAN'T OPEN THIS. YOU HAVE STRONG HANDS. CAN YOU OPEN IT, PLEASE?

LET ME TRY.

Rather than feel sorry for the disabled child and look only at her weaknesses, **it is better to recognize and encourage her strengths.**

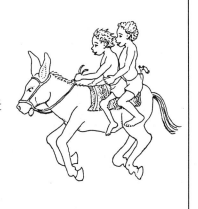

A LETTER TO ALL CHILDREN:

A handicapped child needs friends, play, and excitement — just like you. Try to include the child in your games and adventures. Let him do as much for himself as he can, and help him only when he needs it. But remember, he cannot do everything you can. Protect him from danger. . . but do not protect him too much! Too much protection is dangerous to any child's health. Children need adventure for their minds to grow, just as they need food for their bodies to grow.

Thanks

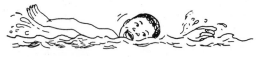

Swimming

Many children with weak or *paralyzed* legs can learn to swim well. Their arms become unusually strong from using crutches, and in the water they easily keep up with other children. But sometimes they have trouble getting to the water, or the other children forget to invite them . . .

A friendly word of welcome to include the child with a special problem, or a little extra time or attention given to him, can make a big difference—and can make everyone feel good.

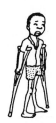

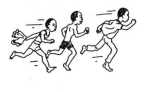

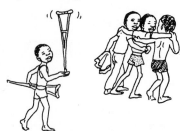

Role playing and children's theater

To help see how much it matters to include a disabled child in their fun, a group of children can act out different possibilities. For example, they might act out (or do a 'role play' of) the pictures at the bottom of the page before this one. After the role play the group can discuss which of the two alternatives made the disabled child, and the other children, feel better, and why.

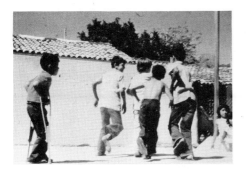
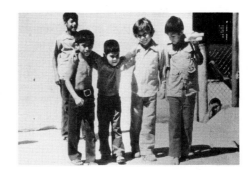

Photos from Ajoya, Mexico

Or they can act out a situation in which they try to solve a particular difficulty, obstacle, or challenge.

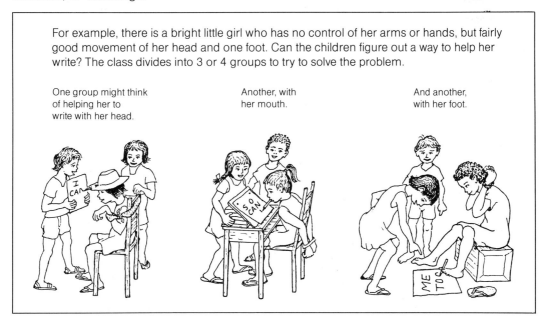

For example, there is a bright little girl who has no control of her arms or hands, but fairly good movement of her head and one foot. Can the children figure out a way to help her write? The class divides into 3 or 4 groups to try to solve the problem.

One group might think of helping her to write with her head.

Another, with her mouth.

And another, with her foot.

In these ways the children will begin to use their imaginations to help solve problems.

If some of the children's role plays turn out especially well, or do an extra good job at demonstrating important points, perhaps they can be developed further. Then the children can present them, in the form of skits or children's theater, to other classes, parent groups, in the health center, or perhaps to the whole village.

(Examples of two skits which schoolchildren, together with health workers and disabled rehabilitation workers, put on in the village of Ajoya, Mexico, are on pages 456 to 461.)

Putting our new understanding into practice

Once the children have developed a greater awareness of the needs and possibilities of disabled children through discussion, games, role plays, and stories, they can begin to put their new understanding into practice.

Ask the children if they know any child in the village (or in a neighboring village) who is disabled or has special difficulties in any way.

Then discuss ways that the children might be able to help each disabled child become as happy, capable, and self-reliant as possible. The children can list their suggestions for each child. Later, after getting to know the child and her family better, they can change and add to their ideas.

If the disabled child is a brother or sister of one of the children in the learning group, starting to do things with the child and the family may be fairly easy. But if none of the children is related to the disabled child, they must be careful in the way they offer their help. Probably only two or three children should make the first visit, perhaps with the help of a teacher, health worker, or rehabilitation worker.

The children, with suggestions from the disabled child and her family, will need to figure out ways that they can help most. However, the following list of possibilities may give you some ideas:

- Become friends—one or more children can become close companions, playmates, and friends of the disabled child.

- Visit the child at home—regularly!

- Help the family by doing errands, 'babysitting' or taking the child on outings.

- Figure out a way to help the child get to and from school.

- At school, one or more children can become the 'buddies' or helpers of the disabled child, making sure her special needs are met.

- If it is impossible for the disabled child to go to school, children may be able to organize an after-school teaching program at the child's home. Ask the teacher to help plan this.

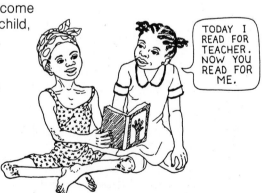

TODAY I READ FOR TEACHER. NOW YOU READ FOR ME.

- Figure out ways to include the child in games.

- Make helpful toys for the child and play together with her. (See p. 467 to 476.)

REMEMBER—
ALWAYS BE FRIENDLY

- Make a 'rehabilitation playground' or 'playground for all children'. Take disabled children regularly to the playground and play together with them there.

- Build simple playground equipment, adapted for the particular child, at her home.

- With advice from a rehabilitation worker or the child's parents, learn to help with the exercises or care that the child needs.

- You may be able to help build special aids for the children, such as crutches, sandbags, braces, or even a simple wheelchair. Try to get advice from a rehabilitation worker. If what you need to make is too difficult, perhaps the children can ask parents who are craftspersons to help. Visit them as a committee.

- Become 'prevention scouts' by following the suggestions on p. 428, or by taking other actions to prevent disability in your village.

- If there is a village rehabilitation center in your village, perhaps a group of children can take turns there as volunteers after school. There are many ways you can help and much you can learn. Those who show most interest can become 'junior rehabilitation workers'.

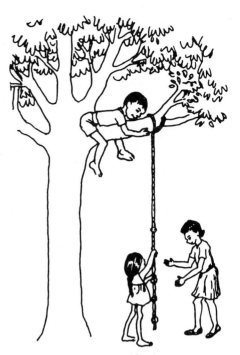

A rope swing like this can help a child with weak legs teach herself to walk—in a way that is fun!

Children with severe disabilities

Some children are very disabled. They cannot walk or swim or play many games. But sometimes these children can learn to play marbles, cards, or guessing games.

Learning is especially difficult for a child who cannot speak or think as easily as other children. This child may be very lonely. Sometimes a child who cannot speak, understands a lot more than people think he does. If there is such a child in your neighborhood, perhaps children could take turns visiting him, to talk or play with him. Let him know you care.

Babies with problems

Sometimes a baby is slower than most to develop. Either her mind may be slow to develop, or her body, or sometimes both. The child will be later than other babies in the village to begin to sit, use her hands, crawl, walk or talk.

Babies who are slow to develop need special care. If possible, their parents should get advice from a rehabilitation worker or *physiotherapist.* However, **there is a lot that brothers and sisters and other children can do.**

More than almost anything else, **these babies need lots of attention.** They need to be **played with** and helped or encouraged to play. They need **simple toys** and **colorful or noisy things** to attract their attention. They need to be **talked to** and **sung to a lot.** These things will help the baby develop faster. And these are all things other children can do.

In the next activity sheet (p. 442) we will talk more about helping a child whose mind develops slowly or who has difficulty understanding.

Helping a disabled child learn to do new things

There are many ways that children can help a baby or young child with a special problem to learn to do new things. Here are some ideas:

- **Make it fun!** If exercises can be turned into games, the child will learn faster and everyone will enjoy it more.

- **Self-help.** Help the disabled child only as much as he needs. Encourage him to do as much as he can for himself and by himself.

- **Little by little.** Remember, some things are especially difficult for the disabled child. Encourage her to do a little more than she already does—and then a little more. If you have her try to do too much, she may get discouraged and stop trying.

- **Show you care.** Show the child how glad you are when he learns to do new things. Praise him when he does well—and when he tries.

- **Mind and body.** Play often with the child, in ways that help her develop not only her body but also her mind. Talk with her and tell her stories. Become her friend.

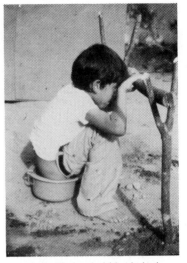

A simple bar held by forked sticks can increase the self-reliance of a child who has difficulty squatting to shit.

AN EXAMPLE: Pablo is having trouble learning to crawl. Using the above suggestions, how can we help him? Perhaps his older brothers and sisters, or other children, can play 'crawling games' with him.

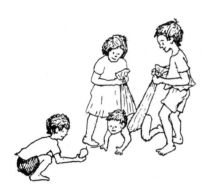

Two children can hold up part of his weight as he tries to crawl. Another child encourages him to crawl by holding out a fruit or toy. Call him to crawl toward the fruit. Praise him when he tries.

Play the game every day. As Pablo grows stronger, less of his weight will need to be held up. In time he may be able to crawl without help.

Note: Many more ideas of ways children can help a child who is slow to develop can be found in PART 1 of this book, especially Chapters 34 and 35.

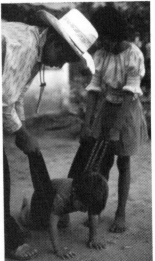

Children in Mexico playing a 'crawling game'.

Story telling

Story telling is another good way to help young people understand the needs and possibilities of disabled children and what can be done to help. You can make up stories. Or better, you can base them on true events where a disabled child has achieved something outstanding, or where a group of children have succeeded in making an important difference in the life of a disabled child. The story that follows is an example.

A Story—to be used with the CHILD-to-child activity,
"Understanding Children with Special Problems"

HOW TOMÁS AND OTHER CHILDREN HELPED JULIA GO TO SCHOOL

At age 7 Julia's world was so small that you could throw a stone clear across it. She had seen almost nothing of her own village. No one ever took her anywhere. The farthest she had ever crawled was to the bushes just outside the small hut where she lived with her family.

Julia was the oldest of 3 children. Her family's hut was at the far edge of Bella Village. The hut was separated from the main footpath by a long, steep, rocky trail. Perhaps for this reason, Julia had missed being *vaccinated* in her first year of life, when health workers had come to the village.

In the beginning, Julia had been a healthy baby, and quick. At 10 months of age she was already able to stand alone for a few seconds, and to say a few words, like 'mama', 'papa', and 'wawa'—which meant water. Her face would light up in a big smile whenever anyone called her name. Her parents took great pride in her, and spoiled her terribly.

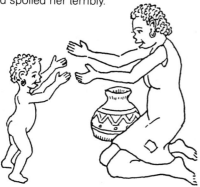

But at 10 months Julia got sick. It began like a bad cold, with fever and diarrhea. Julia's mother took her to a doctor in a neighboring town. The doctor gave her an injection in her left backside. A few days later Julia got worse. First her left leg began to hurt her, then her back, and finally both arms and legs. Soon her whole body became very weak. She could not move her left leg at all and the other leg only a little. In a few days the fever and pain went away, but the weakness stayed, especially in her legs. The doctor in town said it was polio, and that her legs would be weak all her life.

Julia's mother and father were very sad. In those days there was no rehabilitation worker in the village or in the neighboring towns. So Julia's mother and father took care of her as best they could. In time, Julia learned to crawl. But she did not learn to dress or do much for herself. Her parents felt sorry for her, so they did everything for her. She gave them a lot of work.

Then, when Julia was 3 years old, a baby brother was born. This meant her parents had less time for Julia. Her little brother was a strong, happy baby, and her parents seemed to put all their hopes into the new child. They paid less attention to Julia, rarely played with her, and never took her out with them into the village. Julia had no friends or playmates—except for her baby brother. Yet sometimes, for no clear reason, Julia would pinch her baby brother and make him cry. Because of this, her parents did not let Julia hold or play with him often.

Julia became more and more quiet and unhappy. Remembering how quick and friendly she had been as a baby, her parents sometimes wondered if her mind, too, had been damaged by her illness. Although the doctor had explained that polio weakens only muscles, and never affects a child's mind, they still had their doubts.

When Julia was 6 years old, a third child was born—a baby sister. This seemed to make Julia even more unhappy. She spent most of her time sitting outside behind the hut drawing pictures in the dirt with a broken stick. She drew chickens, donkeys, trees, and flowers. She drew houses, people, waterjugs, and devils with horns and long tails. Actually, she drew remarkably well for a child her age. But no one noticed her drawings. Her mother was busier than ever with the new baby.

Julia was 7 years old when the village school teachers, guided by a health worker from a nearby village, began a CHILD-to-child program in the school. The first and second year children (who were in the same class) studied an activity sheet called "Understanding children with special problems."

Most of the children knew of only one seriously disabled child in their village. This was Tomás. Tomás walked in a jerky way, with crutches. He had one hand that sometimes made strange movements. And he had difficulty speaking clearly, especially when he was excited. But Tomás did not seem to need any special help—or at least not anymore. He was already in the fourth grade of school and doing well. He had lots of friends. He managed to go anywhere and do almost anything for himself, if awkwardly, and nearly everyone treated him with respect. It was easy to forget he was disabled.

Then one little boy remembered, "There's a girl who lives in a house at the far end of the village. She crawls around on her hands and knees, and spends a lot of time just sitting outside. She always looks sad. I don't know her name, but she looks old enough to be in school."

"Let's invite her to come to school with us," said one of the children.

"But how," asked another, "if she can't walk?"

"We could bring her in a push cart!"

"No! The path from her home is too steep and rocky."

"Then we'll carry her! If we all help, it will be easy."

"Let's go to her house this afternoon." "Good idea!"

———————•———————

That afternoon after school, 6 of the school children, together with their teacher, visited Julia's home. Julia, who was out back, was too shy to come in. So they started talking with her mother.

"We want to be her friends," they said. "And to help her go to school."

"But she can't go to school," her mother said with surprise. "She can't even walk!"

"We can carry her," offered the children. "We'll come for her every day and bring her back in the afternoons. It's not far, really!"

"The whole class is ready to help out," said the teacher. "And so am I."

"But you don't understand," said her mother. "Julia's not like other children. They'll tease her. She is so shy she doesn't open her mouth around strangers. And besides, I don't see how school could help her."

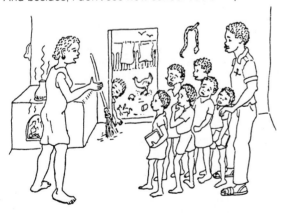

The teacher tried his best to explain to the mother the great importance of school for a child like Julia. The children promised that they would all be friendly and help her in any way they could. But her mother just shook her head.

"Do you think Julia would like to go to school?" asked the teacher.

Her mother gave a tired sigh. Then she turned to Julia, who was hiding outside the door but peeping in at the visitors. "Julia, darling, do you want to go to school?"

Julia's eyes opened wide with fear. She shook her head in a terrified NO and disappeared behind the doorway.

"There, you see!" said Julia's mother. "For Julia, school just wouldn't make sense. . . . Now I have a lot of work to do, please excuse me. But thank you for thinking of my poor little girl."

"Please give it more thought," said the teacher as he and the children went out the door, "And thank you for your time."

"Have a nice day," said Julia's mother, and went back to work.

———————•———————

At school the next day the teacher met with the whole class to discuss their visit to Julia's home.

"This CHILD-to-child stuff sounds so easy and fun when we pretend," said one of the children. "But when we try to use it in real life, it ain't so easy."

"Isn't!" said the teacher.

"Still," said one little girl who had visited Julia's home, "we have to keep trying. Did you see the way Julia looked at us? She was so scared she was shaking. But she was interested, too. I could tell. She looked so . . . lonely!"

"But what can we do? I don't think her mother wants us to come back."

There was a long silence. Then one little boy said, "I've got an idea! Let's talk to Tomás. He's handicapped, too. But he's in school and is doing fine. Maybe he can help us."

After school, several of the first and second year students waited for Tomás, who was in the fourth year. They told him about Julia, and what happened when they visited her home.

"How was it when you began school, Tomás?" asked the children. "Were you afraid? Did your parents want you to go? How did the other children treat you?"

Tomás laughed. "One question at a time!" He spoke slowly, with a twisted mouth and a sort of jerky speech that sometimes made him hard to understand. "Help me sit down under that tree." Tomás moved forward on his crutches. The children helped him sit down. (He explained that his hips and legs wanted to stay straight when he wanted to bend them.) He sat leaning against the tree, and began to answer the children's questions.

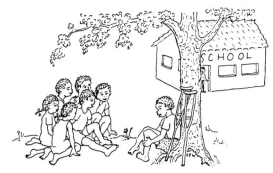

"Sure, I was afraid to go to school, at first," said Tomás. "And my mom and dad didn't want to send me. They were afraid kids would tease me or that it would be too hard for me. It was grandma who talked us all into it. She said if I couldn't earn my living behind a plow, I'd better learn to earn it using my head. And I intend to."

"What do you want to be when you grow up?" asked one boy.

"Maybe a health worker," said Tomás. "I want to help other people."

"Did other kids tease you when you started school?" asked the children.

Tomás frowned. "No . . . not much. But they didn't know what to do with me, so usually they didn't do anything. They would stare when they thought I wasn't looking. And they would imitate the way I talk when they thought I wasn't listening. But when they thought I was looking and listening, they would pretend I wasn't there. That's what was hardest for me. They never asked me what I thought, or what I could do, or if I wanted to play with them. I felt lonelier when I was with the other children than when I was by myself."

"But now you have lots of friends. You seem like one of the gang. What happened?"

"I don't know," answered Tomás. "The other kids just got used to me, I guess. They began to see that even though I walk and talk funny, I'm not really all that different from them. I think it helps that I do well in school. I like to read. I read everything I can find. Sometimes when kids in my class have trouble reading or understanding something, I help them. I like to do that. At first they gave me the nickname 'Crabfoot' because of how I walk. But now they call me 'Professor' because I help them with their lessons."

"The first nickname was about what's wrong with you," observed one little girl. "And the second is about what's right. I guess you showed them what's most important!"

Tomás' mouth twisted into a smile and his legs jerked with pleasure. "Tell me more about Julia," he said.

They told him all they could, and finished by saying, "We tried as hard as we could, but Julia's mother doesn't want her in school and Julia doesn't want to go either. We don't know what to do. Do you have any ideas, Tomás?"

"Maybe if I visit the family—with my parents. They can try to convince her parents, and I'll try to make friends with Julia."

The next Sunday, when Tomás' father was not working in the fields, Tomás asked his parents to go with him to Julia's home. They arrived in the early afternoon. Julia's mother and father, together with the 2 younger children, were all sitting in the shade in front of the hut. Julia's father was sharpening an ax while her mother picked lice from the children's hair. They all looked up in surprise to see the boy on crutches approaching, followed by 2 adults.

The path near the hut was steep and rocky. A few meters from the hut, Tomás tripped and fell. Julia's father ran forward to help.

"Are you hurt?" asked Julia's father, helping him up.

"Oh no," laughed Tomás. "I'm used to falling. I've learned to do it without hurting myself. . . . We've come to talk to you about Julia. These are my parents."

"Come in," said Julia's father. They all exchanged greetings, and everyone went inside.

While Tomás' parents were talking with Julia's, Tomás asked if he could speak with Julia.

"She's outside," nodded her mother, pointing to the back doorway. "But she doesn't speak to strangers. She's too afraid."

"She doesn't have to speak if she doesn't want to," said Tomás gently, yet loudly enough so that Julia could hear, if she was listening.

Tomás went out and found Julia bent over a drawing in the dirt. She glanced up at him as he approached, and then looked down at her drawing, but without continuing it.

There were several drawings on the ground of different animals, flowers, people, and monsters. Julia had just been drawing a tree with a big nest in it and some birds.

"Did you draw all these?" asked Tomás. Julia did not answer. Her small body was trembling.

"You draw very well!" said Tomás, admiring and commenting on each of her drawings. "And with just a stick. Have you ever tried drawing with pencil and paper?" No answer. Tomás continued. "I bet that nobody in school can draw this well!" Julia, still staring at the dirt, trembled and said nothing. Tomás also was silent for a moment. Then he said, "I wish I could draw like you do. Who taught you?"

Julia slowly lifted her head up and looked at Tomás, or at least at his lower half. She looked first at his turned-in feet and the tips of his crutches. Then she looked at his knees, which had dark calluses on their inner sides where they rubbed together when he walked.

"Why do you walk with those sticks?" she asked.

"It's the only way I can," he said. "My legs don't like to do what I tell them."

Julia lifted her head and looked up into Tomás' face. Tomás tried to smile, but knew his mouth was twisting strangely to one side.

"And why do you talk funny?" asked Julia.

"Because my mouth and lips don't always do what I want either," said Tomás. And it seemed he had even more trouble speaking clearly than usual.

Julia stared at him. "Do you really like my drawing?"

"I do," said Tomás, glad to change the subject. "You have a real gift. Real talent. You should study art. I'll bet some day you could be a great artist."

"No," said Julia, shaking her head. "I'll never be anything. I can't even walk. Look!" She pointed to her small floppy legs. "They're even worse than yours!"

"But you draw with your hands, not your feet!" exclaimed Tomás.

Julia laughed. "You're funny!" she said. "What's your name?"

"Tomás."

"Mine's Julia. Do you really think I could be an artist?—No, you're only joking. I'll never be anything. Everybody knows that!"

"But I'm not joking, Julia," said Tomás. "I read in a magazine about an artist who paints birds. People come from all over the world to buy his pictures. And you know something, Julia, his arms and legs are completely paralyzed. He paints holding the brush in his mouth!"

"How does he get around?" asked Julia.

"I don't know," said Tomás. "People help him, I guess. But he does get around. The magazine said he has been to several countries."

Julia said, "Wow! Do you really think I could become an artist?"

Tomás looked again at the drawings in the dirt—and truly wished he could draw as well. "I know you could!" he answered.

"How do I start?" asked Julia, sitting up eagerly.

"First," said Tomás, "you should probably go to school."

"But how?" said Julia, looking at her legs.

"That's easy," said Tomás. "All the school children want to help. But you have to want to go."

"I . . . I'm afraid . . ." said Julia. "Do you go to school, Tomás?"

"Yes, of course," he answered.

"Then I want to go, too!"

Inside the house, Tomás' parents were trying to convince Julia's parents of the importance of sending her to school. They explained how they had had the same doubts about Tomás, and how much school had helped him.

"It's not only what he is learning that's important," said Tomás' mother, "but what it has done for him personally. He has more confidence—a whole new view of himself."

"And we've come to look at him differently, too," said Tomás' father. "He's a good student—one of the leaders in his class!"

Julia's father coughed. "Even if all you say is true, Julia doesn't want to go. She's afraid. You see, the same illness affected her . . ."

His sentence was cut off by Julia, who came bursting in the back doorway on hands and knees. "Mama! Papa!" she shouted. "Can I go to school? Will you let me? Pleeeease?"

Her father's mouth fell open for a moment. And then he smiled.

The next day Julia began school. The other children learned from Tomás that Julia was ready to go, and they worked hard Sunday evening making a 'sitting stretcher' for her. One of the children had seen a similar stretcher when an injured man had been carried down from the high mountains. It was a simple wooden chair, tied firmly between two poles. The children finished making it by sunset and the next morning arrived with it at Julia's house. Tomás went with them to give Julia courage. He was so excited that he fell 3 times!

Julia was so frightened when she saw the children that she almost decided not to go. But when they brought her special chair to the door, she lifted herself onto it with her strong arms. And before she knew it, she was on her way — to school!

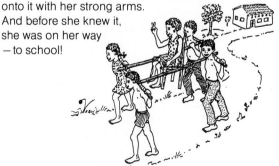

The first day of school went well. Everything was so new, and the children were all so friendly, that Julia almost forgot she was afraid. On the way home, she smiled and laughed as the children carried her.

Six months have now passed since Julia started school. Although she began 2 months late, she is already able to read and write letters and words as well as most of her classmates. But drawing is what she likes most. The other children often ask her to draw pictures for them.

Julia has made many friends. The children in her class who first looked at her as someone 'special', have now accepted her as one of their group. They include her in many games and activities, and treat her as just another child.

Some problems have arisen. At first, carrying Julia to and from school each day was fun. But after awhile, many of the children got lazy and stopped helping. This meant more work for those who were left.

The children got a new idea and asked their fathers for help. One Sunday a group of about 15 men and 20 children worked on improving the steep path from Julia's house to the main walkway leading to school. They made the curves wider so that the trail would be less steep, removed all rocks, leveled the surface, and pounded the dirt into a hard, smooth surface.

One of the children's father had a small repair shop in the village. Another was a carpenter. With the help of their children, these 2 craftsmen made a simple wheelchair out of an old chair, 2 casters, and some bicycle wheels.

Julia was excited when she saw the wheelchair. Her arms and hands were already strong, and with a little practice she learned to wheel her new chair up the long winding trail to the village.

"Now you can come and go to school on your own," said Tomás. "How do you feel?"

"Free!" laughed Julia. "I feel like writing a declaration of independence!" Then she thought a moment and frowned. "I know I'm not completely independent—but that's all right. We all depend on each other in some ways. And I guess that's how it should be."

"It's being equal that counts," said Tomás. "It's knowing that you're worth just as much as anybody else. Nobody's perfect!"

Things also began to go better at home. As Julia's self-respect grew, so did her parents' appreciation of her. Suddenly both Julia and her mother realized that there were many things that Julia could do. She began to help with preparing meals, washing clothes, and taking care of her younger brother and sister. She treated them more lovingly and never pinched or made them cry (except, of course, when they deserved it!).

Julia's mother wondered how she had ever managed to get along without Julia's help. She missed her during the long hours she was at school. And when she realized she was going to have another baby, she thought Julia would have to stop going to school to help more at home.

Julia's father shook his head. "No," he said. "School is more important for Julia than for any of our other children—if she is going to learn skills to make something of her life. And besides," he reminded his wife, "if we hadn't sent her to school, she would probably still be sitting outside in the dirt. It took the schoolchildren to teach *us* what a wonderful little girl we have."

Julia's mother smiled and nodded in agreement. "You're absolutely right," she said. "The school-children . . . and especially that wise little boy, Tomás!"

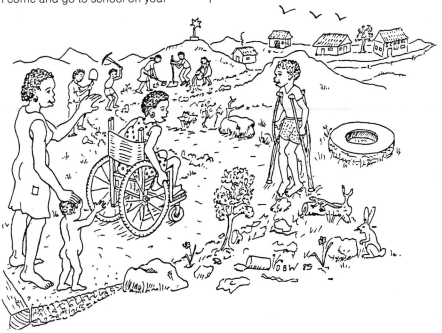

ᴄʜɪʟᴅ-ᴛᴏ-ᴄʜɪʟᴅ ACTIVITY:
CHILDREN WHO HAVE DIFFICULTY UNDERSTANDING

In many communities, a child who is **mentally** slow, or **retarded,** has an especially difficult time. Other children may make fun of him for not being as quick as they are, or for not being able to understand, follow, or remember things as easily as they can. They may not realize that this child has the same need for friendship, play, and respect as they do.

This activity is designed to help children gain more appreciation of both the needs and possibilities of the child who is mentally slow. They will explore possible ways to help the child to feel a part of their group, and to learn new things at his or her own speed.

Talk with the children

You may want to start the activity by asking the children questions such as:

- Do you know a child who doesn't seem to understand or remember things as well as others her age?
- Does this child play much with other children?
- How do other children treat this child?
- How do you think it would feel if you had a similar difficulty?

Games and activities

Begin with games and activities that help the children discover what it may feel like to have difficulty understanding, and to be unfairly blamed for that difficulty. Then the children can look for ways to help a person learn that are easier, friendlier, and more effective.

A GAME TO START WITH: 'ENGLEFLIP'

('Engleflip' is a nonsense word, but let us pretend that it means 'Stand up.')

1. Ask one child in the group to 'engleflip'.

2. Say it louder. Get angry.

3. Ask several other children.

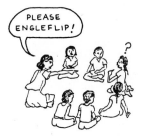

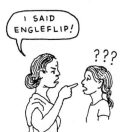

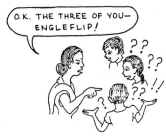

4. Now help the children understand what you mean by showing them, assisting them, or gently explaining.

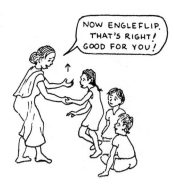

After the activity, discuss . . .

- How did you feel when you could not understand the teacher?
- Was it right for the teacher to get angry? Did it help?
- Did the teacher finally do it better? In what ways?
- In what ways might your difficulty with 'engleflip' be similar to that of a child who has trouble understanding things?

Role playing

You can also use role plays or skits to explore the difficulties of a child who does not understand, and how to help him understand. For example:

Ask 5 children to put on the role play.

They can pretend to be cleaning house. But before they start, ask one child to go out of the room. Tell the other 4 that after they have cleaned for awhile, they should turn to the 5th child and say, "Blah, blah, blah, blah." Tell the 4 children that this means, "Go get some water." But the 5th child will not know this.

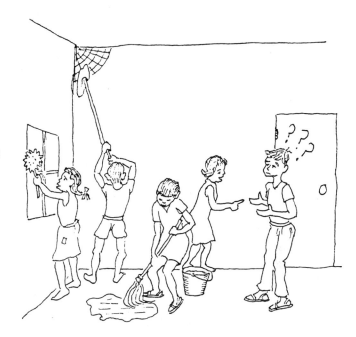

Tell the 4 children to keep saying the words, and then to add other ways to help the 5th child understand.

The 5th child comes back and they begin.

Divide the class in groups of 5 (or more) and repeat the game. Have the children think of different situations and different meanings for "Blah, blah, blah, blah."

Afterwards, discuss with the whole class:

- How did the child feel who did not understand?
- How did the others feel?
- What did the others do to help the child understand?
- What else could they have done?

Follow-up activity: Write or tell a story

The story might begin by one child waking up one morning and not understanding anything anyone says.

Each child in the class writes or tells the rest of the story in his and her own way. Invite them to draw pictures with their stories.

Ask the children to include in their stories ideas for helping the child understand.

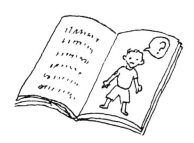

This activity could be done in a language or writing class. After they have written the stories, the children can read them to classes of younger children.

Memory

It is important that the children also realize the importance of remembering things and the difficulties of a child who has an especially hard time remembering. Then they can try to find ways to help that child remember things more easily.

MEMORY GAME #1

Ask the children to do many things, one after the other. Say the list of things in one sentence, very quickly. Do not wait for the children to do each thing before you say the next.

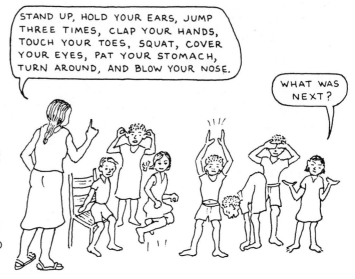

If the children cannot remember all the things, repeat the list louder, but just as fast.

Now do it differently. Say each thing slowly, and wait until they do one thing before you go on to the next.

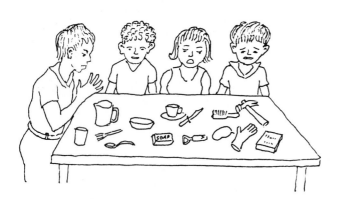

MEMORY GAME #2

Place 14 different things on a table where the children can see them. Let them look at them while you count to 30. Then cover them with a cloth and take 7 things away. Remove the cloth. Have the children write down the things that are missing.

Repeat the game using 6 different things and removing 3. Which is easier?

After the memory games:

- Ask the children why it was easier the second way.
- Explain that children who have trouble understanding are often confused when they are given too many instructions at once. Even 2 instructions at once may be too many for such a child. What suggestions do the children have?
- If the children know a child who has a hard time remembering things, they can help her improve her memory by playing these same kinds of games with her. Start with only 2 or 3 words or things, and as the child's memory begins to get better, gradually add more. Each time the child does well, praise her or give her a prize.

STORY AND DISCUSSION: "I FORGOT"

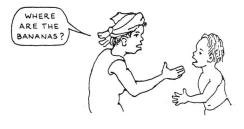

Begin to tell a story about a little boy whose mother asks him to go to the corner store and buy some bananas. He comes back with nothing.

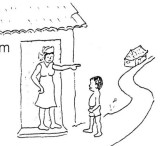

- Why did he not bring the bananas?
- What might have happened?
- How could we help?

Another day the boy goes to buy bananas and comes back with matches. Why? How could we help him remember? Here are some possibilities:

- Another child could go with the boy—not to buy the bananas, but to help him remember, or give him 'clues'.
- He could take a picture to remind him—or sticks to remind him of the number.
- Another child could practice with him at home. Play remembering games. Start with one thing at a time.
- **Praise or reward the boy each time he remembers and does it right.** Do not praise and **never punish** the child when he forgets. Remember: He has difficulty remembering. It is not his fault!

ROLE PLAY—GOING SHOPPING

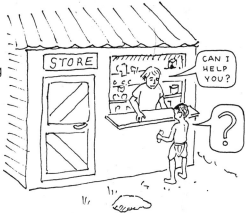

The children can act out a role play something like this:

A mother sends her child shopping. She tells him a long list of things he must buy. He goes around the class 3 times and meets a lot of people who ask him a lot of questions like: 'What time is it?" "Where are you going?" "Which way is the market?"

How much does the child remember when he gets to the store?

Talk with the class about what happened. How might it be made easier for the child to remember what he must buy? (Let us suppose the child cannot read.)

PUTTING INTO PRACTICE WHAT WE LEARN

Do the children know any child in the village or neighborhood who has difficulty understanding or remembering?

Is there something they can do that might help the child to:

- feel he has friends who respect him and with whom he can play?
- remember things better?
- learn to do more for himself?

- go to school, and get the extra help he needs?
- enjoy himself more and fit into the community better?

If there are some children (or grown-ups) in town who make fun of the disabled child or treat him badly, is there anything the children can do? What? What precautions should they take? The story on the next page can give children ideas for helping a child who is mentally slow to learn basic skills. For more ideas, see Chapters 32 to 41.

ZAKI AND NASIR
A Story From Pakistan

This is the story of 2 brothers, Zaki age 9, and Nasir age 7. Their father was a shopkeeper in Peshawar, and their mother was a teacher. They had a big brother and a big sister who were both students, living away from home. Zaki was doing well at school but Nasir had never even started school. There was something different about Nasir from other children. Nasir was mentally disabled. His brain did not work properly. He could only say a few odd words. He could not dress himself, and he made a mess at mealtimes.

Zaki felt ashamed to have such a brother. Neighborhood children made fun of Nasir. They called him nasty names and pushed him about. Nasir would get angry and try to hit them, and then fall flat on his face. Some of the grown-ups would shake their heads and say Nasir had an evil spirit inside him.

The worst of it for Zaki was that he had to take care of Nasir a lot of the time, when there was nobody else at home. It meant that he could not go out to play with his friends from school. And there was nothing to enjoy in looking after Nasir. He could not talk. He did not know how to play any games.

Zaki felt very sorry for himself, and used to hate Nasir for the times he had to stay in the house looking after him. It was so unfair! He had never done anything wrong, so why should he have to have a brother like that, who stopped him from going out and playing with his friends?

One day a visitor came by their house, looking for Zaki's father. It was his cousin, Dr. Daud. Zaki's parents were out. Only Zaki and Nasir were in the house. Dr. Daud noticed that Zaki had been crying. "What's the matter?" he asked. Zaki told Dr. Daud all about his brother Nasir and how his own life was spoiled by having to look after him.

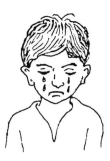

Dr. Daud listened carefully. Then he said, "Yes, you've certainly got a problem. But tell me, what are you doing about it?" "What can I do?" cried Zaki. "Nasir's just as bad now as he was 2 years ago, and he'll be twice as stupid in another 2 years time." Dr. Daud looked thoughtful. "Well, he might be," he replied. "But that depends on how clever *you* are."

"What do you mean?" asked Zaki. "I'm getting good marks at school, while *he* can't even start." "Well," said Dr. Daud, "if you're clever enough for 2 then you could really help Nasir to change for the better. Then you'd both be happier and you'd get more free time to go out and play." "How can I do that?" asked Zaki. Dr. Daud said,

"First, I'll have a talk with your father and mother."

That evening Dr. Daud called again and had a long talk with Zaki's parents. "I can't give you any medicine for Nasir," he said, "because there isn't any that will cure him of mental disability. Not even the best surgeons can do anything. But you have the answer right here in your own home. If you have enough time and patience you can teach Nasir to do a lot more than he can do now." But Zaki's father said, "That's just the problem! We don't have enough time at home. I can't have Nasir in the shop. He pulls everything off the shelves. And his mother is teaching at school and then has to get our food, and then gives private lessons. We can't stop working, or we'll never eat and pay the rent."

"But Zaki has the time," said Dr. Daud. "He could do a lot to teach Nasir. Why not try it for a month. I'll show you where to start."

So Zaki became Nasir's teacher. But he also learned a lot of things himself. He started teaching Nasir to dress himself. Of course, Zaki knew how to put on a shirt. You just pick it up, and put it on! But he soon realized that there was more to it, when teaching Nasir. First you had to find which was the back and which was the front of the shirt. Then you had to find the main hole and get the head through it. Then one arm went into the right sleeve. Then the other arm into the other sleeve. Next you pull the whole thing down over yourself.

Then there was teaching Nasir to feed himself. You would think it was obvious, how to eat! But Nasir had to find out step by step how to pick up a piece of chapati, get some curry on it, put it into his mouth and remember to chew and swallow. It took dozens of repetitions and lots of encouragement and rewards before Nasir learned each step. Zaki began to realize what Dr. Daud had meant. He needed to be clever enough for 2 in order to puzzle out how to teach Nasir. But when Nasir succeeded in some small step, they were both so delighted that it made all the effort worthwhile.

A few months later Dr. Daud was passing Zaki's house. Zaki came rushing out. "Quick, Doctor, you must come in!" Dr. Daud hurried in, thinking he would find someone at the point of death. But all he saw was Nasir, grinning broadly in his chair. "What is it? What's the matter?" demanded the doctor. Zaki was so excited he could hardly speak. "He said a whole sentence, Doctor. Nasir did. He's never said more than 2 words together before now. He just said 'Zaki give sweets to Nasir'. I've been trying for months to get him talking. He did it! He did it!"

Doctor Daud smiled. "I think you like your brother better than you used to," he said.

CHILD-to-child ACTIVITY:
LET'S FIND OUT HOW WELL CHILDREN SEE AND HEAR

Background discussion

Some children cannot see or hear as well as other children. Often we do not know about this and the child says nothing. But because the child does not hear the teacher or see the blackboard, he may not learn as quickly as others. So he may try to hide in a corner. **We can help him by letting him sit close to the teacher.**

Also, babies who cannot hear well do not learn to talk or understand as early as others.

In this activity, the school children try to find out which young children and babies do not see or hear well, and need help.

HELPING CHILDREN UNDERSTAND THE PROBLEM

One way to get children thinking about these problems is to ask questions like:

- Do you know anybody who does not see or hear well?
- Do you act differently with these people? Why?
- How would you feel if you did not see well? Or hear well?

Games to help children understand *the difficulties of poor hearing*

GAME: LISTEN LISTEN

All the children are completely silent for 3 minutes. They listen very carefully to the noises around them. Afterwards, they write down or draw everything they heard.

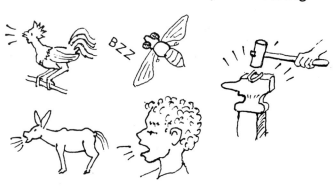

GAME: WHAT DID YOU SAY?

One child plugs his ears while another tells a funny story to the group. Then one of the children plays 'teacher' and asks everyone, including the child who had his ears plugged, to answer questions about the story. Finally, they ask him what it felt like, not being able to hear the story well.

Ask the children what they can do to help a child to hear better. Their suggestions might include:

- Have the child sit 'up front' close to the teacher.
- Everyone can take care to **speak slow, clear,** and **loud** (but do not shout).
- **Use gestures or 'sign language'** (if the child hears very little or not at all).
- Watch people's mouths and try to understand what they say. This is not easy if you do not hear the words. Have the children try it.

GAME: TALKING WITHOUT WORDS

Children who hear very poorly or not at all often cannot speak. This is not because they are stupid, but because they need to be able to hear in order to learn how to speak. This game will help children appreciate the difficulties of a child who cannot speak, and give the children ideas of how to 'talk' without words to a child who does not hear.

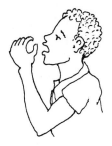

Play a game where someone explains something to others through acting *only,* without words. The others must guess what it is he is trying to say. The leader can start by acting out a simple phrase like: "I want a glass of water." The children try to guess what the leader is doing. Next have the children take turns acting out different things and ideas. Start with easy phrases like:

- I want to go to sleep.
- Give me the ball.

And work toward more difficult ideas like:

- I'm lost and can't find my house.
- I had a bad dream.

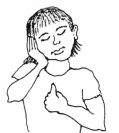

Discussion after the game:

- Was it difficult to explain something without talking?
- How did you feel when no one understood you?
- What did the other children do to help you tell them what you wanted to?
- Could they have done more? What?
- How might you help children who cannot speak to communicate?

Explain to the children about **sign language for the deaf.** This is like the game in which children 'talk' with their hands. One form of sign language uses mostly the alphabet. Another form, which deaf persons prefer for 'talking' with each other, uses symbols for different actions and things.

If there is a deaf child in the school, or in the village or neighborhood, perhaps the children would be interested in finding a way to help that child learn to 'sign'. Or they may want to learn themselves, in order to be able to 'talk' with the deaf child.

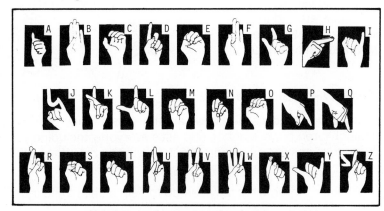

Alphabet sign language used in the USA. More discussion of sign language is on p. 266.

If 1 or 2 children in the class can learn to sign and then help translate spoken language into sign language, this can allow the deaf children to learn and take part more fully in the school and in the community. (For books to learn sign language, see p. 639-640). Also see Chapter 31.

Games to help children understand *the difficulties of poor sight*

GAME: CATCH A THIEF

This game can help children understand both the **importance of good hearing** and the **difficulties of not seeing.**

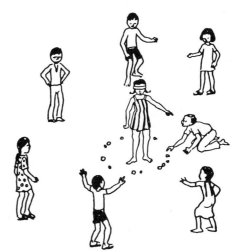

- The children form a circle. One child stands in the middle with her eyes covered. Around her feet are small stones, nuts, or other small objects.

- The other children, one by one, try to creep up and steal these things.

- If the child in the middle hears the 'thief', she points to him and he is out of the game.

- The goal is to see who can steal the most objects without being heard.

GAME: BLURRED VISION

One or more children are temporarily given poor or blurred vision in one of several ways:

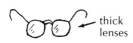
thick lenses

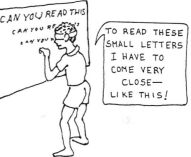

Put somebody's *powerful* eyeglasses on a child who needs no glasses.

Or, cover his eyes with a piece of tracing paper, wax paper, or other material that you can see through slightly.

CAN YOU READ THIS

TO READ THESE SMALL LETTERS I HAVE TO COME VERY CLOSE— LIKE THIS!

Have the child try to read from a book with letters of different sizes. Do the same on the blackboard. What trouble does he have? How close does he have to get? Does he read aloud from his book as well as the other children?

GAME: BLINDFOLDED PARTNERS

The children are in pairs. One is blindfolded, the other is her guide. The guide takes the blindfolded person for a walk, letting her feel different things and taking care of her.

After the game, discuss:

- How did it feel not to be able to see?
- What did your guide do that was helpful? Not helpful? What might she have done better?
- Did you trust your guide?

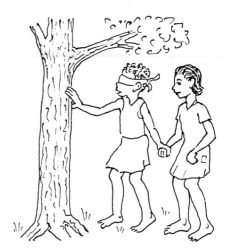

GAME: FEEL A FRIEND

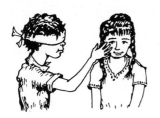

One child is blindfolded. He tries to recognize his friends by feeling them.

Similar feeling games can be played trying to identify different things by feeling them.

GAME: WHAT'S THE SMELL?

Blindfold the children and have them identify things by their smell: things such as orange, tea leaves, banana, and local herbs.

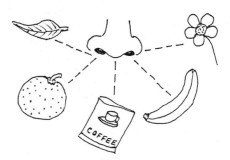

> After the children play these different games, explain to them that because **blind people** cannot see, they **often develop outstanding ability to identify things through hearing them, feeling them, and smelling them.**

FINDING OUT WHICH CHILDREN HAVE PROBLEMS WITH HEARING AND SEEING

It is important to find out **as early as possible** if a child cannot hear or see well. Older children can do some simple tests with their baby brothers and sisters. A class or group of children can also test the seeing and hearing of younger children, such as those in nursery school or the first year of elementary school.

Testing the hearing of babies (4 months old and older)

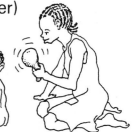

- Children can notice if their baby sister responds to different sounds, high and low, loud and soft. The baby may show surprise, make some movement, or turn her eyes or head toward the sound. Notice if the baby responds to her mother's voice when the baby does not see her.

- Or make a rattle from seeds or small stones. Creep up and shake it behind the baby's head, first on one side and then the other. See if the baby is surprised.

- Then call the baby's name from different places in the room. See if the baby responds.

- To test if a baby hears some kinds of sound but not others, do this. Sit at arm's length from the baby, and to one side. When she is not looking, make different kinds of sounds. Say "Ps" and "Fth" to test for high-pitched sounds, then "Oooo" for low-pitched sounds. For other high-pitched sounds, crinkle a thin, stiff piece of paper or rub a spoon inside a cup. For other low-pitched sounds, watch if the child notices the noise of a passing truck, a train whistle, a cow's 'moo', or low notes on a musical instrument or drum.

If the baby does not show surprise or turn her head with any of these sounds, she may have a severe hearing problem. If she responds only to certain sounds, but not to others, she has some hearing. But she may not be able to understand language well because she cannot tell certain words apart. As a result, she may not speak as early or as clearly as other children and will need special help. (See Chapter 31.)

Testing the hearing of young children (a game)

- An older child stands several meters from a line of younger children.

- Behind each young child stands an older child with pencil and paper.

- The first child says the name of an animal VERY LOUDLY.

COW
DOG
CAT
HEN

- The young children whisper the word to their older partners.

- The older children write it down.

- Then the first child names other animals, each in a softer and softer voice, until he is whispering.

- After about 10 animals have been named, and the words that the younger children heard have been written down, compare the different children's lists.

- Repeat this 2 or 3 times.

- **Any child who has not heard as many words as the others, or has not heard them correctly, probably has a hearing problem.**

What to do for the child with a hearing problem

- Let the child sit at the front of the class where he can hear better.

- Be sure everyone speaks clearly and loudly enough. But **do not shout** because shouting makes the words less clear. Check often to make sure the child understands.

- Have one child who hears well sit next to the one who hears poorly—to repeat and explain things if necessary.

- Always try to look at the child while you are speaking to him.

- If possible, the child should be examined by a health worker—especially if he has pus in an ear or frequent earache.

HOW CAN CHILDREN HELP CARE FOR THEIR BROTHERS' AND SISTERS' EARS?

They can regularly look to be sure that there is no pus or small objects inside. If they see anything wrong they should tell an older person, who should take the child to a health worker.

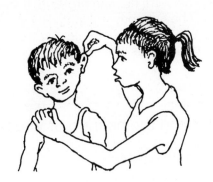

HEARING GAMES THAT CHILDREN CAN PLAY WITH BABIES

Most babies who are 'deaf' hear something. They need help in learning to listen. The children may think of games to help babies listen and learn.

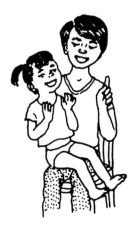

For example:

● Sing to babies, and teach songs to young children.

● Tell them stories and change voices to sound like different people in the story—loud, soft, angry.

Testing if a baby sees (for a child over 3 months old)

● Children can notice if the baby begins to look at things held in front of him, to follow them with his eyes, to smile at mother's face, and later to reach for things held out to him.

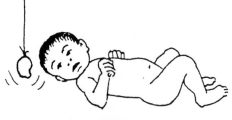

● Hang a bright colored object in front of the baby's face and move it from side to side. Does the baby follow with his eyes or head?

● If not, in a fairly dark room, move a lighted candle or torch (flashlight) in front of the child's face. Repeat 2 or 3 times.

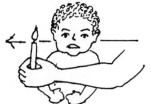

If the baby does not follow the object or light with his eyes or head, probably he does not see. He will need special help in learning to do things and move about without seeing. Other children can help. (See Chapter 30.)

Testing how well children see (4 years old and older)

A group of older children can make an eye chart. They can cut out black 'E's of different sizes and paste them on white cardboard.

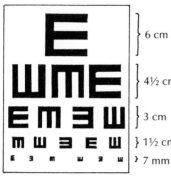

} 6 cm high

} 4½ cm

} 3 cm

} 1½ cm

} 7 mm

Also make one large 'E' shape out of cardboard or other material.

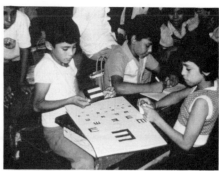

Children making an eye chart. (Mexico)

First let the children test each other. Hang the chart in a place where the light is good. Then make a line about 6 meters from the chart. The child to be tested stands behind the line, holding the cut-out 'E'. Another child points at different 'E's, starting from the top.

Ask the child being tested to hold the cut-out 'E' so that its 'legs' point the same way as the 'E' on the chart.

If the child can easily see the 'E's on the bottom line, he sees well. **If he has trouble seeing the second or third line, he sees poorly.**

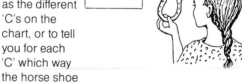

6 m or 20 feet

- To make the testing more fun, you can use horses in the shape of 'E's.

- Make 5 cards using different size horses. Make the sizes the same as those shown for the letter 'E' in the chart at the top of this page.

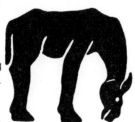

- Or use a chart with 'C's. Ask the child either to hold a horse shoe in the same position as the different 'C's on the chart, or to tell you for each 'C' which way the horse shoe is going.

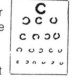

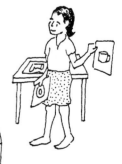

To test children who are mentally slow, deaf, or have trouble communicating, you can use pictures of different things they recognize. Hold up one picture at a time and have the child either name it or point to a similar picture— or the real object. For example, you can make a set of cards with pictures like this:

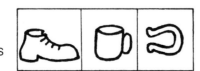

After the children practice testing each other, they can test the eyesight of those in the younger grades and the children who will be starting school soon.

WHAT TO DO FOR THE CHILD WHO SEES POORLY

- Be sure he sits in front, close to the blackboard.

- Write large and dark on the blackboard, and check often to make sure he can read what is there.

- If possible, the child should go to a health worker for more tests. He may need glasses.

- If he cannot get glasses, try to find a magnifying glass. This may help him read small letters.

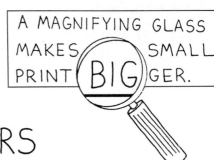

- If he has not learned to read and write because he does not see well, teach him with

EXTRA BIG LETTERS

- If the child still has trouble reading, have another child read his books and lessons to him aloud.

Looking at each other's eyes for signs of problems

Start with questions to get the children interested. For example:

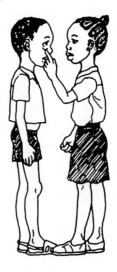

- Are your eyes the same as your classmates? Shiny? Clear?

- How about the eyes of your younger brothers and sisters?

- Can you see well in the dark? Or do you often stumble at night?

- Do a child's eyes look dull? Are there any unusual spots or wrinkles? If so, see a health worker.

Many children in different parts of the world become blind because they do not eat foods that make their eyes healthy. **Eating yellow fruits or dark green leafy vegetables helps protect the eyes.** Some extra cooking oil added to food also helps.

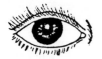 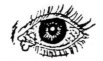

If children's eyes are red or sore, you can suggest that they wash them often with clean water with a little salt in it (no saltier than tears). This may help eyes get better and keep the flies away. If they do not get better soon, see a health worker.

For more information on eye problems and blindness, see Chapter 30.

Popular Theater

Community theater can be an excellent way to raise awareness about specific needs of disabled persons or to gain greater participation of local people in a community *rehabilitation* program. It is also a good method for educating people about important preventive measures. Actors can be disabled persons, parents of disabled children, health workers, rehabilitation workers, school-children, or any combination of these.

No special place is needed. However, some sort of raised area is helpful, with a plain wall or curtain behind. But effective popular theater has also been carried out in the street, the village square, and the marketplace.

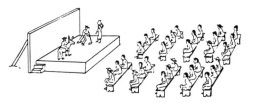
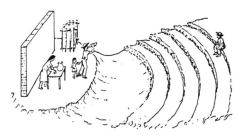

Simple outdoor stages for popular theater.

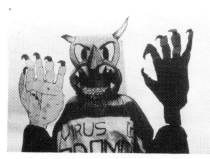

The Measles Monster street theater skit in Nicaragua. The head of the monster is a mask painted on heavy paper, glued to a cardboard carton.

For example, **measles** *is especially dangerous to poorly nourished children, leaving many with blindness, deafness, fits, retardation, or cerebral palsy. Preventing measles helps prevent disability.* In Nicaragua a group of health workers and local children put on a street theater skit called *'The Measles Monster'.* Popular participation is high, for as watchers gather, the monster runs through the crowd looking for unvaccinated children. At the end of the skit, when all the children are protected by *vaccination,* the children in the audience join the children in the skit in beating-up the monster.

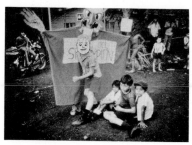

An unvaccinated child actor (wearing a white 'happy' mask) is caught by the measles monster, who closes his huge claws around him.

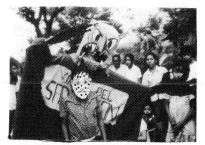

Under the monster's claws, the child rapidly changes masks. When the monster uncovers him, he is wearing a 'sad' mask speckled with red spots. The child nearly dies.

The announcer of the skit asks the children in the audience why the boy was attacked. They shout back, "Because he wasn't vaccinated." At the end, after all the children are vaccinated, the loudspeaker asks, "Why can the children now overcome the monster?" They shout back, "Because we have all been vaccinated!"

To give another idea of what can be done through popular theater, we will show you photos from 2 theater skits organized by Project PROJIMO, the villager-run rehabilitation program based in Ajoya, Mexico.

In order to increase community involvement in PROJIMO and to help local people understand its activities better, the program uses popular theater. The skits were put on soon after the school children had helped build the rehabilitation playground. They tell the story of how PROJIMO began and how the playground was built and is used. The actors are local school children, disabled workers of PROJIMO, and village health workers from neighboring villages who were in town for a refresher course. The health workers' participation in the skits gave them experience working with disabled persons, and also gave them ideas for simple rehabilitation activities and aids in their own villages.

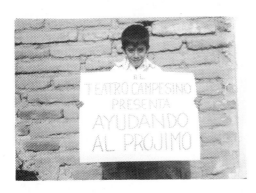

The Farm People's Theater presents:
"HELPING YOUR NEIGHBOR"

—the story of how Project PROJIMO got started and how village school children built a playground for disabled and non-disabled children.

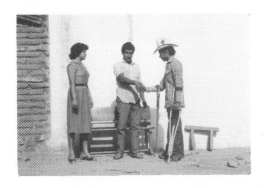

A disabled young man (played by Marcelo, see p. 76) arrives at Ajoya and asks directions to the village health center (Project Piaxtla).

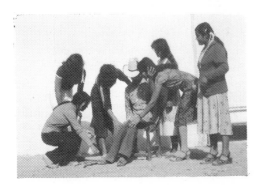

The health workers examine him, find he is disabled by polio and think he may need braces. But they lack the knowledge about what to do for him. So they send him away without helping him.

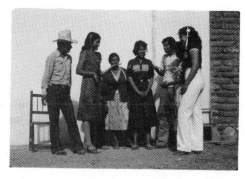

The health workers are concerned: "So many disabled children come to us. Most of them don't need hospitalization or surgery, but simpler things like braces or special exercises. Yet we don't have the knowledge or skills to provide these things for them. Why don't we try to get more training and start a rehabilitation program for disabled children here in our village? We can focus on what parents can do for their children in the home."

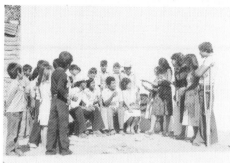

The health workers meet with villagers to discuss the new program. The villagers respond enthusiastically. Men offer to help fix up the center. Women offer to provide room and food for visiting children and their families. And the schoolchildren offer to help build a rehabilitation playground—on condition that they can play there too.

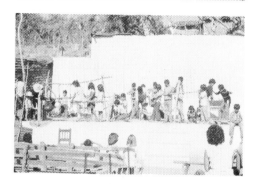

The schoolchildren—who had already built the actual 'playground for all children' in the village—quickly rebuild the playground on stage.

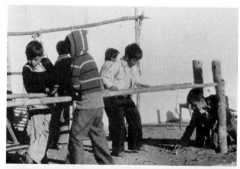

Because they had already dug the holes for the poles, and had practiced over and over again, they were able to set up the playground on stage in about 3 minutes.

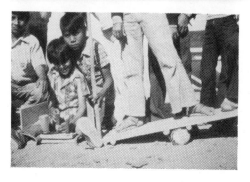

In this way villagers have a chance to see how different equipment in the playground is used—like this 'rocker board' to help children with balance problems, and the sitting frame to help a child with spasticity keep his legs apart while he plays with homemade educational toys.

The second skit is a continuation of the first.

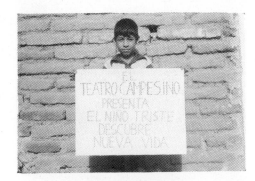

This is the disabled child, Tristín.

His role is played by Inés—one of the disabled village workers. In fact, the skit comes close to telling Inés' own story. Like Tristín in the skit, Inés is an orphan disabled by polio who was helped by PROJIMO to get braces, and then stayed on as a rehabilitation worker.

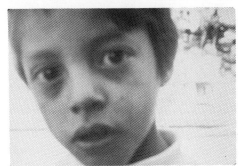

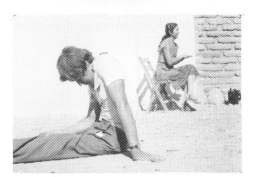

Marcelo, a village rehabilitation worker, finds Tristín in a village hut. The boy is unhappy because he cannot walk and has no friends. Marcelo invites Tristín to come with him to PROJIMO.

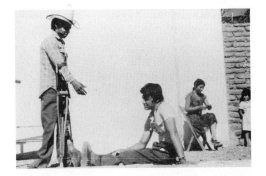

They arrive at PROJIMO, and Marcelo shows Tristín the playground.

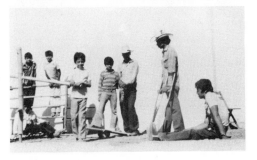

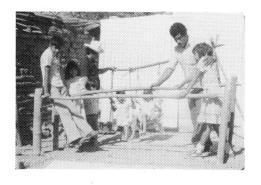

Tristín (and the audience) have a chance to see how the playground equipment is used to help disabled children learn to walk and do other things.

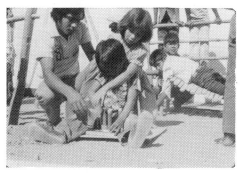

They see how the sitting frame and homemade games are used; also how a child who cannot sit lies on a sloping platform so he can lift his head and use his hands.

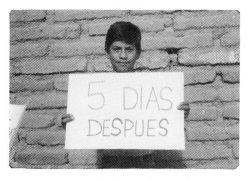

5 days later

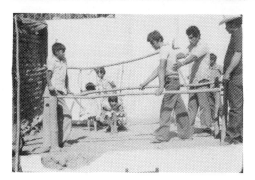

The village rehabilitation workers have made a brace for Tristín, and here fit it onto his leg.

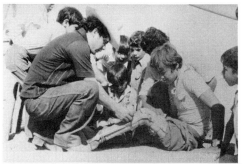

Then they help him learn to walk with the brace, using the parallel bars.

Tristín learns quickly and soon begins to walk with crutches.

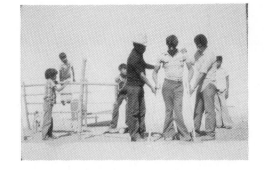

The time comes when PROJIMO has done as much as it can for Tristín, in terms of *physical* rehabilitation. "Where do you go from here?" they ask him. "I don't know," he answers. "I have no family to go to. I've never gone to school. Work is hard to get even for the physically fit." "Why don't you stay with us and help in the rehab program? You can learn some skills and help other children like yourself."

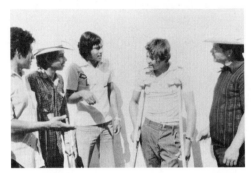

Tristín decides to stay, and begins to learn rehabilitation skills. Here a mother arrives with the first child for whom Tristín becomes responsible as a 'rehabilitation helper'.

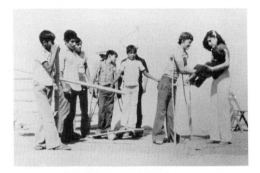

Together the team examines the child, who appears to have cerebral palsy affecting mainly his legs. The team believes he has a good chance of learning to walk.

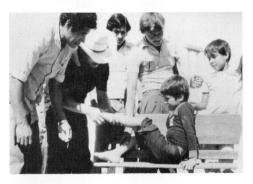

Tristín shows the child's mother how she can help him learn to walk using the parallel bars.

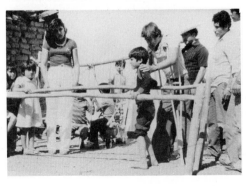

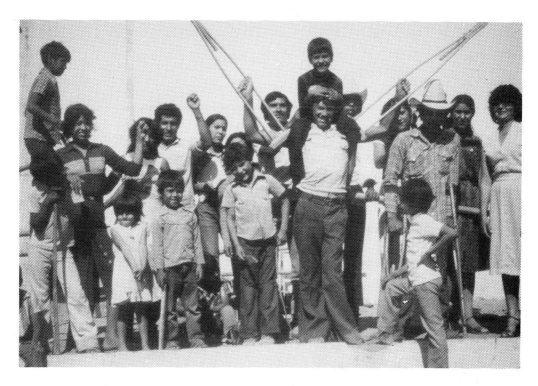

At last the little boy learns to walk. But just as
important, he has new hope, new friends and new self-
confidence. He sees other disabled persons like
himself who are not only leading full lives, but who
are working hard to serve others in need. As the skit
ends, Tristín lifts his young friend onto his
shoulders and raises his crutches in a sign of victory.

The ending of this skit was even more impressive for the village audience because
they had seen Inés (who acted as Tristín) when he first came to their village. They knew
that his transformation from a very disabled, withdrawn youth to a fast-moving,
capable young man was not just acted — it was real.

And because PROJIMO is the village's program, everyone felt proud.

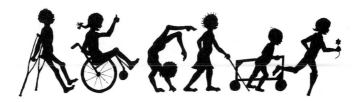

Though not directly related to disability prevention, a
slide set with written script "Small Farmers Join
Together To Overcome Exploitation" is available from
the Hesperian Foundation.

Other skits are mentioned in this book on p. 443 and 445.

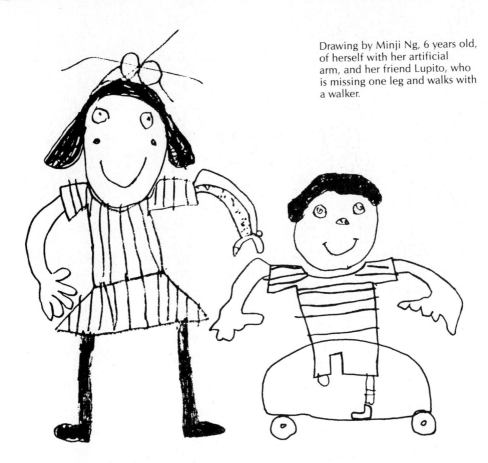

Drawing by Minji Ng, 6 years old, of herself with her artificial arm, and her friend Lupito, who is missing one leg and walks with a walker.

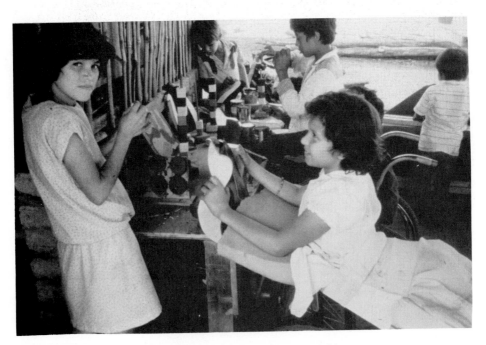

Disabled children together with school children, at work in the toymaking shop at PROJIMO.

A Children's Workshop for Making Toys

If a *rehabilitation* program is to achieve a strong base in the community, it needs to involve large numbers of local children. There are many important ways in which village children of various ages can take part, playing and working together with disabled children. We have already discussed how children can help build a low-cost 'playground-for-all children'.

Another way that village children can contribute to a rehabilitation program is by helping to make special toys for disabled babies and children.

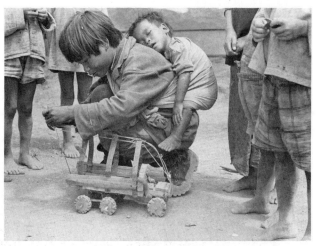

Children often design and make excellent toys. This child from Vietnam puts the last touches on his homemade truck. (Photo: UNICEF/Jacques Danois)

In Project PROJIMO in Mexico, village children help out in this way—and enjoy doing it. In addition to the toys that this voluntary 'labor' produces, it also brings together non-disabled and *disabled* children in a creative work-play relationship.

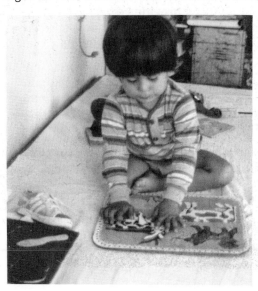

Animal puzzles, like this one made by village children, help a child learn to use his hands, and to match shapes. (PROJIMO)

At first the children at PROJIMO made toys in the same workshop where the disabled staff was busy making braces, wheelchairs, and other *orthopedic* equipment. But soon things got too crowded. The children often played while they worked (which is natural), and a few important tools got broken or 'lost'. While there were advantages to letting the children work in the same shop with skilled disabled craftspersons, the team finally decided to create a separate 'children's workshop' equipped with its own basic tools.

In this workshop, children are invited to make educational and useful toys —'useful' in the sense that they help with a child's early development, providing *stimulation,* exercise, use of the senses, and learning of skills.

As the children or disabled workers become more skillful at making toys, some can be sold to help bring in money to the workers or program. Some of the toys and dolls made at PROJIMO are sold to visitors. In Jamaica, disabled young people run an economically successful factory, making wooden toys. Toys made at the Life Help Center for the Handicapped, Madras, India, are sold world-wide. (See booklet, p. 641.)

PROJIMO has an agreement with the children. **The first toy they make is for the rehabilitation center** or for a particular disabled child. **The second toy they make they can take home** for a younger brother or sister. In this way PROJIMO and the school children also contribute to the development of non-disabled children in the village.

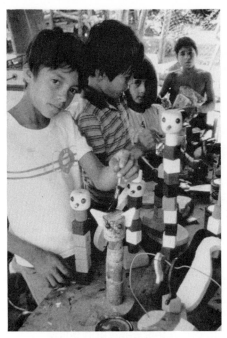

School children making toys.

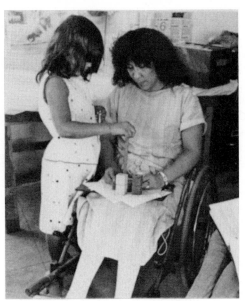

Mari, one of the rehabilitation workers at PROJIMO, uses one of the child-made toys to test the ability of a girl who is developmentally delayed.

Another advantage to the children's workshop is that it **provides experience, fun, productive activity, and skills training for visiting disabled children.** Thus a child who needs to spend a few days in the village, while a brace or limb is being fitted or a joint is being straightened, can spend part of his free time in the workshop.

The orthopedic workshop is not strictly off-limits for the children. Occasionally a child who proves to be a responsible and serious worker will be allowed to help in the 'adult workshop' — perhaps helping to make crutches, braces, special seats, and other orthopedic equipment. But to gain working privilege in the 'big persons' shop, a child must usually first prove himself in the children's workshop. This helps reduce problems. But, of course, some problems do occur — as with any community action that is worthwhile.

Guiding and coordinating the children's workshop (we prefer 'guiding' to 'supervising') is an important job. It can be shared by different persons: rehabilitation workers, volunteer village craftspersons, or even some of the older, more responsible children as they gain experience. What is most important for such a coordinator is (a) that she like children, (b) that she be able to provide direction and keep order effectively without being bossy, and (c) that she be very patient.

Whether parents of visiting or local disabled children are invited as coordinators or helpers in the children's workshop can be decided depending on the particular parent and child. Some parents do a fine job. It may be an opportunity for a parent to relate to and work with his child in a completely new way. However, some parents may continue to overprotect and over-direct their own child or other children in the workshop. Many children need a chance to do and make things with other children independent of their parents' supervision or help. For such children, it may be best *not* to ask their parents to be present in the workshop.

Tools and equipment for a children's workshop

Here are some suggestions for basic equipment. You will want to consider what tools are commonly used and least expensive in your area, and equip the shop accordingly.

- **Workbenches.** You will probably need at least 2, at different heights. One should be just high enough for the local size of children's wheelchairs to fit under. (Unfortunately, many children are given adult-size wheelchairs with high armrests. These often do not fit under a bench at a good height for working.) Make workbenches strong enough so they do not move a lot.

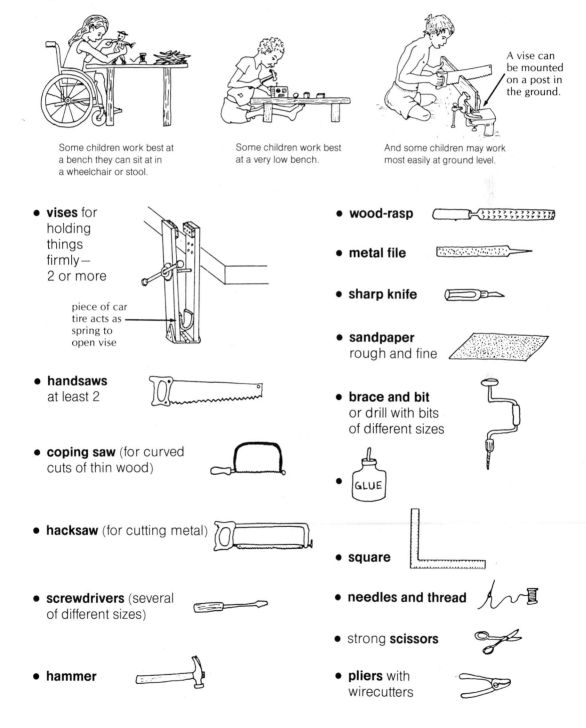

Some children work best at a bench they can sit at in a wheelchair or stool.

Some children work best at a very low bench.

And some children may work most easily at ground level.

A vise can be mounted on a post in the ground.

- **vises** for holding things firmly — 2 or more

  piece of car tire acts as spring to open vise

- **handsaws** at least 2

- **coping saw** (for curved cuts of thin wood)

- **hacksaw** (for cutting metal)

- **screwdrivers** (several of different sizes)

- **hammer**

- **wood-rasp**

- **metal file**

- **sharp knife**

- **sandpaper** rough and fine

- **brace and bit** or drill with bits of different sizes

- GLUE

- **square**

- **needles and thread**

- strong **scissors**

- **pliers** with wirecutters

More expensive tools

If electricity is available and the program or community can afford it, a few **power tools** will make work faster, more fun, and more productive for the children. Clearly, care must be taken to avoid highly dangerous equipment. **Make sure children take the necessary precautions.** Here are some examples of electrical equipment that can make work much easier and faster:

- **an electric jigsaw** for making puzzles, wood animals, and so on

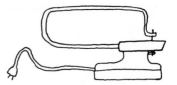

- **grinding wheel** (hand or electric)

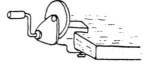

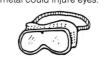

> CAUTION: Be sure children and all workers use goggles (protective glasses) when using tools where bits of wood or metal could injure eyes.

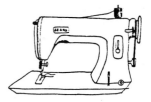

- **an electric drill** with attachments for sanding and grinding

sander   grinder

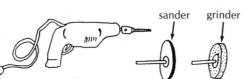

- **A sewing machine** (foot-powered or electric) will also be helpful in making many toys, dolls, and clothing. If the program can afford it, this machine can speed up sewing greatly, and help children learn an important skill.

Gathering materials and supplies

Explore every opportunity to obtain low- or no-cost materials and supplies for making toys. Here are a few possibilities:

- Many materials for making toys can be gathered from local forests—branches of trees, reeds, bamboo, wild kapok (cotton). Also various nuts, seedpods, and sea-shells can be used.

- Broken fruit-packing boxes often have thin wood that is excellent for toy-making. Even the nails can be pulled out, straightened and re-used.

- Old tubes of car and bike tires provide elastic bands for many toys.

- Scraps of wood, wire, and other supplies left over by lumber stores, builders, etc. will often be donated if you explain why you want them.

- Clothing makers and factories may have scraps of cloth left over.

- Cardboard cartons, especially thick ones (even if broken) provide material for making many toys. Ask in local shops.

- Old cans, tins, plastic bottles, thread spools, and so on are also useful.

Ask members of the community to look for and collect these and other supplies.

TOYS CHILDREN CAN MAKE

In a community rehabilitation program it is essential to have lots of toys—different playthings for children at different levels of development who have different strengths, weaknesses, and interests.

There is an old saying . . .

"THEY WHO CHOP THEIR OWN
FIREWOOD WARM
THEMSELVES TWICE!"

We have a new saying . . .

"THE FAMILY THAT MAKES
ITS OWN TOYS HAS
TWICE AS MUCH FUN!"

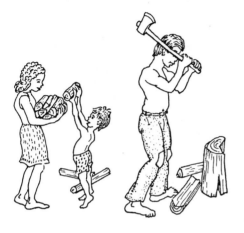

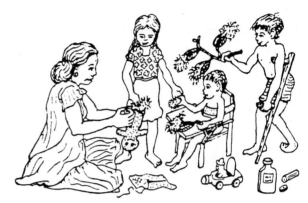

stuffing a homemade doll with wild kapok

Many of the most fun, most educational toys can be made from scrap materials by members of the family or community. Disabled children with good hands can learn skills and take pride in making toys for other disabled children. So it makes sense to **make toys rather than to buy them.**

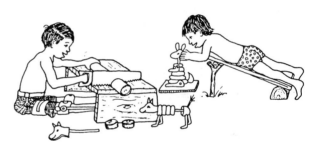

Helping to make toys for other children can be just as educational—and fun—as playing with them.

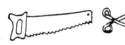 **Spend money on TOOLS, not toys.**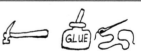

The following pages show a number of toys that children will enjoy making in a children's workshop. Or disabled children or their families can make them at home. We start with very simple toys for babies or children at an early developmental level. Gradually, the toys become more advanced. More skills will be needed by the children who make them, and by those who play with them.

IMPORTANT: Please don't just copy the ideas for toys shown here. Be creative. And **encourage the children making the toys to be creative.** Help them use the examples shown on these pages as triggers to the imagination. Have fun!

TOYS TO ENCOURAGE LOOKING AND LISTENING

small mirrors or pieces of tin foil or shiny paper

colorful objects that move in the air

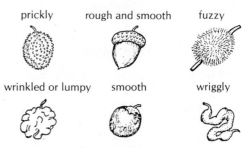

small bells

from UPKARAN manual (See p. 642.)

TOYS THAT HELP DEVELOP USE OF HANDS AND SENSE OF TOUCH

You can make beads and chains out of wild fruits and nuts.

prickly   rough and smooth   fuzzy

wrinkled or lumpy   smooth   wriggly

> *CAUTION:* Be sure not to use things that are poisonous, harmful, or that might get stuck in the child's throat, nose, or ears.

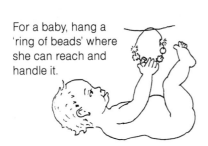

For a baby, hang a 'ring of beads' where she can reach and handle it.

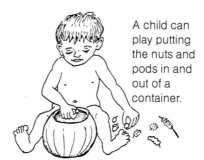

A child can play putting the nuts and pods in and out of a container.

Later he can learn to sort them—first by seeing them, and then blindfolded.

As the child develops more hand control, she can begin to make chains and necklaces by stringing the nuts on a cord.

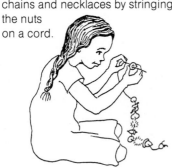

'**Snakes**' can be made by stringing nuts, 'caps' of acorns, bottle caps—or any combination of things.

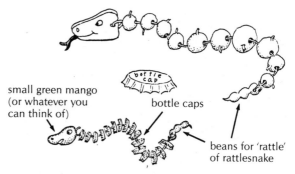

small green mango (or whatever you can think of)

bottle caps

beans for 'rattle' of rattlesnake

'**Hedgehogs**'

acorn

'papache' (woody fruits from wild bush)

guasima fruit

knobby sticks from papache bush →

← cloves →

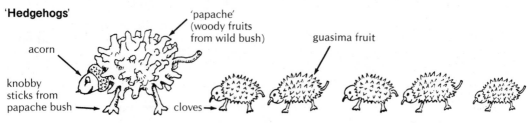

If you use your imagination, there are all kinds of toy animals you and your children can have fun making.

RATTLES AND OTHER 'NOISE TOYS'

Gourd rattle

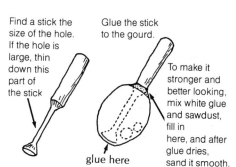

Find a small gourd (wild gourds or 'tree gourds' may work).

Cut a round hole at the stem and clean out the seeds and flesh. Let it dry out well.

Put 2 or 3 small rocks, nuts or other objects inside.

Find a stick the size of the hole. If the hole is large, thin down this part of the stick

Glue the stick to the gourd.

glue here

To make it stronger and better looking, mix white glue and sawdust, fill in here, and after glue dries, sand it smooth.

Paint it colorfully.

Plastic bottle rattle

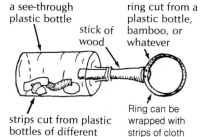

a see-through plastic bottle

stick of wood

ring cut from a plastic bottle, bamboo, or whatever

strips cut from plastic bottles of different colors, colorful stones, nuts, etc.

Ring can be wrapped with strips of cloth or tire tubing for easier grip.

Bamboo rattle

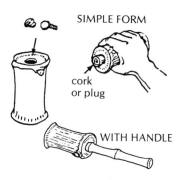

SIMPLE FORM

cork or plug

WITH HANDLE

Tin can rattle

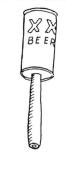

XX BEER

Cowhorn rattle

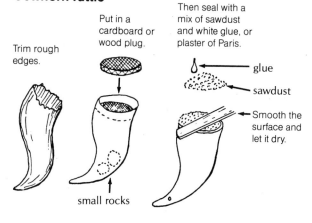

Trim rough edges.

Put in a cardboard or wood plug.

Then seal with a mix of sawdust and white glue, or plaster of Paris.

glue

sawdust

Smooth the surface and let it dry.

small rocks

If the child drops or throws his toys, try attaching strings and help him learn to get them back by himself.

IDEAS FOR HOMEMADE 'MUSIC' (from *How To Raise a Blind Child*, see p. 639)

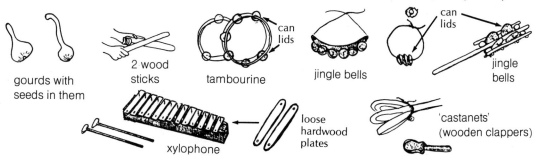

gourds with seeds in them

2 wood sticks

tambourine

can lids

jingle bells

can lids

jingle bells

xylophone

loose hardwood plates

'castanets' (wooden clappers)

Soft rattle

Use a small
can or bottle
with a small
stone inside,

or use
2 small
bells.

Cut a colorful
soft cloth
(flannel)
this shape.

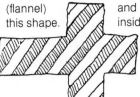

Sew it into
a square
and turn
inside out.

Place can or bells
in cloth square and
pack wild kapok,
cotton or bits of
sponge around it.
Sew it shut.

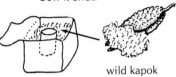

wild kapok

Doll rattle

Draw a doll on
2 pieces of cloth,
and cut them out.

Sew the
2 dolls
together.

Turn the doll
inside out.

Sew or draw
on a face.

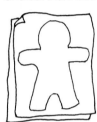

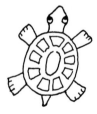

Leave a
small
opening.

Put small bells
or a rattle
inside and
stuff with
kapok, cotton,
or sponge and
sew shut.

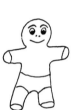

Animal rattles

can be made in
the same way

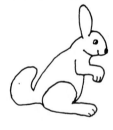

Ball rattle

Cut 3 pieces
of cloth of
one color.

and 3 pieces
of another
color.

Sew them together
except for a small
hole. Turn inside
out and stuff.

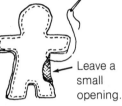

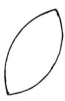

Push-a-long noise toy

Make hole in
lid and bottom
of tin.

Put bottle tops,
small stones,
etc. inside.

Put loop of stiff
wire through holes
with knot inside tin.

Bamboo push-a-long

Cut here.

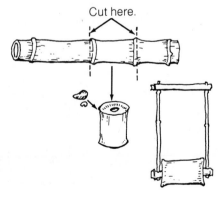

Plastic bottle pig

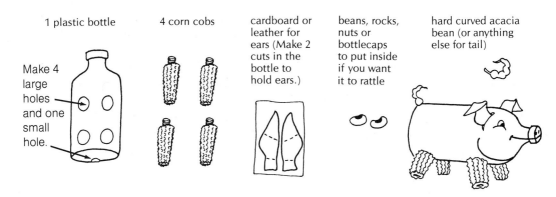

1 plastic bottle

Make 4 large holes and one small hole.

4 corn cobs

cardboard or leather for ears (Make 2 cuts in the bottle to hold ears.)

beans, rocks, nuts or bottlecaps to put inside if you want it to rattle

hard curved acacia bean (or anything else for tail)

Papier-mâché piggybank

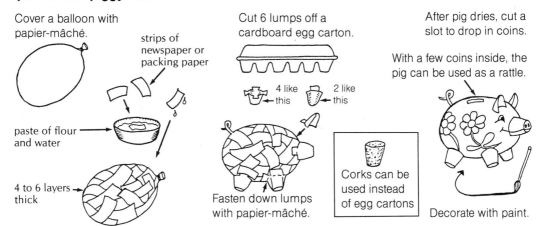

Cover a balloon with papier-mâché.

strips of newspaper or packing paper

paste of flour and water

4 to 6 layers thick

Cut 6 lumps off a cardboard egg carton.

4 like this   2 like this

Fasten down lumps with papier-mâché.

Corks can be used instead of egg cartons

After pig dries, cut a slot to drop in coins.

With a few coins inside, the pig can be used as a rattle.

Decorate with paint.

Children can improve hand control, learn to count, and learn about money by playing with coins and the piggybank.

Papier-mâché frog

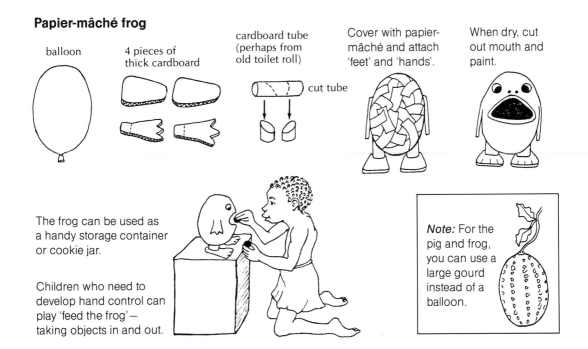

balloon

4 pieces of thick cardboard

cardboard tube (perhaps from old toilet roll)

cut tube

Cover with papier-mâché and attach 'feet' and 'hands'.

When dry, cut out mouth and paint.

The frog can be used as a handy storage container or cookie jar.

Children who need to develop hand control can play 'feed the frog' — taking objects in and out.

Note: For the pig and frog, you can use a large gourd instead of a balloon.

Games fitting pegs or blocks into holes help develop better hand control and 'hand-eye coordination'. They also help the child learn to compare sizes, shapes, and colors.

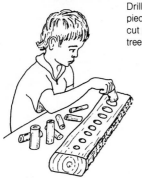

Drill holes in a piece of wood and cut pegs from tree branches.

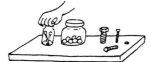

Or you can cut holes in a cardboard box. Glue an extra layer of tough cardboard on the top.

Or make a 'size box' by pouring cement, plaster of Paris, or clay into a mold. Or, make a 'plaster' box out of cow-dung or mud mixed with sand (and lime if you have it). Press pegs into the wet plaster, and remove when almost dry.

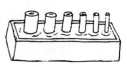

For pegs, use bottles, scraps of pipe, pieces of broom handles, bolts—or whatever.

Also, make games that help the child develop a twisting motion in her hands and wrists.

Other ideas

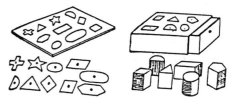

Blocks for building a tower on pegs

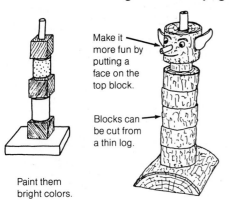

Make it more fun by putting a face on the top block.

Blocks can be cut from a thin log.

Paint them bright colors.

'Animal stackers'

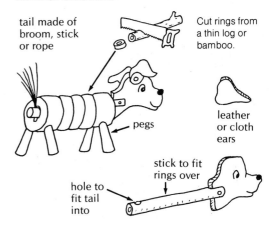

tail made of broom, stick or rope

Cut rings from a thin log or bamboo.

leather or cloth ears

pegs

stick to fit rings over

hole to fit tail into

Slide-on wire toys

To help develop fine control of hand movement, blocks, beads or animal figures can be moved along a wire. Children with poor control need only move the figure from one side to the other. Children with good control try to move the figure without touching the wire. The more bends you put in the wire, the harder it is.

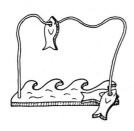

To make it more interesting, match the animal figures with wooden bases in the form and colors of the place the animal lives: fish in water, squirrels in trees, birds in flowers.

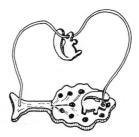

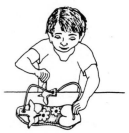

Gourd racing car

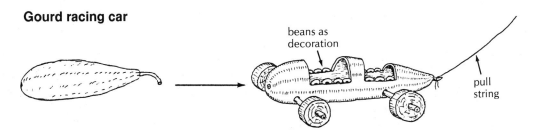

beans as decoration

pull string

Gourd baby

The gourd baby is fun because it can be given drinks and then 'go to the latrine'. Thus it can be a good tool for 'toilet training' children. For other ideas and dolls for toilet training, see p. 341.

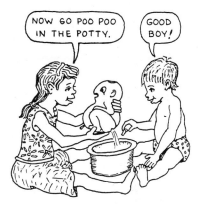

plug   plug

NOW GO POO POO IN THE POTTY.

GOOD BOY!

Shapes on pegs*

With these, children learn about matching colors, shapes, and sizes.

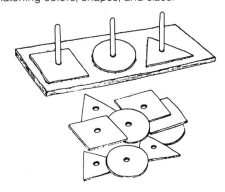

Figures with posts for easy gripping*

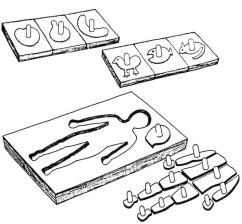

Building blocks*
(of wood, clay, or layers of cardboard)

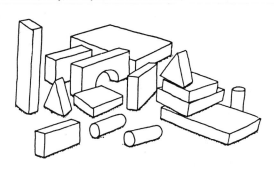

cubes and sticks

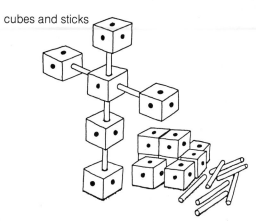

*These are from the UPKARAN Manual (See p. 642.)

Biting donkey

This wooden donkey or horse with a clothes-pin head is fun to make and to play with.

It can also be used as a note or reminder holder. Perhaps disabled children at the rehabilitation center can make this to sell for pocket money.

Trace the donkey onto a piece of wood about as thick as the clothes-pin (1 cm). Cut it out with a jig saw. Also make a base, as shown. Sand pieces smooth and glue together.

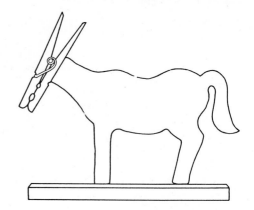

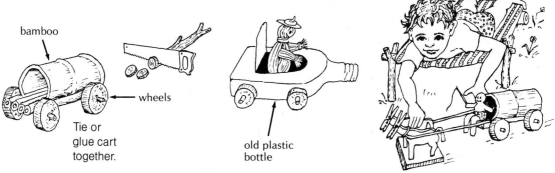

Donkey carts

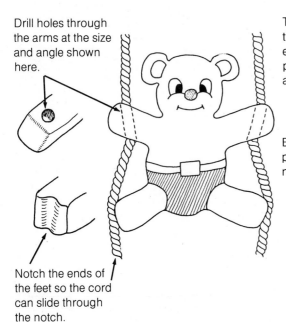

bamboo

wheels

Tie or glue cart together.

old plastic bottle

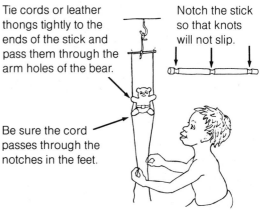

Climbing bear

Cut a pattern of the bear out of a wood board about 2 cm. (3/4 inch) thick.

Drill holes through the arms at the size and angle shown here.

Notch the ends of the feet so the cord can slide through the notch.

Hang a stick from the roof or a tree limb.

Tie cords or leather thongs tightly to the ends of the stick and pass them through the arm holes of the bear.

Notch the stick so that knots will not slip.

Be sure the cord passes through the notches in the feet.

By pulling one cord and then the other, the bear will climb the ropes! Children love it!

Good for developing use of both hands together.

RUBBER BAND WIND-UP TOYS

Steamroller

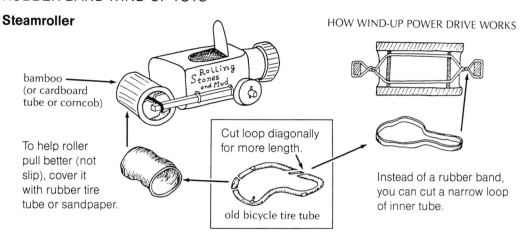

HOW WIND-UP POWER DRIVE WORKS

bamboo (or cardboard tube or corncob)

To help roller pull better (not slip), cover it with rubber tire tube or sandpaper.

Cut loop diagonally for more length.

old bicycle tire tube

Instead of a rubber band, you can cut a narrow loop of inner tube.

Paddle wheel boat

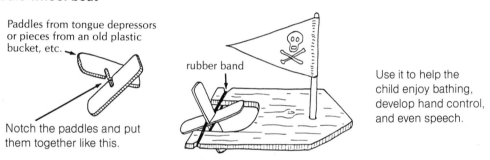

Paddles from tongue depressors or pieces from an old plastic bucket, etc.

Notch the paddles and put them together like this.

rubber band

Use it to help the child enjoy bathing, develop hand control, and even speech.

Corncob creeper

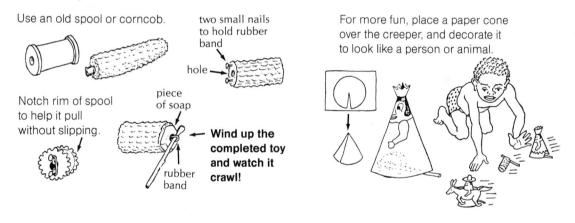

Use an old spool or corncob.

two small nails to hold rubber band

hole

Notch rim of spool to help it pull without slipping.

piece of soap

rubber band

Wind up the completed toy and watch it crawl!

For more fun, place a paper cone over the creeper, and decorate it to look like a person or animal.

Whirlygig screech plane

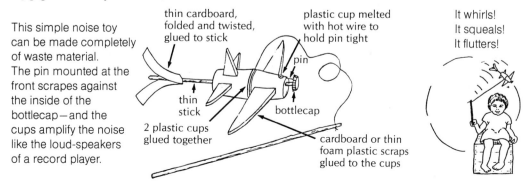

This simple noise toy can be made completely of waste material. The pin mounted at the front scrapes against the inside of the bottlecap—and the cups amplify the noise like the loud-speakers of a record player.

thin cardboard, folded and twisted, glued to stick

plastic cup melted with hot wire to hold pin tight

pin

thin stick

bottlecap

2 plastic cups glued together

cardboard or thin foam plastic scraps glued to the cups

It whirls!
It squeals!
It flutters!

PUZZLES

Puzzles can help a child learn how shapes, forms, and colors fit together. Puzzles can be made by glueing a picture on **cardboard, wood, plywood,** or other material. Cut out the pieces with a coping saw. Puzzles can be made in various styles:

Flower puzzles

Children can first learn to form one flower.

Later, they can play 'sorting games' with flowers of different colors.

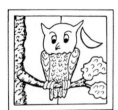 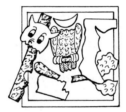

Several children can play to see who can complete a flower first—using dice with different colored sides. ➝

Figure puzzles

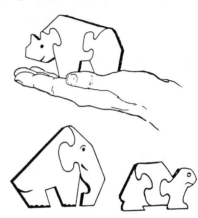

Puzzles with cut-out pieces that follow the forms and lines of the drawing

First have the child build the main object (here, the owl) with a few pieces. Later, she can learn to fill in the background.

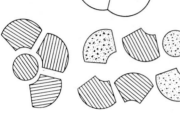

An outer frame helps hold the pieces together.

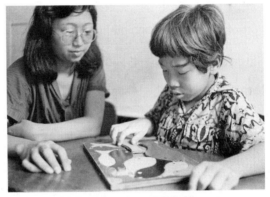

A retarded child in Indonesia learns to fit together a fish puzzle. (Photo: Christian Children's Fund, Carolyn Watson)

Puzzles with interlocking pieces

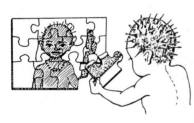

Suggestion: If you have a large photo of the child or a family member, glue it on cardboard and cut out the puzzle. Or use a picture from a magazine or calendar.

Block puzzles

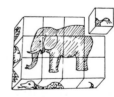

Glue 6 different pictures to the sides of a thick board or sheet of foam plastic, and cut it into blocks. You can also make blocks from cubes of clay or small match boxes.

Ideas for the toys shown in this chapter are from many sources, including books. For books on toys and games, see p. 641. Other toys are on pages 253, 317, 318, 341, 347, and 392.

Organization, Management, and Financing of a Village Rehabilitation Program

CHAPTER 50

ORGANIZATION AND MANAGEMENT— A 'PEOPLE-CENTERED' APPROACH

In Chapter 45 we spoke of top-down and bottom-up approaches to a community program. Programs that are 'bottom-up', or begun by disabled persons, family members, and concerned members of the community, tend to be organized and managed very differently than top-down programs.

A sense of equality among all persons taking part in or benefiting from the program is basic to the organization of bottom-up or 'people-centered' programs:

- Everyone is considered equal.

- Leaders are coordinators, not bosses.

- Decisions are either made by the group or can be openly challenged by the group or by any of its members.

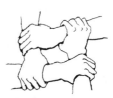

- Everyone has the same rights and deserves the same respect. The ideas and opinions of a *disabled* child or her parents are just as important as those of the village *rehabilitation* worker or visiting professional. All are equal and valuable members of the rehabilitation team.

In a people-centered program, goodwill, friendliness, and a feeling of shared pleasure in meeting each other's needs are often given more importance than polished floors, arriving on time, exact records, number of hours worked, or how many wheelchairs are produced by each worker each month. Success of the program is measured not so much by formal *evaluation* as by the '**smile factor**': how good everyone— workers, parents, and children—feels about what they have put into and received from the interaction.

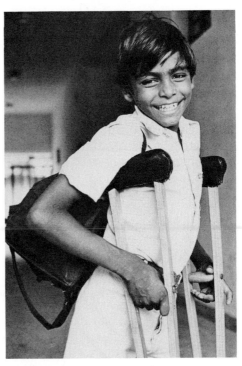

THE SMILE FACTOR—perhaps the best measurement of a program's success. (Photo: UNICEF/T.S. Satyan)

The PROJIMO approach: Informal organization and team management

We who work at PROJIMO are in no position to speak with authority about 'organization and management'. Sometimes we wonder if our achievements are due more to our **disorganization.** Whatever organization and management we have is informal and more or less cooperative. Not only are there no clear-cut divisions between 'managers' and 'workers', but even the division between 'workers' and 'patients' is unclear. (In fact, we avoid words like 'patient' and 'client'.) Parents, children, visitors, and everyone else are invited and expected to help out in whatever way they can. Most members of the PROJIMO team are disabled young persons who first came for rehabilitation or aids. They began to help out as best they could, and finally decided to stay to learn and work. Some stay a few weeks or months, learn new skills, gain confidence, and then go on to something else. Others stay for years. Some come and go, and return again.

PROJIMO is like a big family, mainly of young people, growing up together. Most of the work team is made up of young persons who are themselves benefiting from rehabilitation, learning to work, and learning to relate to each other. It would be a mistake to use the same goals and measure of 'production efficiency' as you would for a shop that employs already trained and experienced workers. There is no boss to give orders. Yet the needs of the disabled children place a demand on the group to work relatively hard, and to accomplish what they can. Hours are flexible. There are quiet afternoons where half the workers suddenly decide to go swimming in the river. And there are busy days when several team members work until midnight to finish a brace or limb or wheelchair for a family that needs to return home on the morning bus. They choose to work overtime, not because someone tells them to, or because they get extra pay, but because a child's father explains that he cannot afford to miss another day's work or a mother is worried about a sick child she left at home.

When a situation arises that will require extra work and responsibility, the group as a whole decides if they think they can handle it. For example, one time a teenage boy named Julio arrived who was almost completely *paralyzed* (quadriplegic). He had severe pressure sores, and was totally dependent for all his daily needs. The team, which had no one specially trained in nursing care, met and discussed whether they could accept Julio in PROJIMO, since no family member was prepared to stay with him. Some argued against accepting him. Others argued in favor, pointing out that his home situation was miserable. (His stepfather resented his mother spending time with the boy.) At last the majority decided to accept Julio, even though a few team members said that they would not be willing to help in his care. It turned out, however, that some of those who had at first been unwilling became those who spent the most time with Julio. Not only did the group do an excellent job in healing his pressure sores and tending his personal needs, they became his close friends.

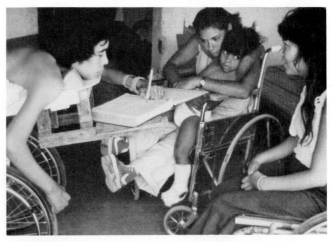

Today Julio is one of the leaders of PROJIMO. Every evening he records the work done by each member of the team.

The team invited Julio to take part in *evaluating* the needs of other disabled children, so that he could learn history-taking and advisory skills. They also gave him the job of chief 'work checker'. His job was to keep a list of the various jobs that needed to be done each day and who was responsible for doing them. He would check to see that the jobs were getting done and speak to those who needed reminding. Since he could not get around easily, the group agreed that when Julio asked anyone to send someone to him, he or she would do so. Thus Julio, as the most severely disabled team member, was given the most power in terms of program management. This is in agreement with the politics of the program, that **only through a just redistribution of power will the weak and marginalized gain a fair place and voice in our society.**

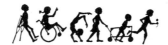

The fact that PROJIMO has no 'boss' creates certain problems while it avoids others. Individual concern, group pressure, children's urgent needs, and parents' appreciation are the main motivations to do a good job. Some team members work much harder than others. When someone is not working enough or other problems arise (such as rudeness to families) the group meets with the person. In extreme cases the person may be asked to meet the group's expectations or to leave. So far, however, those who have left have done so by their own choice.

Different team members are able to work at different speeds and effectiveness, depending on their *disabilities.* Therefore, the group judges a person's work not by how much he produces, but by whether or not he is doing the best he can. A person who works responsibly gets higher pay, even if unable to work fast. Within the limitations of money available, the group decides how much different team members will receive. New team members who are learning work habits and skills begin as volunteers, with only their room and food paid. Later, they earn more, depending on how responsibly and steadily they work. The group decides.

The team meets regularly to plan activities and to decide who will take responsibility for what jobs. Different persons take charge of different aspects of the program: consultations, record keeping, accounting and different shop activities, such as aids making or wheel-chair making. Playground maintenance, housekeeping, cooking and clean-up is usually done by turns. One person keeps track of the hours worked each day by different participants and this is used as a guide for monthly wages.

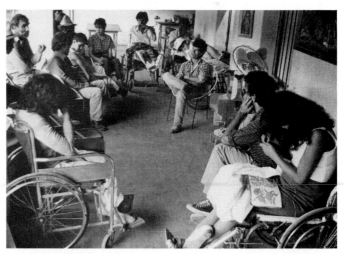

Members of the PROJIMO team at a weekly meeting.

This whole organizational approach is informal and loosely structured. It is a process of ongoing experimentation and change. In short, a group of people are learning how to work and live together as equals. Sometimes things seem to work out better than others. It is the adventure of it all that keeps everyone going — the challenge to create a friendlier and fairer social order, if at first within only a small group.

EVALUATION

An **ongoing process of evaluation** by the members of a community program is necessary if problems are to be corrected and improvements made.

Evaluation is a tool for problem-solving and planning.

Informal evaluation can take place often: the group sits down together once a week (or even for a few minutes once a day) to discuss successes and failures, what seems to be working well, and what does not. Together the group looks for solutions and makes plans.

A somewhat more **formal evaluation** might be done at the end of each month and each year.

The PROJIMO team, at the end of each month, makes an effort to fill out an evaluation form that outlines the following information:

- numbers and names of workers involved, the responsibilities of each, hours worked, and pay received
- number of children seen (new and returning) at the center and in their homes. Also their ages, type of primary disability, and secondary disabilities.
- number of children who stayed at PROJIMO for more than one day, for how long, and with what family members
- attention received by children and families: hours of instruction or *therapy,* number of braces, limbs, wheelchairs, and other aids or equipment made or provided
- accounting for costs of the above, including what portion was paid by each family and how much was paid by the auxiliary fund (See p. 484.)
- summary of financial accounts with lists of all monies gained and spent
- summary of evaluations of individual children by the PROJIMO team and by their parents (This includes a list of children who have made return visits, with comments on their progress and response to suggestions, home therapy, or aids.)
- volunteer help or participation by members of the community (children and adults)
- number and profession of 'special visitors' or visiting instructors
- new relations or interactions with other rehabilitation centers, programs, and communities
- feedback based on parent questionnaires, what they and their children have gained from PROJIMO, how they feel they were treated, what criticisms they have, and suggestions for improvement
- outstanding problems and successes in each of the main activities of PROJIMO
- conclusions and recommendations

To help in the evaluation of PROJIMO, **parent questionnaires** are given to each family at the end of their first visit. Another questionnaire is sent several months later, to learn more about how the child has (or has not) benefited.

The PROJIMO workers are still not happy with the forms and questionnaires they are using, and have revised them several times. For this reason, we do not include samples here. However, we would be glad to send our forms, such as they are, to anyone who thinks they might help in designing their own.

In addition to the monthly written evaluation, at the end of each year the PROJIMO team has an 'evaluation dinner'. The team invites some disabled children, their parents, and some members of the community to participate. The activities of the past year are reviewed, along with problems and successes. The long-range 'vision' and direction of PROJIMO is discussed. Based on this discussion, plans, changes, new activities, and goals are outlined for the coming year.

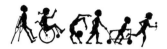

When families first arrive at PROJIMO, they are given a leaflet which describes the program. It describes or lists:

- the reason for the program
- who the workers are
- how the family can help (work that can be done)

- suggestions for donations such as blankets, wood, rope, food
- the services provided
- the disabilities that are attended

This is the way the leaflet starts:

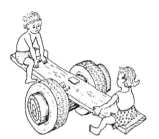

WELCOME TO PROJIMO

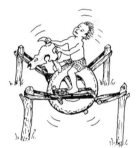

Most of us who work in PROJIMO are disabled villagers. We understand the difficulties disabled children face in our society, just as we understand how hard it is for many families to find adequate rehabilitation counseling and services. *Orthopedic* aids as well as physical therapy are very expensive. The few free services that do exist reach only a small fraction of the children who need them. Therefore, many disabled children, especially in rural areas, lack even basic rehabilitation services.

We formed PROJIMO to provide friendly advice, therapy and orthopedic aids to disabled children whose families could not obtain, for economic or other reasons, the services that their children need.

Family members as rehabilitation workers

For most disabled children, we believe that the best place for rehabilitation is in the home, and that the best 'therapists' are those who most love and understand the child: the members of his or her own family.

Our goal in PROJIMO is to help you, the parents and relatives, to provide the best rehabilitation and opportunities you can for your child.

Here in PROJIMO we live together as a family. We invite you and your child to participate in our work and activities. We ask you for your suggestions and opinions. We appreciate your assistance with exercises or making aids for your child (or other children), as well as your help in the daily maintenance and work of PROJIMO.

PLEASE HELP US TO HELP OTHERS

FINANCING

The myth of self-sufficiency

It is a goal of many community programs to become as financially self-sufficient as possible. Only when a program does not depend on outside funding, can the community and participants of the program have a full sense that "The program is ours. We run it. We control it. We make the main decisions ourselves."

Realistically, however, for health programs in general and for rehabilitation programs in particular, economic self-sufficiency is difficult to accomplish. This is especially true if the program aims to serve mainly those who are poorest and whose needs are greatest. The poor earn barely enough to feed and clothe their children, and then sometimes not adequately. The additional expenses of trying to meet the needs of a disabled child may be too much for the poor family to bear, even when the costs are kept low.

The biggest obstacle to economic self-sufficiency of any community program is poverty.

In a country where social injustice causes widespread poverty, it is not fair to expect the poor to pay for more than a small part of the cost of rehabilitation services or aids. Nor is it fair to ask a busy rehabilitation team to try to make their program self-sufficient through separate 'income-producing activities'. (However, 'income-producing activities' can help meet some expenses and prepare disabled persons to work and earn independently. We discuss this on the next page.)

True self-sufficiency of a community service program may only be possible through a process of social change and fairer distribution within the whole structure of the society. Only when enough jobs are available and nearly every family earns enough to be self-sufficient in terms of meeting its basic needs, can program self-sufficiency become a realistic goal. In the meantime, some sort of outside funding, government or private, is usually necessary.

Funding—government or non-government?

Ideally, governments should help meet the costs of people-centered community-run service programs. Unfortunately, **government funding** often brings with it a high degree of outside control, including pre-defined (often disabling) limitations regarding local planning and how much community workers are taught or permitted to do. The disabled and their families tend to become the objects of program objectives, to be worked upon, rather than the leaders in their own struggle for dignity and self-reliance.

Also, it is usually difficult for a local village or community group to ask for and obtain funding from the government. The red tape, 'preliminary investigations', restrictions, and delays are often endless. More promises are made than are kept. Thus to speak of a government-financed community-oriented program usually makes little sense.*

*One exception to this is the ORD (Organization of Disabled Revolutionaries) in Nicaragua, a non-government, people-centered program for which the Sandinista government had set up a red-tape-free 'auxiliary fund' to help poor families meet costs (see next page). Such restriction-free aid may only be possible in countries where popular governments have a strong political will to serve the people fairly.

NON-GOVERNMENT FUNDING

This can come from a variety of sources, including volunteer agencies, charitable foundations, and religious charities. To permit greater independence, it is a good idea to have several sources of funding. (Some government assistance may possibly be included without sacrificing community control, if the amount is relatively small.)

In Pakistan, a religious (Islamic) law each year takes two and a half percent of the money people have in banks, to be used by local committees for the benefit of widows, orphans, and disabled persons. Since this law was passed in 1981, it has become a growing source of support for community rehabilitation centers.

LOCAL FUNDING

It is also a good idea that a fair part of program costs—if possible at least half—be met within the **community.** Possible local sources for meeting costs include:

- **Fees or contributions from families served:** Some families will be able to pay more than others. Therefore, the fee should depend on their ability to pay. When families come from outside the community, their ability to pay may be hard to judge. Project PROJIMO has tried an 'honor system' for payment of services. They ask the family to make whatever donation they can afford. So as not to shame the family who gives little, or make proud the family who gives more, each family puts whatever they can in a closed box in the corner. Only the family knows how much they gave.

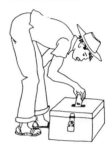
Nobody knows how much the individual family gives.

- **Service 'in kind' or with work:** The community's contribution does not have to be in money. People can donate materials (sand and rock for building), do volunteer work, or provide food and lodging. All this reduces program costs.

- **Income-producing activities:** Production of things for sale is another way to help meet program costs. It also provides skills training for older children and temporary workers in the program. We will discuss this further on p. 509.

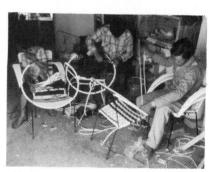
Weaving of chairs with plastic ribbon on a metal frame brings in income and provides skills training. (PROJIMO)

Although production of items for sale may not bring in much money, the extra income may mean that more disabled persons can be employed on the program staff. They can learn rehabilitation skills and at the same time learn income-producing skills, both of which they may put to good use then they return to their own village.

Some programs that are run for and by disabled persons have succeeded in meeting a large part of their costs through production and sale of goods. For example, the Centre for the Rehabilitation of the Paralysed in Bangladesh creates a wide range of orthopedic and hospital equipment, much of which they sell to orthopedic hospitals. (See p. 518.) The Disabled Revolutionaries of Nicaragua has succeeded in developing a nearly profitable business out of making low-cost, rough-terrain wheelchairs. (See p. 519.) In Paraguay, a group of disabled workers has also made wheelchair making a small but profitable business.

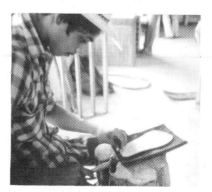
Sandal making produces income and teaches a skill for later self-employment. (PROJIMO)

- **Repair services:** In addition to producing items for sale, a team of disabled village rehabilitation workers can provide a wide variety of repair services. The PROJIMO team in Mexico repairs plows, welds broken machinery and tools, repairs bicycles, solders holes in buckets and car radiators, re-soles boots and sandals, and sharpens axes. (They have even repaired broken plaster saints from the church!) All these services they provide using the same skills and equipment that they use in making wheelchairs and rehabilitation aids. No one else in the village provides these skilled repair services. They have therefore done a lot to increase the villagers' respect and appreciation for disabled persons in the community.

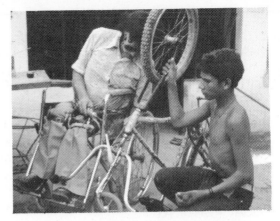

A PROJIMO wheelchair builder welds the broken frame of a village boy's bicycle.

- **An 'auxiliary fund' to help poor families pay for aids and services:** As we have discussed, many families cannot pay for the services or aids their child needs, even though a community program provides these at low cost. Some kind of economic assistance is needed if the disabled child's needs are to be adequately met.

To provide such assistance, PROJIMO has arranged for an 'auxiliary fund' provided by outside donors. The fund, which is kept in a separate bank account, pays to PROJIMO the difference between what a poor family pays and the actual cost of aids or services received. Thus the workers get full payment for the services and aids they provide. In effect, the fund aids poor families, not the program directly. This allows the team to have a better measure of its accomplishments. If the team works efficiently and gains the necessary management skills, in time the program should need no more direct outside funding. The payments from the auxiliary fund, together with whatever families are able to give, should cover the cost of wages, supplies and maintenance. This will mean that the program has in a sense become self-sufficient—even though poor families still need financial aid. Project PROJIMO began to approach self-sufficiency on these terms in its third year.

An argument can be made for trying to obtain government financing for the 'auxiliary fund'. (This is in fact being done in Nicaragua. See footnote on p. 482.) The fund could even be managed by a local official (if honest) or another administrator outside the rehabilitation program. At the end of each month, the team could give the administrator an accounting of the services and aids provided, their calculated value, and the amount paid by families, with receipts. Payment would be made, as if by contract.

Below is a form that can be used for keeping records for money to be paid by the auxiliary fund (adapted from Project PROJIMO).

| RECORD OF SERVICES, COSTS, AND PAYMENTS | | | | | Cost | | | Payment | |
Date	Service or aid provided	By whom	To whom	Record #	Labor at $____ per hour	Materials cost $____	Total (+ 30% overhead) $____	Amount paid by family $____	Amount to be paid by Auxiliary Fund $____

Month of _____, 19____.

Adapting the Home and Community

CHAPTER 51

ADAPTING THE HOME

The kind of *adaptations* needed in the home will partly depend on the *kind of disability* a child has, the *severity of the disability,* and the *age* and *size* of the child. Adaptations for a child who is blind are very different than those for a child who is *paralyzed* and uses a wheelchair. A child who is completely dependent will need aids and adaptations to help the family care for him and move him—especially as he gets older and heavier. However, the disabled child who can do a lot for herself may be helped by adaptations that make self-care and work in the house easier.

The kinds of adaptations needed will also depend on the **local living situation, style of house,** and **customs.** For example:

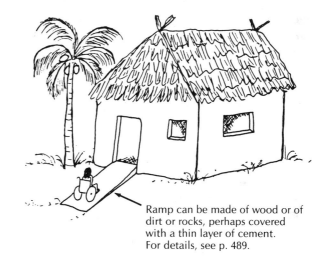

A simple ramp may work well for a wheelchair entrance to a house near ground level.

Ramp can be made of wood or of dirt or rocks, perhaps covered with a thin layer of cement. For details, see p. 489.

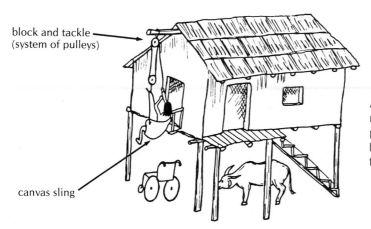

block and tackle (system of pulleys)

canvas sling

A system of ropes and pulleys may be the best way for a person with strong arms to lift herself without help to a 'house on stilts'.

The 'lift' can be made with a platform so that the whole wheelchair can be lifted. But if the house is small and people cook and eat at floor level, it may be best to leave the wheelchair outside.

Adaptations for the child who is learning to walk and balance

HAND RAILS

These can be fixed to the walls and furniture. If necessary, pathways with rails can be put up so that the child can walk with support almost anywhere in the house, and also outside to the latrine (toilet) or garden (see p. 507).

Before attaching hand rails firmly, test the child with a temporary rail at different heights to find out what works best. As the child grows, you may need to place the rails higher. Or you may want to remove rails little by little to help the child improve her balance and walk more independently.

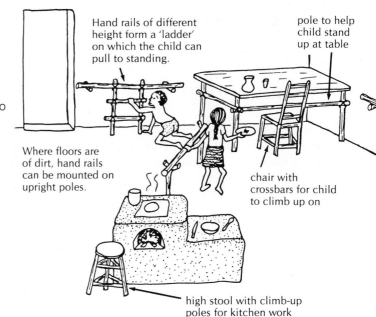

Hand rails of different height form a 'ladder' on which the child can pull to standing.

pole to help child stand up at table

Where floors are of dirt, hand rails can be mounted on upright poles.

chair with crossbars for child to climb up on

high stool with climb-up poles for kitchen work

MATS

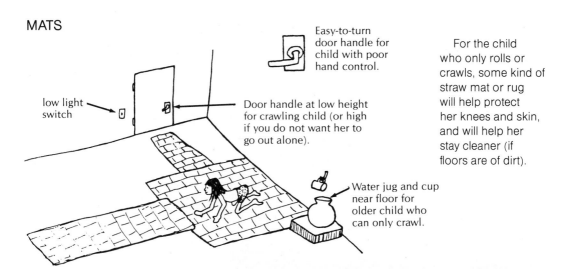

low light switch

Easy-to-turn door handle for child with poor hand control.

Door handle at low height for crawling child (or high if you do not want her to go out alone).

Water jug and cup near floor for older child who can only crawl.

For the child who only rolls or crawls, some kind of straw mat or rug will help protect her knees and skin, and will help her stay cleaner (if floors are of dirt).

The 'model home' in PROJIMO is a guesthouse. It has features that make it easier to care for a disabled person, or for a disabled person to care for herself and do housework. Visiting families can find out what is useful for their child and can adapt their own home. Here PROJIMO workers split wild cane to make screens to keep out the animals.

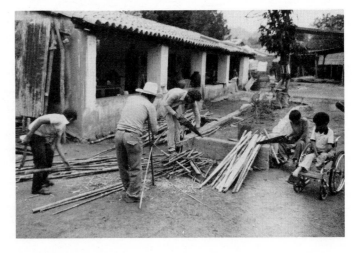

Home adaptations for wheelchair riders

FLOORS

For almost any disabled person—but especially those who use wheelboards or scooters with small wheels, the floor should be as **smooth and firm** as possible (but not slick or slippery). Packed, smoothed clay-and-cow-dung surfaces (as used in India) work well. Cement is even better for long-lasting use of a trolley or wheelchair. Although expensive, a smooth cement floor makes getting around a lot easier.

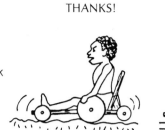

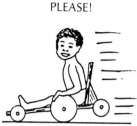

DOORWAYS

Make all **doorways extra wide.** Remember, your child will grow and may need a bigger, wider wheelchair.

In a house that already has very narrow doorways, be sure the wheelchair you buy or make is narrow enough to fit through easily. Most commercial chairs are much wider than necessary, especially for a child.

Try to avoid any rise or bump at the doorway. If it already has a raised sill and you cannot remove it, build a small ramp to go over it. (This will be of special help for children with weak arms and hands.)

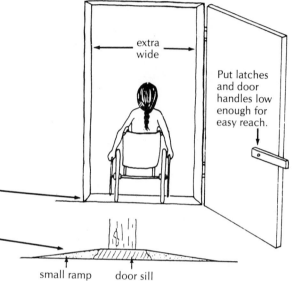

extra wide

Put latches and door handles low enough for easy reach.

small ramp   door sill

BATHROOM OR OUTHOUSE (LATRINE)

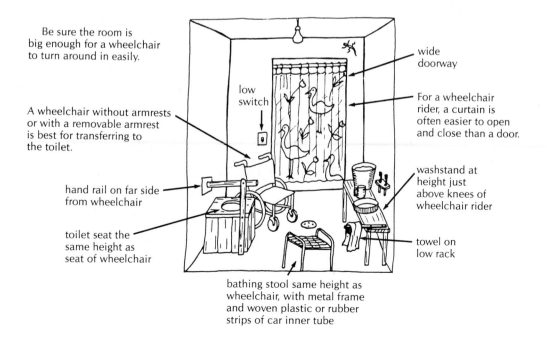

Be sure the room is big enough for a wheelchair to turn around in easily.

A wheelchair without armrests or with a removable armrest is best for transferring to the toilet.

hand rail on far side from wheelchair

toilet seat the same height as seat of wheelchair

low switch

wide doorway

For a wheelchair rider, a curtain is often easier to open and close than a door.

washstand at height just above knees of wheelchair rider

towel on low rack

bathing stool same height as wheelchair, with metal frame and woven plastic or rubber strips of car inner tube

KITCHEN AREA

The stove, work areas, and tables should be as low as possible, but high enough so that the legs of the wheelchair rider can fit under them.

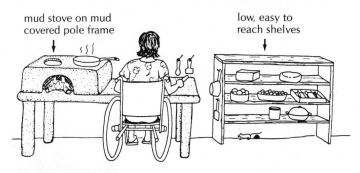

mud stove on mud covered pole frame

low, easy to reach shelves

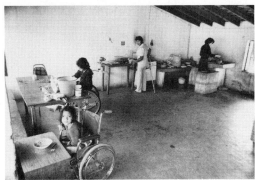

The cooking and eating area in the model home at PROJIMO has a lot of adaptations.

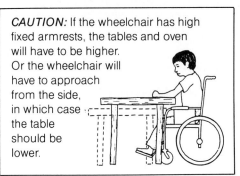

CAUTION: If the wheelchair has high fixed armrests, the tables and oven will have to be higher. Or the wheelchair will have to approach from the side, in which case the table should be lower.

BED OR COT

The bed or cot should be the same height as the wheelchair for easier transfer.

One or more hanging bars or other supports may help the child to transfer or to sit up in bed.

Cot height can be adjusted by drilling new holes and changing the position of the bolt.

WASHING AREA (outdoor)

cement wash stand with ridged bottom

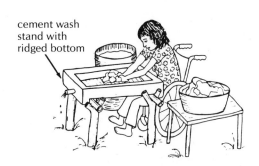

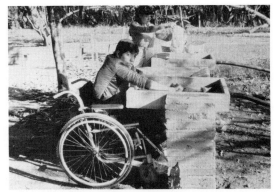

Outdoor washing area at PROJIMO— designed for work from a wheelchair.

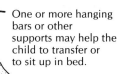

IMPORTANT: Before building fixed-height stoves, tables, and wash areas, **set up something temporary to figure out what works best.** Remember that the child is growing, so try not to make things too fixed or permanent.

ADAPTING THE COMMUNITY

In many villages, disabled persons have a hard time going places because streets or paths are rough, rocky, or sandy. Also, there may be high steps for getting into stores, the cinema, and even the town meeting hall, school, and health center.

A village rehabilitation program can encourage the villagers to make it easier for disabled persons to go places and to participate in community activities.

For example, ask storekeepers to build ramps so that wheelchairs can enter their stores. Disabled persons and their families can promise to give their business to those who cooperate in this way, and if necessary, can boycott (refuse to buy from) those who do not.

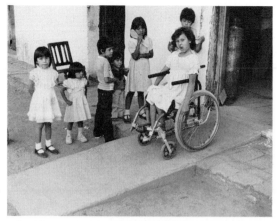

In Ajoya, Mexico, the rehabilitation team convinced store owners to build ramps so that the wheelchair riders could enter the stores. The store owners provided the materials and local masons volunteered the labor.

RAMPS

The more gentle the slope of the ramp, the easier it is for a wheelchair rider to go up it.

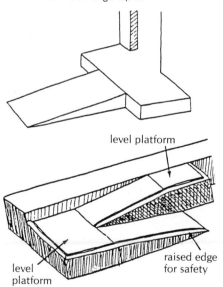

level platform

level platform

raised edge for safety

One or more ramps can be put parallel to the edge of the raised area. Be sure to leave large level platforms for turning.

Addition of hand rails will add safety and make going up ramps easier for persons who walk with difficulty.

HOW STEEP YOU MAKE THE RAMP DEPENDS IN PART ON WHO IT IS FOR.

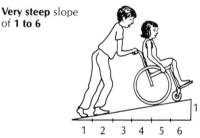

Very steep slope of **1 to 6**

1 2 3 4 5 6

Only possible with electric wheelchair or with help. Rarely possible for rider alone. Chair may tip backwards.

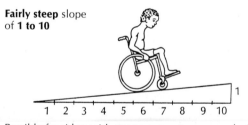

Fairly steep slope of **1 to 10**

1 2 3 4 5 6 7 8 9 10

Possible for riders with strong arms; strong paraplegics

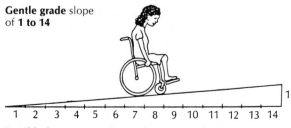

Gentle grade slope of **1 to 14**

1 2 3 4 5 6 7 8 9 10 11 12 13 14

Possible for average riders and strong quadriplegics. This is the best slope for public buildings and rehabilitation centers.

Improvement of walkways and trails

Community work parties or groups of schoolchildren can organize to help fix up **smooth, hard-packed pathways** through the village so that crutch users and wheelchair riders can go places more easily.

Also, if possible, easy-to-use pathways can be set up so that disabled children and adults can get to play areas, bathing areas, and family work areas.

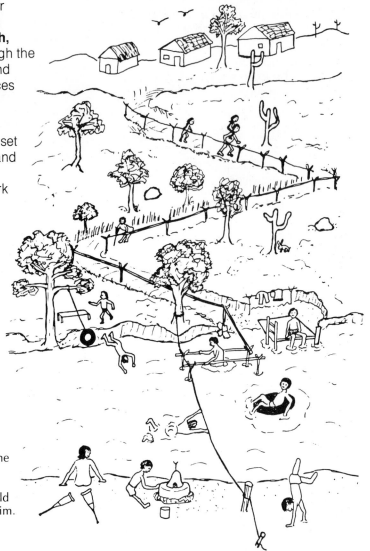

HAND RAILS (or ropes)

When placed along steep trails, these may permit children who are blind, who have balance problems, or who have difficulty walking to reach areas such as swimming or fishing holes.

In one village a rehabilitation team together with some of the village children improved the steep trail down to the river, so that disabled children would have a chance to play and swim.

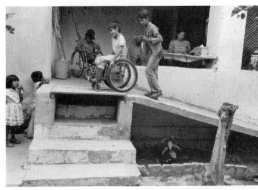

The health workers of Project Piaxtla built this ramp so the wheelchair riders could come into the clinic easier. (Photo: John Fago)

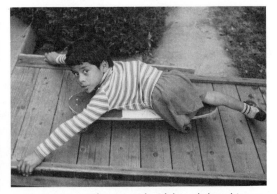

A narrow wood ramp with sideboards lets this child pull himself up it on his skateboard.

Love, Sex, and Social Adjustment

CHAPTER 52

In the village of Ajoya, the home of Project PROJIMO, disabled young men and women happily go to dances and outdoor movies together. They are not ashamed to let people know that they have a close or loving relationship. Some of the disabled young persons who have grown to know and care for each other through the Project have married and now have children.

All this is fairly much accepted as natural and normal and 'right' by most of the local villagers.

But things were not always this way. A few years ago, when PROJIMO had just begun, many people believed that a *severely* or even *moderately disabled* person should not and could not have a loving relationship, get married, or have children.

I remember one evening in the spring, a few years ago. An old woman watched a group of young couples listening to guitar players at the village square. One young man, who had a clubbed foot and used a cane stood close to a young woman in a wheelchair. When the musicians started playing a romantic song, the disabled couple gently put their arms around each other. The old woman was shocked. Angrily she pointed to the pair and cried, "Isn't that disgusting! People like that have no right to behave like that! It's not natural! They're cripples!"

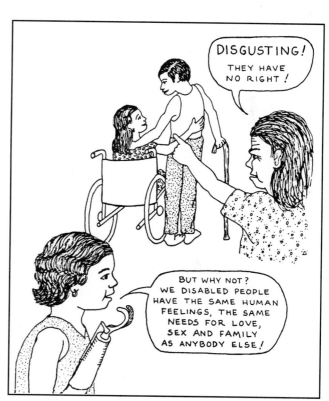

Disabled persons and their families must educate the public about their rights.

When PROJIMO first began, unfortunately the villagers were not the only ones who thought that disabled persons should and could not get married or have loving relationships. Many disabled young people half-believed it themselves, and in their personal lives were often depressed, frustrated, or confused. While society told them one thing, their hearts and their bodies told them another. Most believed they could never be attractive to another person in a sexual way. Yet through adolescence, they felt increasingly attracted. Many had serious doubts about their own sexual ability. Some had discovered that they did, in fact, have fully developed feelings and functions. But they had no acceptable way to express them.

Some visiting advisers to PROJIMO were older disabled persons who had learned to understand their own feelings, had married, or had formed loving relationships. Slowly, the disabled young people at PROJIMO began to accept their own desires, needs, and dreams. More important, they began to discover they were not so alone, not as different from other people, as they had thought. Above all, they discovered that they were attractive to other persons. Soon the romances began.

At first, things sometimes got out of hand. The bottled-up feelings of the young people came flooding out. There were occasional mistakes and abuses. When the disabled group discovered that the rules society had set for them were unfair, often their first response was to break the rules recklessly. But then, faced by the sometimes cruel results of their own hurry, passion, and inexperience, they discovered the need for a few precautions and guidelines determined by the group. They had been hurt often enough themselves not to want to cause additional hurt. And now with the HIV/AIDS epidemic, they are also aware they must have "safe sex" if and when they have sex.

Little by little, the PROJIMO team members have discovered their ability to live fuller lives and have more complete relationships than they had previously believed possible. Also, little by little, the local community has begun to accept this. For the first time, romances have begun to develop openly between non-disabled and disabled villagers. A new level of awareness and acceptance is slowly being achieved.

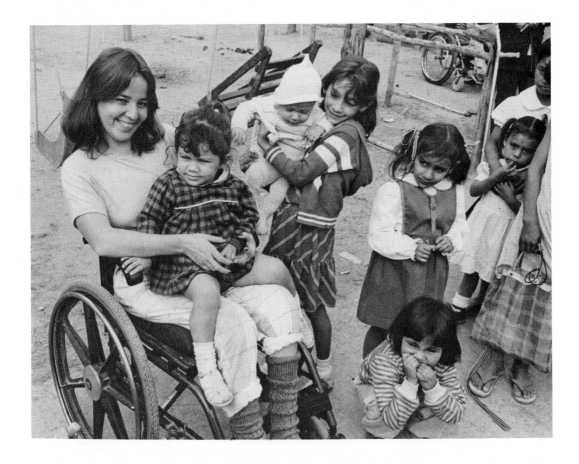

Conchita, who is paraplegic, was sure she could never marry. She came
to PROJIMO for *rehabilitation* and later became one of the workers.
She is now happily married to one of the able-bodied villagers.

The personal and sexual needs of young persons

Every child, whether disabled or not, has the same basic needs for food, protection, and love. The child who is treated consistently with love, respect, and understanding has a greater chance of becoming a loving, respectful, and understanding adult.

Every child has a need to be touched and held. Small children learn about themselves by exploring and touching different parts of their bodies. A child whose disability makes touching and exploring her body more difficult may have an even greater need than other children to be held and hugged.

Most societies have rules and taboos that attempt to limit and govern sexual behavior. And within most societies, young people (and old) usually find ways of getting around some of those rules, usually more or less secretly. The best answer to sex education may be to look for informal and unsupervised ways for disabled adolescents to spend time with and share the secrets of other adolescents.

But it is also important to make sure that disabled children understand how to resist sexual abuse. Adults can take advantage of their power and trust and enter into sexual relations with children, especially disabled children. It should be explained to children that these kinds of "secrets" are not all right and that they should let others know. See *Helping Children Who Are Blind* (Chapter 12) or *Helping Children Who Are Deaf* (Chapter 13) for ideas on how to prevent sexual abuse and ways to talk with children about this difficult topic.

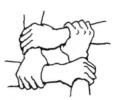

LOVING RELATIONSHIPS, MARRIAGE, AND FORMING A FAMILY

It is important that disabled people and everyone else in the community realize that most disabled persons are capable of getting married and having children. Except for a few *inherited disabilities*, the children born to disabled parents have just as great a chance of being normal as do children of non-disabled parents.

For most disabled persons, a close, loving partnership is possible. This is true even when the disability makes having children unlikely, as in some men with *spinal cord* injury. Persons who have no feeling in their sex parts can discover sexual satisfaction through meeting of lips or other parts of the body that feel. If the couple wants children, perhaps they can adopt them.

In some societies, nearly everyone is expected and able to marry, including disabled persons. But in cultures that put great importance on an 'ideal' or complete *physical* appearance, it may be difficult for the disabled person to find a partner. The biggest barrier is sometimes the feeling by the disabled person that he or she can never be attractive to anyone. To overcome those feelings, disabled persons can sometimes advise one another. Those who have overcome their own fears of unacceptability and have formed loving relationships can do much to help others realize that inner beauty and gentleness of spirit can also make a person attractive.

Often it takes someone with a disability to see beyond the outside of another disabled person to the unique qualities inside. So it often happens that disabled persons take other disabled persons as partners—although their disabilities may be quite different. However, as disabled persons gain greater acceptance and participation in the community, loving relationships and marriage between non-disabled and disabled persons become more common.

Often there are not many chances for disabled young persons to get to know and become close to other youth. Therefore, such opportunities can and should be sought or arranged. The types of opportunities and how they can be arranged will of course differ from one community to another.

Chances should be provided for disabled young people, even in wheelchairs, to go to ceremonies, dances, and public events that other young people attend. A community rehabilitation program can arrange games, parties, and other activities to which both disabled and non-disabled young people are invited, and in which they can participate equally.

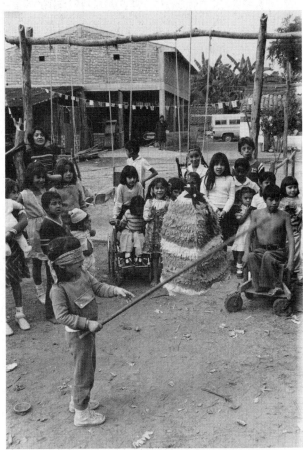

The need for full integration

It must be remembered that opportunities for a close, loving relationship are only one aspect of leading a full, accepted, and participating life in the community. The more that can be done to bring about greater integration and participation of disabled persons in the life of the community, the more everyone will learn to look beyond a disability and see the person. When this happens, it opens up many new possibilities.

A community rehabilitation program finds enjoyable ways to bring disabled and non-disabled children together. Here the village children have been invited to the birthday party of a disabled child. They take turns, blindfolded, trying to break a 'piñata' (a papier-mache toy filled with candy and nuts). (PROJIMO/Richard Parker)

Family Planning

Disabled girls and boys should be given the same information and opportunities as non-disabled young people to avoid unwanted pregnancy and sexually transmitted infections such as HIV/AIDS. Making such information and methods available may be of special importance for participants in a self-run community rehabilitation program. (For different methods of family planning, see *Where Women Have No Doctor,* Chapter 13, or *Where There Is No Doctor,* Chapter 20.)

The mentally retarded child and sex

Mentally retarded children, like others, as they grow up take increased interest in sex. In fact, they may take more interest in bodily experiences because opportunities for other activities are more limited.

Because the complex messages that the retarded child gets from other people are often confusing or contradictory, the child may develop unacceptable patterns of *behavior.* Often parents do not know how to handle this. For example, a mother may be afraid to take her retarded boy with her to the market because he tries to touch every girl he sees.

It is important that retarded children are helped to understand clearly what behavior is acceptable and what is not, and where. To accomplish this, a **behavior approach to learning** can be used. The family can consistently reward good behavior and carefully avoid giving the child special attention or in any way rewarding bad behavior. This approach is discussed in Chapter 40. In children with behavior difficulties, if possible, the family should start using a behavior approach to learning long before the child grows up sexually. The younger the better.

A common mistake is to pretend that retarded young people do not have a need for loving personal relationships. The need exists, and if unanswered, can lead to difficulties both for themselves and for others.

In most communities, it is very difficult for the retarded person to have a close, loving relationship. In some countries, programs arrange for retarded persons to live together in special homes or to come together for social activities. As a result, some of them form couples, and sometimes marry.

Trying to protect retarded girls against sexual abuse, and undesirable pregnancy, and at the same time respect the girls' rights, can be difficult. Some programs try to solve the problem through sex education, or by providing retarded young women with family planning methods to prevent pregnancy. Check with your local health worker to see what family planning methods are available and acceptable in your area.

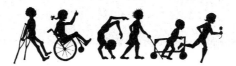

Marriage and family

In countries where the disabled have achieved greater acceptance and involvement in the community, an increasing number of disabled persons, including some with fairly severe disabilities, are getting married and having families of their own.

The ability of a married disabled person to bring up a family depends a lot on economics. Thus, an effort to help young disabled persons learn the skills necessary to work and earn a living or maintain a home is an important part of the preparation for marriage and family.

Sex education

On the average, disabled children begin to mature sexually around the same age as non-disabled children. Girls may begin to have monthly bleeding (menstruate) at about age 11 or 12 (or earlier or later). Boys begin to release semen at age 12, 13, or 14 (sometimes earlier or later). Often these new bodily functions take the child by surprise, and may fill the child with confusion or even guilt unless he or she is informed about their naturalness and purpose.

Because disabled children often do not have the same opportunity to mix with other children in an unsupervised way, they can miss out on one of the most common forms of sex education: children's games, jokes, stories, songs, and private discussions. Therefore, older persons should make a special point to share basic 'facts of life' with these children in a relaxed, trustful way, inviting questions and answering them honestly.

Equally important, of course, is to make arrangements for disabled children to mix with, play with, and join in the secrets of other children.

The need to accept a range of social relationships

Disabled persons have as much right to sexual relationships as non-disabled persons. But opportunities for close relationships may not arise as often or as easily for disabled persons as for non-disabled persons. Many of the ways that young men and women traditionally meet may not be open.

It is therefore not surprising that some disabled people enter into love relationships that are less traditionally accepted—sometimes 2 members of the same sex, or 2 persons from different castes, races, social levels, or other social groups between which relationships are not locally approved.

Before condemning such a relationship, it is important to consider what benefit or harm it is providing for each of the partners. If both partners have entered the relationship willingly and seem happier and more whole because of it, those concerned should perhaps be supportive—even if the relationship is not socially approved. This should be the case whether or not the persons are disabled.

Many groups and organizations of disabled persons are outspoken in defending the rights of persons to live in ways that are different from the norm, as long as no one is being forced or hurt. They know from personal experience that society is often cruel and unfair in its treatment of those who happen to be 'different'. So they try to take the lead in the re-education of the community toward a more flexible and accepting attitude with regard to human variation.

On the other hand, disabled children or young people are sometimes in a position where they can more easily be taken advantage of or abused. The very loneliness of some disabled young people or the innocence of the retarded child often makes them easy targets for abuse. Necessary precautions need to be taken.

What is important when 2 people live together or have a sexual relationship is not who they are, but that they truly care for and respect each other.

Education
At Home, At School, At Work

Guided learning to help a child gain skills and understanding for meeting life's needs is called 'education'. In Chapters 34 to 43 we talked about ways to help disabled and delayed children learn to control and use their bodies and minds, and to master early basic skills for daily living. But as a child grows up many additional skills and knowledge are needed.

For nearly all children, **education begins in the home.** For some it continues in school; for others in the fields, in the forest, at the marketplace, on the riverbank, or in the streets.

In the cities of most countries, a school education has become almost a 'basic need' for getting a job or being accepted by society. In many villages and farming communities, however, 'book learning' still is much less important than the skills children learn through helping their families with daily work.

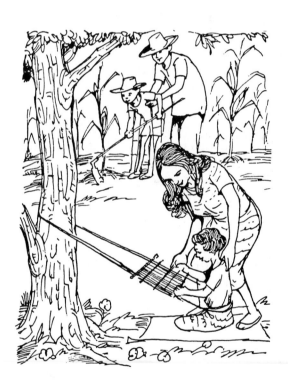

In some rural areas, therefore, it may be a mistake to think that 'every child' should go to school. For the child who is *physically* strong but *mentally retarded,* schooling may be a frustrating and unrewarding experience, especially if no 'special education' is available. The child may be happier and learn more skills for meeting life's needs by helping father in the fields, or mother in the marketplace, than by going to school.

For many children in rural areas, the most important parts of their education do not take place in school.

However, for some retarded children in rural areas, schooling can be important. If the teacher and other children can be helped to understand the special needs of the child, treat him with respect, and give him encouragement, the slow learner may benefit greatly from school, both educationally and socially.

Whatever the case, it is important to consider the local situation carefully. **Do not just follow the recommendations from the outside about the importance of schooling.** Some school situations are better and some are worse than others. So before deciding for a particular child, look carefully at the good and the bad things about the local school and consider the other choices.

For the physically disabled child in the rural area, schooling may be especially important–more so, perhaps, than for able-bodied children. Physically disabled children often cannot do hard physical farm work as well as the able-bodied. Therefore, they need to learn skills using their minds, so that they can work or take part in community activities. It may help them to go as far in school as possible.

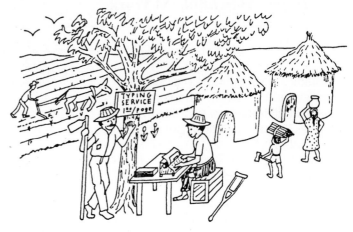

In a village, skills learned through schooling can be be more important for the disabled person than the non-disabled.

Regular school or special schools?

Today, leaders in rehabilitation generally feel that **disabled children should attend the same schools as other children, whenever possible.**

For mildly or moderately disabled children this should not be a big problem, if the parents, school director, and teachers cooperate. In some communities, however, and especially in rural areas, parents may not even think of sending their disabled child to school. They may fear that their child will be teased or have too hard a time. And in some places, school directors or teachers refuse to accept even a moderately disabled child with a quick mind. Distance and other problems getting to school also add to the difficulties.

Wherever possible, try to overcome these problems. Village *rehabilitation* workers can talk to teachers, parents and other schoolchildren and try to work out the best situation. At times parents may need to organize and put pressure on the schools to change their policies. In some countries, laws exist requiring government schools to accept and make special provisions for disabled children. Rehabilitation workers and parents can find out about the laws, and try to have them enforced. Or they can work to get laws passed if they do not exist.

Every effort should be made to make regular schooling easier and more enjoyable for the disabled child. Some possibilities that involve other schoolchildren have already been discussed in Chapter 47 (CHILD-to-child).

For more severely disabled children, attending regular schools often may not be possible, at least as schools exist today. Yet, sometimes if you talk with the teachers and other children, they will become more understanding and make special arrangements.

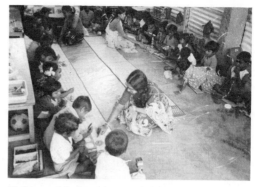

Children with developmental delay get a 'head start' in a pre-school program near Bangalore, India.

For example, we know a boy with spina bifida who lacks *bowel* control and therefore never went to school. But after his parents talked with the teacher and schoolchildren, an agreement was reached. Now the boy goes to school. When he has an accident in his pants, he quietly gets up and goes home to bathe and change. (Fortunately his house is very near the school.)

In cases where some disabled children cannot attend regular school, other alternatives may be possible. In cities of some countries there are '**special education**' programs for children with certain *disabilities.* Such schools, if private, are usually very expensive and if public, are often overcrowded or have long waiting lists.

In the rural areas, with rare exceptions, there are no special education programs. However, parents of disabled children may be able to organize and form their own 'special school'. The group helps each child to learn at her own pace and in her own way. An example of such a school is 'Los Pargos' in Mazatlan, Mexico, described briefly on p. 517. Also, the Centre for Community Rehabilitation Development in Pakistan has helped organize parent-run special education programs in many towns (see p. 520).

If no opportunity for regular or special schooling can be worked out—or even if it can—perhaps some arrangement can be made for **study at home.** Children who do go to school, either non-disabled or disabled, may be able to help teach the severely disabled children at home after school. A community rehabilitation program can also include a study program for disabled children and youths. Project PROJIMO has arranged at the local village school for attendance of children with special needs who have had difficulty in schools elsewhere. In addition, the disabled rehabilitation workers assist the children who need special tutoring in the evenings.

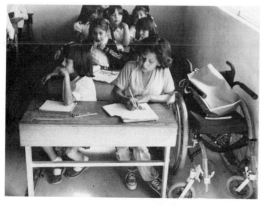

Regular school

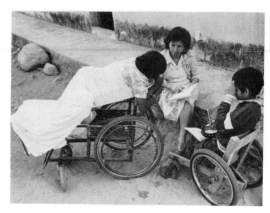

Extra help with a tutor

This book does not cover the details and methods of special education. It is important that the methods used be adapted to the local customs and situation—not just borrowed from Europe or the USA, as is often done. An excellent book on *Special Education For Mentally Handicapped Pupils,* by Christine Miles has been developed for the program in Pakistan, and has many ideas for adapting to the local culture. (See p. 640.)

Meeting the special physical needs of children at school

When physically disabled children are in school or studying, it is important to remember their special needs, and try to meet them.

For example, children who cannot get up and run around should usually *not* spend all day sitting in a wheelchair. This tends to lead to *contractures,* swollen feet, weak leg bones, *spinal* curve, and other deformities.

So try to arrange for the children to spend at least part of the day with their bodies in a straight position.

Part of the day this can be done in standing frames (but usually not for more than half an hour at a time).

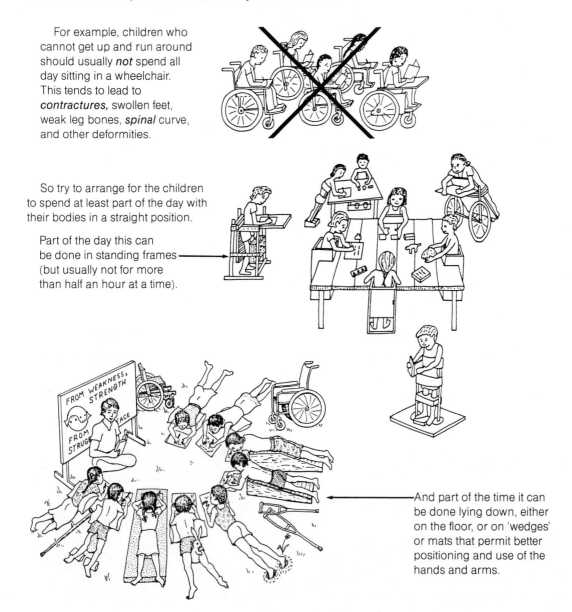

And part of the time it can be done lying down, either on the floor, or on 'wedges' or mats that permit better positioning and use of the hands and arms.

For design details, see pages 571 to 575.

AIDS FOR READING, WRITING, AND DRAWING

PENCIL HOLDER FOR A WEAK OR PARALYZED HAND

For children who have difficulty holding a pen, pencil, or brush, or turning the pages of a book, you can think of all sorts of *adaptations.* Here are a few examples:

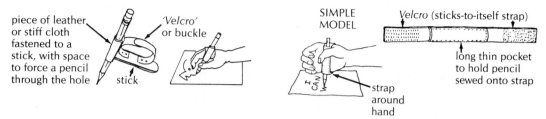

piece of leather, or stiff cloth fastened to a stick, with space to force a pencil through the hole

'Velcro' or buckle

stick

SIMPLE MODEL

strap around hand

Velcro (sticks-to-itself strap)

long thin pocket to hold pencil sewed onto strap

AIDS FOR HOLDING PENCILS, PENS OR BRUSHES

A thick handhold gives better grip and control.

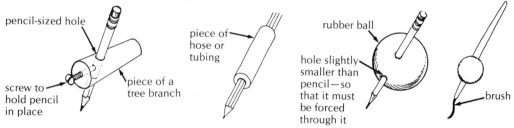

pencil-sized hole

screw to hold pencil in place

piece of a tree branch

piece of hose or tubing

rubber ball

hole slightly smaller than pencil—so that it must be forced through it

brush

For other ideas, see pages 223 and 330.

PAGE TURNER (Design for head)

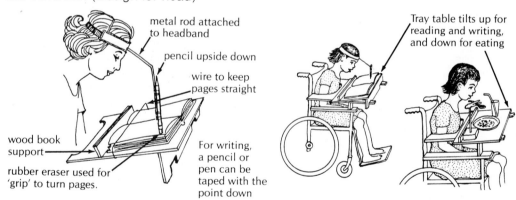

metal rod attached to headband

pencil upside down

wire to keep pages straight

Tray table tilts up for reading and writing, and down for eating

wood book support

rubber eraser used for 'grip' to turn pages.

For writing, a pencil or pen can be taped with the point down

Many children who have poor hand control and cannot write clearly by hand can learn to write well on a **typewriter**—using their hands or a stick attached to their heads. A typewriter may be a wise investment for an intelligent but severely disabled child—and may in time provide a way for her to earn money.

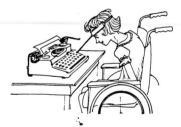

A **pocket calculator** is much cheaper than a typewriter. A disabled person who is good with numbers can do many different kinds of accounting jobs.

For more ideas on special aids and adaptations, see Chapter 27 on amputations, Chapter 9 on cerebral palsy, and Chapter 62 on special aids.

Lupito's family was afraid to let him go to school. They thought the other children would tease him. Village rehabilitation workers convinced his family to let him go to school, and to also lead a CHILD-to-child activity with the schoolchildren. Lupito now attends school happily and does very well.

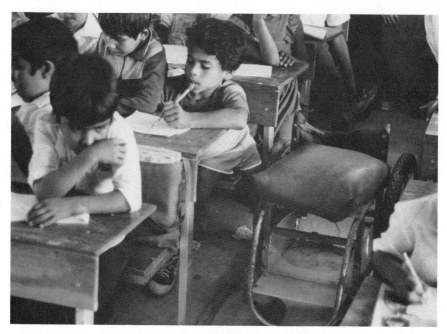

Lupito at school . . .

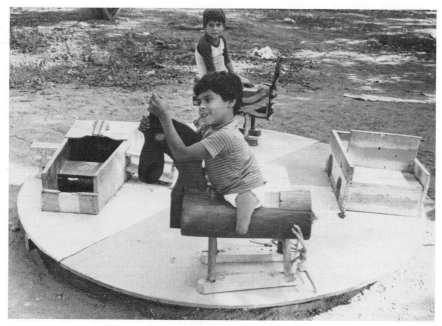

and at play.

CHAPTER **54**

Work
Possibilities and Training

For most people, some kind of work is necessary in order to eat and have a place to live. In rural areas, the main work of many families involves farming, fishing, hunting and gathering, or other forms of food production. Equally important is the work of 'keeping house' and bringing up the family.

Who does most of the work within a family depends on local customs and the family's situation. In most poor rural families nearly everyone—women, men, and children—help with the work of survival. By the time they are 5 or 6 years old, children may be helping to take care of the babies, feed the chickens, herd the goats, shell and clean the grain, and to carry out other tasks so that the older members of the family are free to do other work. In many societies, children by age 8 or 10 bring in more income (food or money) than it costs their families to take care of them.

Work that frees people and work that makes them slaves

Work—whether it is done by adults or children—can be either a good or bad experience. It can help persons gain dignity and independence. Or it can take away their dignity, freedom, and health. How workers are affected depends on work conditions, on the fairness of wages, on workers' rights, and on how much respect and equality exists between workers and bosses.

In some situations, especially in cities, many children are forced to work long, hard hours in unsafe or unhealthy work conditions for very low pay. Such 'child labor' is cruel, and may result in permanent damage to the child's body or spirit.

In some rural areas, children from the poorest families must also work long, hard hours under difficult conditions. But for many rural children, the opportunity to help their families with the labor of production and survival is a greater adventure than is 'play'. The chance to take care of a real baby (not just a doll) or to help grow the family food, gives many farm children a feeling of importance, self-confidence, and personal worth that is not often seen in city children.

As a child grows up, to be wanted and well cared for is not enough. **A young person needs to feel that he or she is needed.** To become 'independent' can be important. But just as important is **to develop an ability to do things for and with others, to contribute toward meeting the needs of family, friends, and community.**

Too often disabled children are not given the opportunity to become helpful or needed, or to learn the skills to contribute in an important way to the family or community. The family and community need to look ahead to the disabled child's future. They need to find ways to build on whatever strengths she has, so that she can have a full and meaningful role in the community.

A money-earning job is not the only meaningful role in society

In some cultures, especially in Europe and the United States, great importance is placed on work to earn money. Often it seems that a person's worth is measured by how much money he or she makes. Where such a value system exists, a standard goal of *rehabilitation* is to prepare disabled persons to work at some kind of money-earning job.

But **caution!** This goal of a paid job may not be appropriate in some parts of the world. Traditions and local values differ from place to place. Some societies are more accepting of persons who do not earn or 'produce', as long as they contribute and take part in other ways.

Also, we must remember that in poor countries the unemployment rate (people without work) is often very high, even for the non-disabled. It may be very difficult for a disabled person to get a job, even if well-trained.

There are many ways, other than by working for money, that disabled persons can contribute to their family and community. They may be able to learn skills to help with daily activities in the home. Or they may become leaders for community action. As we discussed in Chapter 45, disabled villagers who are unable to do hard physical farm work, often make outstanding health workers (paid or volunteer), rehabilitation workers, popular organizers, or defenders of human rights.

It is important that rehabilitation programs have a broad view of how disabled persons might work or fit into the community. Too often 'skills training' prepares a *physically disabled* person to do jobs that able-bodied persons could do just as well. **The challenge, whenever possible, should be to build on the unique strengths, experience, and qualities of the disabled person:** help her to find a role in society that she can do better than most non-disabled persons. Disability does make a person different in certain ways, for better and for worse. Rather than pretending that the difference does not exist, it is wiser to accept the differences and look for ways that

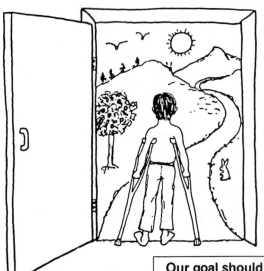

being disabled helps to deepen or strengthen the person. Help the person to have not just an ordinary role in society, but one that is in some ways outstanding. Persons like Helen Keller (a blind and deaf woman who became a social leader and agent for change) can be our role models.

Rehabilitation programs and families should avoid planning a child's (or adult's) life work, or role in the community, for him. Rather, we should help make available as wide a range of opportunities as possible.

Our goal should always be to open doors for the child, not to close them.

ACCEPT THE CHILD'S WEAKNESSES
AND DEVELOP HER STRENGTHS

Children with certain areas of weakness or disability often also have other areas of strength or ability. When deciding what work skills a child should be helped to develop, it is generally wise to pick those in areas where the child is strongest. For example:

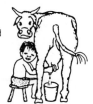

A child who is *mentally retarded* but physically strong . . .

. . . may be happier and do better at learning certain physical skills . . .

. . . than at spending a lot of time trying to learn mental skills.

He will probably make a better farm worker than a writer or bookkeeper.

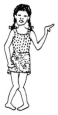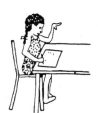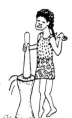

A child who is physically disabled but has a quick, intelligent mind . . .

. . . may be happier and do better learning mental skills . . .

. . . than trying to learn physical skills that will always be more difficult for her.

She may make a better health worker or school teacher than a farmer or grain grinder.

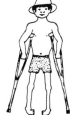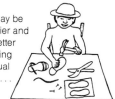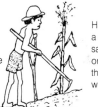

A child who has weak legs but strong arms and hands . . .

. . . may be happier and do better learning manual skills . . .

. . . than trying to learn skills that require use of his legs and feet.

He may make a better sandal maker or welder than a field worker.

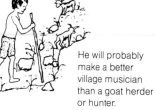

A child who cannot see but has a good sense of hearing, touch, and rhythm . . .

. . . may be happier and do better learning skills that depend mainly on hearing and touch . . .

. . . than trying to learn jobs that are much more difficult without eyesight.

He will probably make a better village musician than a goat herder or hunter.

CAUTION: It usually makes sense to help a child develop specialized work skills in the areas where she is strongest. But it is also important for her to develop self-care and daily living skills as best she can, even though this may be difficult. Thus the child who is mentally retarded needs to learn basic communication skills. The girl with *spasticity* needs to learn, if possible, how to prepare food and keep house. The weak-legged boy or blind child needs to learn how to get from place to place.

LEARNING SKILLS FOR AN ACTIVE OR PRODUCTIVE ROLE IN THE COMMUNITY

Development of the mind

Learning skills that require more mental than physical activity can help the physically disabled child to gain a place in the community.

For development of skills such as reading, writing, and arithmetic, **when possible, it is usually best that the disabled child go to school.** Ideas for helping the child get to school and be accepted there are discussed in chapters 47 and 53. **If the child cannot go to school, figure out ways for her to be taught at home**—perhaps by school-children.

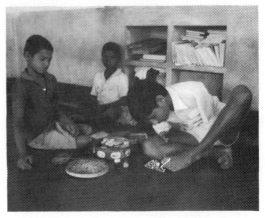

In Melkote, India, the Janapada Seva Trust teaches disabled village children many productive skills. Here, a boy without hands uses his foot to draw greeting cards, which are later sold.

As soon as the child learns to read and write, try to buy or borrow simple, interesting, and educational books. With these the child can develop her mind further.

Starting a village library is often an excellent idea. In fact, a disabled young person may be able to become the village 'librarian'—and a non-formal educator.

To open up other possibilities, help your village recognize both the needs and value of disabled and other disadvantaged persons (such as single mothers). **When deciding who to choose for public service jobs and community responsibilities, try to make it a village policy to consider choosing persons who have disabilities or special needs.**

Although they are sometimes unable to do hard physical farm work, disabled persons can often make outstanding health workers, cooperative administrators, shop keepers, librarians, 'cultural promotors', or child care center coordinators—if they are given the chance.

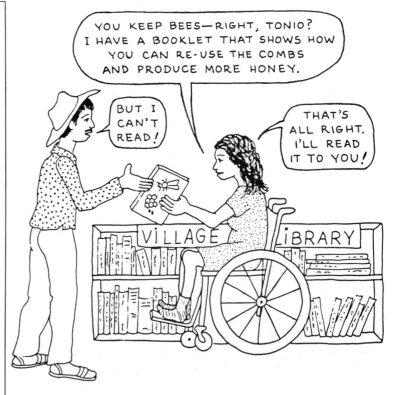

In a village, a young person who learns to read and write can become a 'librarian' and sharer of information.

Adaptations for farm work and gardening

Persons with weakness in their lower bodies but who have strong arms and hands can learn a wide variety of work skills where they can sit and use their hands. (See list of skills on p. 509.) However, for many villagers, the growing of food is central to their lives.

If certain *adaptations* are made, disabled villagers can often help with farming and gardening. Here are a few suggestions.

AIDS FOR CRAWLING

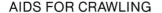
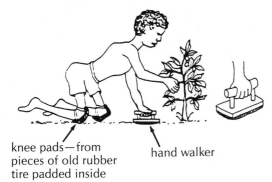

knee pads—from pieces of old rubber tire padded inside

hand walker

hand walker attached to garden trowel

ELEVATED GARDENS

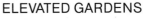
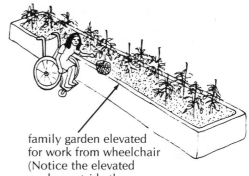

family garden elevated for work from wheelchair (Notice the elevated garden outside the 'model home' in the photo on p. 486.)

OFF-ROAD TRANSPORT

Getting to distant fields over rough trails may be difficult for the young person who cannot walk. A simple carrying frame can be used to carry the child and also the tools and grain.

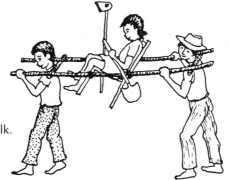

GUIDELINES OR RAILS

For the child who is blind, or has difficulty with balance, hand rails may make it easier to get from the house to the garden, the latrine, and the well or water hole.

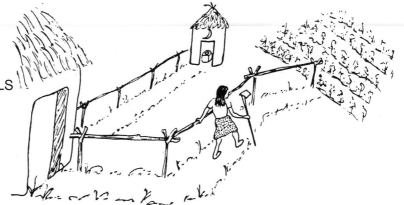

Alternatives to farm work

Many disabled villagers will need to learn skills other than farm work. **If unemployment is high it may not be wise to train disabled persons for jobs where there is a lot of competition.** In fact, any sort of paid job may be hard to get. Therefore, it often makes more sense **to teach young disabled persons skills so that they can become self-employed.** Or perhaps several disabled and non-disabled persons can become partners in a small 'home industry'.

A village-based rehabilitation center with a shop can teach young disabled persons different manual skills such as leatherwork, clothes making, woodworking or welding. While they are with the program, they can use these skills to make a wide range of rehabilitation and *orthopedic* equipment. They can also make toys, chairs, leather goods, clothes, and other objects for sale. The income from the sale of these things can help cover some of the costs of the rehabilitation program and training. When the learners have gained enough skills, perhaps the community program can help them set up their own small 'shop' in their home, village, or neighborhood.

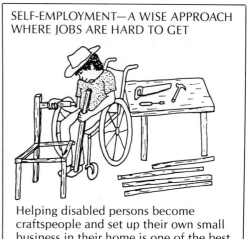

SELF-EMPLOYMENT—A WISE APPROACH WHERE JOBS ARE HARD TO GET

Helping disabled persons become craftspeople and set up their own small business in their home is one of the best approaches to employment for disabled persons with good minds and hands.

In several countries, organizations for the disabled have started **revolving loan plans** that provide the disabled craftsperson with the basic equipment to start his or her own small business. The loans are paid back little by little over a reasonable time, so that the same money can be used to help another disabled person get started.

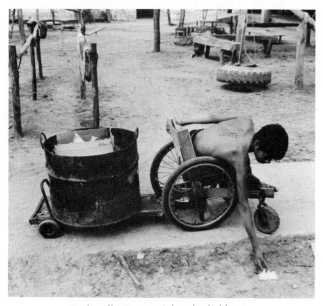

Trash collection—a job nobody likes but everyone must help do. (PROJIMO)

In the West Indies, the Caribbean Council for the Blind provides a guarantee to local banks which give 'start-up' loans to disabled persons. So far, 97 percent of the disabled persons who have received loans have met their payments on time. This record is better than that of able-bodied persons. It helps convince bankers not only that disabled persons can run their own small businesses responsibly, but that they are a good investment. By involving local banks in the loan program, the public is being educated toward a new respect and appreciation for disabled persons.

Disabled villagers can become skilled in a wide variety of manual skills. Here we list some skills that are taught in different rehabilitation programs, training programs, and special workshops.

* skills marked with a star are sometimes taught to blind persons
☐ skills marked with a box are sometimes taught to mentally retarded persons

leatherwork ☐
sandal and shoe making and repair
metal work of a wide variety
welding
radio and television repair
electrical and mechanical repairs
weaving of cloth, blankets, etc. *
sewing and clothes making ☐
toymaking *
basketweaving * ☐
dollmaking ☐
carpentry * ☐
cabinet and furniture making *
hospital equipment making
making rehabilitation equipment
   and aids
wheelchair making
prosthetic limb making
drawing, painting, sculpture and
   design, wood or ivory carving
production of simple marketplace
   gadgets, cages, utensils and
   nicknacks (see p. 510)
designing and making greeting cards
printing and silk-screening
pottery making *
broom making * ☐
chalk making * ☐
candle making *
artificial flower making ☐
typing and secretarial skills
bookkeeping, accounting
bee keeping
knife, scissor, and saw sharpening ☐
gardening and vegetable raising * ☐
animal raising (chickens, ducks, goats,
   rabbits, pigs, fish) * ☐
managing a small store or street shop *
cooking and restaurant management
health work
jewelry making
rope and string making * ☐
landscaping, grounds maintenance ☐
janitorial service (cleaning and
   maintenance) ☐
fish net making and repair *
teaching *
playing music *
laundry work, pressing
hair cutting, dressing
dental work

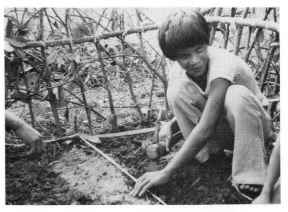

A blind boy in the Philippines plants a vegetable garden. (Photo by Robert Jaekle for Helen Keller International)

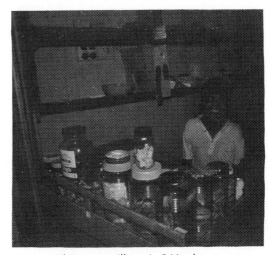

This young villager in Sri Lanka became quadriplegic at age 14. The Sarvodaya CBR program helped him set up this small store in front of his home.

The above list includes only a few of the activities that disabled persons have learned in order to run their own small business or set up shop in their home. As much as is possible, let the disabled person decide what skill or skills she wants to learn. Choices that are possible will depend on the person's combination of disability, abilities, and interest as well as on the local situation, resources, market, training opportunities, and other local factors.

Making craft goods out of old junk — an experiment in Pakistan

Leaders in the Community Rehabilitation Development Project (see p. 520) in Peshawar, Pakistan realize that in their country it is very difficult for disabled persons to 'earn a living'. Most either live by begging, are cared for by their families, or die of neglect. Since chances of employment are so limited, it is more realistic to help disabled persons learn simple craft skills for self-employment at home (if they have a home) or in the marketplace. They can make small things at low cost and sell them in the marketplace. If their small business helps the family a little or covers part of their daily expenses, something has been gained.

In the marketplace of Pakistan there is a variety of clever, simply made cages, tools, utensils, toys and other objects, mostly made out of very low-cost or waste materials. The Project has hired a self-taught craftsperson to collect, study, and make design plans for some of these marketplace things, so that disabled persons can learn to make and sell them. To follow are a few examples. For more complete instructions, write to Mental Health Centre, Mission Hospital, Peshawar, N.W.F.P. Pakistan

Marketplace crafts for self-employed production by disabled persons

These examples and the examples on the next page are from FAMN/UNICEF Community Rehabilitation Development Project, Peshawar, Pakistan.

WIRE BIRD OR SMALL ANIMAL CAGE

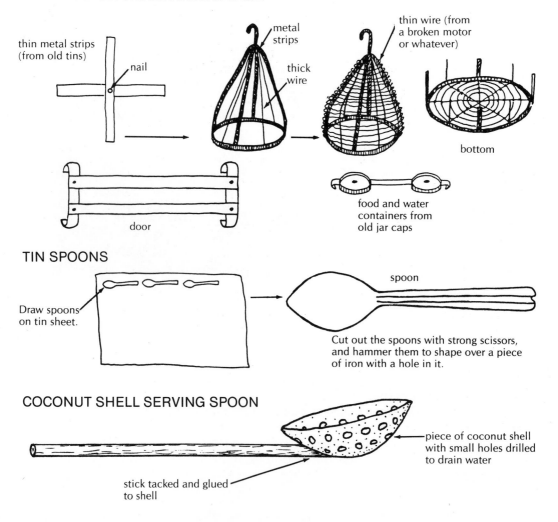

thin metal strips (from old tins)

nail

metal strips

thick wire

thin wire (from a broken motor or whatever)

bottom

door

food and water containers from old jar caps

TIN SPOONS

Draw spoons on tin sheet.

spoon

Cut out the spoons with strong scissors, and hammer them to shape over a piece of iron with a hole in it.

COCONUT SHELL SERVING SPOON

piece of coconut shell with small holes drilled to drain water

stick tacked and glued to shell

TIN CUPS

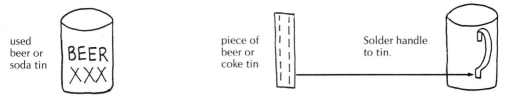

used beer or soda tin

BEER XXX

piece of beer or coke tin

Solder handle to tin.

BROOM

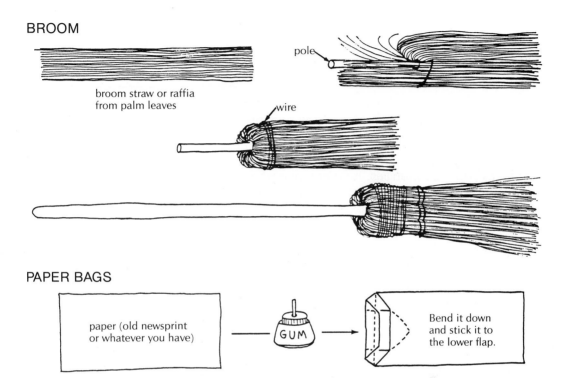

broom straw or raffia from palm leaves

pole

wire

PAPER BAGS

paper (old newsprint or whatever you have)

GUM

Bend it down and stick it to the lower flap.

CANDLES

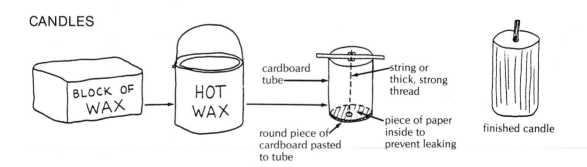

BLOCK OF WAX

HOT WAX

cardboard tube

string or thick, strong thread

round piece of cardboard pasted to tube

piece of paper inside to prevent leaking

finished candle

FLY SWATTER

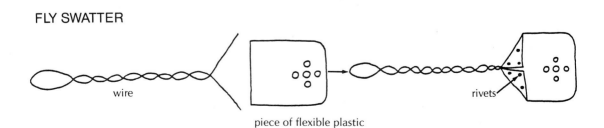

wire

piece of flexible plastic

rivets

TRAINING

The integrated approach

When possible, it is usually best that skills training for disabled persons take place together with skills training for non-disabled persons. For example:

- A disabled girl can go to the river to learn to wash clothes with other girls and their mothers.

- A disabled boy can go to the fields to help plant, weed, and harvest alongside his able-bodied brothers, sisters, and father.

- A disabled child can go to the same school as other children, and then go on to some specialized training course.

- A disabled young man or woman may enter a shop or production team as an apprentice just as non-disabled young persons often do.

For a *mildly or moderately disabled* child, there are many possibilities to prepare for life's work together with non-disabled children — especially if parents encourage the child and explore opportunities. A community rehabilitation program can help by encouraging schoolteachers, schoolchildren, training program instructors, crafts-persons, and possible employers to be more open to giving disabled young people an equal chance.

For more *severely disabled* young people, opportunities for integrated education or skills training will be much more limited. Alternatives need to be looked for, or arranged, especially in communities that are still not open to giving them an equal chance.

Special training possibilities

Different approaches have been tried to help disabled persons learn specific skills. In cities, special training centers are sometimes set up for children with similar disabilities. These include programs for deaf children, centers for retarded young persons, and programs for blind children. Each program chooses skills and activities suited to the particular limitations and abilities of the group. For example, a skills training and production program for the blind may focus on skills that depend largely on touch, such as weaving or chalk making.

In smaller villages, it is often not possible to bring together enough persons with the same kind of disability to create a specialized training program just for them. However, a community rehabilitation program can, in its workshop, include a variety of skills training opportunities which can be adapted to persons with a wide range of disabilities.

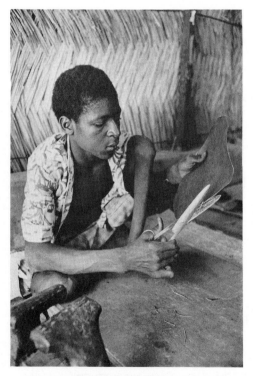

This young man in Niger, Africa, learned to make leather goods together with other disabled young people. Later he can work out of his own home and sell his goods in the marketplace. (Photo: Carolyn Watson)

'Sheltered workshops' — yes or no?

Sheltered workshops are special training and production centers for disabled persons. The idea is to provide a work opportunity and a little pay to those who would find it difficult to get training and employment 'on the outside'.

At best, these workshops can be a very valuable experience for participants, and may serve as a step toward greater independence. They help participants gain the technical and social skills, work habits, responsibility, and self-confidence needed for outside employment or self-employment.

At worst, sheltered workshops can (and often do) actually hold back the development and crush the spirit of participants. Too often they are run by persons who treat the workers like babies or slaves, giving them simple, repetitive tasks. The workers are not involved in the planning, organization, or running of the program. They are simply told what to do. They become increasingly dependent on the center and fearful of their inability to make it on their own in the outside world.

Perhaps the key difference between these two kinds of sheltered workshops is the question of **control and equality.** If the participants are involved in the direction and decision making of their own program, then they will grow and mature along with the program. Perhaps they will make more 'mistakes' than a program that is controlled and run by 'superiors'. But they will learn from those mistakes. At the same time they learn crafts, they learn skills in decision-making, problem-solving and small-group democracy — essential skills for improving life in the 'real world'.

A community-based rehabilitation program run by disabled persons may have some features of a sheltered workshop. It may provide special training and work opportunities adjusted to the pace, abilities, and limitations of each participant. It may provide such an enjoyable 'home' and 'family' setting that some persons may choose to keep working rather than to 'move on' into the 'outside world'. But because it is a program run by disabled persons, and major decisions are made at all-group meetings, it tends to be a dignifying and liberating experience.

A program where disabled and non-disabled persons work side by side, sharing equally in decisions and responsibility, may be even more liberating.

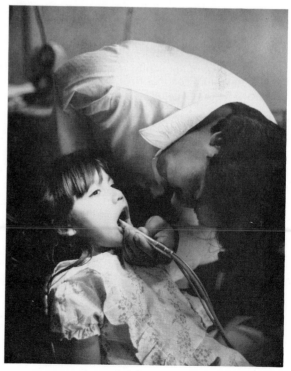

A one-armed young man who works as a village dental worker in Project Piaxtla drills a tooth before filling it. (Mexico)

Children with *paralysis* in their bodies often develop strong arms and hands—and can do many kinds of work as well as anyone.

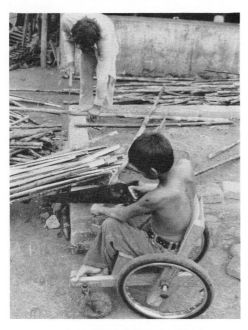

Here 2 boys who had polio build cane blinds for the model home at PROJIMO.

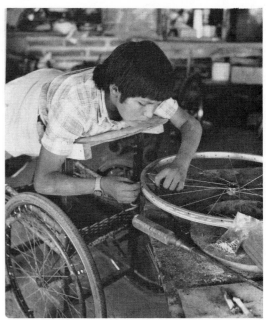

This boy, who is paraplegic from tuberculosis, spokes a wheel for a wheelchair. He rides a wheeled lying board because of pressure sores on his *butt*.

Combining work with therapy

Whenever possible, look for work that will help a disabled person fit into the life of his or her community, and that will also provide needed exercise or therapy. Here is one example from the Sarvodaya community-based rehabilitation program in Beruwala, Sri Lanka.

With the help of her family and a village rehabilitation volunteer, this girl with cerebral palsy learned to make rope from coconut fiber (jute). This is a common village craft, so she can work with other villagers.

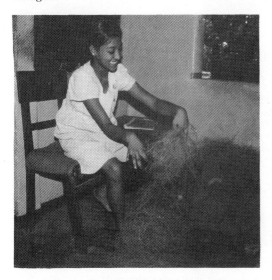

Separating and preparing the fibers is good therapy for her spastic hands.

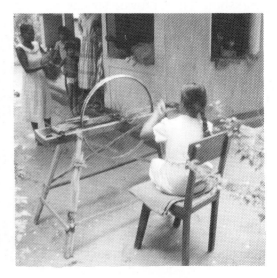

Twisting the fiber with this wheel to make rope helps her move her stiff arms in a smooth circle—providing excellent, active therapy while she works.

Examples of Community-Directed Programs

In this chapter we give examples of 6 *rehabilitation* programs in 5 countries. Each is quite different, yet all are similar in that they are largely or completely run by *disabled* persons themselves, or by their families. Although they all work closely with the local community, each has a small 'center' of some kind where disabled persons or their families can help meet each other's needs.

We do not claim that the examples given here are the most outstanding or successful programs. Rather, they are the ones with which we are personally most familiar.

Our description of each program must be brief. We will, therefore, try to focus on their most interesting and original features, especially those that could serve as examples for other programs. Also, we describe how these have grown and spread to new communities. This kind of grassroots seeding from community to community, although slower and less orderly, may be more effective than is 'planting' of pre-designed programs from on top.

1. PROJIMO—RURAL MEXICO

Project PROJIMO is a rural rehabilitation program in western Mexico, run by disabled villagers, to serve disabled children and their families. It was started in 1982 by disabled village health workers from an older community-based health program (Project Piaxtla).

PROJIMO's goal is to help disabled children and their families become more self-reliant. It aims to provide low-cost, high-quality services to poor families who cannot obtain or afford services elsewhere.

The PROJIMO team provides a wide range of rehabilitation activities and equipment. These include: family counseling and training, *therapy,* work and skills training, brace making, artificial limbs, wheelchair making, special seating, and therapeutic aids.

PROJIMO is based in one small village but serves children and their families from neighboring towns and villages, and even from the closest cities (over 100 miles away). Local villagers cooperate by taking visiting disabled children and their families into their homes. Schoolchildren help make the **playground-for-all-children** and toys for disabled children.

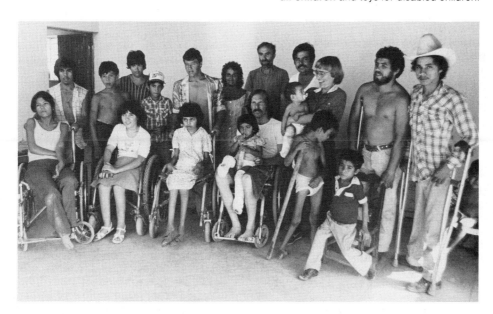

Part of the PROJIMO team

PROJIMO DIFFERS FROM MANY
REHABILITATION PROGRAMS IN
A NUMBER OF WAYS:

1. **Community control.** Unlike many
'community-based' programs, which are designed
and run by outsiders, PROJIMO is run and
controlled by local disabled villagers.

2. **De-professionalization.** The village team,
although they have mastered many 'professional'
skills, is made up of disabled persons with an
average education of only 3 years of primary
school. Their training has been mostly of the non-
formal, learn-by-doing type. There are no titled
professionals on the PROJIMO staff. However,
therapists, brace makers, limb makers, and other
rehabilitation professionals are invited for short
visits to teach rather than to practice their skills.

> The PROJIMO team believes that only by
> simplifying rehabilitation knowledge and skills
> to make them widely available in the
> community, can the millions of unserved
> disabled children in the world receive the basic
> assistance they need.

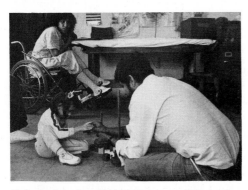

Roberto Fajardo and Mari Picos, two of the leaders
of PROJIMO, *evaluate* a child's developmental
level. Both Roberto and Mari first came for
rehabilitation, then stayed in order to help others.

3. **Equality between service providers and
receivers.** When asked how many 'workers' they
have, the PROJIMO team has no easy answer.
This is because there is no clear line between
those who provide services and those who receive
them. Visiting disabled young persons and their
families are invited to help in whatever way they
can. Most of the PROJIMO workers first came
for rehabilitation themselves. They began to help
in different ways, decided to stay, and gradually
became team members.

4. **Self-government through group process.**
The PROJIMO team has been trying to develop
an approach to planning, organization, and
decision-making in which all participants take part.
They are trying to free themselves from the typical
'boss-servant' work relationship and form more
of a 'work partnership'. The group elects its
coordinators' on a one-month rotating basis so
that everyone has a turn. This leads to a lot of
inefficiency and confusion, but to a much more
democratic group process. (See p. 478.)

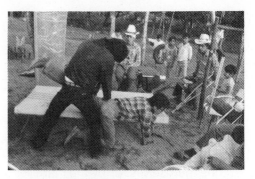

Most of the training of the PROJIMO team
members is through guided 'learning by
doing'. Here, PROJIMO workers practice
exercises under the guidance of a visiting
physiotherapist. Parents, children, and
anyone who wants to learn are welcome.

5. **Modest earnings.** The PROJIMO team
believes that they should work for the same low
pay as that of the farming and laboring families
they serve. They can see that the high pay
demanded by professionals and technicians is one
reason that the children of the poor often cannot
get the therapy and aids they need.

6. **Unity with all who are marginalized.** The
PROJIMO team sees society's unfair attitudes
toward the disabled as only one aspect of an unjust
social structure. They feel that disabled persons
should join in solidarity with all who are rejected,
misjudged, exploited, or not treated as equals.
This feeling has led the team to become more self-
critical and to seek greater equality for women
within their own group.

Thus the PROJIMO team views its role not only
as one of helping disabled children and their
families gain power, but as part of the larger
struggle for social change and liberation of all who
are 'on the bottom'.

7. **Grassroots multiplying effect.** The PROJIMO
approach has been spreading in various ways.
Locally, families of disabled children in a number
of towns and villages have begun to organize,
build playgrounds, and form their own special
education programs, as more or less 'satellites'
of PROJIMO. PROJIMO has also invited visitors
from rehabilitation and community health
programs in other parts of Mexico and Latin
America to visit and take ideas back with them.
Some programs have sent disabled representatives
to work and learn at PROJIMO for several months
so they can start similar programs in their own
area.

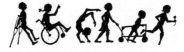

The PROJIMO experience has been the basis
for writing this book. Different examples or
descriptions from PROJIMO are discussed in
various chapters. For further references, see the
Index. A 64-page report on PROJIMO with many
illustrations is available from The Hesperian
Foundation (see p. 637).

2. LOS PARGOS—URBAN MEXICO

Los Pargos is an organization of families of disabled children in Mazatlán, a city on the west coast of Mexico. The program was started privately by Teresa Páez, a local social worker. While she was working in a public hospital, Teresa became concerned that although disabled children were given basic medical treatment, they received almost no rehabilitation. Most did not go to school because of non-acceptance by teachers, difficulties in transportation, or overprotection by parents.

Teresa began by bringing a group of concerned parents together, and they invited others. Today Los Pargos includes about 60 families with disabled children, and it continues to grow.

Los Pargos has set up its own special education program and has convinced the local university authorities to make space available in a local prep school after school hours. Some of the teachers, who are volunteers, are also disabled. This makes them good role models for the children.

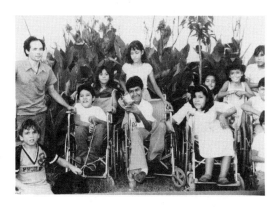

A few of the children of Los Pargos with one of their teachers, on the left. The teacher, severely affected by cerebral palsy, has a personal understanding of the children's needs.

The word 'Pargos' is the name of a large, colorful fish! The children picked the name. It is perhaps appropriate, since much of the money for running the program and transporting the children comes from fish scales! On weekends the children and their parents visit the beach where fishermen dock their small boats and clean their fish for the market. The group collects the large fish scales, which they clean, bleach, color, and use to make artificial flowers. The children and parents set the flowers in attractive bouquets and designs together with small seashells, seaweed, and other dried sea life. In the tourist city of Mazatlán, selling the flowers has become a good business. When we last visited Los Pargos, parents and children were working very hard to fill a rush order for 2000 bouquets!

Los Pargos, located about 100 miles from PROJIMO, often takes groups of 'parguitos' (disabled children) to PROJIMO for rehabilitation services that they have trouble getting in the city. Also, their visit to PROJIMO is an adventure into the country for these city children and their parents.

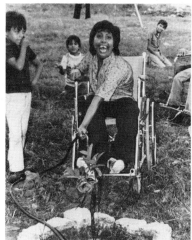

One of the children of Los Pargos waters a young tree—part of an orchard the parents and children are planting together.

One of the goals of Los Pargos is to convince the government, the public schools, and society in general to accept, respect, provide opportunities, and help meet the needs of disabled children. Some things are changing, but slowly. As one of the parents explains, "The best way to get something done is to do it ourselves!"

The idea of Los Pargos has begun to spread to other communities. Families of disabled children in Culiacán, the next biggest city to the north, are trying to organize a similar program. The key to success seems to be a few persons with energy, commitment, and an ability to get people working together.

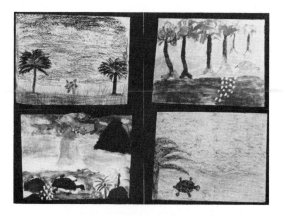

Four pictures of sea turtles, painted by Los Pargos children, as a part of their "Save the Turtles" campaign.

3. CENTRE FOR THE REHABILITATION OF THE PARALYSED (CRP)—BANGLADESH

Located in the capital Dhaka, CRP is run by a local team, with the help of a British physiotherapist. Four of the staff members have *spinal* injuries themselves.

The CRP provides short- and long-term 'participatory rehabilitation' to severely *paralyzed* persons. Almost from the day of arrival, newly paralyzed persons begin to do jobs to help the Centre bring in some income. Those who must lie on stretcher trolleys (wheeled cots) work on jobs ranging from making paper bags to be sold in the local marketplace, to welding and painting of orthopedic equipment. The group produces orthopedic and hospital equipment, not only for those it serves directly, but also for sale in hospitals and in the community.

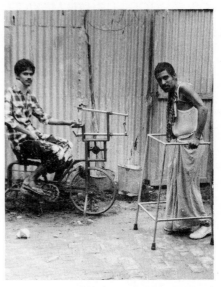

Badd, who is quadriplegic, pedals a CRP-made 'exercycle' while Delwar, paralyzed by tuberculosis of the spine, practices walking.

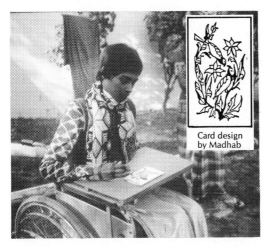

Card design by Madhab

Madhab, who is quadriplegic and who has been employed as the Centre's counselor since 1980, paints by means of a simple hand splint. Disabled workers print his paintings as greeting cards and sell them to bring in money. Madhab is responsible for the education program. He supervises those who read and write, who teach classes to those who do not.

CRP teaches practical skills through 'learning by doing'. The work that participants do not only brings in money for the program, but also teaches them ways to earn money after they return home. Skills learned are mostly those that will let persons have their own small home business—a roadside stand, sewing and tailoring, weaving, welding, and metalwork.

CRP has developed a wide range of low-cost *orthopedic* and rehabilitation equipment adapted to the needs and lifestyle of local villagers. Examples are ground level wheelchairs, or 'trolleys', for those who cook and eat on the floor (see p. 590), and simple metal frame beds that can be easily lowered to near ground level for easy transfer into the low trolleys (see p. 572).

Although CRP is much loved by disabled persons and their families, it has suffered attacks—sometimes physical—from opposition groups. (Many successful community-directed programs have faced similar difficulties—partly because they provide friendly, flexible, effective care that differs so much from the services provided by many large institutions.)

The Centre for the Rehabilitation of the Paralysed is financed mainly from outside grants and partly from the sale of its products.

For more information on this center and its equipment, see p. 199, 483, and 509.

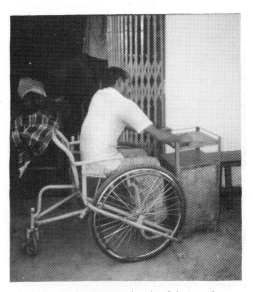

A worker in the CRP-made wheelchair makes a bedside stand to be sold to a local hospital.

4. ORGANIZATION OF DISABLED REVOLUTIONARIES—NICARAGUA

The Organization of Disabled Revolutionaries (ORD) was started after Nicaragua's liberation from the Somoza dictatorship, by a group of young persons who had become paralyzed by *spinal cord* injuries. Some had been boys of 13, 14, or 15 years old when they first joined the struggle against Somoza.

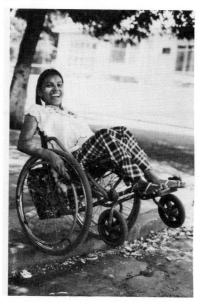

ORD was begun because of concern for a common need: wheelchairs. With the increase in disabled persons from the war, the lack of a local wheelchair factory, and the difficulties of importing wheelchairs due to the United States' embargo, the shortage was severe.

Two young North Americans who both have spinal cord injuries, one a peer counselor for the disabled and the other a wheelchair designer and engineer, helped ORD organize and set up a small wheelchair factory.

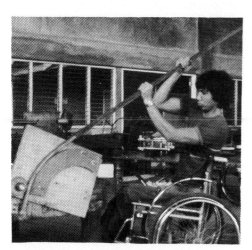

The ORD team of disabled workers produced its own high-quality metal tubing wheelchairs, adapted for rough ground (see p. 622) at a cost far lower than standard commercial wheelchairs.

Although ORD started with wheelchairs, it grew to become a group that represented and stood up for the rights of all disabled people. It pressured the Health Ministry to respond more to the disabled and their needs. The government, which tried to represent the people much more than most governments, responded well. It allowed ORD 'time' for short educational programs on public radio and television. And it agreed to help pay the cost of wheelchairs made by ORD for families too poor to pay. ORD was in close communication with the head of rehabilitation for the nation. In this way, the disabled organization had some voice in national policy making.

These are some of the advantages experienced by a community-directed program in a country with a revolutionary popular government. On the other hand, ORD suffered from the embargo and other difficulties imposed by the United States government. At times, the wheelchair production almost stops for lack of metal tubing, bearings, and other basic materials.

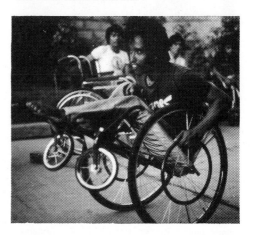

ORD had a far-reaching influence. It helped organize groups of disabled persons in other parts of Nicaragua. Also, members have helped conduct training workshops in Central American and Caribbean countries to teach representatives from other disabled groups how to make wheelchairs.

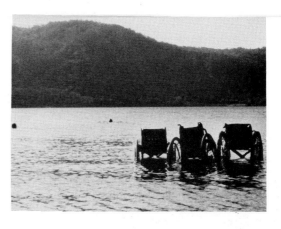

5. COMMUNITY-DIRECTED REHABILITATION DEVELOPMENT—PAKISTAN

The program began in Peshawar in the Northwest Frontier Province of Pakistan as a small play group for 8 *mentally* handicapped children. In 1978 the 3 Pakistani staff were joined by a Welsh special education teacher and her husband. During the next 7 years the play group grew to become a community rehabilitation and resource center with daily participation of 70 physically and 40 mentally and multiply disabled children.

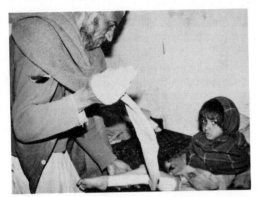

Splinting a leg to straighten a knee contracture.

Local staff persons are trained by the few professionals in special education, physical therapy, brace making, parent counseling, and planning services.

An important part of the program is the **Community Rehabilitation Development Project.** The big, largely rural area surrounding Peshawar is very underserved. To accomplish as much as possible with limited resources, disabled children in towns were considered first. Volunteer college students went door-to-door to find and bring together parents and relatives of disabled children. Public meetings were held and an Association was formed in each town with the aim of starting rehabilitation activities. People (sometimes young disabled persons) were chosen and sent to learn basic skills at the Peshawar center. Meanwhile, the Association committee raised funds and found a place that could serve as a modest rehabilitation center.

Although the parent program has had UNICEF and other outside funding, the neighborhood rehabilitation centers have mostly been funded locally, some with a government subsidy. Management is entirely in the hands of local people.

In addition to providing daily special education and physical therapy, the neighborhood centers act as a resource within their districts. They distribute advice, pamphlets, and books to families for home rehabilitation. Where possible, going to normal schools is encouraged.

12-minute radio broadcasts about home rehabilitation started in 1984. (The scripts for these, which are excellent, are available at the website of Disability World, www.disabilityworld.org/01-03_02/arts/afghan.shtml. An article on handicrafts by which disabled young people can contribute to their family's income is at www.independentliving.org/docs3/milesm1987a.html. (See examples on p. 510.)

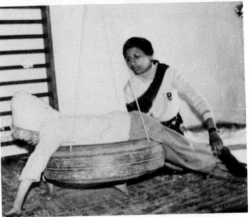

Helping a child begin to learn to move.

Also available is an excellent book by Christine Miles, called *Special Education for Mentally Handicapped Pupils: A Teaching Manual.* It points out the importance of re-thinking special education to meet local needs and customs in developing countries. (See the reference section, p. 640.)

M. Miles, Christine's husband, has also written many excellent and critical papers on rehabilitation efforts – and problems – in developing countries (see p. 641).

The Peshawar program has succeeded in promoting community-directed rehabilitation activities in much of the Northwest Frontier through organizing an already motivated group (parents of disabled children). One of their keys to success is to: "Do the easy thing first!"

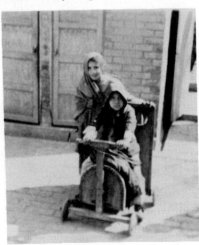

Going for a ride.

6. OPERATION HANDICAP INTERNATIONALE'S (OHI) ARTIFICIAL LIMB PROGRAM—THAILAND/KAMPUCHEA

It is estimated that in the last 8 years of the war in Kampuchea (Cambodia) more than 12,000 men, women, and children have lost their legs from stepping on land mines. A lot of the injured are evacuated for hospital care to a large refugee camp, called Khao-i-dang, close to the Thai border.

At first the hospital had no way of making or obtaining artificial *limbs.* For this reason a French relief agency (at that time SOS, or Enfants Sans Frontières, now Operation Handicap Internationale) began making low-cost artificial legs.

The workers in the large workshop are almost all refugee amputees. Some start learning by helping to make their own leg.

The team (run by Frenchmen, some of whom are professional limb makers) has developed different models of very low-cost limbs using local materials. The bamboo limb described on p. 628 is one example.

Bamboo is in fact the main building material for the shop itself, the rehabilitation center next door, and for most of the beds, aids, and equipment. The rehabilitation playground (which served as a model for PROJIMO) is made completely of bamboo. (See p. 425.)

One of the most outstanding features of the program is the way it has spread to other areas. Many of the amputee workers trained in Khao-i-dang have gone back into Kampuchea and opened small artificial limb shops. The program therefore trains the amputees not only in the technology of limb making, but also in basic management. Some of the 15 'satellite shops' now have teams of several amputees working in them. The most remote shops are run in make-shift shelters deep in the forest near the fighting.

The spirit of hard work and friendship in shops run by amputees does much to help recent amputees accept the loss of their limbs and get back into the adventure of survival.

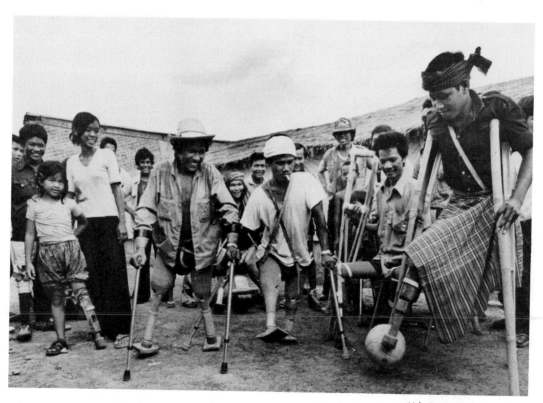

Aids For Living (AHRTAG)

Photos from the OHI Limb Program, Thailand

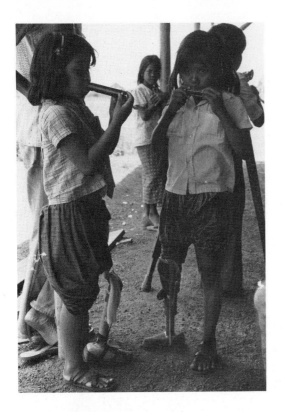

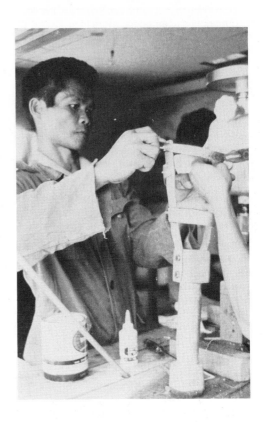

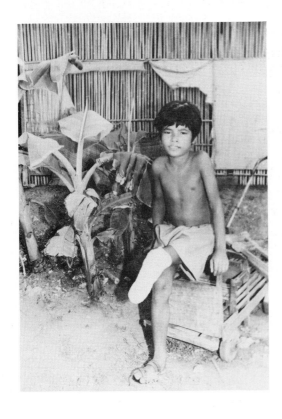

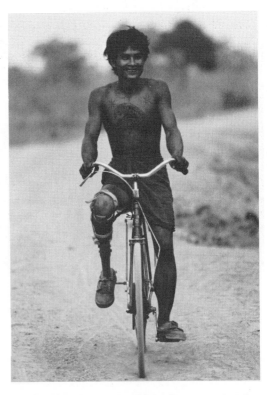

PART 3

WORKING IN THE SHOP

Rehabilitation Aids
and Procedures

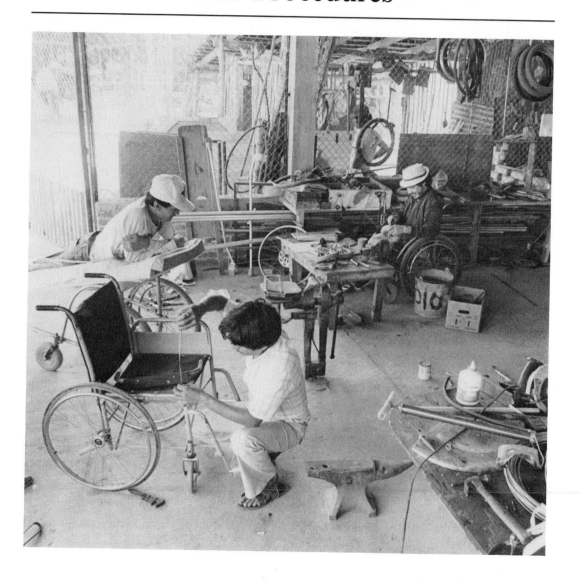

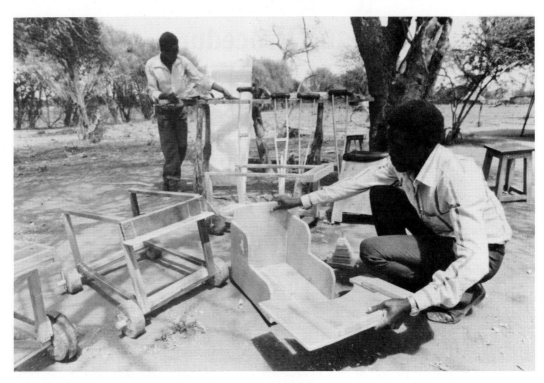

A lot of 'shop work' can be done outside. Here young men in Kibwezi, Kenya (Africa) learn to make low-cost aids. (Photo: *Aids for Living*, AHRTAG)

CHAPTER 56

Making Sure Aids and Procedures Do More Good than Harm

When I (David Werner) was about 10 years old, I was taken to a doctor because I was having problems with my feet. I kept falling over things and spraining my ankles. No one knew yet that these were early signs of a *progressive muscular atrophy.*

The doctor examined my feet. They were somewhat weak and floppy, so he prescribed arch supports. An *'orthotist'* across town would make them.

When the arch supports were ready, the orthotist put them on my feet. "Do they hurt?" he asked. "No," I said. So I was sent home with instructions to wear them every day.

I hated the things! — not because they hurt, but because it was harder for me to walk with them than without them. They pushed up on my arches and bent my ankles outward. I fell and sprained my ankles more than ever.

I tried to protest, but nobody listened to me. After all, I was only a child. "You have to get used to them!" I was told. "Who do you think knows best — you or the doctor?"

So mostly I suffered in silence. I took the arch supports out of my shoes and hid them whenever I could. But when I was caught I was punished. I was made to feel naughty and guilty for not doing what was 'best' for me.

Several years later, as my walking continued to get worse, I was prescribed a pair of metal braces. They held my ankles firmly, but they were heavy, uncomfortable, and made me feel more awkward than ever. I hated them, but wore them because I was told to.

One holiday I took a long walk in the mountains. The braces rubbed the skin on the front of my legs so badly that deep, painful sores developed. I refused to wear them again.

It was not until many years later, long after I had begun to work with *disabled* children, that a brace maker and I figured out what kind of ankle support would best meet my needs. So now I use lightweight, plastic braces that provide both the flexibility and support that best suit me.

When I look back, I realize that **the doctor did not know more about what I needed than I knew**. After all, I was the one who lived with my feet! True, at age 10, I could not explain the mechanics and anatomy for what was happening. But I did have a sense of what helped me manage better and what did not. Maybe if the adults who were so eager to help had included me in deciding what I needed, I might have had aids that better met my needs. And I might not have felt so guilty and naughty for expressing my opinion.

I learned something from these childhood experiences. I learned how important it is to listen to the disabled child, to ask the child at every stage how she feels about an aid or an exercise, and to include the child and her parents in deciding what she needs. **The child and her parents may not always be right. But doctors, therapists, and *rehabilitation* workers are not always right either. By respecting each other's special knowledge and looking together for solutions, they can come closest to meeting the child's needs.**

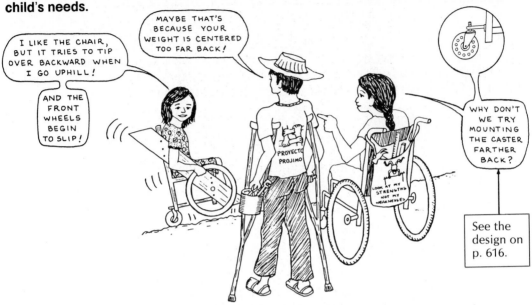

I LIKE THE CHAIR, BUT IT TRIES TO TIP OVER BACKWARD WHEN I GO UPHILL!

AND THE FRONT WHEELS BEGIN TO SLIP!

MAYBE THAT'S BECAUSE YOUR WEIGHT IS CENTERED TOO FAR BACK!

WHY DON'T WE TRY MOUNTING THE CASTER FARTHER BACK?

See the design on p. 616.

Some of the best design improvements in aids and equipment come from the ideas and suggestions of the children who try them out.

PRECAUTIONS IN PROVIDING A CHILD WITH AIDS, EQUIPMENT, AND PROCEDURES

To make sure aids and equipment really meet the child's needs, consider the following:

1. **How necessary are the aids or equipment? Might it help the child more to learn to manage without them?** For example:

Elena has arthritis. Her thighs have become too weak to support her body weight. You can fit her with braces and crutches. But watch out! These aids will not make her thighs stronger. They may even make them weaker, since she could then walk without having to use her thigh *muscles.*

A better solution might be exercise to strengthen her thighs. For example, walking in water will make it easier for her legs to support her weight.

Also, using a cane instead of crutches helps her to use and strengthen her thigh muscles (see p. 587).

AVOID MAKING THE CHILD TOO DEPENDENT ON AIDS!

LESS APPROPRIATE

MORE APPROPRIATE

2. As any child grows and develops, his needs keep changing. **Frequent re-*evaluation* is necessary to find out if an aid should be changed or is no longer needed. Ask the child what he wants.** For example:

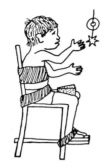

Misha has been slow to develop balance for sitting. At first, straps helped him sit in a stable, upright position.

But as he continues to develop, keeping him strapped in a chair may keep him from improving his balance more or from learning to sit without help.

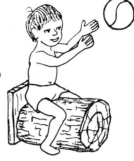

Misha might be helped more by a seat that gives support to his legs and hips but lets him balance the top part of his body without help (see p. 573).

APPROPRIATE ONLY AT FIRST   APPROPRIATE LATER

3. **A simple, low-cost aid** that is designed and made to meet the needs of a particular child often works better than an expensive commercial one. For example:

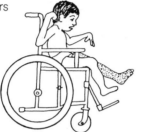

Commercial wheelchairs are often too big for children, and hard to adapt to their positioning needs. Repairs are difficult and expensive; replacement parts are hard to get.

A simple wood or plywood chair can be easily made to fit the child's size and positioning needs. Repairs and replacements are easy because bicycle wheels and other standard parts are used. (See p. 620.)

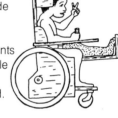

LESS APPROPRIATE   MORE APPROPRIATE

4. **Consider the economic limitations of the family and community.** Growing children will frequently need larger sizes of aids such as leg braces, artificial limbs, and special seating. **Use either aids that are cheap enough to replace often, or that can be easily made bigger.** For example:

Poor families sometimes spend as much as a year's earnings on an expensive, modern brace with knee and ankle hinges and special shoes.

When the child outgrows the brace, or it breaks, the family cannot afford to repair or replace it—so the child goes back to crawling, develops *contractures* and may never walk again.

A cheap brace without hinges will not let the child bend his knee to sit. But the brace can be cheaply replaced, so the child is able to stay on his feet. Up to 20 low-cost braces can be made for the price of one expensive one.

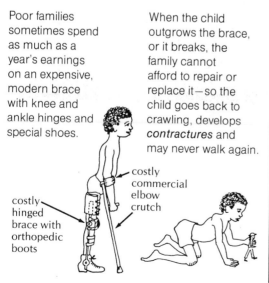

costly commercial elbow crutch

costly hinged brace with orthopedic boots

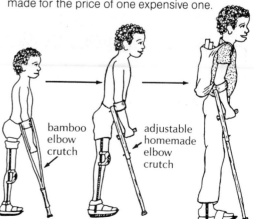

bamboo elbow crutch

adjustable homemade elbow crutch

LESS APPROPRIATE   MORE APPROPRIATE   (See p. 543 and 586.)

5. **Make use of the special opportunities in rural areas.** Look for ways that a child can do her exercises as part of daily work and play with other people—not as a boring chore that keeps her separate and different. For example:

If a child needs a special aid to strengthen her weak arm,

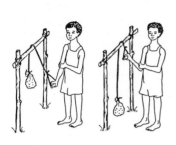

avoid making her do the exercises in a way that isolates her.

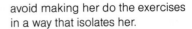

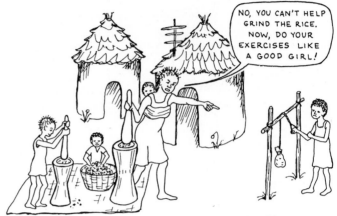

LESS APPROPRIATE

Instead, find ways for her to do her exercises while taking part in activities with others.

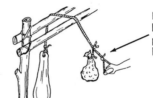

If the grinder is too heavy to lift, you can put another weight here.

Another child can help lower the grinder.

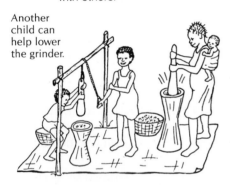

MORE APPROPRIATE

In places where people grind grain with a handmill, this can also be used for exercises. So can grinding grain on a stone dish. A mill can be adjusted from 'easy' to 'hard'. (Also see pages 6 and 377.)

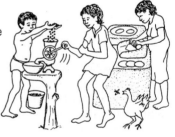

6. Whenever a choice can be made, **keep orthopedic aids as light and unnoticeable as possible.** For example:

Tina is from a village where most children wear sandals. A rehabilitation center in the city fitted her with a heavy metal brace and boots like this. She hated them and refused to leave the house with them on.

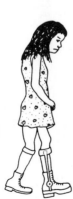

Six months later, Tina's father took her to a village rehabilitation center where they fitted her with a lightweight plastic brace. She could wear it under stockings, and still use her old sandals. She was happy to wear it anywhere.

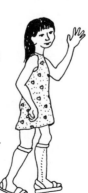

Note: In areas where children do not wear shoes and socks, a brace with a wood clog, leaving most of the foot open to the air, may be preferred (and may be cleaner).

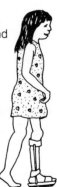

7. **Try to adapt aids and equipment to the local culture and way of life.** An example of adaptation to the local situation is the 'Jaipur limb' (see also Chapter 67):

In India, villagers squat a lot. They cook and eat at ground level. A person with a standard artificial leg cannot squat because the leg does not bend enough in the knee and ankle. Also, the standard leg is not made to be used when barefoot, or in water.

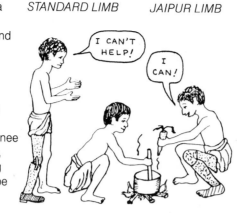

STANDARD LIMB   JAIPUR LIMB

LESS APPROPRIATE   MORE APPROPRIATE

The 'Jaipur limb' was designed for the needs of villagers in India. It has a knee with a joint that bends all the way. The foot piece is made mostly of rubber and is very flexible, allowing the person to squat. It is the color and shape (including toes) of a normal foot. It is waterproof, so that people can work in water or rice fields without harming it. The leg is low cost and quick to fit.

(For more information on the Jaipur limb, see p. 636.)

8. **Make aids and equipment as attractive and enjoyable as possible.** To test the attractiveness of an aid, find out:

- Does the child take pleasure or pride in his aid?

- Do the parents like it?

- Do other children want to use it or play with it?

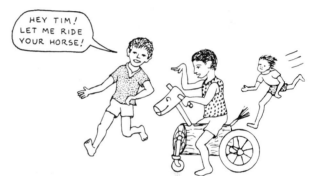

9. A common error is to provide children with more bracing than they need. Often a child will come to the rehabilitation center already fitted with big heavy braces that he never needed or no longer needs. They may actually slow him down. **Always check to see what a child can do with and without his aids. Try smaller, lighter aids, or none at all. Above all, ask the child what he prefers.**

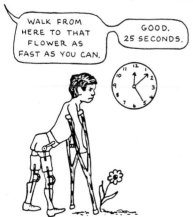

LESS APPROPRIATE

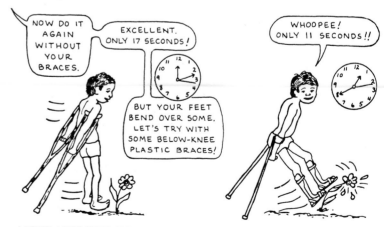

MORE APPROPRIATE

STILL MORE APPROPRIATE
(for this child)
(See p. 550.)

EVALUATING WHICH DEFORMITIES SHOULD BE CORRECTED AND WHICH SHOULD NOT

PART 3 of this book, in addition to aids and equipment, also discusses methods for correcting joint contractures, which are discussed in Chapter 59. Just as you need to decide if a brace is appropriate, **you need to decide whether correcting a contracture will actually help a child.** Although many contractures increase difficulty for a child, some may actually help and should be left uncorrected. For example:

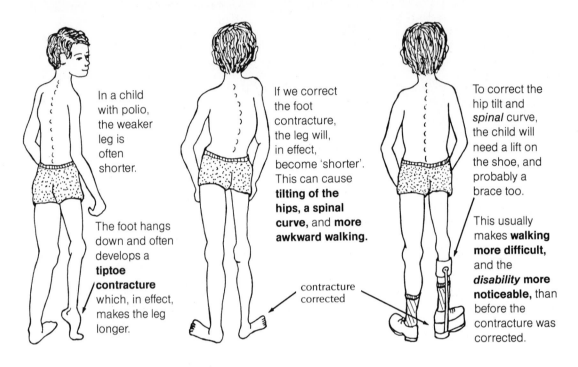

In a child with polio, the weaker leg is often shorter.

The foot hangs down and often develops a **tiptoe contracture** which, in effect, makes the leg longer.

If we correct the foot contracture, the leg will, in effect, become 'shorter'. This can cause **tilting of the hips, a spinal curve, and more awkward walking.**

contracture corrected

To correct the hip tilt and *spinal* curve, the child will need a lift on the shoe, and probably a brace too.

This usually makes **walking more difficult,** and the *disability* **more noticeable,** than before the contracture was corrected.

For this child it may be best NOT to correct the contracture.

Other examples of contractures that are sometimes more beneficial than harmful are finger contractures in persons with hand *paralysis* (see p. 183) and tightness of back muscles in persons with *spinal cord* injury or muscular *dystrophy* (see p. 375).

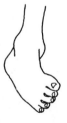

CAUTION: In children with *spastic* cerebral palsy, sometimes orthopedic surgeons perform operations to correct contractures or awkward positions, without completely evaluating the effects on the children. Often children find it harder to walk or function after the surgery. **Always seek the opinion of therapists and other orthopedists before deciding to have the operation.**

Before deciding to correct any contractures or deformities, try to be sure that the correction will help the child to do things better.

WHAT IS MORE IMPORTANT—APPEARANCE OR FUNCTION?

When a choice needs to be made between an aid that is more useful and one that is more attractive (or perhaps no aid at all), it is important to **consider the cultural factors** and to respect the **wishes of the child and her parents.** Here is another story.

A HELPING HAND FOR SRI

When Sri was 13 years old, one day she was helping her father at a small sugar-cane mill that was pulled round and round by a mule. Her hand got caught in the gears of the mill and was crushed. It had to be cut off at the wrist.

The stump healed quickly, but Sri's spirit did not. It seemed as though it, too, had been crushed. She had been a happy girl. Now she just sat around. She did not help with house-work, and refused to go outside. She kept her stump hidden in her clothing or behind her back.

Sri's family worried about her. They took her to a specialist in the city who examined her and suggested an artificial limb. She gave Sri the choice between hooks, which would be useful, and an artificial hand, which looked more natural but would be less useful. The specialist encouraged her to choose the hooks, and explained how well she could learn to use them. But Sri picked the hand.

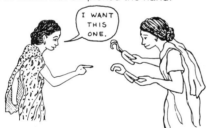

The hand was very expensive, but it looked almost real, and the family agreed. Her father had to sell his mule to pay for it, and was in debt for more than a year.

As time went by, however, Sri never really used her new hand. She tried it on a few times, but it seemed cold and dead. One day when her mother took her to the market wearing the hand, Sri thought everyone was looking at her. Two little boys, who had been her friends, pointed at the hand and laughed. She never wore it again.

One day a village health worker visited Sri's home. She saw that everyone was busy working and doing things except Sri, who sat quietly in the corner.

After talking with her family, the health worker suggested that they make an effort to treat Sri just like the other children. "Encourage her to help with work, and to take part in all your activities," she said. "Don't pretend that Sri's hand isn't missing. Just accept her as she is. Let her know that you love her and need her help as much as before."

So instead of feeling sorry for Sri, or letting her just sit and feel sorry for herself, her family began to treat her as they had before the accident. They asked her to help with the housework, prepare the meals, and care for the baby. At first Sri was unwilling and found everything difficult. But soon she learned how to do many things by using her good hand and her stump. She began to gain new confidence in herself, and in time started going to the market alone. At first, people took notice of her missing hand, or whispered, "Oh, poor thing!" But when they saw how well she did things, they soon stopped feeling sorry for her and began to treat her like any other person.

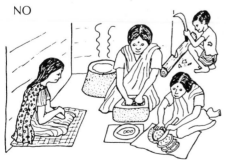

NO

It is important that the family not let the disabled person be separated from daily work and activities.

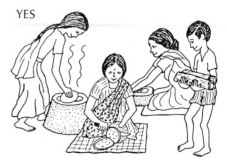

YES

Instead, look for ways to let the disabled person help as best she can.

When trying to decide about an aid, we need to seek the balance between usefulness and attractiveness that helps the child fit in best with his or her family and community.

Rehabilitation experts often place great importance on usefulness, or 'function'. But acceptance in the community is also very important. In some places it may be *more* important. So, before trying to convince a child like Sri to accept an aid that will make her deformity more noticeable, we must consider how this could affect her. In some communities, people will soon accept both the child and her aid. But in some societies, people have beliefs or deep fears about a person whose body is 'incomplete'. In other societies, amputation of a hand has traditionally been the punishment, and sign, of a thief. Or a girl who is seen as defective

---

APPEARANCE CAN BE IMPORTANT

For example, one of the most useful solutions to amputations of both hands is an operation which uses the two bones of the lower arm to create 'pinchers'. The operation is fairly simple for an orthopedic surgeon, and once completed no aids are needed for grasping and handling a wide variety of things. The biggest advantage is that **the person can feel what he handles**. But few people choose this alternative because, they say, it looks so strange.

---

may not be likely to find a husband. So, it may be socially very important for her to have an aid that looks real or is less noticeable, even if it does not function. (If the family can afford them, sometimes the best solution is 2 artificial limbs—hooks for home use or work, and a 'hand' for 'dressing up' and going out.)

It is, of course, unfortunate that a child feels ashamed or thinks she has to hide her disability. We must work for greater understanding. But people do not change their attitudes quickly. Often the child and her parents have good reasons for their fears, and we must learn to accept them. However, we must also help the child, her family, and the community to become more accepting of the child's disability and to provide as many opportunities for the child as possible.

We need to help the child find courage. A child with a new disability will often be afraid to go out into the community, or back to school. And other persons or children may at first take notice and 'feel sorry' for her—or even tease her. But if she can be helped through this first difficult period, usually other people and children will soon get used to her 'difference' and accept both it and her. As more disabled persons find the courage to go out into the community, it will be easier for those who follow, because people will become more open and accepting.

In the story of Sri, the rehabilitation specialist tried to solve her problem by giving her an artificial limb. Her family spent a lot of money on it. But the new 'hand' did not solve her problem. She never really accepted or used it. Her problem, which was partly emotional, was finally solved by the whole family helping her to join them again in daily activities, and to gain new confidence in herself.

This is very important. **Too often we try to find technical answers to problems that are mostly personal, social, or emotional.** So we turn to special aids and equipment. Sometimes these are needed. But sometimes they are unnecessary, too costly, or make life more difficult for the child (even though they may be of some help physically). So . . .

> Before deciding if a child needs special aids, braces, surgery, or equipment, and what kind, carefully consider the needs of the whole child within her family and community.

A 'Shop for Making Aids' Run by Disabled Villagers

CHAPTER **57**

In PART 2 of this book we talked about the value of village-based rehabilitation centers run by local disabled village workers.

One important feature of such a center is a simple but adequately equipped shop for making basic *orthopedic* equipment and *rehabilitation* aids at low cost. The shop also gives disabled persons a chance to learn useful skills, to earn some money, and to be good examples for other disabled children and their families.

There is no formula for how big the shop should be or what it should include. **Often it is best to start small but to leave room for growth.**

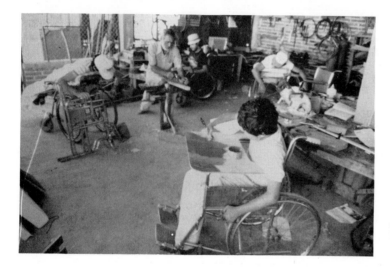

Disabled villagers at work in shop— PROJIMO, Mexico.

A 'rehab shop' might include areas and equipment for any or all of the following activities:

- **plaster casting** for correcting contractures and club feet

- **brace (caliper) making** using metal, plastic, or both

- **woodworking**—for making crutches, walkers, lying and standing frames, special seating, wooden wheelchairs

- **welding and metalwork** for making and repairing wheelchairs and other metal aids

- **leatherwork** for making brace straps, *adaptations* for shoes and sandals, and knee pieces

- **sewing** (with machine if possible) for wheelchair seats, straps, special clothes, and other articles

- **artificial limb making**—for making simple bamboo or leather limbs and perhaps more complex ones of wood, aluminum, or resin

- **game and toy making** (or this can be done in a separate 'children's workshop'. See Chapter 49).

Income-producing activities as a part of the shop function

The skills and tools for welding, woodworking, sewing, and leatherworking can also be used to make things other than those needed for rehabilitation. The village shop and its workers can make things that can be sold to help pay for program costs.

For example, disabled workers in the shop of PROJIMO in Mexico make metal framed chairs with woven plastic seats, sandals with auto tire soles, and silk-screened goods such as bags, T-shirts, and aprons. The shop also provides welding or repair services for plows, bicycles, machinery, shoes, and many other things. Selling these things and asking small charges for repair services brings in some money to the program, helping it toward self-sufficiency. It also provides training and work experience for disabled workers who may later choose to work independently.

However, caution **must be taken not to try to do too many things in one workshop**— especially if space is limited. It can easily become too disorganized.

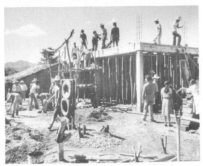
Villagers and visiting students building the PROJIMO workshop.

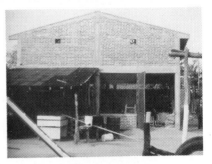
The completed workshop—at the edge of the playground.

The building

You may have to start with whatever space or building you can find. If you have enough funding or community cooperation (or both) you may be able to build a shop. However, **it is often best to start in some old rented or borrowed building, and not build your own shop until you have experience and a better idea of just what you need.**

Three things are important:

1. Try to put the shop close enough to the rest of the rehabilitation center for convenience, yet **far enough** away so that shop **noise** does not disturb discussions and therapy with children and their families.

2. In hot climates especially, make sure the shop is **well ventilated** (allows air movement). A roof with one or more walls that are open, except for bars or fencing, works well.

3. Be sure there is plenty of **storage space.** This is especially important if old braces, wheelchairs, bicycles, and other used equipment are collected for used parts, to save money.

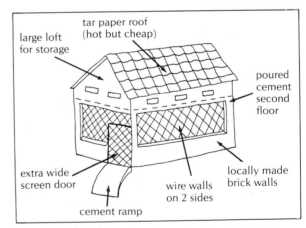

The PROJIMO workshop first opened on the back porch of an old house. A year later a new shop was designed and built with community participation, and some outside funding. It is 8 x 12 meters. Two walls are screened, on the sides the rain is least likely to blow in. A large loft provides storage space and helps to keep the work area below cooler. The new shop is already too small!

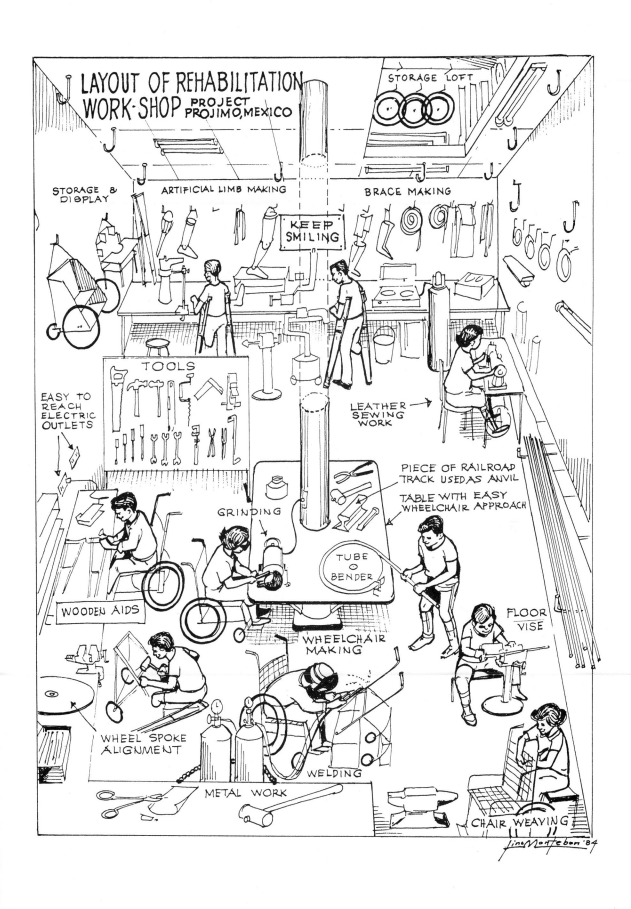

LAYOUT OF REHABILITATION WORK-SHOP PROJECT PROJIMO, MEXICO

STORAGE LOFT

STORAGE & DISPLAY

ARTIFICIAL LIMB MAKING

BRACE MAKING

KEEP SMILING

TOOLS

EASY TO REACH ELECTRIC OUTLETS

LEATHER SEWING WORK

PIECE OF RAILROAD TRACK USED AS ANVIL

TABLE WITH EASY WHEELCHAIR APPROACH

GRINDING

TUBE O BENDER

FLOOR VISE

WOODEN AIDS

WHEELCHAIR MAKING

WHEEL SPOKE ALIGNMENT

WELDING

METAL WORK

CHAIR WEAVING

Arrangement of work space

Each program needs to plan its own use of space. However, a few things are important if persons in wheelchairs will be workers:

- Enough **space** should be allowed everywhere for 2 wheelchairs to pass each other.

- At least some of the **workbenches** should be low enough to work at from a wheelchair or stool. Build them so that wheelchairs can get close to or under them with as few obstacles as possible.

- **Tools and supplies** should be stored **within easy reach of** workers in wheelchairs. Also, switches and power outlets.

The drawing on p. 535 shows how the workshop of PROJIMO is arranged. We include it as an example, not as a model.

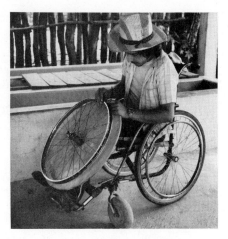

Photo: Richard Parker, PROJIMO

Tools and Equipment

What is needed will depend on what activities the shop includes, how simple or complex is the technology used for each activity, and whether or not electric power and tools are available. **Nearly all aids can be made of local materials with hand tools,** and without electricity. Even wheelchairs, if made of wood, can be built with few tools or equipment. The small amount of welding required for axles could perhaps be done by the nearest welding or auto repair shop. However, **having a few time- and effort-saving tools can make work easier, faster, and more enjoyable:** a sewing machine, a grinding wheel (whether hand crank or electric), and a gas or electric stove (to heat plastic for braces). Welding equipment or a blacksmith's forge and bellows makes possible the production of many things.

Basic tools and equipment for the shop will be discussed in more detail in this section of the book, PART 3, the chapters of which describe making different kinds of aids.

> One very expensive but important piece of equipment is an **electric cast cutter**. It is an extremely useful tool for removing plaster casts and for cutting molded plastic braces from plaster forms. It is also a relatively safe tool, because the blade vibrates but does not turn, so it cuts hard things like plaster more easily than soft things like skin and flesh.

Training for shop skills

Possible ways for learning different shop skills were discussed in Chapter 54. Here we will only repeat that **one of the best ways to learn shop skills is through 'apprenticeship'**, or learning-by-doing under the guidance of someone with more experience. Perhaps local craftspersons, such as carpenters, welders, and shoemakers would be willing to help teach members of the team. If the team has one or two persons with basic crafts experience, they can teach the others. For brace and limb making, it may help if one of the rehabilitation team has a chance to visit and learn in an orthotics and *prosthetics* shop. Or perhaps a skilled brace or limb maker can come for a few weeks to help set up shop, obtain basic materials, and teach the local team.

With an active, learning-by-doing approach, together with hard work to meet daily needs, team members can quickly become relatively skillful. On the other hand, if the team is made up, at least in part, of young disabled persons who have never worked before or cooperated as members of a team, both learning and work may at first progress more slowly.

Management and job assignment

How work is organized in the shop, and who organizes it, are decisions that need to be carefully discussed and decided by the group. Some programs have someone acting as 'boss' or 'foreman' who assigns each person a job. This may be more efficient. But programs that are 'people centered' prefer a more cooperative approach, where the whole group is involved in making key decisions. With such an approach, a coordinator may be chosen (or different coordinators can be chosen for different responsibilities). The coordinator does not give orders, but rather takes orders from the group. This approach is usually less efficient and more confusing. However, it is more enjoyable. Workers tend to take more interest, responsibility, initiative (and time off) than they do under a boss.

Also, the team needs to decide about how work is divided, and who does what jobs. Some workshops employing disabled persons use an 'assembly line' approach. Each person does a simple, repetitive job, such as cutting out one piece of tubing time after time or putting spokes into wheels. This approach requires relatively little training for each worker. Mentally retarded workers who learn by repeating something over and over again often do well working this way.

However, **most people work better when they are able to make something from beginning to end.** Then they can share the satisfaction of a child and her family when a wheelchair or brace or toy they made looks nice and works well. In PROJIMO, whenever possible, workers (individually or in pairs) are responsible for the complete production of an aid. They start by helping to evaluate the child's needs and end by seeing how well the finished aid meets those needs. This way, each worker can see the personal value of each aid that he or she makes. This approach may be less efficient, but it is more satisfying. Thus the team watches the results rather than the clock, and works first for the people, not the money. This personalized approach is very important to a program designed to serve those in greatest need.

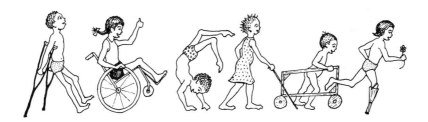

PART 3 of this book provides information on two main areas: (1) non-surgical orthopedic procedures (straightening contractures and club feet with casts), and (2) the production of low-cost rehabilitation aids. All of these things can be done in a village-based workshop such as the one just described. However, many of the aids can also easily be made at home by the family of the child.

To encourage family participation in making aids, and later repairing them, mothers, fathers, sisters, or brothers can be invited to the shop to help build the aid. Or disabled children can help make their own aids. Some of the best workers in the PROJIMO workshop today began as young people who helped make their own crutches or wheelchairs—and then began to help make aids for others.

The ideal is that everyone does what they can to help and learn from each other: one big, human family working together and enjoying each other.

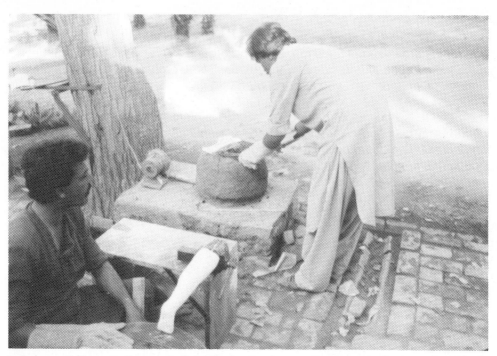

In Peshawar, Pakistan, the Community Rehabilitation Development Program makes leg braces from plastic bus windows. Here a worker heats the plastic over an outdoor mud stove.

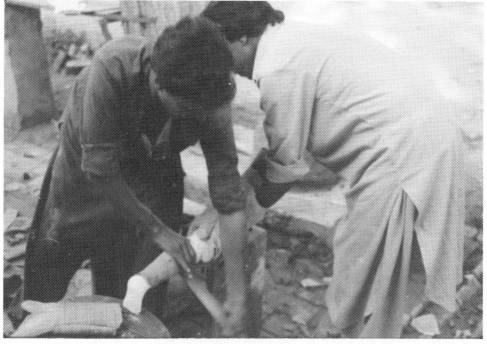

When the plastic is hot and soft, workers drape it over the plaster leg mold. Then they wrap it tightly with strips of rubber inner tube until it hardens. (See p. 552.)

Braces (Calipers)

Braces are aids that help hold legs or other parts of the body in useful positions. They usually serve one or both of **2 purposes:**

1. To provide support or firmness to a weak joint (or joints). For example, this child had polio:

His leg is too weak to support his weight without help.

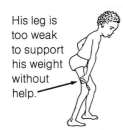

This brace keeps his knee from bending forward

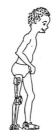

2. To help prevent or correct deformity or *contracture*. For example, this child had a club foot:

He was born with a club foot.

His club foot was corrected with a cast.

After correction, his foot is kept in a good position with a brace.

> *CAUTION:* The need for braces should be carefully evaluated. Braces should be used only if they will help the child move better and become more independent. Too much bracing may actually weaken *muscles* and cause greater *disability*. As a general rule, **try to use as little and as light bracing as possible to help the child *function* better.** (See Chapter 56.)

Different braces for different needs

The main lower-limb brace types are:

Foot brace

usually made of molded plastic

for deformities in the foot (not ankle) such as severe flat foot

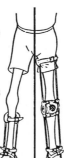

Below-knee braces (ankle brace)

for weakness or deformities in the lower leg, ankle, and foot

Above-knee brace (long-leg brace)

for weakness in the upper leg and knee— possibly also ankle and foot

Above-knee brace with a hip-band

for severe weakness in hips and legs

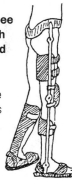

Less commonly used types (described on p. 547 and p. 558) include:

Leg-separating braces

for *dislocated* hips or damaged head of thigh bone (See p. 158.)

Foot-*positioning* night brace

for holding the feet, legs, and hips at a set angle when they tend to turn in

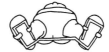

Body brace or corset

for curve of the spine

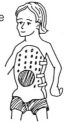

Body brace with leg braces

for body and back weakness together with hip and leg weakness

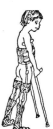

Different materials and ways to make braces

As we discussed in Chapter 56, **an ideal brace should:**

- serve its purpose well (help the child walk or function better)
- be comfortable
- be lightweight yet strong
- be as attractive as possible
- be easy to put on and take off
- do no harm

- be low cost
- be easy and quick to make with local tools and limited skills
- use local or easily available materials
- be easy to repair and adjust as the child grows or develops
- be long lasting

Unfortunately, no brace will meet all these requirements. As much as possible, **try to put the child's needs first.**

In this chapter we give ideas for making different braces using various materials. When deciding how to make a brace, carefully evaluate both the child's needs and the available resources (see Chapter 56).

Sometimes it is wise to start with a simple low-cost temporary brace or splint to see how well it works and what the problems are.

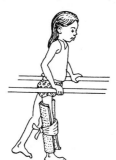

Keep old and outgrown braces for testing on new children before final braces are made.

But take care not to discourage the child by making him use braces that do not fit him well.

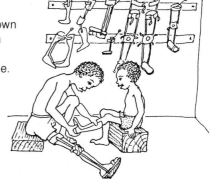

Examples of very simple, low-cost braces and splints:

A temporary leg splint of cardboard, folded paper, or the thick curved stem of a dried banana leaf, or palm leaf.

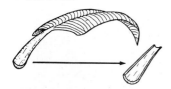

Aluminum tube finger splint

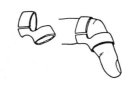

Mango seed finger splint

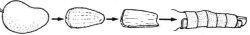

Remove the woody coat of a mango seed, and wrap the coat firmly onto the finger. It will dry into a firm splint. To change its shape, first soak it in water.

Bamboo ankle splint
A piece of seasoned bamboo can be heated and bent.

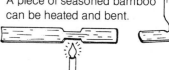

Plastic cup ankle braces for night or temporary use on a small child.

For a small baby:

plastic cup   Cut like this.   padding

rivets

straps of leather, canvas, or *Velcro,* if possible

piece of wood

Rivet or nail wood to cup.

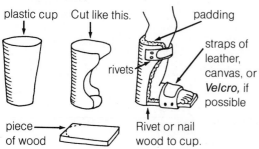

For a child:

3 cups cut and riveted together

Make a flat inner sole out of cloth or wood.

Or cut the foot piece from a flat plastic bottle.

Add straps to fasten the brace around leg.

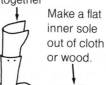

Metal or plastic braces

Modern, high-quality braces are usually made out of metal or molded plastic.

The best metal is a mix or 'alloy' of aluminum and steel which is both light and strong. However, this is very costly and often hard to get. Pure aluminum is very light, but breaks easily, especially when you try to bend it. Steel is cheaper and easier to bend and weld, but is much heavier.

The best plastic for braces is probably polypropylene, which is strong, light, and fairly easy to shape when hot.

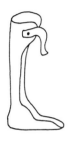

Pre-formed metal parts for making these braces are sold at *orthopedic* supply stores. Unfortunately, they are usually much too expensive for a community program. However, sometimes you can get large orthopedic centers to donate old braces, from which locking knee joints and other pieces can be used to build high-quality metal or plastic braces. Also, many broken or outgrown braces are lying in the corners of thousands of homes. A campaign to get families to donate these can greatly reduce the costs of making high-quality braces.

plastic
below-knee
brace

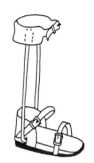

metal below-knee
brace with wood
clog

Low-cost metal or plastic braces can be made in a village shop. They can be made simply, with or without joints. Since children grow quickly, they often need a larger brace every 3 to 6 months. Therefore, keeping cost low and work simple is essential. (See Chapter 56, p. 527.)

Metal and plastic braces each have advantages and disadvantages. We discuss these on p. 542 and 550.

In Mexico, **we have found that for most children who need below-knee braces, plastic works best. And the children (and parents) like it more.**

However, a child with a lot of muscle tightness (due to *spasticity* or contractures) which pulls his foot a lot to one side, like this,

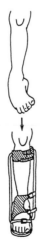

may need a metal brace with an ankle strap. After the brace is on, the strap is tightened to pull the foot into a better position.

Above-knee braces can be made using a combination of plastic and metal.

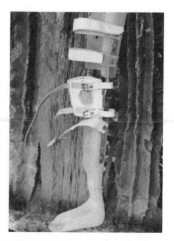

> **Whenever possible, equip your village shop to make both plastic and metal braces. That way, you can make what seems most appropriate for each child.**

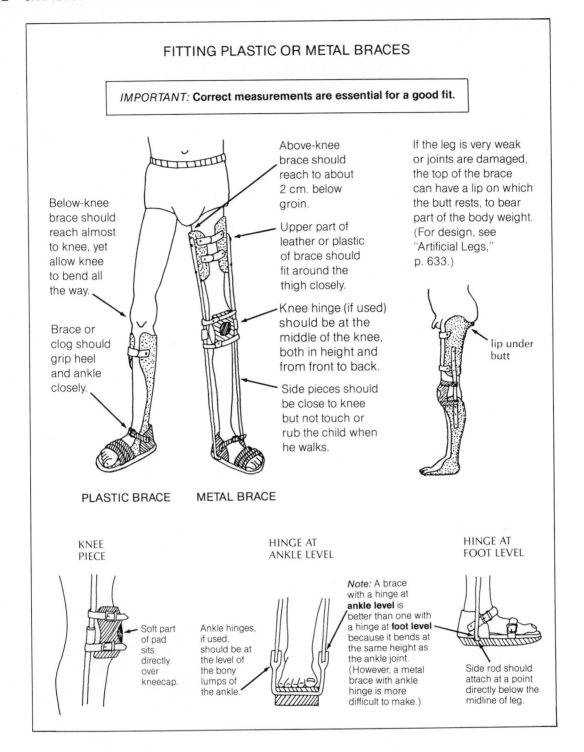

FITTING PLASTIC OR METAL BRACES

IMPORTANT: **Correct measurements are essential for a good fit.**

Below-knee brace should reach almost to knee, yet allow knee to bend all the way.

Brace or clog should grip heel and ankle closely.

Above-knee brace should reach to about 2 cm. below groin.

Upper part of leather or plastic of brace should fit around the thigh closely.

Knee hinge (if used) should be at the middle of the knee, both in height and from front to back.

Side pieces should be close to knee but not touch or rub the child when he walks.

If the leg is very weak or joints are damaged, the top of the brace can have a lip on which the butt rests, to bear part of the body weight. (For design, see "Artificial Legs," p. 633.)

lip under butt

PLASTIC BRACE   METAL BRACE

KNEE PIECE

Soft part of pad sits directly over kneecap.

Ankle hinges, if used, should be at the level of the bony lumps of the ankle.

HINGE AT ANKLE LEVEL

Note: A brace with a hinge at **ankle level** is better than one with a hinge at **foot level** because it bends at the same height as the ankle joint. (However, a metal brace with ankle hinge is more difficult to make.)

HINGE AT FOOT LEVEL

Side rod should attach at a point directly below the midline of leg.

METAL BRACES

The **advantages** of simple metal braces are that they are quick, easy, and cheap to make. They often last longer, and, if used with sandals or clogs, in hot weather they are cooler than plastic. However, they also have **disadvantages:** because a shoe, sandal, or wood 'clog' must be built or attached to the brace, there is additional work and cost. Also, they are heavy, clumsy, and more noticeable. In hot or wet weather, leather or cloth, or even the metal starts to rot. Shoes or boots which the child cannot change, even when they get wet, begin to stink.

METAL ROD BRACES* using 're-bar' (reinforcing rod for use in cement building construction)

For a brace shorter than 50 cm. (20 inches) you can use rod that is 5 mm. thick. For a longer brace, the rod should be thicker — up to 8 mm.

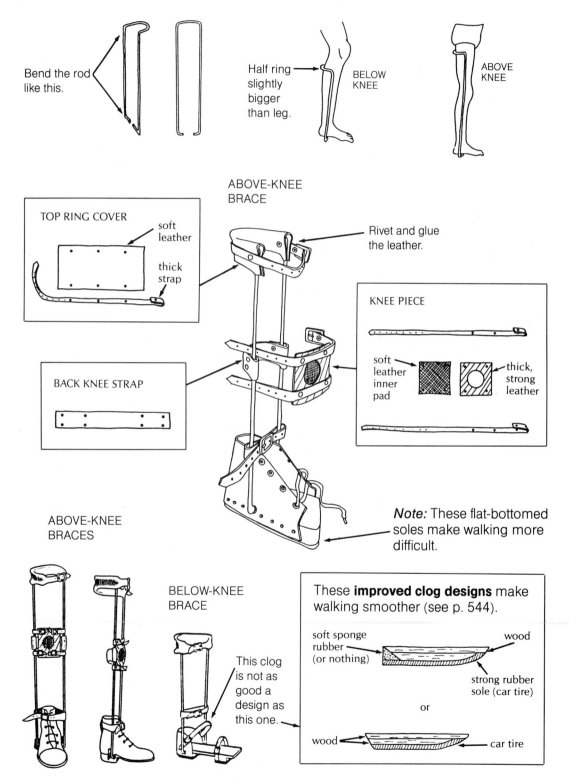

Bend the rod like this.

Half ring slightly bigger than leg.

BELOW KNEE

ABOVE KNEE

ABOVE-KNEE BRACE

TOP RING COVER
soft leather
thick strap

Rivet and glue the leather.

KNEE PIECE
soft leather inner pad
thick, strong leather

BACK KNEE STRAP

ABOVE-KNEE BRACES

Note: These flat-bottomed soles make walking more difficult.

BELOW-KNEE BRACE

This clog is not as good a design as this one.

These **improved clog designs** make walking smoother (see p. 544).

soft sponge rubber (or nothing)
wood
strong rubber sole (car tire)

or

wood
car tire

*Much of the information on metal braces, on this and the following pages, is taken or adapted from *Poliomyelitis* by Huckstep, and *Simple Orthopaedic Aids* by Chris Dartnell.

SHOES AND CLOGS FOR METAL BRACES

High-top leather shoes often work best, especially in communities where children usually wear shoes.

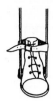

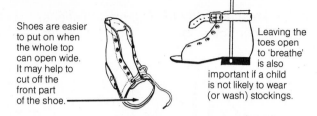

Shoes are easier to put on when the whole top can open wide. It may help to cut off the front part of the shoe.

Leaving the toes open to 'breathe' is also important if a child is not likely to wear (or wash) stockings.

For adding thicker soles and making other changes, it helps to buy shoes **with soles that are sewed on.** (Today, many shoes have plastic or rubber soles that are glued on or molded with the shoe. These are much harder to work with.)

Unfortunately, leather shoes are costly. Also, they may not last long in rain and mud. So, you may want to make simple, low-cost wooden-soled shoes, or clogs. This design is from *Simple Orthopaedic Aids.*

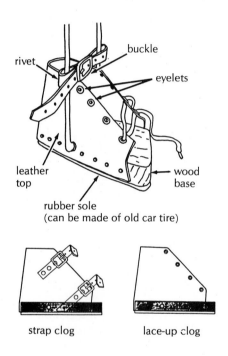

rivet
buckle
eyelets
leather top
wood base
rubber sole (can be made of old car tire)

strap clog   lace-up clog

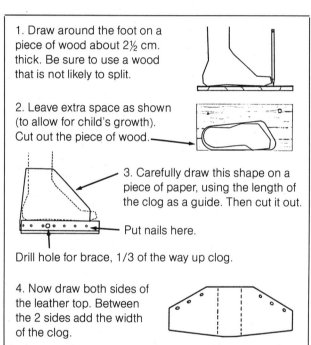

1. Draw around the foot on a piece of wood about 2½ cm. thick. Be sure to use a wood that is not likely to split.

2. Leave extra space as shown (to allow for child's growth). Cut out the piece of wood.

3. Carefully draw this shape on a piece of paper, using the length of the clog as a guide. Then cut it out.

Put nails here.

Drill hole for brace, 1/3 of the way up clog.

4. Now draw both sides of the leather top. Between the 2 sides add the width of the clog.

In communities where most children go barefoot, a disabled child may prefer more open clogs. This design is adapted from Huckstep's *Poliomyelitis*, and the 'Jaipur Sandal'.

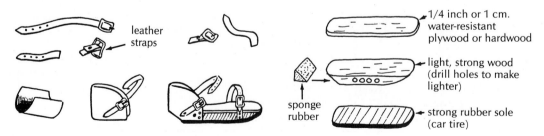

leather straps

1/4 inch or 1 cm. water-resistant plywood or hardwood

light, strong wood (drill holes to make lighter)

sponge rubber

strong rubber sole (car tire)

Note: These open clogs are hard to fit on deformed feet or feet with tiptoe contractures. In such cases, high-top clogs or boots work better. Or use plastic braces molded to fit the foot.

HOW TO CONTROL UP AND DOWN MOVEMENT OF FOOT

CONTROLLING FOOTDROP AND TIPTOE DEFORMITIES

A child with 'footdrop' or a floppy foot that hangs down so that she has to lift her leg high with each step,

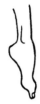

needs a brace that holds the foot up. Use a plastic brace,

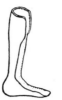

or a metal brace with a backstop that lets the foot bend up, but not down.

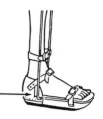

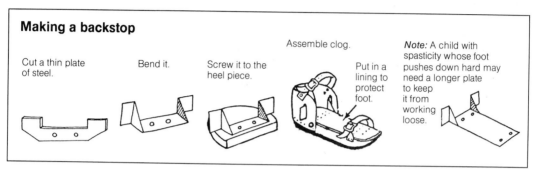

Making a backstop

Cut a thin plate of steel.

Bend it.

Screw it to the heel piece.

Assemble clog.

Put in a lining to protect foot.

Note: A child with spasticity whose foot pushes down hard may need a longer plate to keep it from working loose.

Toe-raising spring

Another way to help prevent footdrop is with a toe-raising spring.

This is a more complicated design.

wire spring

This is a simpler design.

piece of car tire inner tube

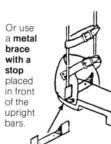

CONTROLLING FOOT-RISE AND UNWANTED KNEE-BEND

A child who walks with knees bent and feet bent up,

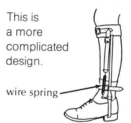

may (or may not) be helped by a brace that prevents the foot from bending up as much. If possible, use a stiff **plastic brace.**

Or use a **metal brace with a stop** placed in front of the upright bars.

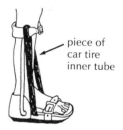

A strong stop with a long plate will be less likely to work loose or damage the clog.

A child whose weak leg bends at the knee when he tries to put weight on it,

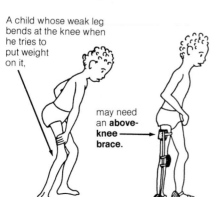

may need an **above-knee brace.**

But sometimes a **below-knee brace** that stops the foot from bending up will help push the knee back enough so that the child can support his weight on it. (See p. 557.)

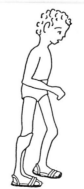

The brace can be of stiff plastic, or metal with stops to prevent foot-rise.

If a brace with an ankle joint is used to prevent the ankle from bending up, the base piece will need a long, strong, forward plate.

The joint can be adjusted to allow only the desired range of motion.

KNEE HINGES

Braces with locking knee hinges permit the child to bend her knees for sitting or squatting.

Non-bending knees are satisfactory for most children. The child can sit with her leg straight.

NON-HINGED BRACE

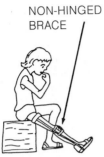

However, in some communities, a child may 'fit in' better if he can squat.

However, hinged braces have disadvantages: they are more costly and take longer to make. A child outgrows them quickly—unless they are adjustable. So use your judgment.

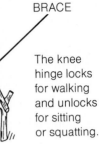

HINGED BRACE

The knee hinge locks for walking and unlocks for sitting or squatting.

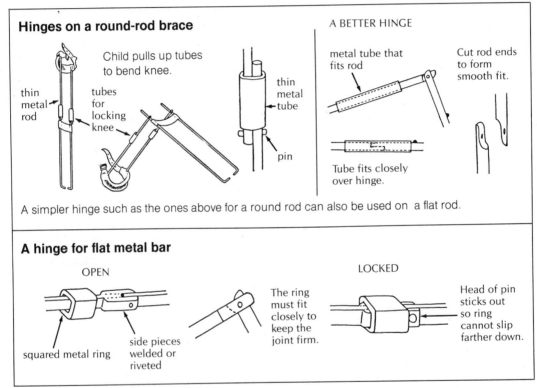

Hinges on a round-rod brace

A BETTER HINGE

Child pulls up tubes to bend knee.

thin metal rod

tubes for locking knee

thin metal tube

pin

metal tube that fits rod

Cut rod ends to form smooth fit.

Tube fits closely over hinge.

A simpler hinge such as the ones above for a round rod can also be used on a flat rod.

A hinge for flat metal bar

OPEN

LOCKED

squared metal ring

side pieces welded or riveted

The ring must fit closely to keep the joint firm.

Head of pin sticks out so ring cannot slip farther down.

BRACES THAT FOLLOW THE SHAPE OF THE LEG

Flat metal bar can be bent to fit the shape of the leg more closely. This is not always necessary but if done well the brace will fit better—especially when the bar is used with molded plastic.

Instructions for bending and fitting the rod are on p. 557.

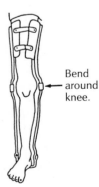

Bend around knee.

ADJUSTABLE BRACES

As the child grows, a brace made like this can be lengthened. Teach family members how to do this.

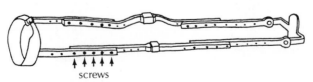

screws

HIP BANDS

Braces with a hip band may be needed for the child:

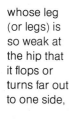

whose leg (or legs) is so weak at the hip that it flops or turns far out to one side,

WITHOUT HIP BAND

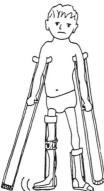

or whose legs tend to twist too much inward (or outward).

WITHOUT HIP BAND

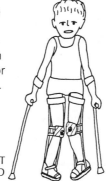

Put hinges at height of hip bone.

WITH HIP BAND

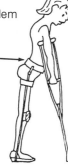

A common problem with hip bands is that the low back bends forward and the butt sticks out. This can cause back problems, and hip contractures.

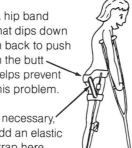

A hip band that dips down in back to push in the butt helps prevent this problem.

If necessary, add an elastic strap here.

The back of the hip band can be made of thin metal lined with leather, or of strong plastic.

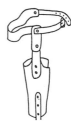

On plastic braces the side bars and hinges can also be made of thick, strong plastic. This adds some flexibility, which will be better for some children but not provide enough support for others.

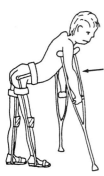

A child who tends to flop forward at the hips, may need a hip band with a locking hinge. You can use the design on p. 546.

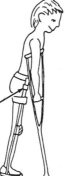

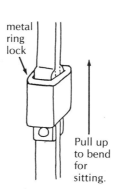

metal ring lock

Pull up to bend for sitting.

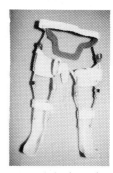

Braces with plastic hip band and locking plastic hip hinges. (PROJIMO)

Hip band without lock

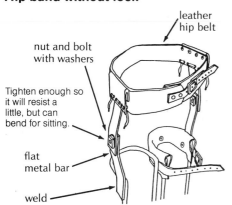

leather hip belt

nut and bolt with washers

Tighten enough so it will resist a little, but can bend for sitting.

flat metal bar

weld

Hip band with lock

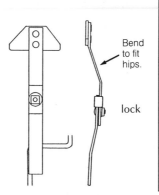

Bend to fit hips.

lock

For a young child whose feet turn in a lot, **a night brace to hold the feet (and hips) turned outward** may help. It can be made from a thin metal bar or from wood.

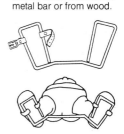

KNEE PIECES (Use the design on p. 543.)

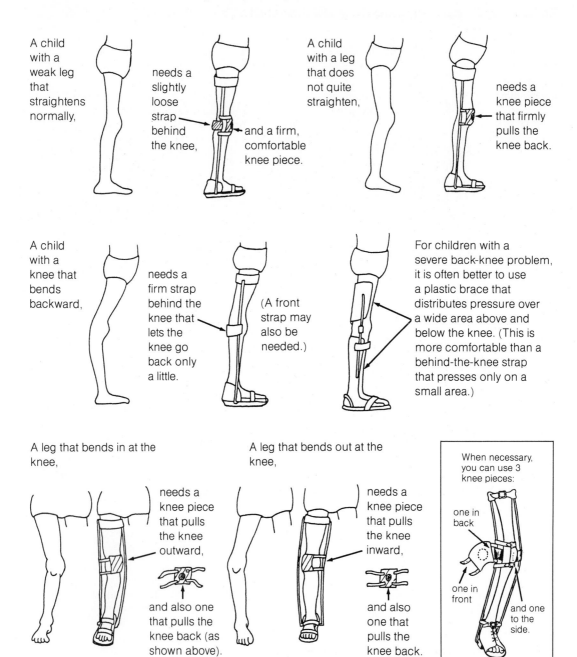

A child with a weak leg that straightens normally, needs a slightly loose strap behind the knee, and a firm, comfortable knee piece.

A child with a leg that does not quite straighten, needs a knee piece that firmly pulls the knee back.

A child with a knee that bends backward, needs a firm strap behind the knee that lets the knee go back only a little. (A front strap may also be needed.)

For children with a severe back-knee problem, it is often better to use a plastic brace that distributes pressure over a wide area above and below the knee. (This is more comfortable than a behind-the-knee strap that presses only on a small area.)

A leg that bends in at the knee, needs a knee piece that pulls the knee outward, and also one that pulls the knee back (as shown above).

A leg that bends out at the knee, needs a knee piece that pulls the knee inward, and also one that pulls the knee back.

When necessary, you can use 3 knee pieces:
one in back
one in front
and one to the side.

ANKLE STRAPS

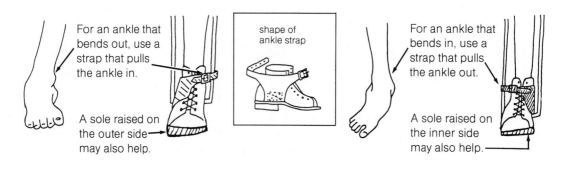

For an ankle that bends out, use a strap that pulls the ankle in.

A sole raised on the outer side may also help.

shape of ankle strap

For an ankle that bends in, use a strap that pulls the ankle out.

A sole raised on the inner side may also help.

RAISED SOLES OR 'LIFTS' for one leg that is shorter

(For instructions on measuring leg length difference and for homemade measuring instruments, see p. 34.)

For a child who has one leg shorter than the other:

Measure the difference in leg length.

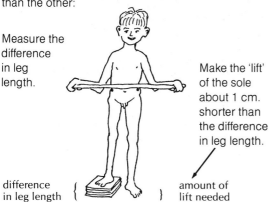

Make the 'lift' of the sole about 1 cm. shorter than the difference in leg length.

difference in leg length { } amount of lift needed

> *Note:* Almost all children have one leg that is a little shorter than the other, and this does not usually affect how they walk. Raised soles ('lifts') are usually not needed if the difference in leg length is less than 2 cm.
>
> However, a child who drags a foot because his hips tilt down on that side may be helped by a small lift on the other side—even if that leg is the same length or longer. (See p. 163.)

IMPORTANT: Before putting a permanent lift on a shoe or sandal, test it by tying or taping on a **temporary lift.** Watch the child walk and ask how he likes it. You may want to try several heights before deciding on the one that works best.

Tie on a temporary lift with string, tape, or a loop of inner tube.

Material used for lifts should be as lightweight as possible. You can use cork or a light, porous rubber. If the material is heavy but strong, to make it lighter you can drill holes through it. Put a thin, strong sole on the bottom.

For a lift with a stiff-ankle brace, the child can often walk more smoothly with a 'rocker-bottom' sole.

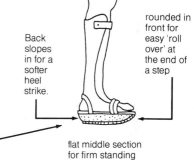

Back slopes in for a softer heel strike.

rounded in front for easy 'roll over' at the end of a step

flat middle section for firm standing

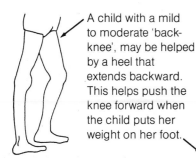

A child with a mild to moderate 'back-knee', may be helped by a heel that extends backward. This helps push the knee forward when the child puts her weight on her foot.

For a more severe back-knee, the child may need a long-leg brace (See p. 67 and 548.)

A high lift, when needed, can be built into a bar brace.

bolt
washer
nut

bolt

height of lift

Design from *Simple Orthopaedic Aids,* by Dartnell.

> Ask a local shoe or sandal maker to teach you how to fasten on the soles and lifts.

PLASTIC BRACES

Below the knee

For most children who need a below-knee brace, plastic braces molded to fit the leg and foot of the individual child have many **advantages:**

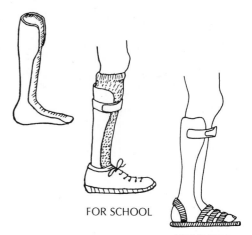

FOR SCHOOL

- They are lightweight and often more comfortable than metal braces.
- They fit the child comfortably and exactly (if made well).
- They can be worn with ordinary shoes or sandals, which can be easily changed when they get worn out or wet. Shoes can be changed for school and for work.
- They are water resistant and easy to clean.
- They are less noticeable than metal braces. If desired, socks can be worn over them to hide them.
- Children usually prefer them and are more likely to keep wearing them.

FOR WORK

Although a little more equipment and skill are needed to make plastic braces, once a village worker has learned the basic technique, they can be made as quickly and easily as a simple metal brace with a clog.

A **disadvantage** to plastic braces is that usually after a year or two the plastic 'gets tired' and breaks. However, growing children need larger braces fairly often. It is wise to **keep the plaster mold of each child's brace so that a new brace can be easily made if needed.**

> **A suggestion to save time and money:**
>
>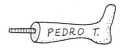
>
> Keep the mold of the child's foot — or have the family keep it.

The biggest expense in making plastic braces is the plaster bandage used for casting a mold of the leg. The cost can be reduced a lot by making your own plaster bandage material (see p. 569).

Plastic braces can feel uncomfortable in hot weather and can lead to skin irritation and fungus *infections* if care is not taken. They can be made cooler by drilling 'breathing holes' in them. Or cut out a hole in the back.

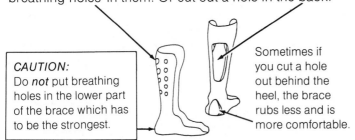

> *CAUTION:*
> Do *not* put breathing holes in the lower part of the brace which has to be the strongest.

Sometimes if you cut a hole out behind the heel, the brace rubs less and is more comfortable.

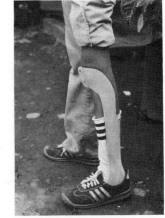

This design of plastic brace supports the knee from the front and pushes it back (see p. 545 and 557).

To prevent skin irritation, it is important to bathe daily. It also helps to wear cotton (not nylon) stockings under the brace and to use clean stockings every day.

How to make plastic braces

Here we describe 2 methods for making molded plastic braces:

The first method uses **old plastic buckets** or containers, and needs less equipment. Unfortunately, these braces tend to break easily when used for walking. However, they make excellent, low-cost **night braces** (to wear while sleeping).

The second method uses sheets of polypropylene plastic. Additional equipment (such as a vacuum sweeper) is needed, and it is a little more expensive. However, the result is a high-quality brace that can last for months or sometimes years.

Method 1: Plastic bucket braces

Equipment and materials needed:

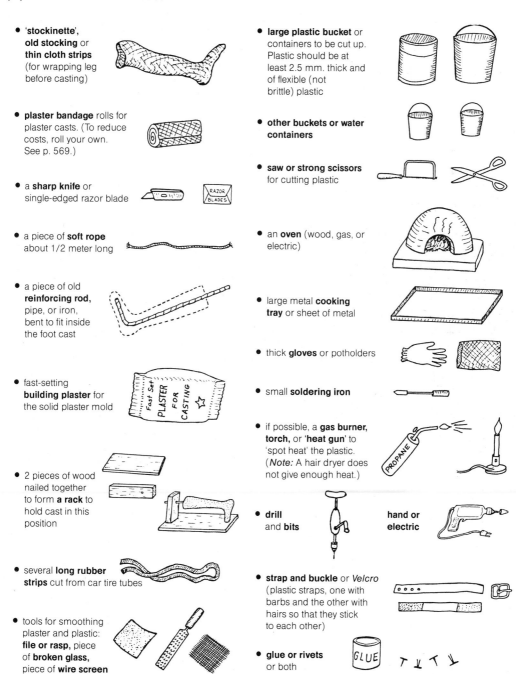

- 'stockinette', **old stocking** or **thin cloth strips** (for wrapping leg before casting)

- **plaster bandage** rolls for plaster casts. (To reduce costs, roll your own. See p. 569.)

- a **sharp knife** or single-edged razor blade

- a piece of **soft rope** about 1/2 meter long

- a piece of old **reinforcing rod,** pipe, or iron, bent to fit inside the foot cast

- fast-setting **building plaster** for the solid plaster mold

- 2 pieces of wood nailed together to form **a rack** to hold cast in this position

- several **long rubber strips** cut from car tire tubes

- tools for smoothing plaster and plastic: **file or rasp,** piece of **broken glass,** piece of **wire screen**

- **large plastic bucket** or containers to be cut up. Plastic should be at least 2.5 mm. thick and of flexible (not brittle) plastic

- **other buckets or water containers**

- **saw or strong scissors** for cutting plastic

- an **oven** (wood, gas, or electric)

- large metal **cooking tray** or sheet of metal

- thick **gloves** or potholders

- small **soldering iron**

- if possible, a **gas burner, torch,** or 'heat gun' to 'spot heat' the plastic. (*Note:* A hair dryer does not give enough heat.)

- **drill** and **bits**   hand or electric

- **strap and buckle** or *Velcro* (plastic straps, one with barbs and the other with hairs so that they stick to each other)

- **glue or rivets** or both

Making the plastic-bucket brace consists of 3 main steps:

A. Making a hollow plaster cast of the child's leg

B. Making a solid plaster mold of the leg

C. Heat-molding the plastic-bucket brace

A. Making the hollow cast

1. Tie a knot in the end of a soft rope.

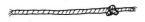

2. Put the rope on top of the leg with the knot between the toes.

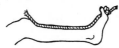

3. Put the stocking tightly on the foot with the rope inside (or wrap it with a thin cloth). Avoid wrinkles.

Make sure the rope stays very **straight.**

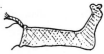

4. Wet a plaster bandage and squeeze out the extra water.

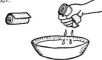

5. Wrap on a thin cast (about 3 layers) while someone else holds the foot in a good position. Be sure the heel is covered with several layers.

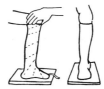

6. While the plaster is still wet, smooth it gently with moist hands, and press the cast gently into all the hollows of the foot.

7. Before the plaster becomes firm, place the foot in exactly the position that you want the brace to hold it in. Sometimes it works well to hold the foot in your hands. But often it works best to have the child step firmly on the floor, or on a padded board.

Be sure to position the leg **straight up,** from side view and front view.

8. Draw some lines over the front of the cast.

9. When the cast is almost firm but still damp (usually in 5 to 10 minutes), carefully cut through the plaster over the rope. Take care not to cut the child.

10. Then gently remove the cast without changing its shape.

11. Quickly (before it is fully hard) close the cast, line up the lines you drew, and tie it shut with cloth or string.

12. Tie a cloth tightly over the opening of the toes.

B. Making the solid plaster mold

1. Put a bent piece of rod into the hollow cast.

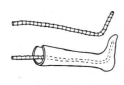

2. Hold the cast in a standing position— perhaps in a box of sand.

3. Mix the plaster: Put water in a container, enough to fill the cast.

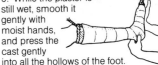

While stirring, sprinkle dry plaster into the water. Keep adding until the mix is just thick enough that wrinkles stay a moment on the surface.

4. Quickly pour the mix into the cast. Jiggle the rod and tap the cast to be sure the mix fills all spaces.

5. Hold the rod in the middle until the plaster is firm.

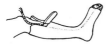

6. After plaster hardens fully (about one hour) remove the solid mold.

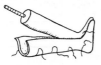

7. Being careful not to change the shape or size of the mold, use fresh plaster to fill in any holes or pits that are not caused by the shape of the foot. Add a little fresh plaster over bony places (so final brace will not rub).

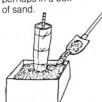

8. Smooth the surface (with a file, piece of wire screen, or piece of broken glass). Do *not* reduce any of the bumps caused by the bones.

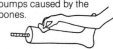

C. Heat-molding the plastic-bucket brace

1. Mark on the child's leg the shape of the brace.
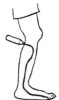

2. Take measurements as shown for the width and length of the brace.
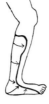

3. Draw an outline on paper, according to the measurements and cut out the pattern.
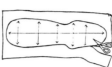

4. Mark the pattern on the plastic.

5. Cut out the pattern with a saw or strong scissors.

6. Make V-shaped cuts here to help bend the hot plastic around heel.
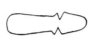

7. Heat the oven to at least 450° F (230° C). If you cannot measure or control heat, put a small piece of plastic into the oven and heat it until the plastic becomes soft and gooey.

8. Heat the plaster leg cast in the hot oven for 15 to 20 minutes.
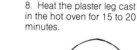
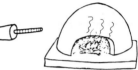

9. Put the hot mold on the rack.
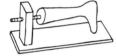

10. Lightly sprinkle dry plaster or talc on a metal sheet or tray.

11. Put the plastic form on tray and put the tray into the hot oven.
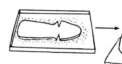

12. Leave it in oven only until plastic becomes somewhat flexible.*

13. Take hot plastic out of oven with gloves. Bend it over the hot mold.
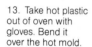
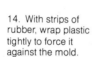

14. With strips of rubber, wrap plastic tightly to force it against the mold.
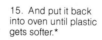
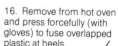

15. And put it back into oven until plastic gets softer.*
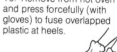

16. Remove from hot oven and press forcefully (with gloves) to fuse overlapped plastic at heels.

17. Also press in any hollows around bones and on bottom of foot. Keep pressing until plastic begins to cool and stiffen.
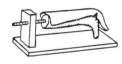
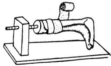

18. While brace is cooling, heat soldering iron.

Heat to moderate heat—*not* red hot.
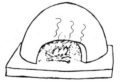

19. Unwrap cloth from brace while still warm and use soldering iron to smooth and weld heel joint.
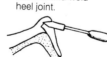

20. When cool, trim and smooth the edges of the brace.
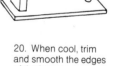
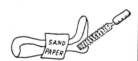

SAND PAPER

21. Glue or rivet a strap near the top of the brace.

For night splints, add 1 or 2 more straps at the ankle and foot.
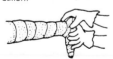
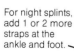
Pad well.

For easier fastening, use *Velcro* straps.
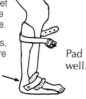

For day use, or use with sandals or shoes, only the upper strap is needed.

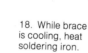

Note: Braces made from plastic buckets or containers tend to break fairly easily if a larger child uses them for walking. It is better to use polypropylene plastic (see next page).

*Take care not to overheat the plastic, because the plastic used for many buckets and containers tends to wrinkle like bacon when it gets too hot.

Method 2: Polypropylene braces

Polypropylene is a special plastic available in large sheets from orthopedic supply stores and some plastic factories. For most braces, sheets 30 cm. by 60 cm. (1 foot by 2 feet) are large enough. Thickness should be 3 mm. (1/8 inch) for thinner, more flexible braces and 4 mm. to 5 mm. (3/16 inch) for stronger, less flexible braces.

Polypropylene, where available, is usually the best plastic for braces. It is flexible but strong. It is easy to stretch and mold when hot. Cost is US $1.00 to $2.00 per brace. *Polyethylene* can also be used but is more likely to wrinkle like bacon if it gets too hot. You can experiment with whatever plastic you find. A program in Pakistan uses **plastic bus windows,** although this hard clear plastic (*Plexiglas*) is more difficult to stretch and shape when hot.

This method is the one used by professional brace makers. Here we simplify it as much as possible. Equipment and materials needed are mostly the same as in Method 1 (see p. 551). However, high-quality braces can be made more easily with a few extra pieces of equipment (they are not absolutely necessary). This **extra equipment** includes:

• special oven*

SIMPLE SHEET-METAL BOX OVEN
(riveted or soldered together)

window for looking at plastic when it is heating, with sliding or hinged door

handles

Box should be at least 70 cm. (28 in.) long, 40 cm. (16 in.) wide, and 10 cm. (4 in.) high.

sheet of metal (preferably aluminum, because it spreads heat best) at least 6 mm. (1/4 in. to 1/2 in.) thick

If you can get it, rivet a piece of *'Teflon'* cloth over the metal sheet. This will help keep the hot plastic from sticking to the metal. Or you can use a *Teflon* spray.

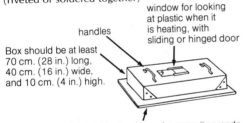

The 'oven' can be placed over any source of heat. Use the cooking fire, or you may want to build a simple fireplace to support it.

Burn wood or cow dung here.

COMPLEX GAS OR ELECTRIC OVENS
(designs from Huckstep's *Poliomyelitis.*

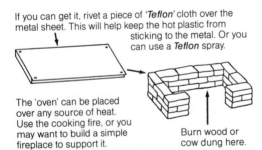

2 kitchen ovens welded together

heat resistant glass or plastic window in door

heating filaments mounted on top

thermostat— for controlling temperature

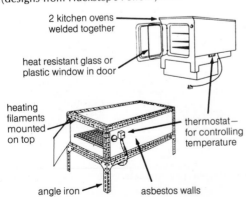

angle iron   asbestos walls

• vacuum sweeper

(if electricity is available) or other form of suction. (The suction pulls the hot plastic tightly against the cast until it cools. However, this is not absolutely necessary.)

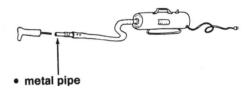

• metal pipe

Tape it to the end of the vacuum sweeper hose.

The pipe should be a little bigger than the rod used in the leg cast. By bending the rod slightly, it will fit very tightly into the pipe.

Figure out some way to clamp or bolt the pipe firmly to a strong bench or table.

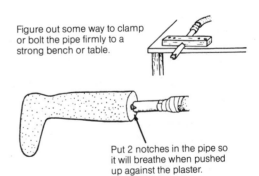

Put 2 notches in the pipe so it will breathe when pushed up against the plaster.

• electric cast-cutter

These are *very* expensive but a great help if you are making a lot of plastic braces.

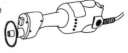

If you do not have a cast-cutter you may have to use a hammer and chisel to cut the plastic. You can heat the chisel so that it will melt the plastic.

---

*Some brace makers in Pakistan use no oven, but simply hold the plastic sheet over a 'chula' (earth pot) of hot coals. See photo on p. 538.

Making the polypropylene (or polyethylene) brace

Steps A and B are the same as described for Method 1 (see p. 552).

Step C. Heat-molding the plastic brace

1. Put the rod of the plaster mold into the vacuum pipe. Be sure it is very tight. (If not, take it out and bend the rod a bit more.)

2. Stretch stockinette or stocking tightly over the cast and tape it to the pipe.

3. Sprinkle dry plaster powder or talc over the entire foot and smooth it with your fingers.

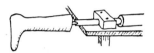
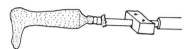
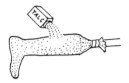

4. Preheat the 'oven' and sprinkle plaster powder or talc evenly over the hot metal sheet.

5. Cut a piece of polypropylene plastic large enough to stretch around the entire foot, and put it into the oven to heat.

6. As the plastic gets hot enough to mold, it will turn clear so you can easily see through it. It often gets clear in the middle first.

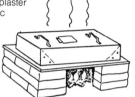
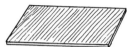
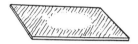

7. To move the hot plastic, 2 persons must wear thick gloves. Sprinkle dry plaster powder, lime, or talc on them.

8. As the plastic is getting hot, turn on the suction (vacuum cleaner) and listen for a hissing sound where the pipe joins the cast. (This means the suction is working.)

9. When the plastic is hot enough (clear and limp), remove the oven lid, lift the hot plastic by its 4 corners, and quickly stretch it over the whole cast.

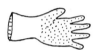
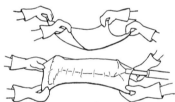
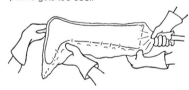

10. Quickly pinch the edges of the plastic together along the bottom side of the leg and around the pipe. Squeeze together all edges to form a seal. You **must work quickly** to complete the seal before the plastic gets too cool.

As soon as the seal is complete, the suction should pull the hot plastic close against the cast. But if necessary, help by pushing it into the hollows.*

11. While the plastic is still hot and soft, cut off the extra with a sharp knife or strong scissors.

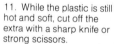
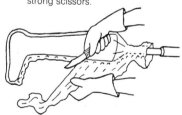

12. After it cools, draw the form of the brace on the plastic,

13. and cut it out either with a cast cutter,

or a hammer and chisel,

or a red hot soldering iron, or however you can.

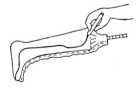
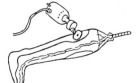
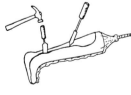

Finish the brace in the way described under Method 1 (steps 20 and 21).

*If no suction equipment is available, you can heat mold the plastic by stretching it over the cast and pushing in the hollows until it cools. With practice, this gives almost as good results, and you only need about half as much plastic.

Making sure plastic braces fit well and are comfortable

The most common problem with plastic braces is that they **press on bony bumps.** To avoid this,

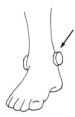

put small pads over bony bumps before casting foot. Or, put the pads on the mold, and add a little fresh plaster to the bony bumps before molding the plastic.

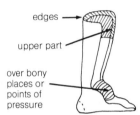

When the child wears the plastic brace, if it presses too much on bony places, or elsewhere,

heat a small area over the spot where the bone presses, and with a smooth, rounded stick push the hollow deeper. (Use a heat gun if you have one.)

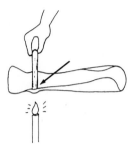

Soft padding inside the brace can make it more comfortable. Places that may need to be padded are:

edges →

upper part →

over bony places or points of pressure →

For padding you can use a product called 'moleskin', or a special foam plastic material available from orthopedic supply stores. Or you can glue in pieces of cotton blanket or car inner tube (but make sure the child wears cotton stockings to avoid skin problems).

The sole of the brace can end at the ends of the toes (or slightly beyond to allow for growth).

The side of the brace at the foot can extend to the toes if necessary for support.

Or the sole can end at the base of the toes.

For better comfort and shoe fit, the side can dip down around the base of the big toe.

AVOID brace edges that stop at middle of toes.

Avoid an edge that curves in (better to heat it and bend it out a little).

AVOID brace edges that pass across the middle of bony bumps. The edge should be either behind or in front of the bump.

Deciding how wide or narrow to make the sides of the brace at different points will depend on the needs of the particular child.

A child whose ankle or foot is floppy or deformed, or who needs a stiff ankle brace to help push back a weak knee (see p. 557) may need a brace with wide sides at the ankle and foot.

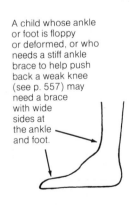

A child who needs only the ankle stabilized may walk better with a brace that lets the front of the foot bend up and down a little.

Many children benefit by a brace that allows some up and down ankle movement but prevents sideways movement.

This can be done by cutting back the sides of the brace here.

This will be the weak point in the brace. So, the plastic must be extra thick here.

Or you can strengthen it by putting extra strips of hot plastic on the back of the plaster mold *before* stretching the whole plastic over it.

Different plastic brace models for different needs

In various places in this book we have shown different brace models and how they meet the particular needs of a child. See, for example, p. 66 to 73 and p. 116. Here are a few more ideas for different plastic braces:

Below-knee brace that gives knee support

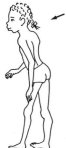

The child with a weak upper leg whose knee cannot support her full weight, may be helped enough by a brace that pushes her knee back.

A strong stiff ankle on the brace, with the foot tilted down slightly (more than 90°), pushes the knee back when she steps.

Front of brace presses against knee.

The simplest way to make this brace is to rivet the seam where the plastic joins in front. (See photo, p. 550.)

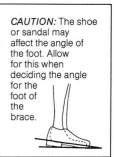

CAUTION: The shoe or sandal may affect the angle of the foot. Allow for this when deciding the angle for the foot of the brace.

A similar brace can be made in 2 parts.

1. Make the lower part, and place it back on the plaster mold.

2. Place the mold like this and form the top part of the brace over the lower part.

When the child grows, this brace can be made longer by removing the rivets and separating the 2 ends more.

rivets

Side-support knee brace

A brace that supports the knee may help a child that has a sideway bend or partial dislocation of the knee.

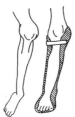

Make the brace higher on the side that needs more support.

Also, make the brace higher on the side of the ankle that needs more support.

Also, in an above-knee brace, you can put extra support on the side of the knee that needs it.

Above-knee plastic braces

The simplest kind of above-knee plastic brace is a single piece without a knee hinge. You can make it in the same way as a below-knee brace, with or without a footpiece. These braces are useful on small children.

To make a jointed above-knee brace:

1. Draw the shape of the child's leg on paper.

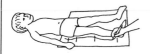

2. Mark the height of the

hip bone
crotch
mid-knee
ankle bone

3. After forming the plastic pieces on plaster molds, bend metal joint pieces so they fit the shape of the leg.

To bend the flat bar, make or buy a bending iron.

steel bending iron

4. Temporarily pin or bolt the plastic pieces to the metal pieces. Then you can adjust the front-to-back angles with the brace on the child.

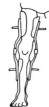

5. When the angles are right, mark the position, and after checking all aspects of fit, rivet the pieces together and add straps and knee supports.

Hinged braces can also be made using the plastic itself for knee hinges,

and even ankle hinges.

However, these hinges may not last long with heavy use.

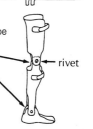

rivet

BODY SUPPORTS

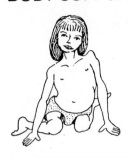

In most cases, a body brace or body jacket probably does little or nothing to correct or prevent further curving of the spine. However, a child with a 'flail' spine that curves so much that it makes sitting difficult or awkward, may sit more comfortably and have more use of her arms if she has a body brace.

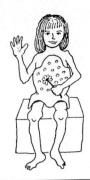

Making a plastic body brace

1. Put small pads over upper outer corners of hip bone.

2. Put a stockinette or old tight-fitting shirt on the child.

Tie a cloth band or soft rope tightly over the hip bones so that it pulls in the waist.

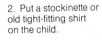

3. Cast the child's body with plaster bandage while holding her in a sitting position.*

Press plaster into groove here.

Bring plaster down to the level of the seat.

While the plaster dries, hold the child as straight as you can.

This 'shelf' over the hip bones becomes a base for the final brace to hold her body upright.

4. Cut the cast into 2 halves and remove.

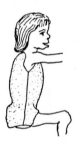

5. Tape or tie the 2 halves of the cast together and put it into a plastic bag.

6. Make a solid plaster mold inside the cast (see p. 552).

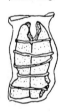

metal rod

You can make it lighter and save plaster by mixing sawdust or bits of plastic foam into the plaster.

7. Remove the plaster mold and smooth it carefully to keep its shape, especially the waist and hip curves.

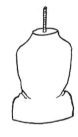

8. Stretch hot plastic over the mold as described on p. 555. If your oven or sheets of plastic are not big enough, you may have to mold it in 2 halves, front and back.

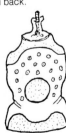

9. Mark and cut the plastic. Leave a little room under arms.

Cut breathing holes and perhaps a large central hole over the stomach.

10. Try it on the child. Make adjustments. Smooth edges. Add padding and straps.

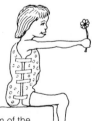

The bottom of the brace should just touch the seat when the child sits.

A body brace attached to leg braces may be needed by a child whose body is weak from the chest down.

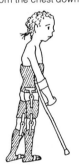

---

*Casting can also be done with the child lying lengthwise over a wide strip of cloth stretched between two points.

Correcting Joint Contractures

In this chapter we discuss different **aids used for gradually straightening limbs** that have joint *contractures*.

Information on contractures, their causes and prevention is in Chapter 8. Exercises to prevent and correct contractures are in Chapter 42. For other references to contractures, see the Index, p. 647.

Joint contractures can often be gradually straightened with casts or braces that **gently** but firmly hold the joint in a stretched position for a long time. We stress **gently** because unless great care is taken **it is very easy to cause injuries.**

To straighten a *limb,* 3 areas of pressure are needed.

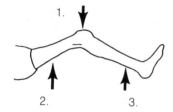

In **theory**, the leg could be straightened like this.

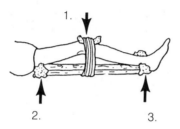

WRONG

In **fact,** this would cause **pressure sores** on the **small areas** where the splint presses.

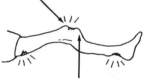

Also, the knee could be *dislocated* if the calf is not supported while stretching.

Always use wide areas of pressure. Avoid pressure on the knee, behind the heel, and over bony areas.

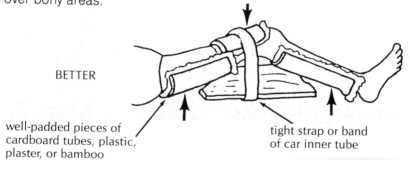

BETTER

well-padded pieces of cardboard tubes, plastic, plaster, or bamboo

tight strap or band of car inner tube

BETTER

If a child stays in bed, a stretching aid like one of these might work. (But try to keep the hip straight, so that the aid does not cause a hip contracture while it straightens the knee.)

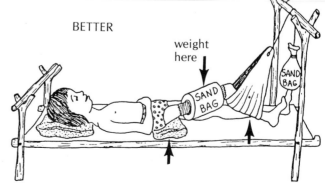

weight here

SAND BAG

SAND BAG

There are several ways to straighten contractures that let the child continue to move about. These include:

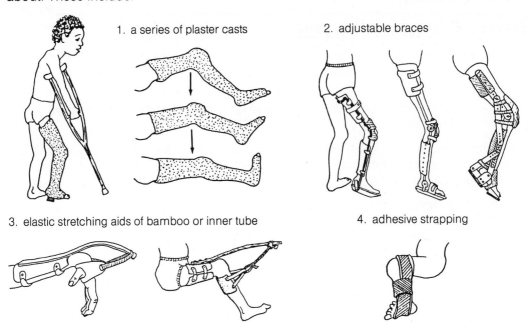

1. a series of plaster casts

2. adjustable braces

3. elastic stretching aids of bamboo or inner tube

4. adhesive strapping

The advantages and disadvantages of the first 3 ways are discussed on p. 85. **It is important that you read this before deciding which one to use for a particular child.** The 4th method (strapping) is used mostly on clubbed feet of newborn babies (see p. 565).

HOW TO CORRECT CONTRACTURES USING PLASTER CASTS

The example we give here is for the knee, but the basic methods are the same for contractures in ankles, feet, elbows, and wrists.

Casting the leg

FIRST WEEK

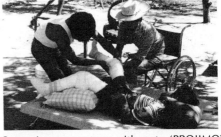

Correcting contractures with casts. (PROJIMO)

1. Put stockinette or a close fitting cotton stocking on the leg. Avoid wrinkles.

3. To protect the knee, it helps to put a soft sponge or piece of sponge rubber over the knee.

5. Put a plaster cast on the leg. Be sure it reaches **high up the thigh.**

7. Holding the calf below the knee, gently straighten the leg as far as it will go, **without using force.**

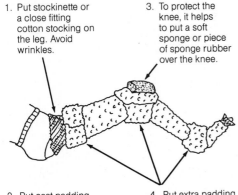

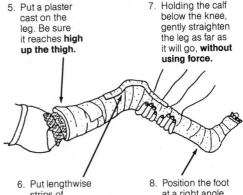

2. Put cast padding or cotton roll (or wild kapok) evenly around the leg.

4. Put extra padding around the thigh, the knee, and the ankle.

6. Put lengthwise strips of plaster for reinforcement over the knee.

8. Position the foot at a right angle (or as near to it as you can without using force).

STRAIGHTENING THE CAST WITH WEDGES

The cast is straightened a little every few days. In a small child or a person with recent contractures, it can be done every 2 or 3 days. In persons with old contractures, progress will be slower. To save on costs, change the cast every week or 10 days.

SECOND WEEK

1. Cut through the plaster behind the knee.

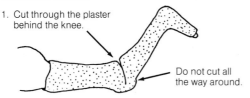

Do not cut all the way around.

2. Use steady, **gentle** pressure so that the leg straightens a little and the cut opens.

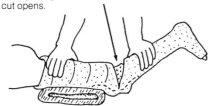

3. Hold the cut open with a small wedge of wood.

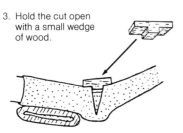

4. Wrap a piece of cloth around the knee.

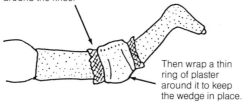

Then wrap a thin ring of plaster around it to keep the wedge in place.

CAUTION: When stretching the leg, use gentle, steady pressure until **it begins to hurt a little**. Do not try to advance too fast, as you may cause permanent damage to *nerves, tendons,* or the joint.

For a day or so after stretching, the child may have some discomfort behind the knee. This is normal, unless it hurts too much. You can give aspirin. If the child complains of pain over pressure points or bony bumps, remove the cast or cut open a window in the cast to check if a sore is forming.

WARNING: When casting a child who does not feel in his limbs, take great caution to avoid pressure sores, and use very little pressure.

THIRD WEEK

1. Cut and remove the ring of plaster.

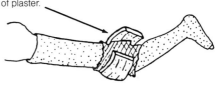

2. Gently stretch the joint and put in a wider wedge.

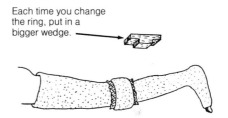

3. And cover it with a new ring of plaster.

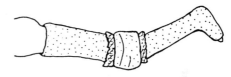

FOURTH WEEK

Each time you change the ring, put in a bigger wedge.

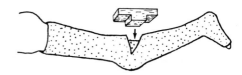

FIFTH WEEK

Continue casting until the knee is completely straight or bends backward just a little. Then use a brace for at least a few weeks (day and night) to keep it straight.

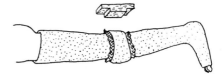

SIXTH WEEK

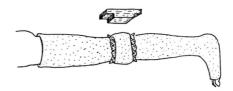

The time to straighten a contracture may vary between 2 weeks and 6 months—or more. If the leg stops straightening for 3 or more cast changes, stop casting and try to arrange surgery.

Straightening a leg that is hard to stretch

In an older child who has a knee contracture with strong *muscles* that bend the knee, it may be hard to straighten the knee more with each cast change.

STRONG MUSCLE HERE

If the leg does not move when you pull it, ask the child to . . .

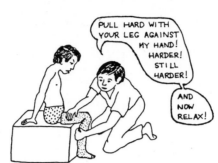

PULL HARD WITH YOUR LEG AGAINST MY HAND! HARDER! STILL HARDER! AND NOW RELAX!

When he relaxes, keep pulling, and the leg should straighten a little.

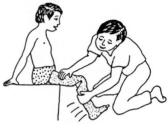

Repeat this several times while you steadily pull the leg. Each time the knee should straighten a little more.

Straightening a tiptoe contracture

A foot with a contracture like this,

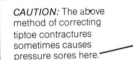

tight heel cord

can sometimes be straightened with casts and wedges.

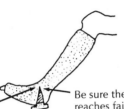

Put lots of padding under the cast on top of the ankle.

Be sure the cut reaches fairly **high** up the ankle (not across the top of the foot).

Try to overcorrect the contracture so that it will rest easily at a (90°) right angle when the cast is removed.

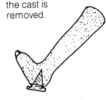

Do not let the child walk on the cast until the day after it is put on—and then only if you put a 'walking heel' on it. Otherwise the sole of the cast will become floppy and will not help. **Active children need very thick plaster on the bottom of the foot.**

wood or rubber walking heel →

CAUTION: The above method of correcting tiptoe contractures sometimes causes pressure sores here.

To prevent pressure sores, it often works better to cut a complete ring out of the cast.

For more precautions, see p. 567, on the casting of club feet.

For the child who lives too far away to have her cast changed every few days, you can try to make an aid that will gradually pull the foot up without needing frequent cast changes. Here is one idea:

strip of car inner tube

Bend the cast edges outward with pliers so they will not dig into skin as foot rises.

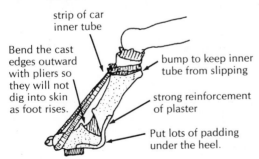

bump to keep inner tube from slipping

strong reinforcement of plaster

Put lots of padding under the heel.

CAUTION: If the child is sent home with a cast, **be sure the family knows the danger signs.** If any of these appear, have them quickly bring the child back or remove the cast themselves.

Danger signs:

● constant, severe pain—especially in areas where pressure sores can occur

● a darkening or change of color in the toes

● numbness or burning

● a smell like rotting meat (a late, very serious sign)

To take off the cast without tools, in an emergency, soak it in warm water and unwrap or tear it apart.

Note: This cast is not as strong as a fully covered one and will not last on a very active child. It will usually only work on a child without much sideways deformity of the foot or ankle. The cast may need to be changed 2 or 3 times as the foot straightens.

HOW TO CORRECT CONTRACTURES
USING ADJUSTABLE BRACES

The advantage of these braces is that children do not have to visit the *rehabilitation* center so often to have them adjusted. The family can adjust them at home.

Orthopedic suppliers in some countries sell special knee and ankle joints that can be locked in different positions. But these are very expensive. However, a skilled village craftsperson can put together something similar:

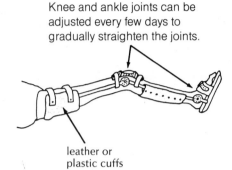

Knee and ankle joints can be adjusted every few days to gradually straighten the joints.

leather or plastic cuffs

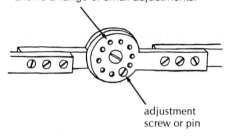

Space the holes on the 2 pieces differently so that lining them up allows a range of small adjustments.

adjustment screw or pin

A much simpler low-cost model can be made of **round or flat metal bar.**

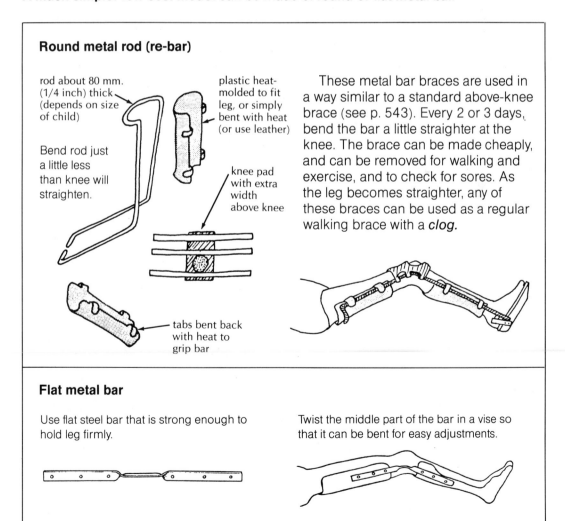

Round metal rod (re-bar)

rod about 80 mm. (1/4 inch) thick (depends on size of child)

Bend rod just a little less than knee will straighten.

plastic heat-molded to fit leg, or simply bent with heat (or use leather)

knee pad with extra width above knee

tabs bent back with heat to grip bar

These metal bar braces are used in a way similar to a standard above-knee brace (see p. 543). Every 2 or 3 days, bend the bar a little straighter at the knee. The brace can be made cheaply, and can be removed for walking and exercise, and to check for sores. As the leg becomes straighter, any of these braces can be used as a regular walking brace with a *clog.*

Flat metal bar

Use flat steel bar that is strong enough to hold leg firmly.

Twist the middle part of the bar in a vise so that it can be bent for easy adjustments.

Two designs for adjustable braces to correct ankle contractures

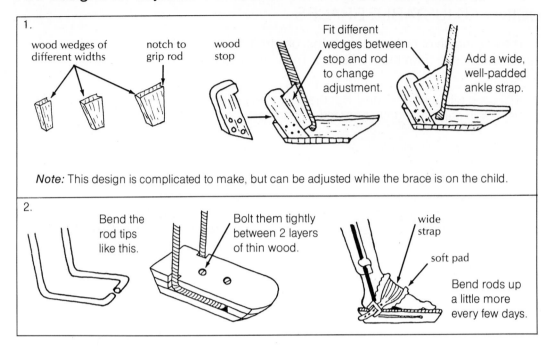

1.

wood wedges of different widths

notch to grip rod

wood stop

Fit different wedges between stop and rod to change adjustment.

Add a wide, well-padded ankle strap.

Note: This design is complicated to make, but can be adjusted while the brace is on the child.

2.

Bend the rod tips like this.

Bolt them tightly between 2 layers of thin wood.

wide strap

soft pad

Bend rods up a little more every few days.

An adjustable wood brace for knee and ankle contractures

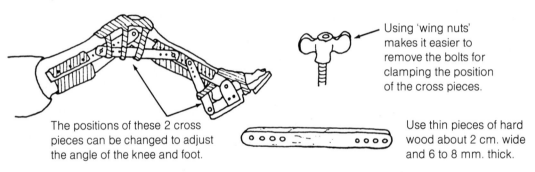

The positions of these 2 cross pieces can be changed to adjust the angle of the knee and foot.

Using 'wing nuts' makes it easier to remove the bolts for clamping the position of the cross pieces.

Use thin pieces of hard wood about 2 cm. wide and 6 to 8 mm. thick.

For **homemade aids to straighten contractures, using car inner tubes and other elastic or springy material**, see p. 85.

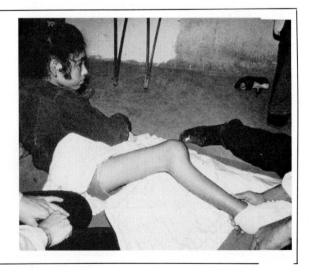

WARNING:

If a knee looks like this, it is probably dislocated. Trying to straighten it could make the dislocation worse. Take great care to put pressure only on the leg just below and behind the knee, not at the foot. Gradually try to correct the dislocation (bring the lower leg forward) before trying to straighten. If possible, get advice or help from an experienced health worker or specialist.

CHAPTER **60**

Correcting Club Feet

Note: **In Chapter 11 we discussed club feet. We suggest you read pages 114 and 116 before trying to correct a club foot.**

The younger a child is when you begin, the more easily and quickly her foot can be straightened. **For best results, begin 2 days after the baby is born.** If the child is over 1 year old, usually a good correction is only possible with surgery. Ways to predict how easy or difficult correction may be for a particular child are listed on p. 116.

club foot

Method 1: STRAPPING

This method works well in a baby with mild to moderate clubbing, especially when the foot can be put into a nearly normal position. The method is easier and cheaper than casting, and sometimes gives better results. You will need:

- tincture of benzoin (to paint on the skin to help the adhesive felt stick firmly. Zinc oxide in the tincture will help protect the skin.)

- cotton wool

- adhesive surgical felt (padding) 8 mm. thick and at least 2.5 cm (1 inch) wide

- adhesive tape (sticking plaster) or zinc oxide strapping 2.5 cm. wide

1. Paint tincture of benzoin on the skin areas to be covered by the tape.

2. Hold the baby's foot like this and gently straighten it as far as you can without forcing.

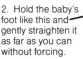

3. With the knee bent as far as possible, stick strips of felt around the foot and over the knee and leg as shown.

SIDE VIEW   FRONT VIEW

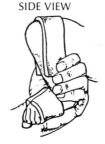

SIDE VIEW   FRONT VIEW

4. Stretch adhesive tape over the felt. Start on the outer side of the foot, go around the foot, up over the knee, and down the other side. Use the tape to pull the foot into a better position.

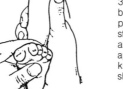

Tape coming down leg ends here.

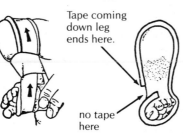

no tape here

FRONT VIEW

5. Put a second piece of tape around the leg twice here, to hold the first tape.

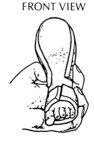

CAUTION: 10 minutes after putting on the tape, check to see if any part of the foot has turned dark. If so, look for the trouble spot and try to adjust the strapping. If it stays dark, take everything off and start again.

Every 2 or 3 days, tighten the correction by stretching new tape over the old, in the same way. On the 7th day, remove everything and leave the leg free until the next day. On the 8th day, apply new felt and tape.

(Continued on next page.)

Exercises during strapping

While the baby's foot is strapped, someone in the family should do stretching exercises on his foot every time he is fed or changed (at least 8 times a day).

1. Hold the baby's leg like this and **turn his whole foot UP and OUT.**

Hold and count to 10. Repeat 10 times.

2. Turn it as if you were trying to touch the little toe to the outer side of the knee.

The strapping and exercises should be continued until the foot is **overcorrected** (bends outward a little).

3. If the foot is shaped like a bean, also do an exercise to stretch the foot in the opposite direction of the deformity, like this.

4. After stretching the baby's foot this way, help the baby to stretch it himself by tickling the outer edge of his foot.

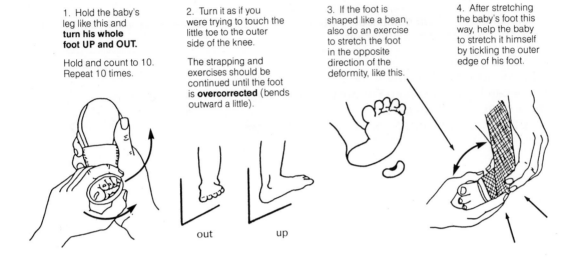

out   up

If the foot is not straightened completely within about 3 months of strapping and exercises, surgery is probably needed.

Method 2: PLASTER CASTS

This method uses a casting technique similar to the one for correcting contractures (see Chapter 59). A club foot is gradually straightened in 3 stages:

Stage A ──────► **Stage B** ──────► **Stage C**

Straighten the inward bend so that the foot points **down**. Do not yet begin to lift the foot.

Overcorrect so that the foot points **down** and **out**. Keep the foot in this position **until the heel no longer turns in** but is straight or turns out just a little.

Now bring the foot **up**, making sure that the outside of the foot is higher than the inside. **Overcorrect**.

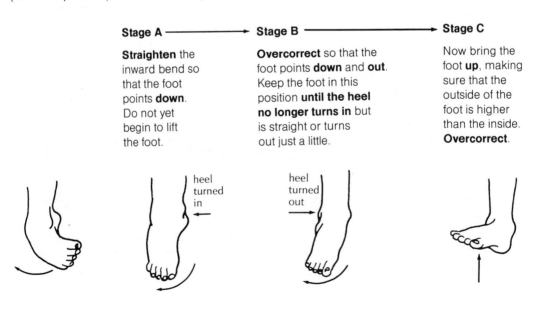

heel turned in

heel turned out

Stage A

1. In a young baby it is often necessary to **cast the whole leg with the knee bent** to keep the cast from slipping down. First, wrap cotton padding evenly around the whole leg.

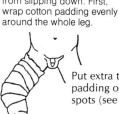

Put extra thick padding over bony spots (see p. 560).

Put bits of cotton between the toes. (Take them out after the foot has been cast.)

2. Cast the leg and foot. Make the cast especially thick around the knee and heel, where he is more likely to bump it.

Make it wider on this side.

3. After the plaster is dry, cut out a wide ring from heel to mid-foot.

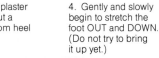

4. Gently and slowly begin to stretch the foot OUT and DOWN. (Do not try to bring it up yet.)

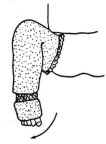

5. To keep edges of cast from hurting the skin, bend them out with pliers.

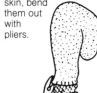

6. Put a ring of cotton or soft gauze over the foot and cover with new plaster bandage.

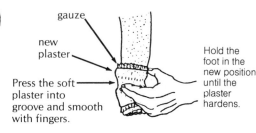

gauze

new plaster

Press the soft plaster into groove and smooth with fingers.

Hold the foot in the new position until the plaster hardens.

7. Once or twice a week take off the outer ring of plaster, bend the foot down and out a little more, and cover with a new ring of plaster.

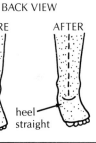

Repeat Step 7 until the foot bends outward a little. This usually takes several weeks.

Stage B

1. Remove the whole cast and check the position of the heel.

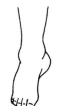

Often the heel still bends in even after the bend of the foot has been corrected.

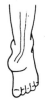

2. If so, keep casting the foot in a **down** and **out** position until the heel is straighter.

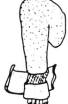

BACK VIEW

BEFORE   AFTER

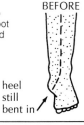

heel still bent in

heel straight

Stage C

1. After the sideways twist of the foot and heel is corrected, begin to raise the foot, using casts.

2. As you wrap the foot with plaster bandage, hold it in a raised position with 2 fingers.

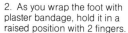

3. Hold the foot up as the plaster dries.

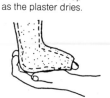

As you hold the foot, keep it turned outward so that the little toe is always higher than the big toe.

Take care to keep the toes straight.

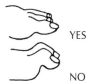

YES

NO

4. Keep raising the foot little by little using the same casting method as before.

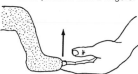

Bend up cast edges with pliers.

(*CAUTION:* Be very careful cast does not pinch or dig into skin here.)

5. Raise the foot a little in this way once or twice a week until it is as high as this, or until it stops raising for 3 or 4 cast changes.

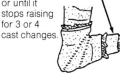

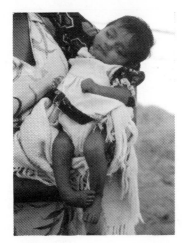

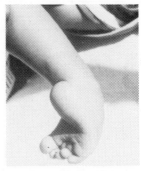

This child was born with a club foot. Village *rehabilitation* workers used a series of casts to straighten it. First they corrected the inner bend of the foot.

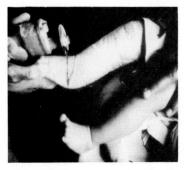

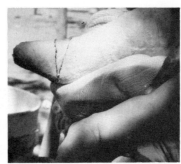

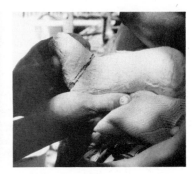

Then they gradually lifted her foot by cutting out rings on the cast, closing the space, and holding it closed with a new strip of plaster. (See p. 567.)

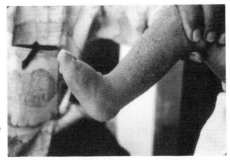

After 4 months of casting, the foot was in a good position.

IMPORTANT

After a club foot has been corrected, great care is needed to prevent it from coming back.

Both exercises and braces are essential. After strapping or casts have been removed, continue the recommended stretching exercises twice a day (see p. 115). Braces for use after correcting club feet are on p. 116.

Many children need to wear braces until they stop growing (age 13 to 18). If the problem keeps returning, surgery is probably needed.

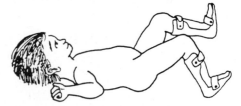

This child who had club feet needs to use braces day and night, at least until he begins to walk, and still at night after that.

Check his feet regularly, for years, for any sign that the foot is beginning to turn in again. Improved bracing may be required.

Homemade Casting Materials

Plaster bandages

Although commercial plaster bandages work best, they are very expensive. You can make homemade plaster bandages for as little as one tenth the cost. Or some of the disabled children can learn to make them. You will need:

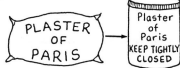

- **plaster of Paris.** If possible, a high-quality type such as dental plaster of Paris. Keep it in a tightly closed moisture-proof container.

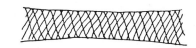

- **gauze cloth or crinoline.** Crinoline, which is a high-quality open mesh cloth, works best. Good quality gauze can also be used. Holes should be about 8 to 10 per cm. (20 per inch). Cheesecloth also works, but not as well.

HOW TO PREPARE:

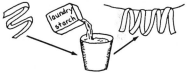

- If you use gauze or cheesecloth, first dip it into a weak solution of laundry starch and let it dry. This helps the bandage keep its shape.

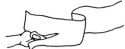

- Cut the cloth into strips of the width you want.

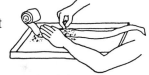

- Rub plaster powder into the cloth and roll or fold it loosely. **Do not roll it tightly** or the inner part will not get wet when dipped for use.

The most common problem is that the gauze does not hold enough of the plaster powder. Even if you put on a lot, some powder always falls out. The test is when you apply the wet bandage. As you rub each layer into the next, the threads of cloth should disappear into the smooth, wet, plaster surface. If not, there is not enough plaster and it will not set hard.

Suggestion: Have some dry plaster powder ready when you are casting. If needed, sprinkle a little powder over each layer of bandage and rub it smooth with wet hands. Add more to the final layer and rub it in to form a polished surface.

Storage: Wrap the plaster bandages in old newspaper or plastic bags and store in an airtight container. Do not prepare too many at a time. They can absorb moisture and spoil.

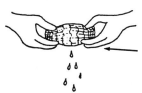

CAUTION: When wetting for use, up to a third of the plaster may be lost in the water. To reduce loss, put bandage gently into water and then let it drip. If you squeeze it, hold the ends of the roll and gently squeeze toward the center.

Homemade plaster takes longer to get hard than commercial 'fast-setting' plaster. **To speed up hardening, heat the water or add a little salt to it.**

Casts made of wax

To prepare a mold of a leg for making plastic braces, the first (hollow) cast can be made of wax instead of plaster. Use either candle wax (paraffin) or beeswax. **Wax can be much cheaper than plaster bandage, especially if the wax is re-used. To make a wax cast:**

1. Melt the wax in a can placed in hot water.

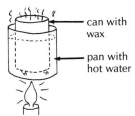

can with wax

pan with hot water

2. Cut several strips of soft absorbent cloth.

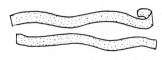

3. Soak the cloth in hot wax.

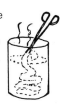

4. When it has cooled enough not to burn, wrap the waxed cloths around the foot.

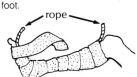

rope

Note: Before putting on the wax, you can cover the foot with 'stockinette'. Also, place a rope or strip of plastic along the top of the leg to make cutting the cast easier. (See p. 552.)

5. While the wax is still warm and soft, rub and press it against the leg.

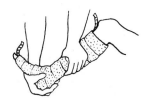

6. Hold the foot in the desired position until the wax hardens. (To speed hardening, you can put the foot in cold water.)

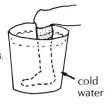

cold water

7. Cut the wet cast along the rope, and carefully remove it. Go on with the other steps as described on p. 552.

Re-using the wax: After the positive plaster mold has been made from the wax cast, the wax can be re-used. Heat up the pieces of waxed cloth and use them to form a new cast. Or boil the waxed cloth in water, holding the cloth under the surface with rocks or metal. The hot wax will rise to the surface. When it cools, lift it off and re-use it.

OTHER POSSIBLE MATERIALS FOR CASTING OR MOLDING

Many materials can be used for casts. **Most have the disadvantage that they take a long time to harden.** Possibilities include:

1. **Papier mâché** (see p. 471). Very slow hardening. Careful use of a heat lamp or 'hair dryer' speeds drying.

2. **Traditional cast materials.** For example:

   ● In Mexico, the juices of certain plants, boiled into a thick syrup and soaked into a cloth, will harden into a cast (see *Where There Is No Doctor,* p. 14).

   ● In India, traditional bone setters make casts using cloth covered with egg white mixed with flour.

3. **Flour** made from cassava (manioc) is also used in India to make casts.

To make the solid (positive) mold of a limb (see p. 552), 'building plaster' works well. (Wax cannot be used because it melts when hot plastic is placed over it.) Clay also works, but takes several days to dry.

CHAPTER **62**

Developmental Aids

In this chapter we look at the design details of aids for **lying, sitting, standing, balance, use of hands,** and **communication.** Aids for walking are in Chapter 63.

Whether or not a particular child needs an aid, and what kind of aid she needs, must always be carefully and repeatedly evaluated. An aid that helps a child at one level of development may actually hold her back at another. When considering aids, we suggest you first read the chapters on child development, those covering the particular *disability* of the child, and Chapter 56.

> *Note:* Many developmental aids have already been shown in PART 1 of this book, especially in Chapter 9 (cerebral palsy), and in Section C, on child development. Aids and equipment for play and exercise are in PART 2, Chapter 46 (Playgrounds). Wheelboards and wheelchairs are in Chapters 64, 65, and 66.

Lying aids

Lying face down is a good position for a child to begin to develop control of the head, shoulders, arms, and hands, and also to stretch *muscles* in the hips, knees, and shoulders. However, some children have difficulty in this position. For example:

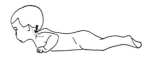 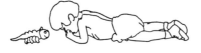 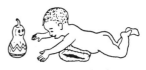

Rosa cannot lift her shoulders. She has to bend her neck far back to lift her head.	Juan does not have enough control and balance to reach out his arms.	A firm pillow under the chest may help both these children to lift their heads better and to reach out.

A 'wedge' or slanting support is often helpful. The height depends on the needs of the particular child.

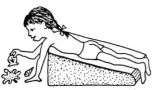

Letting feet hang down helps prevent tiptoe *contractures.*

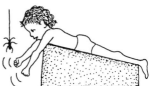

Diana manages best on a wedge high enough so that she can lift herself up a little at arms length. (Height is the length from wrist to armpit.)	Cassio does better on a lower wedge, so he can lift up on his elbows. (Height is slightly less than length from elbow to armpit.)	Carmen and others with little or no arm or hand control do best when their arms can dangle. She can see them moving when she moves her shoulders.

Wedges can be made with:

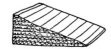 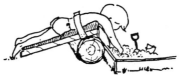 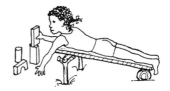

stiff foam plastic or layers of cardboard	a log and a board with a soft foam cover	a stick frame

If necessary, a leg separator can be added (see p. 81).

Or sides can be included for the child who needs to be *positioned* with supports or cushions.

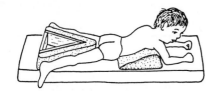

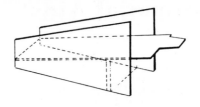

Design from *Functional Aids for the Multiply Handicapped.*

Some children are able to control their shoulders, arms, and hands better when lying on one side.

A side-lying frame may be helpful for some children with severe cerebral palsy. Try cushions or padded blocks of different shapes until you find what works best. Use straps only if clearly needed to keep a good position.

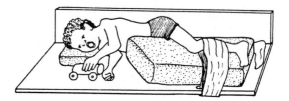

Also see lying frames for straightening hip flexion contractures (p. 81 and 86), and lying frames with wheels (p. 618 and 619).

ADJUSTABLE BEDS

This design from the Centre for the Rehabilitation of the Paralysed in Bangladesh adjusts easily from an upper position to a lower position.

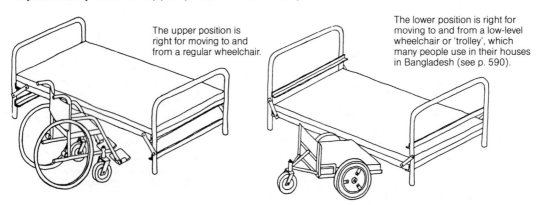

The upper position is right for moving to and from a regular wheelchair.

The lower position is right for moving to and from a low-level wheelchair or 'trolley', which many people use in their houses in Bangladesh (see p. 590).

These metal beds and wheelchairs are welded together by paraplegic workers. For the 'coconut fiber' mattresses they use, see p. 199.

ADJUSTABLE BACK SUPPORT CLAMP

Supporting a severely *paralyzed* person so he lies on his side can be difficult. Pillows easily move or slip. This simple clamp helps solve the problem. It was designed and made by disabled workers at the Centre for the Rehabilitation of the Paralysed, Dacca, Bangladesh (see p. 518).

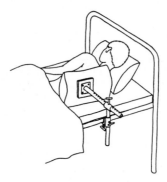

CAUTION: To prevent pressure sores, be sure the child changes position often (see Chapter 24).

Sitting Aids

A wide variety of early sitting aids are included in the chapter on cerebral palsy (see p. 97 and 98). Special seating *adaptations* for chairs and wheelchairs are in Chapter 65. Here we include a few more ideas:

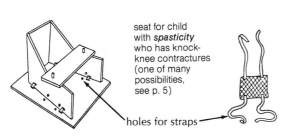

seat for child with *spasticity* who has knock-knee contractures (one of many possibilities, see p. 5)

holes for straps

strap for keeping legs apart (one around each leg and tied through holes in sides of seat)

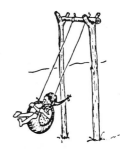

Tire seat or swing bends head, body, and shoulders forward to help control spasticity (see p. 421).

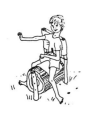

A log or roll seat helps the child with spasticity or poor balance sit more securely with legs spread. Log should be as high as the knees. Leave a little room between the cut-out circle in the table and the child's belly.

seat for a child with spasticity whose body stiffens backward

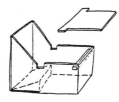

Design from *Handling the Young Cerebral Palsied Child at Home* (see p. 638).

OTHER IDEAS FOR HOLDING LEGS APART

from Don Caston and AHRTAG

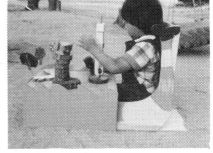

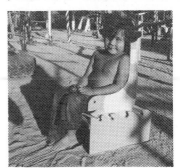

A seat and table like this in the form of a fish on the ocean makes sitting in a special seat fun. So do the village-made toys (PROJIMO, seat design by Don Caston).

from other parts of this book

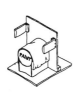   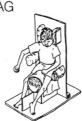

p. 5, 416   p. 5   p. 7

p. 81, 97   p.98   p. 609   p. 329

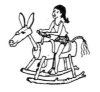

The seat can be used for straight leg sitting, or put on top of the table for bent-knee sitting. Other designs include 'squirrel' seats on 'tree' tables.

For more ideas on adapted seating, see Chapters 9, 35, and 65. Also, see scooters and walkers with roll seats, p. 98.

Standing aids (See also p. 99, 312, and 500.)

Many children who have problems with balance or control for standing may benefit from standing or playing in a 'standing aid'. Even for the child who may never stand or walk on her own, being held in a standing position with weight on her legs helps *circulation* and bone growth and strength.

STANDING BOARD

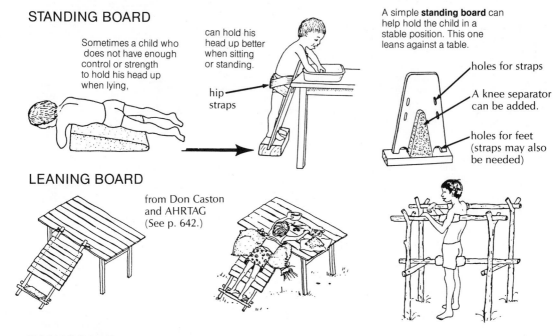

Sometimes a child who does not have enough control or strength to hold his head up when lying,

can hold his head up better when sitting or standing.

hip straps

A simple **standing board** can help hold the child in a stable position. This one leans against a table.

holes for straps

A knee separator can be added.

holes for feet (straps may also be needed)

LEANING BOARD

from Don Caston and AHRTAG (See p. 642.)

BACK-BOARD

This can be used to gradually bring a child to a standing position. It is especially useful for older children who get dizzy if stood up straight too quickly. This can happen after a spinal cord injury or a long, severe illness. The child can be stood up gradually and for longer each day.

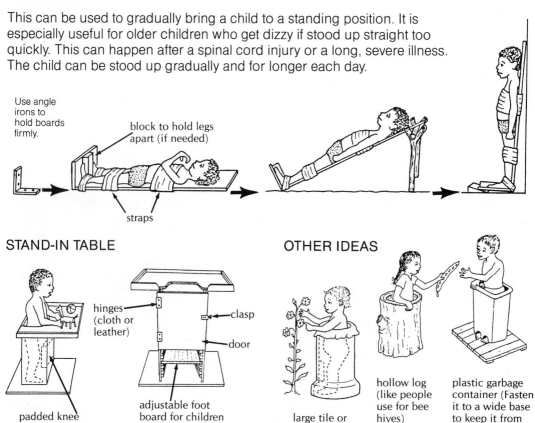

Use angle irons to hold boards firmly.

block to hold legs apart (if needed)

straps

STAND-IN TABLE

hinges (cloth or leather)

clasp

door

padded knee block

adjustable foot board for children of different heights

OTHER IDEAS

hollow log (like people use for bee hives)

large tile or cement pipe

plastic garbage container (Fasten it to a wide base to keep it from tipping over.)

STANDING FRAMES

These are mainly for a child with contractures or painful joints who has difficulty standing straight. The child can gradually be straightened up.

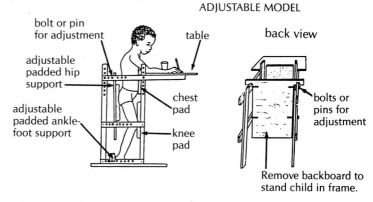

ADJUSTABLE MODEL

bolt or pin for adjustment
table
back view
adjustable padded hip support
chest pad
adjustable padded ankle-foot support
knee pad
bolts or pins for adjustment

Remove backboard to stand child in frame.

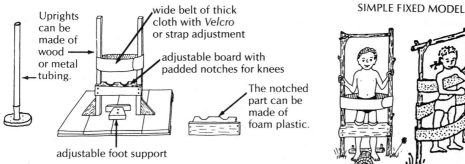

MOVABLE MODEL

Uprights can be made of wood or metal tubing.
wide belt of thick cloth with *Velcro* or strap adjustment
adjustable board with padded notches for knees
The notched part can be made of foam plastic.
adjustable foot support

SIMPLE FIXED MODEL

For some children, a chest belt will also be needed.

STANDING-AND-WALKING FRAME

This is a useful aid to begin standing and walking, for children paralyzed or severely affected below the waist (paraplegia, spina bifida, diplegic cerebral palsy).

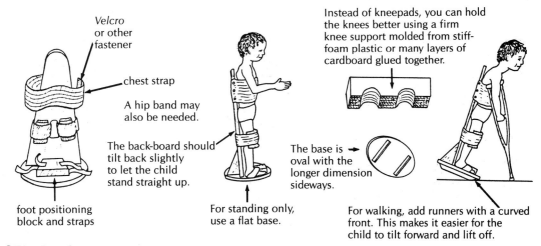

Velcro or other fastener

chest strap

A hip band may also be needed.

The back-board should tilt back slightly to let the child stand straight up.

foot positioning block and straps

For standing only, use a flat base.

Instead of kneepads, you can hold the knees better using a firm knee support molded from stiff-foam plastic or many layers of cardboard glued together.

The base is oval with the longer dimension sideways.

For walking, add runners with a curved front. This makes it easier for the child to tilt forward and lift off.

STANDING-WALKING BRACE

This has the same use as the standing-walking frame above, but is especially useful for children who need to learn how to walk before they are fitted for braces with a hip band or body brace.

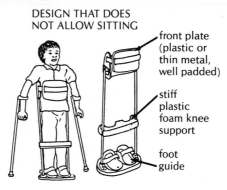

DESIGN THAT DOES NOT ALLOW SITTING

front plate (plastic or thin metal, well padded)
stiff plastic foam knee support
foot guide

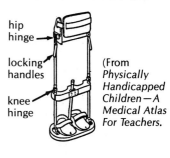

DESIGN WITH HIP AND KNEE HINGES TO ALLOW SITTING

hip hinge
locking handles
knee hinge

(From *Physically Handicapped Children—A Medical Atlas For Teachers.*)

Aids for balancing and body control

Activities for improving balance are discussed on p. 105, 311, and 312. Here we bring together a few of the aids for balancing that are shown in different parts of this book, together with a few new ones.

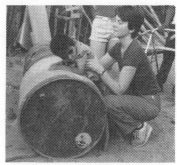

An old drum or barrel makes a good 'roll' for exercise and positioning.

BALANCE BOARDS

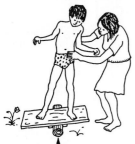

A balance board like this rocks less smoothly because the center rocker is so narrow.

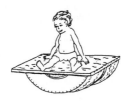

A wider rocker works better.

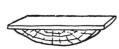

An upright stick can be used at first to help her keep her balance.

padding to avoid injury

BALANCE BEAMS

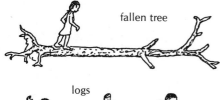
fallen tree

logs

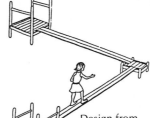
Design from *UPKARAN Manual.* (See p. 642.)

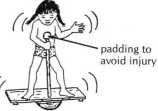
adjustable wide or narrow balance beam

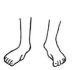
For the child whose ankles bend in,

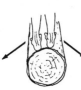
walking on a log helps bend the ankles outward.

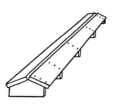
Or the child can walk on slanting boards, like this.

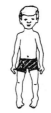
For the child whose ankles bend outward,

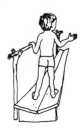
walking on boards like this helps bend the ankles inward.

To improve balance also see **swings, rocking horses** and **merry-go-rounds.**

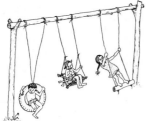
p. 420 and 421

p. 422

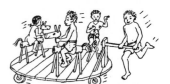
p. 425

Other aids

Many aids not yet described in PART 3 have been described in other parts of this book. Here is a brief summary of some of these to give you basic ideas and tell you where to look. We also give a few ideas of aids not shown before.

EATING AND DRINKING AIDS

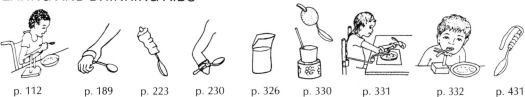

p. 112 p. 189 p. 223 p. 230 p. 326 p. 330 p. 331 p. 332 p. 431

TOILETING AIDS

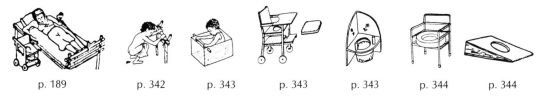

p. 189 p. 342 p. 343 p. 343 p. 343 p. 344 p. 344

HOLDING AND REACHING AIDS (Also see p. 6, 223, 230, 335, 336, 431, and 507.)

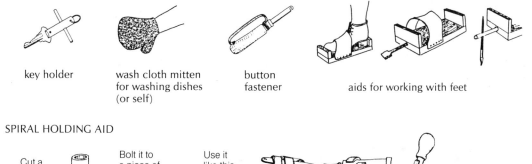

key holder

wash cloth mitten for washing dishes (or self)

button fastener

aids for working with feet

SPIRAL HOLDING AID

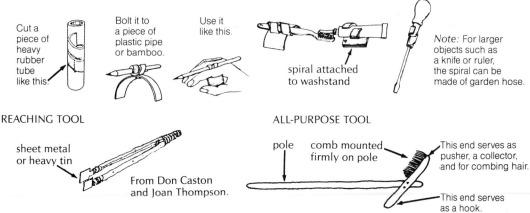

Cut a piece of heavy rubber tube like this.

Bolt it to a piece of plastic pipe or bamboo.

Use it like this.

spiral attached to washstand

Note: For larger objects such as a knife or ruler, the spiral can be made of garden hose.

REACHING TOOL

sheet metal or heavy tin

From Don Caston and Joan Thompson.

ALL-PURPOSE TOOL

pole

comb mounted firmly on pole

This end serves as pusher, a collector, and for combing hair.

This end serves as a hook.

WRITING AIDS (Also see p. 189, 223, 230, and 501.)

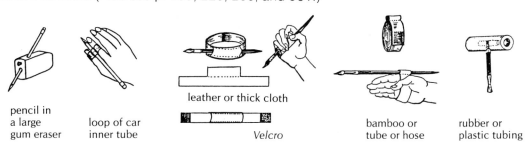

pencil in a large gum eraser

loop of car inner tube

leather or thick cloth

Velcro

bamboo or tube or hose

rubber or plastic tubing

COMMUNICATION AIDS (Also see "Blindness" p. 253 to 254 and "Deafness" p. 259 to 275.)

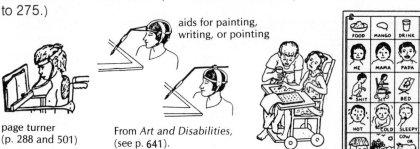

aids for painting, writing, or pointing

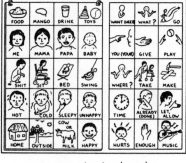

page turner
(p. 288 and 501)

From *Art and Disabilities*, (see p. 641).

communication board

PHYSICAL EXAMINATION, MEASURING AND RECORDING AIDS

INSTRUMENT FOR LEVELING HIPS

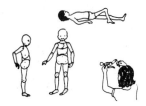

Cut 2 pieces of thin plywood like this. Fasten them together so that they slide back and forth.

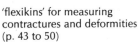

long, thin hole

← 25 cm. →

nut, bolt, and washer

To use, close instrument around child's waist and push down against hip bones. Then raise or lower shorter leg until the instrument is level.

Cut rectangles of 1/4 inch thick boards and bolt them loosely together at one corner.

aid for measuring leg length difference
(p. 34 and 549)

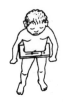 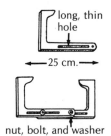 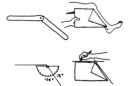 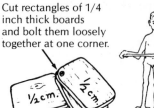

'flexikins' for measuring contractures and deformities (p. 43 to 50)

other methods for measuring contractures (p. 43 and 79)

rib-hump angle measurer (p. 163)

aids for hearing examination (p. 450)

aids for seeing examination (p. 452 and 453)

FOOT CONTRACTURE PREVENTION AIDS

Also see Chapter 59, "Correcting Joint Contractures," and Chapter 58, "Braces."

  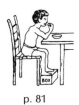 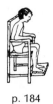

p. 81   p. 81   p. 81   p. 81   p. 184

EXERCISE AIDS

     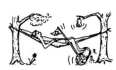

p. 5   p. 71   p. 141   p. 145   p. 146   p. 149

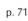

inner tube

p. 186   p. 229   p. 373   p. 388   p. 392   p. 528

CHAPTER 63

Walking Aids

In designing aids for a child, we need to think not only about her type and amount of *disability,* but also the stage of progress she is at. For learning to walk, she may progress through a series of stages and aids. Here is an example:

1. Parallel bars
2. Wheeled walker
3. Crutches modified to form walker

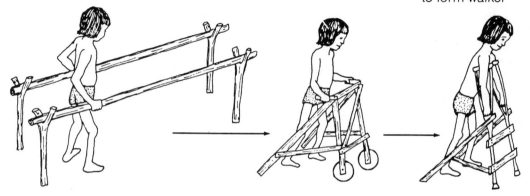

4. Underarm crutches
5. Below elbow crutches
6. Cane with wide base
7. Walking stick (cane)
8. If possible, no aids at all

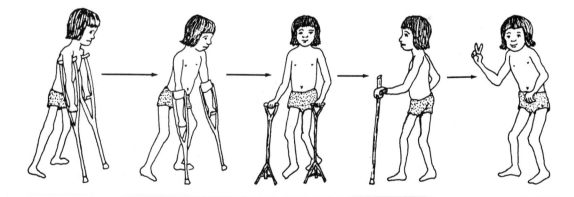

In this chapter we show a variety of aids for walking. Most can be made easily out of tree branches or wood. Some can be made from building construction bars (reinforcing rod) or metal tubing, and may require welding.

We include these ideas not to ask you to copy them, but with the hope that they will 'trigger' your imagination. Take ideas from these designs, and use the materials you have at hand. When possible, make your aids to meet the needs of the individual child.

At a village *rehabilitation center,* it helps to have a wide selection of aids on hand, so that you can try different ones on a particular child to find out what works and what she likes best.

Parallel bars

Simple designs for outdoor parallel bars, both adjustable and non-adjustable, are included in Chapter 46 on playgrounds, p. 417 and 425. On p. 417 we also give suggestions for adjusting the bar height to meet the needs of the individual child. The designs shown are:

OUTDOOR BARS

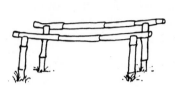
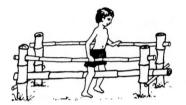
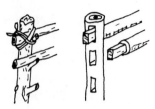

simple, non-adjustable bars
(bamboo, wood, or metal)

bars with a leg separator for a
child whose knees pull together

2 designs for bars
with adjustable height

INDOOR BARS (design details for two of several models)

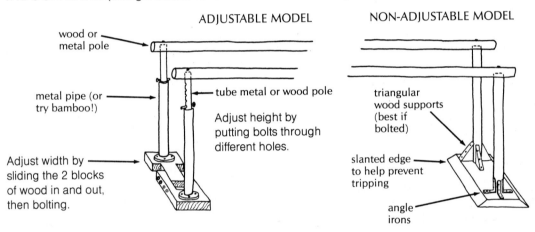

ADJUSTABLE MODEL

NON-ADJUSTABLE MODEL

wood or
metal pole

metal pipe (or
try bamboo!)

tube metal or wood pole

Adjust height by
putting bolts through
different holes.

Adjust width by
sliding the 2 blocks
of wood in and out,
then bolting.

triangular
wood supports
(best if
bolted)

slanted edge
to help prevent
tripping

angle
irons

IRON PIPE BARS

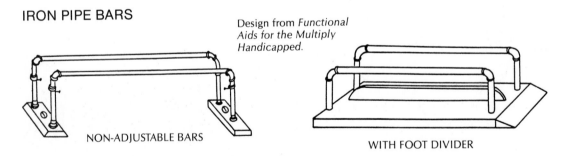

Design from *Functional
Aids for the Multiply
Handicapped.*

NON-ADJUSTABLE BARS

WITH FOOT DIVIDER

METAL CONDUIT TUBING

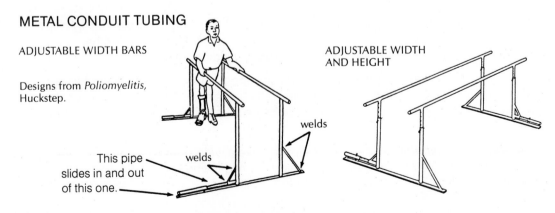

ADJUSTABLE WIDTH BARS

Designs from *Poliomyelitis,*
Huckstep.

ADJUSTABLE WIDTH
AND HEIGHT

welds

This pipe
slides in and out
of this one.

welds

Walkers

There are many ways to make walkers or walking frames. Here we show a range from very simple to more complex. Choose the design and height depending on the child's needs and size.

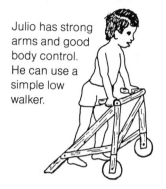

Julio has strong arms and good body control. He can use a simple low walker.

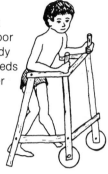

Lico has weak elbows and poor balance or body control. He needs a higher walker with armrests.

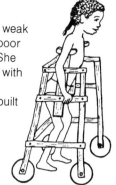

Anna has weak legs and poor balance. She does best with underarm crutches built into the walker.

The above walkers can be made with 2 cm. x 4 cm. boards (such as those used on roofs to hold tiles), or thin trees or branches. The wood or plywood wheels roll easily when little weight is on them (when child pushes walker) but have a braking action when child puts full weight on them (when taking a step).

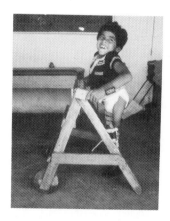

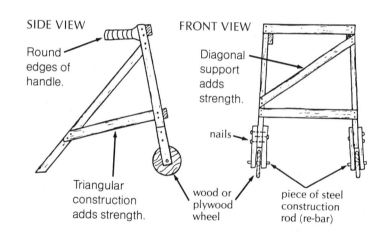

SIDE VIEW

Round edges of handle.

Triangular construction adds strength.

wood or plywood wheel

FRONT VIEW

Diagonal support adds strength.

nails

piece of steel construction rod (re-bar)

Finding the design that works best for a particular child often involves experimenting and changing different features.

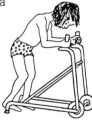

For example, Carlota has poor body and hip control, and tends to 'fall through' the space between her arms when the handgrips are upright.

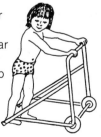

A higher walker with a bar as the handgrip works better for her.

These walkers can be made out of welded or bolted metal tubing.

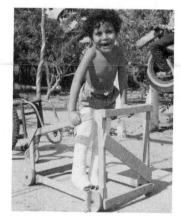

This walker with slanting bars lets a child hold it at the height that he finds works best.

Other walker designs

WALKER MADE FROM CANE, RATTAN, OR BAMBOO

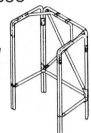

Design from *Rattan and Bamboo Equipment For Handicapped Children,* J. K. Hutt.

Joints can be tied with cane, ribbon, nylon string, strips of car inner tube or whatever.

WOOD WALKER

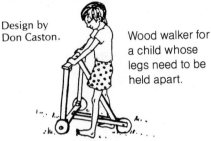

Design by Don Caston.

Wood walker for a child whose legs need to be held apart.

Note: A walker with no wheels is very stable but harder to move.

A walker with 2 wheels and 2 posts is fairly stable but easy to move.

A walker with 3 or 4 wheels is very easy to move but can easily roll out from under the child (unless the child is seated).

seat

WALKER MADE FROM SOLID IRON ROD (RE-BAR) WITH ARMRESTS—WELDING REQUIRED

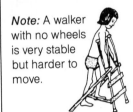

Design from *Simple Orthopaedic Aids,* Chris Dartnell.

Measure child.

elbow height

Cut and bend rod.

Assemble walker.

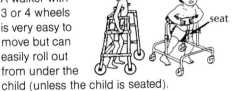

padding or hand-grips from crutches

slider

rubber

wood wheel

SIDE VIEW

FRONT VIEW

ARMREST

Weld curved armrest to rod.

width of forearm

angled toward body

leather, cardboard, plastic, or sponge

80°

wheel

washer

nail

weld

SIMPLE WALKER MADE FROM SOLID IRON ROD (RE-BAR)— WELDING REQUIRED

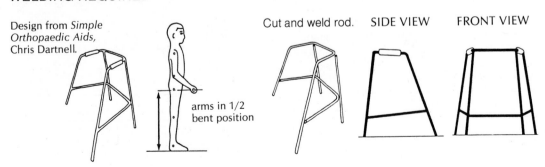

Design from *Simple Orthopaedic Aids,* Chris Dartnell.

arms in 1/2 bent position

Cut and weld rod.

SIDE VIEW

FRONT VIEW

CART WALKERS

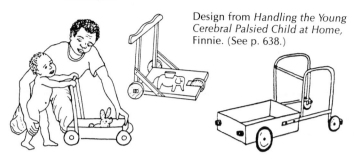

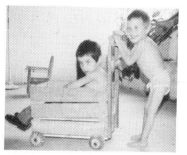

Design from *Handling the Young Cerebral Palsied Child at Home,* Finnie. (See p. 638.)

The added weight in the cart can help the child stand firmly—and makes learning to walk more fun.

As the child progresses, he can change his grip from the front bar to the side bars.

Wheels on this cart walker are made from the round seed pods of a tree in Mexico, called Hava de San Ignacio.

ROLLER SEAT AND TRICYCLE WALKERS

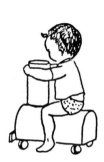

Useful for a child with cerebral palsy who 'bunny hops' (crawls pulling both legs forward together). Seat holds legs apart. The 'chimney' helps child keep his arms up and apart.

Design from *Handling the Young Cerebral Palsied Child at Home,* Finnie. (See p. 638.)

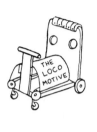

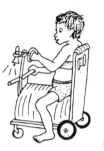

stable for the beginner

WALKERS FOR SITTING AND STANDING

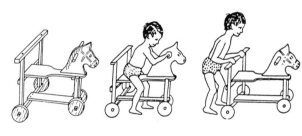

SPIDER WALKER

Useful for the small child severely affected by cerebral palsy.

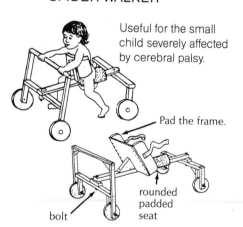

Pad the frame.

bolt

rounded padded seat

SADDLE-TYPE WALKER

Design from *UPKARAN Manual.* (See p. 642.)

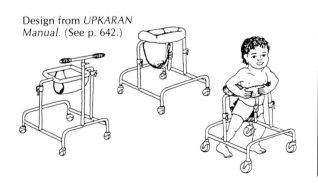

CAUTION: Sitting walkers should usually be used, if at all, as an early and temporary step toward walking. With them, the child does not learn to balance well and the hips are often at an angle which can form *contractures* (see Chapter 8, p. 86).

Crutches

MEASUREMENTS FOR UNDERARM CRUTCH

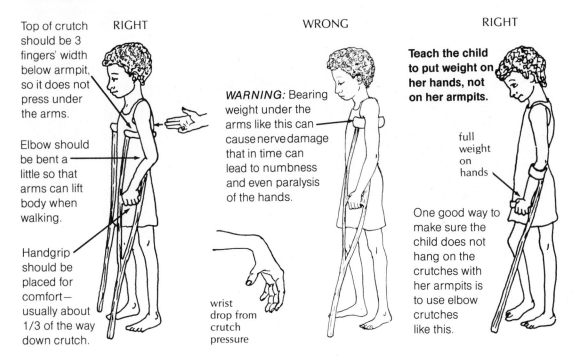

RIGHT

Top of crutch should be 3 fingers' width below armpit, so it does not press under the arms.

Elbow should be bent a little so that arms can lift body when walking.

Handgrip should be placed for comfort— usually about 1/3 of the way down crutch.

WRONG

WARNING: Bearing weight under the arms like this can cause nerve damage that in time can lead to numbness and even paralysis of the hands.

wrist drop from crutch pressure

RIGHT

Teach the child to put weight on her hands, not on her armpits.

full weight on hands

One good way to make sure the child does not hang on the crutches with her armpits is to use elbow crutches like this.

There are many designs for underarm crutches. Here we show a few.

CRUTCHES FROM TREE BRANCHES, padded with wild kapok

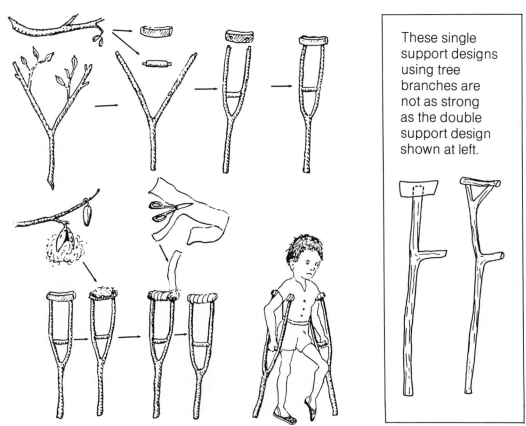

These single support designs using tree branches are not as strong as the double support design shown at left.

WOODEN CRUTCHES

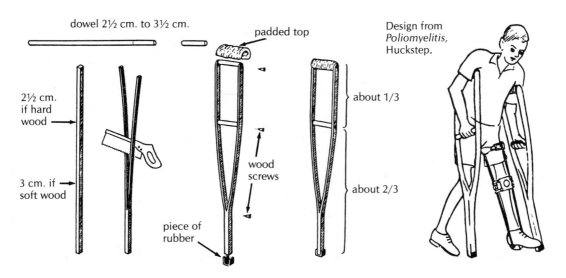

dowel 2½ cm. to 3½ cm.

padded top

Design from
Poliomyelitis,
Huckstep.

2½ cm.
if hard
wood

about 1/3

3 cm. if
soft wood

wood
screws

about 2/3

piece of
rubber

METAL CRUTCH

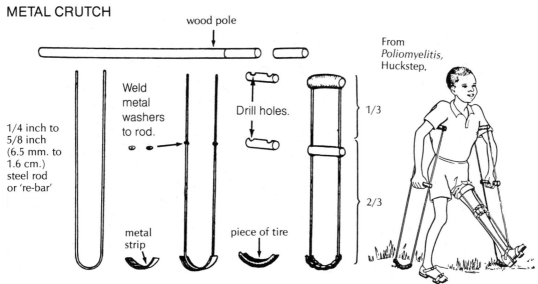

wood pole

From
Poliomyelitis,
Huckstep.

1/4 inch to
5/8 inch
(6.5 mm. to
1.6 cm.)
steel rod
or 're-bar'

Weld
metal
washers
to rod.

Drill holes.

1/3

2/3

metal
strip

piece of tire

ADJUSTABLE WOOD CRUTCH

STANDARD

Handgrip
adjusts by
putting
bolt
through
higher or
lower
holes.

sponge
rubber
padding

wing nut

thin bolt

washers

bolts with
wing nuts

standard
rubber
crutch tip

side view
showing holes
for height
adjustment

LEATHER RING ELBOW CRUTCH

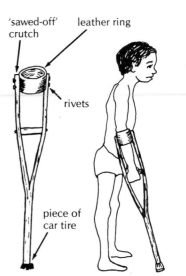

'sawed-off'
crutch

leather ring

These crutches
are easy to make
and work well
for children who
have strong arms
and hands.

rivets

A disadvantage
is that if a
child falls he
may have trouble
getting his arms
out quickly.

piece of
car tire

OTHER ELBOW CRUTCHES

With these open elbow-ring crutches, the child can easily get his arms out if he falls.

STANDARD ADJUSTABLE

USING LOCAL RESOURCES

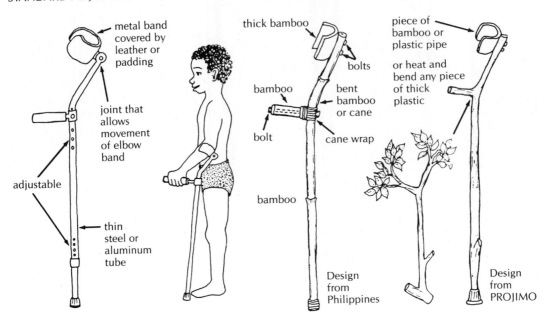

metal band covered by leather or padding

joint that allows movement of elbow band

adjustable

thin steel or aluminum tube

thick bamboo

bolts

bamboo

bent bamboo or cane

bolt

cane wrap

bamboo

Design from Philippines

piece of bamboo or plastic pipe

or heat and bend any piece of thick plastic

Design from PROJIMO

Gutter crutch ('arthritis crutch')
For children who, due to elbow pain or stiffness, cannot use straight-arm crutches.

Crutch for a child with weak elbow-straightening muscles.

STANDARD

USING LOCAL RESOURCES

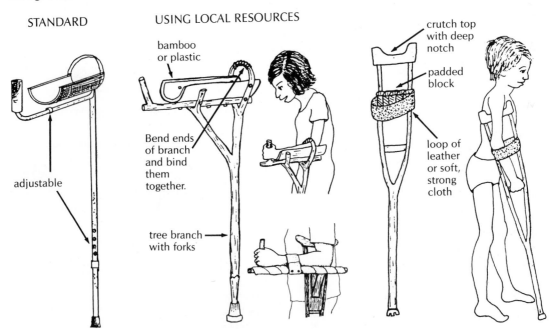

adjustable

bamboo or plastic

Bend ends of branch and bind them together.

tree branch with forks

crutch top with deep notch

padded block

loop of leather or soft, strong cloth

These are only examples. Once you get the idea, you can invent your own. A lot of experimentation is often needed to adapt crutches for children with severe arthritis.

Canes and walking sticks

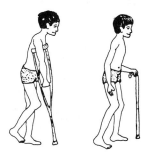

Straight poles can help a child with balance problems.

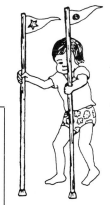

CAUTION: Use poles that are taller than child so if she falls, they will not poke her eyes.

Canes. Simple canes provide some balance and support, but the child has to use the walking muscles in both legs.

For the child who needs to strengthen a weak or painful leg, a cane makes him use his leg. A crutch lets him avoid using his leg, so the muscles that bend his leg get stronger, rather than the ones that straighten it. (See p. 526.)

CANES CUT FROM FOREST PLANTS

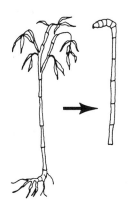

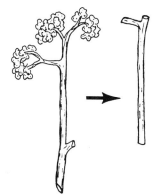

ADJUSTABLE METAL TUBE CANE

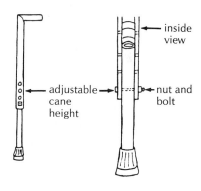

inside view

← adjustable cane height

← nut and bolt

3 OR 4 FOOTED CANE—FOR GREATER STABILITY

STANDARD METAL TUBE

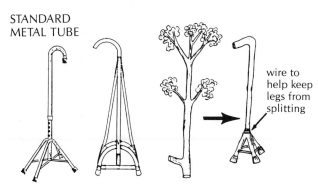

wire to help keep legs from splitting

ALTERNATIVE HANDGRIP

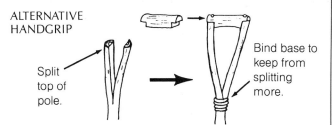

Split top of pole.

Bind base to keep from splitting more.

Rubber tip made from car tire

for metal tube or bamboo crutch or cane

STANDARD CRUTCH AND CANE TIP

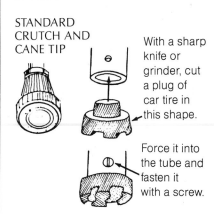

With a sharp knife or grinder, cut a plug of car tire in this shape.

Force it into the tube and fasten it with a screw.

metal ring

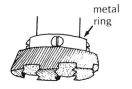

For walking in **sandy places**, make crutch and cane tips extra wide.

Adaptations of walking aids for carrying things and for work

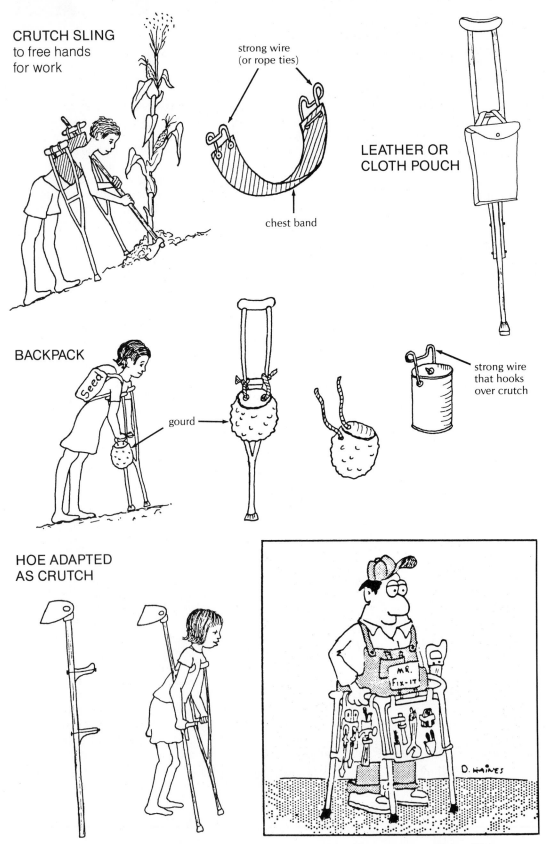

CRUTCH SLING
to free hands
for work

strong wire
(or rope ties)

chest band

**LEATHER OR
CLOTH POUCH**

BACKPACK

gourd

strong wire
that hooks
over crutch

**HOE ADAPTED
AS CRUTCH**

Reprinted from *Accent on Living,* 1984

Decisions about Special Seats and Wheelchairs

CHAPTER **64**

In this chapter we look at the things you will need to consider when buying or building a special seat or wheelchair, to best meet the needs of a child. *Adaptations* of seats and wheelchairs for special *positioning* needs are discussed in Chapter 65. Designs for building 6 basic wheelchairs are in Chapter 66.

Meeting the needs of the individual child, family, and community

Most children who need a wheelchair or special seat have severe weakness in parts of their bodies, or *muscles* that pull them into awkward or deforming positions. Seating should, as much as possible, keep these children in **healthy and useful** positions. It must **provide support,** but also **allow them enough freedom** to move, explore, and develop greater control of their bodies. For example:

1. A child who is 'floppy' and slow to develop ability to sit,

2. may at first need a seat with straps and supports to hold her up.

3. As she develops better head control and then body control, the supports can be removed little by little,

4. until finally— if possible— she is able to sit anywhere, with little or no special supports. Now low back support is all she needs.

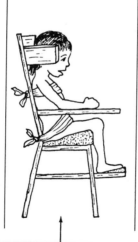

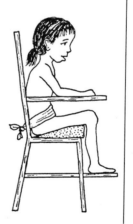

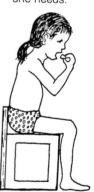

CAUTION: If a child needs to be supported as much as the one in the second picture, **do not keep her strapped in her seat for long.** She also needs periods of free movement and exercise to develop more independent head and body control. Keeping her strapped in for too long, or providing too much support after she has begun to gain more control, may actually slow down her progress. **Seating needs to be changed and supports reduced as the child develops.**

Also, children who do not feel in their *butts* need frequent position changes and 'lifting' (see p. 198), and special cushions (see p. 200).

Special seats and wheelchairs need to be adapted not only to the individual child, **but also to the particular family, local customs, and community situation.** For example:

A '**high chair**' lets the child join the family that eats at a table.

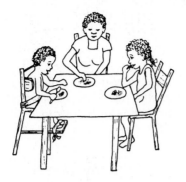

A '**low chair**' lets the child fit in where the family eats at ground level.

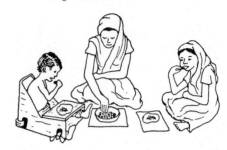

Also, a '**high**' **wheelchair** may be helpful where cooking and other activities are done high up.

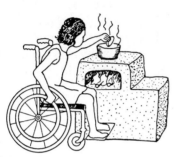

But a **low** '**wheelboard**' **or** '**trolley**' may be better where cooking and other activities are done at ground level.

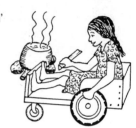

It is also important to consider the type of ground surface on which a wheelchair will be used.

Where land is flat and fairly smooth, and entrance into houses is level, a **chair with a small wheel at the rear** may work well and be less costly to make.

But where there are curbs, steps, rocks, or other obstacles, a chair with small wheels at the front works better.

On rough, sandy surfaces **wide back tires** and relatively large, wide front casters make moving about much easier.

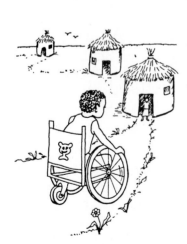

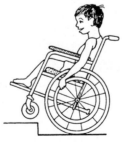

Narrow back tires and small front wheels allow for faster travel on hard smooth roads but are useless on rough, sandy roads.

To jump over obstacles, the child can learn to do a 'wheely' (tilt the chair back with the front wheels in the air).

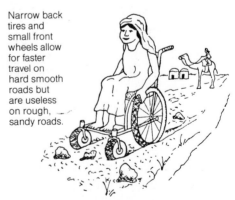

Wide tires, like the wide feet of a camel, help in sandy places.

Having the right wheelchair for the local situation frees the child to move about more easily in the community.

Healthy, comfortable, and functional positions

Whether or not a chair has wheels, **the position in which it allows a child to sit is very important.** (See Chapter 65.)

For most children, the chair should help them to sit more or less like this:

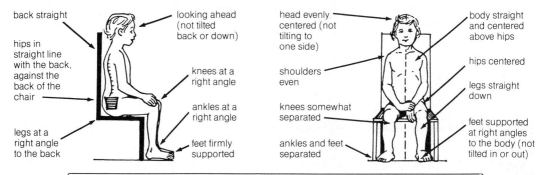

back straight

looking ahead (not tilted back or down)

hips in straight line with the back, against the back of the chair

knees at a right angle

ankles at a right angle

legs at a right angle to the back

feet firmly supported

head evenly centered (not tilting to one side)

shoulders even

knees somewhat separated

ankles and feet separated

body straight and centered above hips

hips centered

legs straight down

feet supported at right angles to the body (not tilted in or out)

> *CAUTION:* **The seat should be wide enough to allow some free movement and narrow enough to give needed support** (see Measurements, p. 602).

Common seating problems and possible solutions

Problem: **Hips tilt back**

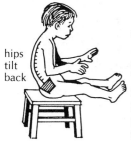

hips tilt back

In children with spastic cerebral palsy the hips often stiffen backward. This triggers spasms that straighten the legs and cause other muscle tightness with loss of control.

Also, children with weak hips or back, from *spinal cord* injury, spina bifida, or severe polio, often sit slumped with their hips tilted back and the back severely curved. This can lead to permanent deformity.

One of the most common causes of backward tilting hips is **a chair like this one that is too big** for the child.

Other causes of backward tilt and bad position are:	A good position can often be gained through:

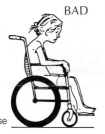

a chair back that tilts far back

and a cloth back that sags.

These let the child lean back and cause the hips to slip forward.

BAD

Also, footrests that are far forward so that knees do not bend enough can increase *spasticity* that tilts hips back.

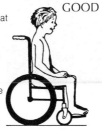

a fairly **stiff, upright back** at a right angle to the seat,

a chair that fits the child so that his hips reach the chair back,

GOOD

the knees at right angles, and **feet firmly supported.**

BETTER

Most children, and especially a child who tends to fall forward in his seat, will sit better and more comfortably if the whole chair tilts back a little. But be sure to keep right angles at hips, knees, and ankles.

> To tilt the chair back, the rear wheel mount can be moved higher **up**. You may also need to move the wheel mount **back** farther to keep the chair from falling backward with going uphill. Be sure the front caster barrel is still straight up or making turns will be harder.

 NO

 YES

Keeping cost down and quality up

For many families, a wheelchair can be a great or even impossible expense. There are many ways to keep costs down. But be careful. Some low-cost choices may make the chair too clumsy, weak, or unsafe. Other low-cost choices may actually increase the chair's usefulness and life. For example, a very useful, long-lasting wheelchair can be made of wood—or from a cheap wooden chair. Even wheels made of wood (if made well) may work well and last a long time. But, making the hubs or bearings of wood usually leads to trouble. Standard wheelchair wheel bearings are very expensive. However, you can often get strong, high-quality, used metal bearings free or very cheap at electrical appliance repair shops or auto repair shops.

Factory-made or homemade wheelchairs?

Often you can save money by making your own wheelchair or by asking a local craftsperson to make one. Also, a homemade chair design can be more easily adapted to your child's particular needs.

On the next pages we give information that may help you decide about different wheelchairs and effective low-cost ways to make them.

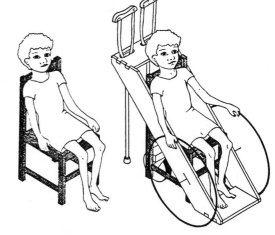

You can make a fairly effective low-cost wheelchair by attaching bicycle wheels or wooden wheels to an ordinary wooden chair. Also, it is easier to attach special aids or supports to a wooden chair than to a metal chair. This design is adapted from AHRTAG's booklet, "Personal Transport for Disabled People" (see p. 604).

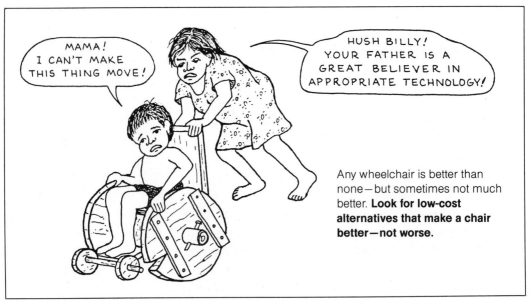

Any wheelchair is better than none—but sometimes not much better. **Look for low-cost alternatives that make a chair better—not worse.**

REMEMBER: A wheelchair needs to satisfy the rider—not just the maker. Before (and after) buying or making a chair, think carefully about the different features that will help it best meet the needs of the particular child and family.

When buying or making a wheelchair (or any other aids), consider:

- **Cost.** Keep **cost low** but **quality high** enough to meet the child's needs (see p. 592).

- **How long will the chair last?** The longer the better, unless it is only for temporary use.

- **How easy and quick is it to make?** The easier and quicker the better, as long as it meets your needs.

- **Availability of materials.** Make use of local low-cost, good-quality resources (local wood, cheap metal, used bearings, bike parts, etc.).

- **What tools and skills are needed to make it?** If welding equipment or skills are not locally available, a wooden chair may be a more practical choice.

- **How easy will it be to adjust or repair?** Wood chairs that are bolted together are often the easiest to adjust or add special supports to.

- **Weight.** The lighter the better, while making sure it is strong enough.

- **Strength.** Heavier persons need stronger chairs and stronger axles. (A small child's chair may be supported by a bicycle axle attached on one side only. A bigger child needs the axle to be supported on both sides, or a stronger axle. See p. 598 and 615.)

- **Width and length.** The narrower and shorter the better while meeting the child's needs (but not so short that it tips over easily).

- **How easily can it be moved** — by the child sitting in it or by someone behind? **How easily can it be tilted back** to go over rough spots? **Lifted** up stairs? **Transported?** (Does it need to **fold** to take up less space?)

- **How well is it adapted to the particular child's wants and needs?** Is it comfortable? Does it allow the child to sit in a healthy position?

- **Fit and growth factor.** How well does it fit the child now? How long will it continue to fit her? Can it be adjusted to fit her as she grows?

- **How well is it adapted to living situations,** the **home,** local **customs,** width of **doorways,** surface of **floors** and **roads,** curbs and other barriers?

- **Appearance.** Is the chair attractive? Does the child take pride in it? Do other children want to ride it?

In considering choices for the design, building materials, and special features of a wheelchair, be sure to carefully consider the above questions.

Design choices for wheelchairs

FEATURE	DESIGN DETAILS	ADVANTAGES	DISADVANTAGES
WHEEL SIZE AND POSITION **2 big wheels** with 1 or 2 small caster wheels INDOOR OUTDOOR one or 2 rear wheels rear wheel set back to avoid tipping backward on slopes Child's weight should be mostly over big wheels.	• Large wheels let rider push herself. • Small caster wheels allow easy turns (on cement, not sand). • For leg amputees, rear wheels must be moved back to prevent tipping over backward.	• Child can move it herself if she has hand and arm control. • Large wheels go over rough surfaces easier.	• takes up more space • harder to get in and out of from the side (because wheels need to be higher than seat so that rider can push herself)
4 small wheels casters for easier turning	Very simple temporary chairs can be made by putting 4 wheels on an ordinary wood chair. chair leg pin rod wheels	• good only on smooth floors for a child who cannot push or help push his own chair • cheaper • takes up less space • easier to move child in and out of	• not good on rough surfaces • Child cannot move it herself. • creates dependency
3 big wheels hand crank and steering	• You can use 3 bicycle wheels. • Some models have removable front wheel so that chair can be easily changed to small front wheels for use inside the home.	• excellent for long distance and rough road travel • can be used by a person with strength in one hand only Some riders have 2 chairs: one like this for road travel, and a smaller one for home or work.	• too big for use inside home • more costly • more difficult to make
BUILDING MATERIAL FOR FRAME **Steel tube** Whirlwind wheelchair See p. 622. AHRTAG design, see p. 604.	• Thin-walled electrical conduit tubing can be used—5/8 inch to 1 inch diameter.	A strong, long-lasting, fairly light chair can be made better and cheaper than most commercial chairs.	• requires welding skills, some design ability, and a fair amount of equipment • a good chair for a well-equipped rehabilitation center workshop to build, but not a family • builders need to be trained
Wood AHRTAG model	For wood design details, see p. 615 and 620 and references on p. 604. wood chair model design p. 615 plywood model design p. 620	• relatively cheap and easy to make—mostly wood, few or no welds • easy to adapt and to add special supports or tray tables	• May not be as stable and long-lasting as other models. (For tighter joints and more adaptability, use nuts and bolts instead of nails.)

FEATURE	DESIGN DETAILS	ADVANTAGES	DISADVANTAGES
Re-bar (metal reinforcing rod used to strengthen cement) 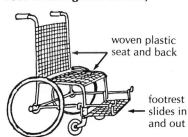 woven plastic seat and back footrest slides in and out	Design can be the same as for metal tube chairs, but it is easier to adapt because the re-bar is easy to bend.	• relatively cheap • easier to bend and weld than steel tubing • can have plastic woven seat and back (easy to clean) • especially good for small chairs	• A heavy person or rough treatment may bend it out of shape. • fairly heavy
PVC pipe (plastic water pipe) 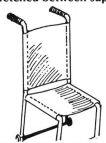	• Use 15 mm. PVC pipe. • comes with joints so that it can be fitted together with a special glue • For details see reference, p. 606.	• lightweight • can be built mostly by glueing pieces together	• costly materials (around $100 US) • Plastic tubing will in time sag or bend in the direction of stress. Therefore it may be necessary to fiberglass the frame—which adds to cost, work, and weight.
SEATS AND BACKS **Soft canvas or leather stretched between supports** 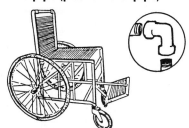	• For child who is likely to pee or shit in the chair, use a cloth that is easy to wash. • Plastic-coated canvas makes cleaning easy but is hot and may irritate child's bottom. Best to use an absorbent washable pad over it.	• easiest seating and back design for folding wheelchairs • Adjustment to shape of butt gives comfort (but cushion is needed to protect against pressure sores). • Curving back may help keep child from falling sideways.	• Soft, curving back lets child bend in an unhealthy position (see p. 591). • hard to attach positioning aids • In children with spasticity or muscle imbalance, this may increase the risk of developing knock-knee *contractures.*
Firm (but padded) back and seat 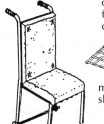 other possibilities for use under cushion metal slats wood slats	• Use wood or thin plywood. • Special designs allow a wood seat to swing up for folding.	• Wood seat and back allow easy addition of supports and adaptations. • Firm wood back and seat help child sit with back straight and knees apart (especially important for children with spasticity).	• may be less comfortable • without cushion may cause pressure sores in child with no feeling in his butt • heavier • difficult or impossible to fold the chair
Woven seat and back 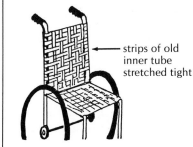 strips of old inner tube stretched tight	• Use natural basket fibers, reeds, or rattan, • or use plastic webbing, • or use tightly stretched strips of car inner tube.	• An open weave is cooler in hot weather. • Plastic or rubber woven seats can be easily washed. Can be used as a chair to bathe in.	• must be kept stretched tight; not useful on folding chairs • may not last long if material is not strong • same sag problems as with canvas or leather

FEATURE	DESIGN DETAILS	ADVANTAGES	DISADVANTAGES
TIRES **Pump-up with air 'balloon' tires**	• Bicycle tires and tubes work well for the large wheels—20 inch (51 cm.), 24 inch (61 cm.), or 26 inch (66 cm.), **wide or narrow.** Puncture-proof inner liners may be available.	• **softer ride** • easy to replace • **wide** tires good for sand and rough ground • **narrow** tires better on smooth, paved roads	• **Puncture** (hole in tire) may occur—especially on rough roads. • more costly than some other tires • wears out sooner than solid tires
Solid tires (standard wheelchair wheels)	Buy from wheelchair supply center to fit diameter and width of rim.	• no flat tires • good for speed on very smooth surfaces	• costly • hard to replace • very hard, bumpy ride on rough surfaces • very narrow—sinks into sand
Rubber hose inside bicycle tire	• Overlap ends and cut at 45° angle. • Fit hose into tire.	• no flat tires • softer ride than with solid tire • cheap	• Flattening of tire where it touches ground means it moves slower, and is harder to push.
Thin strip of old car tire	• Cut strip in wedge shape to fit rim. • Wire ends together.	• no cost • long-lasting Sink bolt head, Wire ends together. and/or bolt the ends.	• bumpy ride • difficult to fit well on rim and to fasten ends firmly
Large machinery fanbelt (discarded)	• Use old power belts or fan belts from industrial machinery or tractors. Cut to fit and wire ends together.	• no cost • long-lasting • wedged to fit wedge rim	• bumpy ride • difficult to fit • may be hard to find at the right width
Piece of old bicycle or scooter tire	• used for middle-sized or small **wood wheels** • Notch edges, glue, and nail to wheel.	• cheap • If heavy tire is used it may last a long time. • Protects edge of wood wheel.	• hard, bumpy ride (but softer than on wood wheel alone) • may tear off
BIG WHEELS **Standard factory-made wheelchair wheels**	• Buy to fit chair. • available from wheelchair dealers • 24 inch (61 cm.) or 26 inch (66 cm.) rims for adults • 20 inch (51 cm.) rims for small children (may be hard to find)	• little work needed (if they are bought to fit standard hubs) • May come fitted with hand push rim.	• costly • may be hard to find • wide-wheeled models often not available • may not hold up on rough ground • poor quality bearings
Bicycle wheels (rims and spokes)	• For children, standard thickness spokes may be enough. • For large persons, heavy-duty spokes may be needed.	• less costly than standard wheelchair wheels • available in different sizes and widths	• Putting on and lining up spokes takes time and skill. • axles weak (but stronger ones can be adapted)
Bicycle rims with wooden spokes	• notched wood cross-pieces on a triangular wood base can be greased and used as the hub	• no need to know how to fit spokes • works with wood hub	• Rim may easily get bent—especially on rough roads. • hard to line up evenly • Hub wears out easily.

FEATURE	DESIGN DETAILS	ADVANTAGES	DISADVANTAGES
Wood wheels—big or small 	• Use boards or plywood. • To avoid splitting, screw and glue 2 layers together with grain running in opposite directions. • Cut notch in rim to hold solid tire.	• relatively cheap • little skill required—mostly carpentry • works with wood axles • heavy-duty bearing can be added	• often heavy • may not hold up long—especially in wet climate or mud (Keeping wood oil-soaked helps them last. Use old engine oil.)
CASTERS AND WHEELS (**Caster** means that the wheel can swing in different directions for making turns.) **Standard wheelchair caster wheels** 	• Casters come with hard or balloon tires in many sizes, weights, styles, and prices. If possible, get (or make) casters with ball bearings.	• little work to attach—especially if standard mount and bearings are used	• usually very costly • may not be locally available
Casters from other (non-wheelchair) equipment (used or new) for mounting into metal tube frame for mounting on wood frame caster welded to metal plate for screwing to wood	• Use 3 inch to 6 inch wheels. • larger, wider wheels for rough ground • Be sure bearings are strong enough and in good condition. • Drill holes in rubber wheels to make them weigh less.	• less costly (especially if not new) • often full wheel and caster bearings come with them	• Poor quality casters make wheelchair much harder and more awkward to use. • Hard-rubber casters make a bumpy ride. • Some used casters are too weak.
Bent and welded steel caster forks 	• Choose bolt width to fit bearings. • A bent steel tube can be used instead of a metal band.	• less costly than factory-made casters • strong (if well made)	• needs special equipment (bending jig) and welding skills
HUBS, BEARINGS, AND AXLES **Standard wheelchair bearings** ball bearings ball bearings at each end of hub	• A standard wheelchair uses 12 bearings: 2 for each wheel axle and 2 for each upright caster bearing. • How a ball bearing works: 	• These bearings come as part of standard wheelchair hubs and wheels. • Most factory-built wheelchairs have unusual sized axles and therefore must be fit with special wheelchair bearings.	• Bearings on most factory-built chairs are costly, of poor quality, and wear out quickly. • Unusual hub size makes it hard to replace commercial wheelchair bearings with other standard machine bearings.
Bicycle bearings and axles front wheel axle hub axle	For mounting alternatives, see wheelchair designs p. 598 and 615. Also, see the AHRTAG Manual (see p. 604).	• cheap—especially if old bicycles are used • easy to get • can be used with complete bicycle wheels	• Axle is too weak to be supported by one end only (except in a small child's wheelchair).

FEATURE	DESIGN DETAILS	ADVANTAGES	DISADVANTAGES
Rear bicycle wheel axle and bearings hub metal plate wheelchair frame	• First take free-wheel mechanism apart and remove ratchets. • Then attach hub to a metal plate as shown and spot weld it. • Other methods for one-end axle support are in the AHRTAG Manual (see p. 604).	• Allows axles to be attached by one end only.	• Needs fairly skilled work and welding. • heavy
Used machinery bearings thin metal pipe 5/8'' bolt holes for spokes narrower tube to hold bearings apart bearing	• Find used high-speed bearings of the size shown (or near the size). *Volkswagen* alternator bearings and certain power tool bearings work well. • Use 5/8 inch steel bolts for axle. For details, see p. 604, 622, and 623.	• no need to adjust, grease, or clean • usually free or very cheap • In wheelchairs they will last a very long time. • If done well, results are better than with commercial hubs and bearings.	• very careful exact work needed for good results
Wood bearing washer bolt (welded to fork) oil-soaked wood tube metal fork wood wheel (oil-soaked hole) bolt spot welded to fork	• Use a hard wood that will not split. • Soak wood in old motor oil. • For more ideas and details on wood bearings, see AHRTAG Manual p. 604.	• cheap and fairly easy to make	• tends to wear out, wobble, or crack quickly unless very well made; not as smooth or easy to ride as with ball bearings
SUPPORT OF AXLES **Axle supported on one side only** nut axle passes through metal tube welded to frame This is the standard mount for factory-built chairs.	• Strong steel axles are needed for support at one side only. Axle should be at least 5/8 inch thick for a large person. • For a very small child bicycle axles can be supported by one side only. One way is to weld bicycle axles to a thin metal pipe.	• Not as wide or heavy as the chair with 2-side support. • easier for user to get a full-length push with hands and arms • narrow size important for doorways and transporting Pass pipe through a wood frame, or weld to metal frame.	• For adults and large children, standard bicycle axles are too weak for one-side support. • Even for smaller children, bicycle axles are weak, and rough use can bend them. Put a sign on chair: FOR SMALL CHILDREN ONLY
Axle supported on both sides This can be done in several ways: metal strips on wood frame metal tube on tube frame 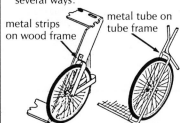	• Place outer bar of axle support so that it allows as much room for hand pushing by the rider as possible. single caster wood on wood frame 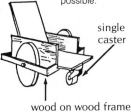	• 2-sided support allows use of standard bicycle wheels and axles. • easy to build and replace re-bar loop on re-bar frame 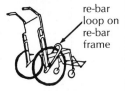	• chair wider, more difficult to get through narrow doors and spaces; more difficult to transport • Wheel supports get in the way of hands when user moves by pushing wheels. • heavy

FEATURE	DESIGN DETAILS	ADVANTAGES	DISADVANTAGES
TO FOLD OR NOT TO FOLD **A typical folding chair** 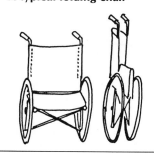	• folding mechanism usually with 2 scissoring flexible cross pieces and cloth or leather seat • For details of a make-it-yourself model, see p. 622.	**Folding:** • narrow when folded for easier transport or storage • smoother ride due to flexibility **Non-folding:** • cheaper and lighter • easier to make • more adaptable • often stronger	**Folding:** • heavier • harder to make • more costly • less adaptable **Non-folding:** • Transport in cars and buses more difficult. Consider how much this will affect the child's ability to go where she wants. • stiff ride
ARMRESTS **No armrests** 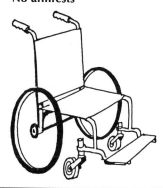	*Note:* Many chairs are built so that armrests are part of the main structure and strength of the chair. The armrests cannot be easily removed, even though this might benefit the child. Carefully consider the child's need for armrests **before** buying or making a chair.	• Many children with strong arms and trunk control prefer a chair with no armrests and a very low back support. • Moving by pushing the wheels is easier. • less weight • Getting off and on from the side is easier — especially important when legs are completely *paralyzed* and when arms are also weak.	• Many small children need armrests for stability, for positioning, or for comfort.
Fixed armrests 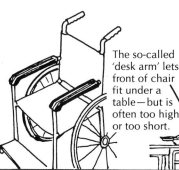 The so-called 'desk arm' lets front of chair fit under a table — but is often too high or too short. 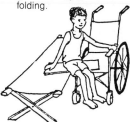	• Armrest height and length should be determined for each child and her needs. • For measurements, see p. 602.	• especially helpful if child cannot use legs to get out of chair • They can help child to sit in a better position and be more comfortable. • They can sometimes be used for attaching a removable table.	• They get in the way for pushing wheels and for getting off chair to the side. • **For many children, fixed armrests get in the way more than they help.**
Removable armrests 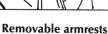 adjustable armrest 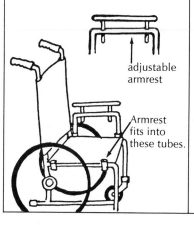Armrest fits into these tubes.	• In folding chairs, armrest attachments must be placed so they do not get in the way of folding. child transferring from a chair on a board — one armrest removed	• Provides arm support when needed, yet can easily be removed for travel and transfer.	• requires more work, materials, and exact fittings • adds slightly to weight • Separate armrests may get lost.

FEATURE	DESIGN DETAILS	ADVANTAGES	DISADVANTAGES
FOOTRESTS **Positions** In adult chairs, footrests often angle legs forward to leave room for casters. For a small child, often footrests can position legs straight down. This is important in many cases (see p. 591). A larger child may need to sit on cushions so that his feet are above the casters.	• Footrest should keep the knees and ankles at right angles and the legs slightly separated. • It should usually not twist them or force them together. 	• Good positioning and support of the feet help the whole body to stay in a better position. A footrest like this, may help feet like these. 	• A footrest that keeps the leg at right angles may cause or increase knee contractures in some children. Children should not stay sitting too long and should do daily exercises to stretch their legs, feet, and hips. To prevent or correct contractures, one or both legs may need to be kept as straight as they will go.
Fixed position footrests The height of the rests should be carefully measured to fit the child who will use them. (For measurements, see p. 602.) *REMEMBER:* Cushions or seating adaptations will change the height needed for the footrests.	• If the footrest is too low, blocks can be placed on it to make it higher. They can be removed as the child grows. • However, fixed footrests that are too high are more difficult to correct. So it is better if they are too low. 	• easiest to build • For a small child who can easily be lifted in and out of the chair, they are fine. • If footrests are screwed or bolted onto a wooden wheelchair, their position can easily be changed as the child grows.	• They often get in the way when the child gets in or out of the chair, or in the way of the person lifting a larger child. (See other methods below.)
Removable or swing-away footrests wood chair swing-away footrest 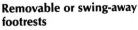 back-stop for feet pin on which footrest swings stops	There are many designs. Here we show one for the wood chair shown above and one designed for a metal chair. Other designs for sliding or swing-away footrests are on pages 616, and 622. 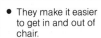 metal chair footrest See p. 622. swing up	• They make it easier to get in and out of chair. • The best footrests are those the child can easily move out of the way herself. 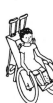	• Removable footrests may get lost. • more work to make them • Unless well-made, they may be less stable than fixed footrests.
Adjustable footrests hand hole for pulling 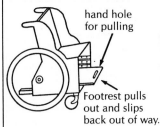 Footrest pulls out and slips back out of way. Also serves as storage shelf.	There are many designs. Here is one of the simplest, for a plywood chair. FRONT VIEW strips of wood to form slots adjustable height 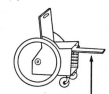 For straight leg sitting, a longer board fits into high slots.	• very adaptable • easy to make • can support a casted leg 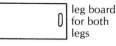 leg board for both legs for one leg	• A cushion or padding should be placed over the leg board (unless leg is casted). • Side supports may be needed to keep leg from slipping off. 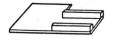
No footrests 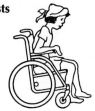	• Seat is mounted low so that feet rest flat on floor.	• useful for persons who can pull their chair along with their legs and feet—especially when one or both arms or hands are too weak to push the wheels	• Feet may drag when someone else pushes the child in the chair. Swing-away footrests may be the best solution.

FEATURE	DESIGN DETAILS	ADVANTAGES	DISADVANTAGES
PARKING BRAKES **Lever brakes** Brake for wooden chair	There are many brake designs. This one is from AHRTAG. Two others are on p. 623. SIDE VIEW push handle out and up catch weld pivot metal plate washer split pin	• takes little space • fairly easy to use if made right (which often they are not)	• needs welding and skill to make • Homemade brakes often give problems—yet it is important that chairs have them if possible.
Parking block	Brakes on wheelchairs are for keeping the chair from rolling when getting in or out, or stopped on a hill. The simplest form of brake is a parking block that keeps the wheel from turning. To 'brake', roll wheel up ramp and into groove.	• easy to make, requires no welding, and is cheap • If the child usually only gets in and out of the chair in one or two places in the home, blocks in these places may be all that is needed.	• a heavy, awkward object to move from place to place • not practical outside the house (or in it) • have to tilt child to one side to 'park' chair
HANDRIMS FOR PUSHING using thin metal tubing (cane or wood have also been used) jig for bending tube Cut down this line before removing from jig. Weld ends. Wrap tube around several times to make several rims at once.	Designs taken from ARHTAG. See p. 604.	• Handrims help keep hands clean. (Otherwise child has to push on tire.) • especially important where there are very dirty paths and roads tire Attach rim with metal brackets like this. bracket rim	• Added width makes it harder to get through narrow doorways. • adds weight
Handrim grip improvers rim pegs wood or rubber tube rim bolt nut Posts can be bolted or welded onto rim.	Cut a piece of rubber hose lengthwise and tape it onto rim. cut rim hose metal post welded onto rim	• For child with weak or paralyzed hands, a smooth rim can be hard to grip—especially if it is chromed or galvanized. • Putting rough cloth tape, a rubber hose or many small handles on the rim will make pushing easier. • Or you can wrap the rim with a long thin strip of car tire inner tube.	• Pegs sticking out from rims increase width of chair. • Pegs sometimes cause hand injuries—especially when going fast downhill. strip of inner tube rim

Fitting the chair to the child: measurements

These measurements are for **wheelchairs** and for **special seating without wheels.**

SEAT WIDTH

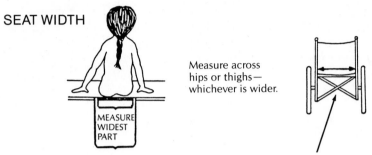

Measure across hips or thighs— whichever is wider.

MEASURE WIDEST PART

Add 1 cm. (1/2 inch) to both sides for seat width.

Note: Some specialists recommend wider seats. But the child gets a better arm position for pushing the wheels if only 1 cm. is added on either side. However, you may want to leave a little more room to allow for the child's growth.

SEAT DEPTH

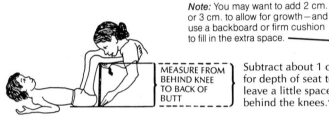

Note: You may want to add 2 cm. or 3 cm. to allow for growth—and use a backboard or firm cushion to fill in the extra space.

MEASURE FROM BEHIND KNEE TO BACK OF BUTT

Subtract about 1 cm. for depth of seat to leave a little space behind the knees.

CAUTION: When measuring, be sure to allow for cushions or backboards that will be added.

SEAT HEIGHT

CAUTION: Be sure to include cushion when measuring height for chair seat.

Note: Raising the seat of a small child higher lets his feet rest above the casters and therefore directly below the knees. The higher seat also helps for eating at the table with the family. Sideways transfers are also easier. Sometimes seats are placed even higher than shown, but this makes pushing wheels with hands more difficult.

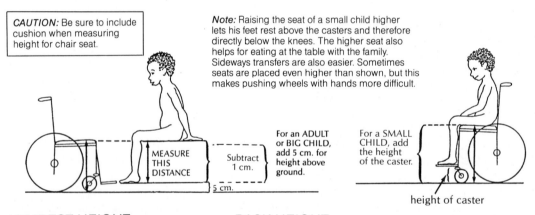

MEASURE THIS DISTANCE

Subtract 1 cm.

5 cm.

For an ADULT or BIG CHILD, add 5 cm. for height above ground.

For a SMALL CHILD, add the height of the caster.

height of caster

ARMREST HEIGHT

MEASURE FROM BOTTOM OF BUTT TO BEND OF ELBOW.

Before measuring, be sure child is sitting as straight as possible.

Put armrest height a little higher than his elbow so that the elbow will be positioned away from the body.

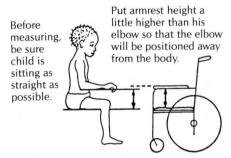

Note: This measurement is standard, but some children need arm support at a higher level. Experiment.

BACK HEIGHT

MEASURE FROM BOTTOM OF BUTT TO ARMPIT.

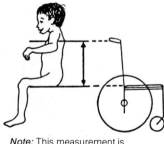

Note: This measurement is standard, but some children need a higher back, and sometimes head support. Others prefer a back that supports only the hips.

IMPORTANT: Also check how much hips and knees bend, as this may affect position of footrests and casters.

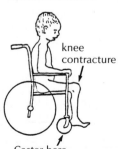

knee contracture

Caster here will not work.

Wheelchair production as a small 'village-industry'

In several countries small groups of disabled persons have started to produce low-cost, good-quality wheelchairs adapted to local needs. Usually this is in places where standard factory-made wheelchairs are very high-priced and are not suited for use on rough or sandy ground.

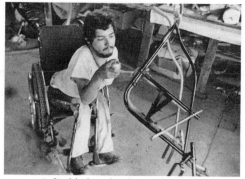

Some of these 'little factories' try to be self-sufficient. A few have even succeeded in making a modest profit, while keeping prices low.

A disabled worker from PROJIMO paints a wheelchair frame.

Sometimes, a small-scale wheelchair making and repair shop is set up as part of a community rehabilitation program. Self-sufficiency (selling the chairs for a little more than it costs to make them) is often a goal. But because families with the greatest need are often least able to pay, the chairs must often be sold below cost.

WHAT KIND OF WHEELCHAIRS TO MAKE

This depends on many factors: cost, skills or training available, tools and equipment needed, amount of money available to start, building materials available, the possible market, the local economy, and needs of the wheelchair user and family.

For example, folding tube-metal chairs are relatively expensive to make and require more skill, training, and equipment. However, they often work smoother, last longer, and are easier to transport than are many other models. These high-quality, good-looking chairs — painted or even chrome plated — may sell the best, even if expensive, and may compete with factory-made chairs (see p. 622).

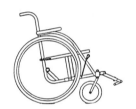

If the wheelchair users will be mostly children and poor families, low-cost wooden chairs may be more appropriate. These can be easily built to size and adapted to the needs of the individual child. The chair may not last as long. But the child is growing and her needs may change. Simple wood chairs also require fewer skills to build — mainly carpentry. They are easier for the family to build, repair, or add changes to at home.

Ideally, a village shop would make a variety of chairs out of different materials and at different prices. Chairs of all models, sizes, and adaptations should be kept on hand to give the child and family a chance to know and try different possibilities. **Be sure to make child-sized chairs. And make chair inserts so that adult-sized chairs can be adapted for children.**

Look for every opportunity to keep costs low. Providing **repair services** for used and broken chairs are good ways to keep children on wheels. Also use as much 'waste', and used and free materials as you can: old bicycle wheels, old machinery bearings, scrap metal, and bolts from junk yards. For basic building materials, check prices of different sellers. Once you are sure of what you need, try to buy large amounts at lower cost. If you explain to the sellers the purpose of your purchase, they may lower prices or give you useful scraps.

Designs for 6 different wheelchairs are in Chapter 66.

How-to-do-it Reference Materials for Wheelchairs, Wheelboards, and Other Seating

It is impossible, in a book such as this, to give detailed building plans for more than a few wheelchairs, scooters, wheelboards (trolleys), and special seats. The following reference materials have more detailed plans. You can send for them at the addresses shown. Some may also be available from TALC, P.O. Box 49, St. Albans, Herts, AL1 4AX, England. With each reference we give one or more drawings of key designs and a few comments about their usefulness and cost.

Personal Transport for Disabled People—Design and Manufacture

AHRTAG
Farringdon Point
29-35 Farringdon Road
London EC1M 3JB
ENGLAND

Also available through TALC

- many good designs and plans for low-cost aids
- does not compare strengths and weaknesses or describe limitations of different designs
- no design for wheelchairs with casters in front (which are needed for many areas)

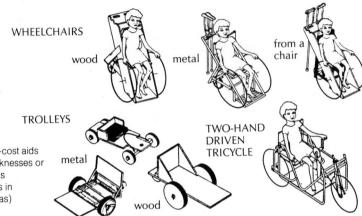

Independence through Mobility: A Guide to the Manufacture of the ATI-Hotchkiss Wheelchair
by Ralf Hotchkiss

c/o Wheeled Mobility Center
Dept. of Engineering SFSU
San Francisco, CA 94132, USA

- design for the 'whirlwind', a high-quality middle-cost steel tube wheelchair that can be built by disabled craftspersons as a village industry
- short training usually needed to build it effectively; welding skills and simple math required
- cost of materials about US $100

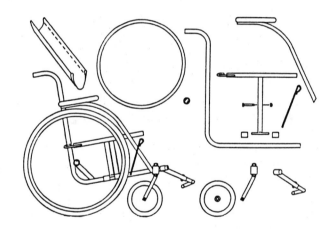

Local Village-made Wheelchairs and Trolleys
by Don Caston

Available upon request.

DON CASTON
202 Cheesman Terrace
London W14 9XD
ENGLAND

- simple, very low-cost aids, made mostly out of wood, using bicycle or wood wheels
- all models are based on one 3-wheel trolley design
- Instead of a standard caster, the front slides on its axle and is pushed back to center by a choice of simple methods. (This method is cheap and clever, but unstable and does not turn as well as designs with casters.)

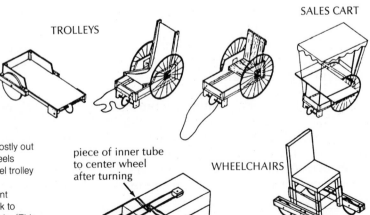

Asia-Pacific Disability Aids and Appliances Handbook, Part 1: Mobility Aids, 1982

ICTA
Box 510 S-162-15
Vällingby, SWEDEN

- brief descriptions and non-technical drawings and addresses for information on many aids

TROLLEYS

ADAPTED TRICYCLE

ONE-HAND POWERED TRICYCLE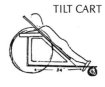

'HOMEMADE' ELECTRIC WHEELCHAIR USING CAR FAN MOTOR AND BICYCLE PARTS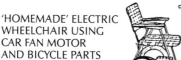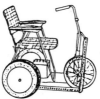

WHEELCHAIR TO BE PULLED OVER ROUGH GROUND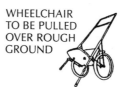

TILT CART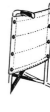

An Accent Guide to Wheelchairs and Accessories

ACCENT
P.O. Box 700
Bloomington, IL 61702
USA

- information about different aids, features, and accessories of factory-made chairs
- basic information on cleaning and repairing
- design and building information limited to a few accessories

LAP TRAYS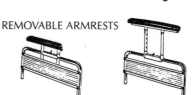

BACKS

REMOVABLE ARMRESTS

UPKARAN—A Manual of Aids for the Multiply Handicapped

The Spastics Society of India
Upper Colaba Road
Near Afghan Church
Bombay 400 005
India

- an excellent resource
- many simple, practical designs for seating, wheelchairs, crawlers, standers, walkers, therapy aids, and toys

SEATS

adjustable

WHEELCHAIRS

toilet adaptation

PUSH-ALONG

TRICYCLE WITH SUPPORT

WALKER-RIDER

TIRE SCOOTER

How to Make Basic Hospital Equipment
by Roger England and Will Eaves

Intermediate Technology Publications
103-105 Southampton Row
London WC1B 4HH
ENGLAND

Also available through TALC and AHRTAG

- simple, attractive designs using tube steel
- welding skill required; fairly costly to make
- no designs for casters-in-front chairs

HOSPITAL WHEELCHAIR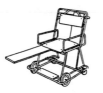

OUT-OF-HOSPITAL WHEELCHAIR (2 wheels only)

BICYCLE AMBULANCE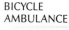

CHAIR MADE WITH WHEELS OF RATTAN (also works as a walker)

ONE-HAND DRIVEN TRICYCLE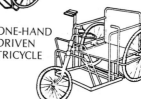

Poliomyelitis—A Guide for Developing Countries
by R.L. Huckstep

Churchill Livingstone
5 S Fontenac Road
Naperville, IL 60563 USA

- detailed designs for 3 models of wheelchairs commonly used in Africa
- only casters-at-rear designs (which often may not be the most appropriate design)

WHEELCHAIRS

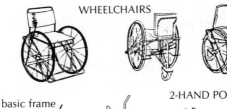

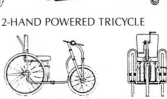

2-HAND POWERED TRICYCLE

basic frame

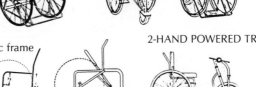

Positioning the Client with Central Nervous System Deficits: The Wheelchair and Other Adapted Equipment
by Adrienne Falk Bergen and Cheryl Colangelo

Valhalla Rehabilitation Publications, Ltd.
P.O. Box 195
Valhalla, NY 10595
USA

- excellent detailed discussion of specific needs of children with cerebral palsy
- many well-illustrated examples
- written for developed countries but many aids and designs are simple and can be made anywhere at low cost

SEAT BELTS

WRONG RIGHT WRONG RIGHT

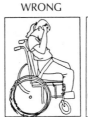 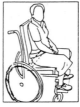 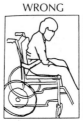 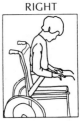

This child, whose hips tilt forward, needs a higher belt.

This child, whose hips tilt back, needs a low belt.

'Build Yourself' Plastic Wheelchair

Directions for assembly available from:

Spinal Research Unit
Royal North Shore Hospital of Sydney
St. Leonards, NSW 2065
Australia

- relatively expensive (materials about US $100)

- plastic frame made of 9 m. of 15 mm. PVC pressure pipe; plastic set of 8 mm. soft PVC tubing; 2 rear 24 inch bicycle wheels; 2 front casters (15 mm.)
- relatively expensive (materials about US $100)
- Plastic will sag with continued use.
- uses standard bicycle axles—which will bend with the weight of an adult or large child
- relatively lightweight
- does not fold
- design plan complicated and difficult to follow

Measuring the Patient

Everest and Jennings, Inc.
Available through Everest and Jennings wheelchair dealers or:

Everest and Jennings
4203 Earth City Expressway
Earth City, MO 63045 USA

- good information on measurements for standard chairs
- illustrated discussion of problems with chairs that do not meet a person's specific needs

SEAT HEIGHT

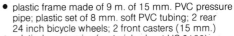

too low

too high

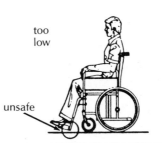 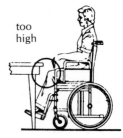

unsafe

Functional Aids for the Multiply Handicapped
by Isabel Robinault

Harper and Collins Sales
10 East 53rd Street
NYC, NY 10022 USA

- mostly factory-built examples but some are simple and well-illustrated enough to serve as design guides
- many good wood special seats
- also support frames, standers, walkers, toys, and eating aids

SMALL-WHEELED ADJUSTABLE WALKERS

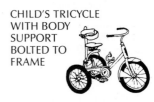

CHILD'S TRICYCLE WITH BODY SUPPORT BOLTED TO FRAME

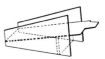

SCOOTER THAT IS ALSO A WHEELED STANDER

 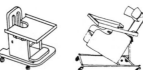

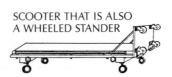

SUPPORT FRAME

Adaptations for Wheelchairs and Other Sitting Aids

Many children need more support or special *positioning* than is usually provided by a regular chair or ordinary wheelchair. So we should try to **get or make a chair designed to fit the individual child.** Unfortunately, many children get wheelchairs that are much **too big.** Often no others are available. Here are 3 ways to adapt them.

(CP)

---

1. **If a folding chair is too wide,** make the cloth seat and back narrower. The chair will not open as wide (but may be too high).

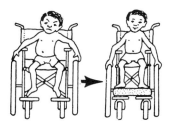

TOO WIDE   NARROWER (BUT HIGHER)

Be sure to check how well the child can reach to turn the wheels.

---

2. **If the chair is too big from front to back,** or if the child needs a better position, try a wedged cushion and padded backboard.

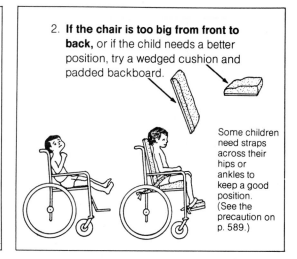

Some children need straps across their hips or ankles to keep a good position. (See the precaution on p. 589.)

---

3. **If still more help is needed** for positioning the child, make a **sitting frame** designed to meet her needs. Here is an example.

CAUTION: Not all children will need all the special features shown here. Some will need still other features. Adapt special features to the needs of the particular child, and **test them before making them permanent.**

adjustable head support (padded)

holes for chest support strap and hip support strap

hip support pads

lift for tilting seat back

lower-back support pad

notch for removable table-board

knee separator

removable footrest with holes for foot straps

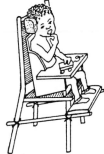

The sitting frame can be used on the ground.

It can be placed in a chair (or strapped into the seat of a car).

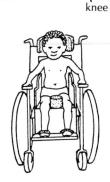

It can be fitted into a wheelchair.

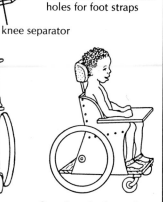

Or make a simple wood wheelchair with all the features of the sitting frame (see p. 620 and 621).

Seating adaptations for specific children

The various *adaptations* discussed here are designed to meet specific needs of individual children, especially children with cerebral palsy. Remember that **each child's needs are different,** and adaptations that are not carefully fitted to the needs of the child may do more harm than good.

1. **Carefully consider the child's specific needs before** including any adaptation or special seating.

2. After making an adaptation, **evaluate how the child uses it.**

3. **Check often** to see if it continues to help the child. An adaptation for a growing child may help her progress at one stage of development but hold her back a few weeks or months later.

General position

We have talked about this a lot, but it is worth repeating:

Most children who require special seating sit best with their hips, knees, and ankles at right angles.

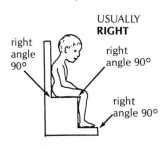

USUALLY **RIGHT**

right angle 90°

right angle 90°

right angle 90°

USUALLY **WRONG**

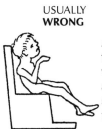

A chair shaped like this may cause a child with *spasticity* to stiffen and straighten, or cause a severely *paralyzed* child to slip forward and slump.

ANGLE OF BODY AND HEAD

A slight backward tilt helps most children sit in a better, more relaxed position.

If the child still falls or stiffens forward,

it may help to tip the chair back even more.

A head pad may help position him to look forward, and may decrease some spasticity. It can also reduce spasticity in the eye muscles.

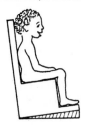

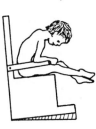

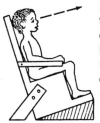

However, this may cause his head to lean back so his eyes look upward.

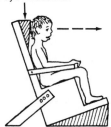

The heads of babies and small children may be so big that the headrest tilts them forward so their eyes look down.

Putting the headrest behind the level of the backboard lets the child hold her head in a better position.

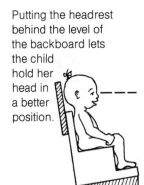

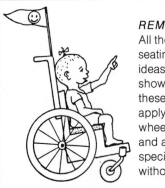

REMEMBER: All the seating ideas shown on these pages apply to wheelchairs, and also to special seats without wheels.

Other ways to help keep hips at a right angle

(CP)

HIP STRAPS

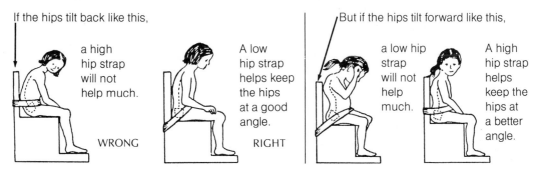

If the hips tilt back like this,

a high hip strap will not help much.

WRONG

A low hip strap helps keep the hips at a good angle.

RIGHT

But if the hips tilt forward like this,

a low hip strap will not help much.

A high hip strap helps keep the hips at a better angle.

Notice that in both of these children with cerebral palsy, supporting the hips in a better position helps the whole body take a more normal position.

SPECIAL CUSHIONS

For the child whose hips tilt back, or whose upper body is 'floppy', a **padded support across the lower part of the back** may help her keep a good position.

> Good cushions sometimes make straps unnecessary.

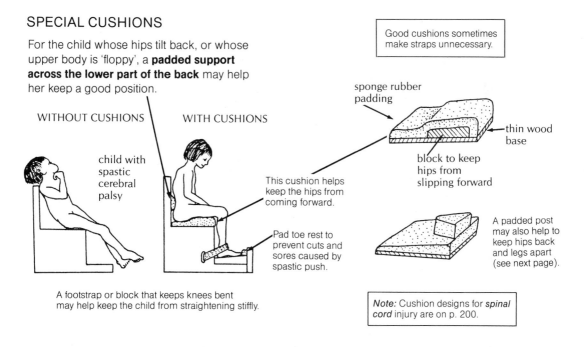

WITHOUT CUSHIONS

child with spastic cerebral palsy

WITH CUSHIONS

This cushion helps keep the hips from coming forward.

Pad toe rest to prevent cuts and sores caused by spastic push.

sponge rubber padding

thin wood base

block to keep hips from slipping forward

A padded post may also help to keep hips back and legs apart (see next page).

A footstrap or block that keeps knees bent may help keep the child from straightening stiffly.

> *Note:* Cushion designs for *spinal cord* injury are on p. 200.

Keeping the body straight from side to side

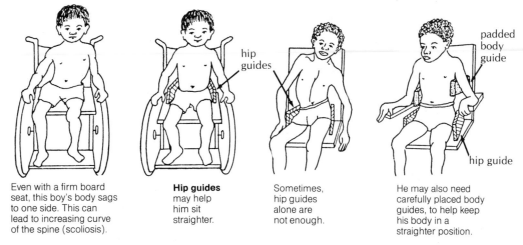

Even with a firm board seat, this boy's body sags to one side. This can lead to increasing curve of the spine (scoliosis).

Hip guides may help him sit straighter.

hip guides

Sometimes, hip guides alone are not enough.

padded body guide

hip guide

He may also need carefully placed body guides, to help keep his body in a straighter position.

Deciding where to place body guides

(CP)

1. Look carefully at how the child sits.

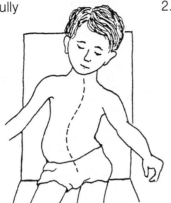

2. Draw a sketch of how he sits. Then draw arrows where you would need to push to help him sit straighter.

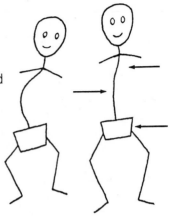

3. While someone holds the child in his best position, mark where you think the guides should be placed.

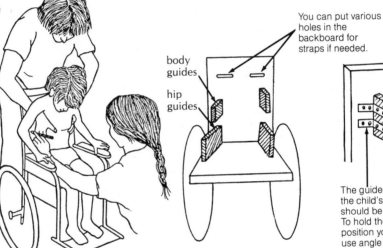

4. First, build in the guides in a temporary way.

You can put various holes in the backboard for straps if needed.

body guides

hip guides

The guides under the child's arms should be thin. To hold their position you can use angle irons.

5. See how well the child sits in the adapted seat. When you cannot improve it more, fasten the guides firmly and pad them so they do not hurt him.

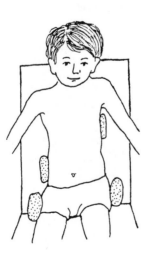

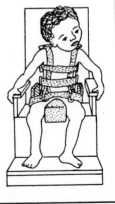

An 'H' harness, with straps that pass through slots in the backboard, is another way to help hold steady the body of a severely disabled child.

Carefully evaluate what kinds of support each child needs.

(CP)

Maria's legs straighten, press together, and turn inward. Her whole body position is affected.

Pedro is a heavy child whose body stiffens and his knees push open.

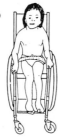

A **hip strap** holds her hips back some but does not help her overall position much.

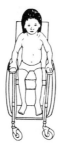

However, a **backboard** that bends her hips more, plus a **knee post,** help improve her whole body position— **without straps!**

A combination of a **backboard** with guides, a special **cushion** and a **knee block** does not help him.

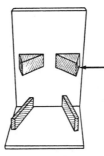

However, a **hip strap** together with **blocks** outside his knees gives him a much better position (He may also need foot straps.)

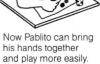

SHOULDER-BLADE WINGS

Pablito's spastic muscles pull his shoulders back and make it hard for him to bring his hands together in front of him. The village team had an idea.

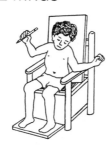

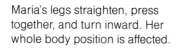

They put 'wings' behind his shoulder blades, like this, to help keep his shoulders forward.

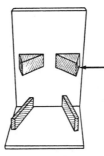

Now Pablito can bring his hands together and play more easily.

LAP BOARDS

These can be made from thin wood, plywood, or fiberboard. They should be easy to take off, but grip firmly when in place.

You can make a simple instrument out of cardboard or stiff paper to measure the child's body for cutting out the lap board.

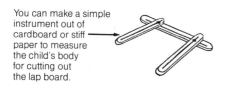

Extra holes for changing peg position.

Raised edges help keep toys from falling.

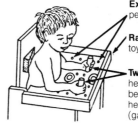

Two pegs to hold onto may help him sit, or move into a better position. They also help him develop hand control (games with rings, etc.).

A **lap board** can help keep shoulders, arms, and body in a better position, especially if it has a part cut out measured to fit around the child.

Height of the lapboard is usually the same as for armrests (see p. 602). Experiment to find out what works best.

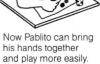

'*Velcro*' (stick-to-itself tape) can be used to fix the board to the chair for easy removal— and to adjust it forward or backward.

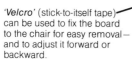

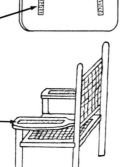

Be sure to put the softer part of the *Velcro* on the chair arms. The rough parts could scratch the child when the board is not used.

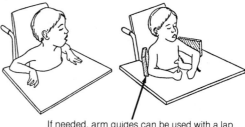

If needed, arm guides can be used with a lap board to keep a child's shoulders forward and his arms in a better position to use his hands.

(CP)   **DESIGN FOR A WHEELCHAIR INSERT**

This insert, from *Positioning the Client with Central Nervous System Deficits,*
provides a lot of control, and is especially useful for some children with spasticity.
Although it was designed as an insert for a wheelchair, you can use it as the frame
of a wooden wheelchair, or chair without wheels built for a specific child.

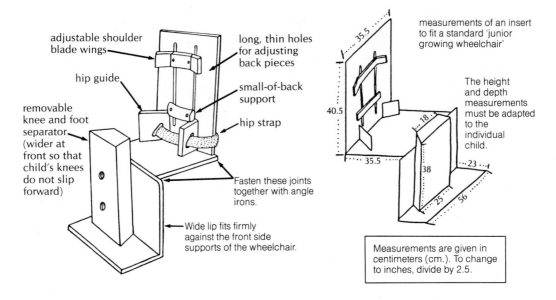

adjustable shoulder blade wings

long, thin holes for adjusting back pieces

hip guide

small-of-back support

removable knee and foot separator (wider at front so that child's knees do not slip forward)

hip strap

Fasten these joints together with angle irons.

Wide lip fits firmly against the front side supports of the wheelchair.

measurements of an insert to fit a standard 'junior growing wheelchair'

The height and depth measurements must be adapted to the individual child.

Measurements are given in centimeters (cm.). To change to inches, divide by 2.5.

DESIGN FOR A STRAIGHT-LEG SITTING FRAME
(mostly for very young children)

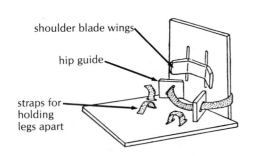

shoulder blade wings

hip guide

straps for holding legs apart

To seat the child, the frame can be put on the ground, a table, a chair, or into a wheelchair.

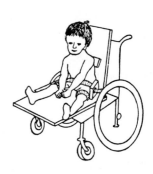

DESIGN FOR AN ADAPTED CASTER CART (WHEEL BOARD)

Use the same suggestions for supports, guides, and straps.

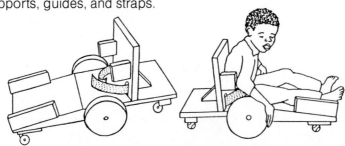

Note: The child's weight is over the large wheels. He can rock from one caster to the other. For travel over rough ground, he will learn to balance on the center wheel and barely touch down with the others.

> **CAUTION: Be sure to add cushions or adequate padding to all seating designs. Children whose bodies push in uncontrolled ways can very easily develop pressure sores (see Chapter 24).**

Designs for 6 Basic Wheelchairs

CHAPTER **66**

There are dozens of designs for low-cost, 'appropriate technology' wheelchairs. Some are lower cost and more generally useful than others. In PROJIMO, we have built many different wheelchairs. In this chapter we give designs for 6 of the ones that we have found most useful. Each has advantages and disadvantages.

AHRTAG wood wheelchair
made from a child's chair, bicycle wheels and axles at front, one rear caster

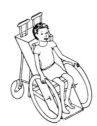

Advantages: the simplest and one of the cheapest chairs to make; easy to modify or adapt; very little welding needed; can be built in one day by someone with some carpentry skill; low cost.

Disadvantages: Single, small rear wheel makes it difficult for either the child or helper to push over rough ground or up curbs. Fixed footrest makes it hard for child to climb in and out without tipping chair forward when weight is on footrest. Sideboard makes *transfers* to side and lifting child from behind difficult.

Re-bar and woven plastic wheelchair
steel construction rod frame with woven plastic seat, back, and footrest

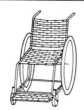

Advantages: simple design; fairly low-cost re-bar is easy to bend; plastic woven seat is comfortable and easy to clean; slide-away footrest makes getting in and out easier.

Disadvantages: Builder needs welding skills; relatively heavy and not as strong as tubing chairs. Big bumps may bend the chair out of shape.

Square metal tube wheelchair
frame bolted together

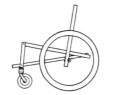

Advantages: strong, stable metal chair that can be built with nuts and bolts (welding needed only to attach front wheels). Flat surfaces make it easier to put on wood *adaptations;* fairly low cost.

Disadvantages: more work and skill needed than for above chairs; design more complex; slightly higher cost than wood chairs.

Wheelchair with lying board
made of steel tubing, with removable wood lying board

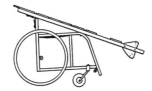

Advantages: useful for active child who must lie face down to heal sores or stretch *contractures*. When board is removed, it is a regular wheelchair; low cost; very adaptable.

Disadvantages: requires welding (but a simpler model can be made of wood); does not fold; board takes up a lot of space; stiff ride.

Plywood frame wheelchair
with 20 inch bicycle wheels and axles, and 2 front casters

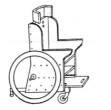

Advantages: attractive; lightweight; low cost, easy to make and adapt. Caster wheels in front (not in back) make it easier to go over rough ground and curbs. Adjustable push-away footrest makes *positioning* and getting in and out easy.

Disadvantages: Plywood and double casters increase cost (although it is still a cheap chair). Plywood (if not marine grade) may come apart in wet weather. Bicycle axles may bend or break with a heavy child or rough use.

Metal tube folding wheelchair
made from thin-wall steel tubing; strong axles with machinery bearings

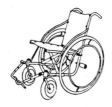

Advantages: Chair folds for transporting or storage; very tough; flexible design good for uneven surfaces; good for side transfers; a very high-quality chair if well-made.

Disadvantages: needs more skill (tube bending, welding, exact fittings, wheel spoking, etc.) to build; relatively costly; hard to adapt.

Tools needed for making wheelchairs

Ideas for setting up a workshop for *disabled* workers are discussed in Chapter 57 and p. 603 of Chapter 64. How you equip your workshop for making wheelchairs will depend on (1) how much money you have (or can borrow) to do it, (2) the kinds of chairs you hope to build (metal or wood), (3) the skills, *physical* and *mental* abilities, learning potential, and responsibility (regarding safety) of the workers, (4) the availability of electricity and power tools, (5) how many persons will be working, and (6) how many chairs you hope to produce.

Here we list the basic equipment you will need for making the 6 wheelchairs described in this chapter. Many choices are possible. More specialized parts of the work can be done by outside craftspersons. For example, in a wheelchair production center in Belize, axles must be machine tooled on a metal lathe. Local machine shops cooperate by doing this free.

CODE		TYPE OF CHAIR					
AN — Absolutely necessary **N** — A big help, but you might do without it **(N)** — Necessary only for axles **?** — Depends on model		wood chair	re-bar and woven plastic	square metal tubes with wood seat and back	wheelchair with lying board	plywood	round metal tube
TOOLS REQUIRED							
bench vise		N	AN	N	AN	(N)	AN
tubing bender					AN		AN
welding (brazing) equipment		(N)	AN	N	AN	(N)	AN
metal saw		(N)	AN	AN	AN	(N)	AN
wood saw		AN			AN	AN	
hammer		AN	AN	AN	AN	AN	AN
wrench (set or adjustable)		N	N	AN	AN	N	AN
metal file and/or grinder		(N)	AN	AN	AN	(N)	AN
screwdriver		AN	AN	AN	AN	AN	AN
sewing equipment (hand or machine)				?	N?		N?
drill (hand or electric)		N	?	AN	AN	N	AN
drill bits for metal				AN	AN		AN
drill bits for wood		AN		AN		AN	
spoke wrench		?	?	N	N	?	N
bicycle pump		?	?	?	?	?	?
center punch		N	N	N	N	N	N
tape measure		N	N	N	N	N	N
carpenter's square		N	N	N	N	N	N

Terms for metal tube or bar used to build wheelchairs

- *Thin-wall* refers to thin steel tubing often used for electrical wiring work and sometimes for lightweight metal furniture.

- *Thick-wall* refers to heavy weight pipe such as the one used in plumbing.

- *Re-bar* refers to solid metal rod, usually used to reinforce cement.

Jigs or guides for more exact welding

For making the metal tube chairs and the welded wheel mounts and handrims of any of the chairs, your work will be easier and more exact if you make or purchase certain 'jigs' or guides to hold parts in the right place while you weld them. For example, to weld the front caster fork you can make a 'jig' like this. Details on 'jigs' and other techniques for making different wheelchair parts are well described in Ralf Hotchkiss's book *Independence Through Mobility* (see reference on p. 604). We strongly recommend it to any group planning to make wheelchairs.

Notes on measurements
For some of the wheelchair designs in this chapter, we give the measurements for a standard child's or adult's model. **Be sure to adapt the measurements to the size and needs of the particular child.**

In many countries inches (") are used for measurements of certain things, and centimeters (cm.) for others. We therefore also use both. **Centimeters** is abbreviated **cm.** and **inches** is abbreviated **"**. Two inches is written **2"**.

1" equals 2.54 cm. You can use the scale on the edge of this page (and on the inside back cover) to change inches to cm.

AHRTAG WOOD WHEELCHAIR

(Somewhat modified from AHRTAG manual, see p. 604.)

The AHRTAG wheelchair is built onto an ordinary **child's wood chair.** Measurements should be adjusted to the child's needs.

A webbed plastic seat lets air move through it and can be easily cleaned.

It uses standard 20" x 1 3/4" bicycle wheels and axles.

Basic carpentry tools are needed to build this wheelchair. It can be made in one day by someone with basic carpentry skills. The local blacksmith may be able to help weld together the wheel supports if you cannot. It is easy to add positioning aids or make other adaptations. The cost in Mexico using new materials is about US $40.00.

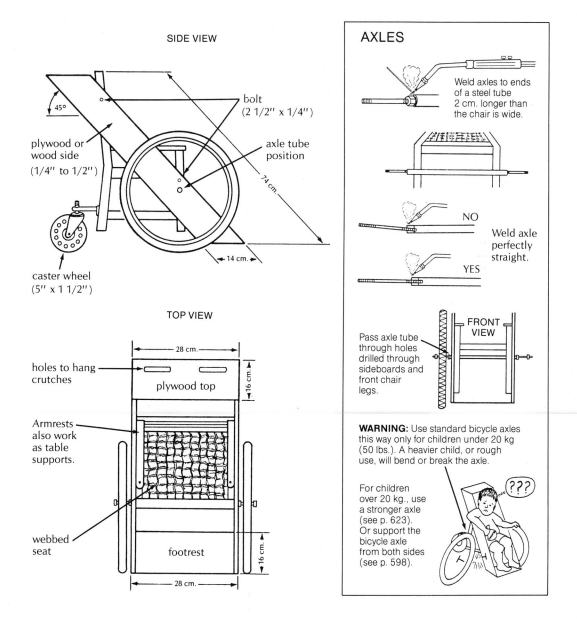

SIDE VIEW

- 45°
- plywood or wood side (1/4" to 1/2")
- caster wheel (5" x 1 1/2")
- bolt (2 1/2" x 1/4")
- axle tube position
- 74 cm.
- 14 cm.

TOP VIEW

- holes to hang crutches
- plywood top
- 28 cm.
- 16 cm.
- Armrests also work as table supports.
- webbed seat
- footrest
- 16 cm.
- 28 cm.

AXLES

Weld axles to ends of a steel tube 2 cm. longer than the chair is wide.

NO — Weld axle perfectly straight.

YES

Pass axle tube through holes drilled through sideboards and front chair legs.

FRONT VIEW

WARNING: Use standard bicycle axles this way only for children under 20 kg (50 lbs.). A heavier child, or rough use, will bend or break the axle.

For children over 20 kg., use a stronger axle (see p. 623). Or support the bicycle axle from both sides (see p. 598).

???

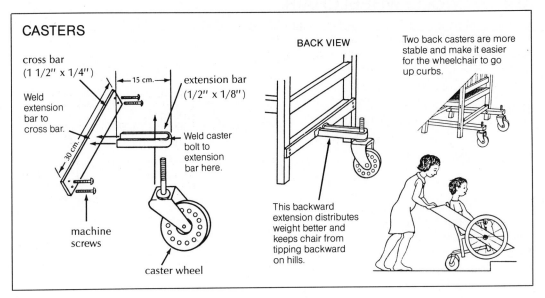

CASTERS

cross bar
(1 1/2" x 1/4")

Weld
extension
bar to
cross bar.

← 15 cm. →

extension bar
(1/2" x 1/8")

30 cm

Weld caster
bolt to
extension
bar here.

machine
screws

caster wheel

BACK VIEW

Two back casters are more
stable and make it easier
for the wheelchair to go
up curbs.

This backward
extension distributes
weight better and
keeps chair from
tipping backward
on hills.

For **brake designs,** see p. 601 and 623. For other pictures and models of the AHRTAG wheelchair, see p. 526, 592, 600, 601, 604, and 624.

RE-BAR AND WOVEN PLASTIC WHEELCHAIR

Total cost using new parts is about US $40.00.

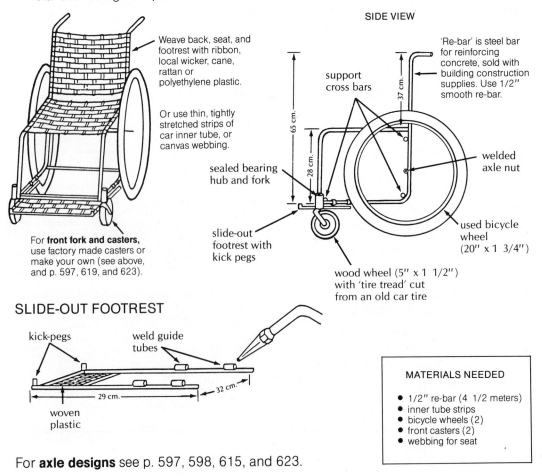

Weave back, seat, and
footrest with ribbon,
local wicker, cane,
rattan or
polyethylene plastic.

Or use thin, tightly
stretched strips of
car inner tube, or
canvas webbing.

For **front fork and casters,**
use factory made casters or
make your own (see above,
and p. 597, 619, and 623).

SIDE VIEW

'Re-bar' is steel bar
for reinforcing
concrete, sold with
building construction
supplies. Use 1/2"
smooth re-bar.

support
cross bars

65 cm.

37 cm.

28 cm.

welded
axle nut

sealed bearing
hub and fork

slide-out
footrest with
kick pegs

wood wheel (5" x 1 1/2")
with 'tire tread' cut
from an old car tire

used bicycle
wheel
(20" x 1 3/4")

SLIDE-OUT FOOTREST

kick-pegs

weld guide
tubes

← 29 cm. →

32 cm.

woven
plastic

MATERIALS NEEDED

- 1/2" re-bar (4 1/2 meters)
- inner tube strips
- bicycle wheels (2)
- front casters (2)
- webbing for seat

For **axle designs** see p. 597, 598, 615, and 623.

SQUARE TUBE WHEELCHAIR

This wheelchair, like other steel tube chairs, should use only thin-wall tubing. Total cost in Mexico using new parts is about US $40.00. To keep costs down, check with various sources of materials and ask at small fix-it shops for advice and possibly even some free scrap material. Metal scrap heaps are great for materials.

FRONT VIEW

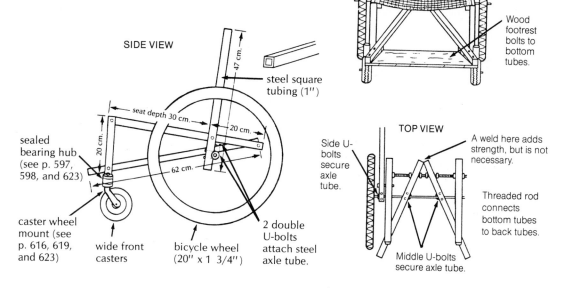

canvas back and seat

Wood footrest bolts to bottom tubes.

SIDE VIEW

47 cm.

steel square tubing (1")

seat depth 30 cm.

20 cm.

20 cm.

62 cm.

sealed bearing hub (see p. 597, 598, and 623)

caster wheel mount (see p. 616, 619, and 623)

wide front casters

bicycle wheel (20" x 1 3/4")

2 double U-bolts attach steel axle tube.

TOP VIEW

Side U-bolts secure axle tube.

A weld here adds strength, but is not necessary.

Threaded rod connects bottom tubes to back tubes.

Middle U-bolts secure axle tube.

SIDE VIEW

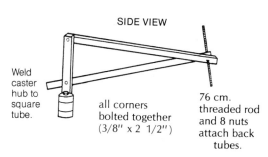

Weld caster hub to square tube.

all corners bolted together (3/8" x 2 1/2")

76 cm. threaded rod and 8 nuts attach back tubes.

MATERIALS NEEDED

- thin-wall square tubing (1" x 3.64 meters)
- thick canvas cloth (1 square meter)
- galvanized steel tube (1/2" x 66 cm.)
- bicycle wheels (2) (20" x 1.75")
- caster wheels (2) (wood or rubber)
- threaded rod (3/8" x 38") (Use extra 20" to bend 4 U-bolts.)
- 2 front casters
- 21 3/8" nuts and 12 screws for seat and back supports

HOW TO MAKE YOUR CHAIR

1. Review drawings. Adjust measurements to fit child.
2. Cut all sections of square tubing. Make sure that matching tubes are equal in length.
3. Drill holes in bottom tubes and pass the threaded rod through them. Adjust nuts until a 'V' is formed. (Weld tip of 'V' for extra strength.)
4. Drill all holes in seat tubes. Pass threaded bolt through seat holes.
5. Drill holes in back support tubes and front caster tubes. Bolt to frame.
6. Weld axle nuts to ends of axle tube. Drill holes for U-bolts and bolt axle tube to frame.
7. Weld front caster forks to front tubes.
8. Sew cloth back and seat supports. Screw into place.
9. Cut out and bolt wood footrest to frame. (Use wedges to get the angle right.)
10. Attach axle tube with U-bolts and put on the wheels.
11. Paint frame to help keep tubes from rusting (if not galvanized).

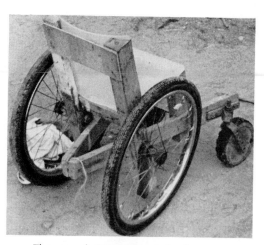

The same design can be made of wood.

WHEELCHAIR WITH LYING BOARD

This is useful for an active child who must lie face down to heal pressure sores or to stretch hip and knee contractures.

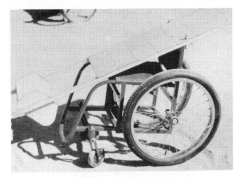

The board is sloped so that the child can play, look ahead, and move about more easily. If necessary, you can make the lying board adjustable so that the child can rest lying flat. This helps to improve *circulation* and to prevent swelling of the feet.

After the pressure sores heal, the lying board can be removed and the frame is easily adapted to form a lightweight wheelchair. The cost for materials in Mexico is about US $40.00.

The design we show uses a simple, non-folding steel tube wheelchair frame with a wooden lying board mounted on top. However, many other designs are possible. (See, for example, the photo of a lying and standing wood wheelchair on p. 190.)

WITH LYING BOARD

Lying-board should be well padded with thick foam rubber. If necessary, cut out a hole for urine to pass through (line hole with thin plastic so the foam rubber stays dry).

angle iron

bicycle wheels

6" casters

footrest (height and angle adjustable)

For tall persons, place the casters farther from the big wheels to help prevent tipping.

WITHOUT LYING BOARD
and with other additions

3/4" round thin-wall tubing (or 1" tubing for adults) or use square tubing

removable handle for pushing

shopping or book basket

heel strap

front bar forms footrest

3/4" square tubing. Use 1" for persons over 150 lbs (70 kg.).

THE LYING BOARD

SIDE VIEW

Attach thin wood or plywood boards with small screws so that they can be easily adjusted to leave open spaces under bony parts or sores.

strong wood pole (or 1" square tubing)

rack to hold urine pot (if needed)

adjustable footrest

TOP VIEW

urine hole

height adjustment pin

angle adjustment pin

footrest

Make the board and wheelchair just a little wider than the child's hips.

The board attaches to the chair with angle irons or **wing bolts.** You can make wing bolts by brazing a stiff bent wire to a bolt.

wire

bolt

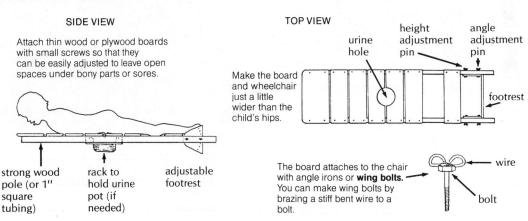

FOOTREST

Use thin wood or plywood. (Pad sides and bottom well to prevent sores. Examine feet daily.)

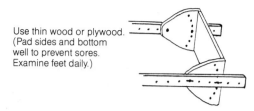

REMOVABLE HANDLE

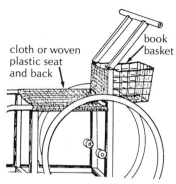

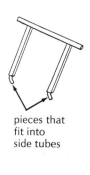

cloth or woven plastic seat and back

book basket

pieces that fit into side tubes

FRONT CASTER WHEEL

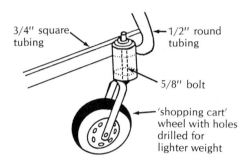

3/4" square tubing

1/2" round tubing

5/8" bolt

'shopping cart' wheel with holes drilled for lighter weight

You should now have enough information to make a wheelchair with a lying board without step-by-step instructions. Adapt it, and make it the size to fit the child that needs it.

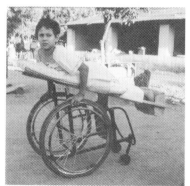

Wheelchair with lying board. A wide strap holds the child in place (but take care it does not press on sores).

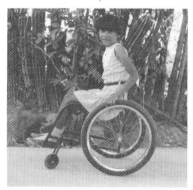

Wheelchair without lying board.

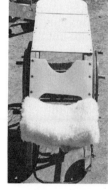

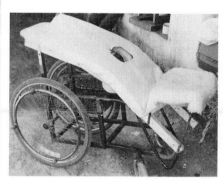

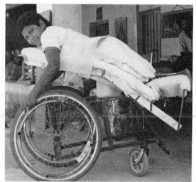

A variation of the wheelchair with lying board (p. 618) adapted for a paraplegic child with both contractures and pressure sores of his hips and knees. Urine is collected in a plastic container. The wheelchair seat has been converted into a basket.

CAUTION: Remember that a child who has some pressure sores can easily get new ones. Be sure the child lies and sits so that there is little or no pressure over bony places. **Examine her whole body at least once a day and try to keep her dry.**

(CP) PLYWOOD FRAME WHEELCHAIR

This can be easily built by someone with basic carpentry and welding skills. (Cost in Mexico using new materials is about US $40.00.) Positioning aids (head rest, hip pads, etc.) can be easily added. The chair can be designed to meet a child's particular needs. For example, if the child sits well without extra support, the tops of the side pieces can be removed to allow more freedom of movement.

A plywood frame is a low-cost alternative to metal. However, if not made well, or if left out in the rain, the chair may weaken and the plywood can split. As with any wheelchair, it must be protected from misuse, periodically examined for weaknesses, and promptly repaired.

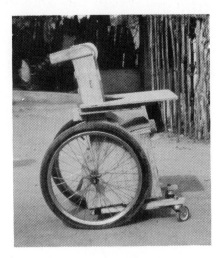

See model on p. 621 ————————————➤

For active children the wheelchair can be strengthened by reinforcing all joints and by adding strong hubs and axles (see p. 623).

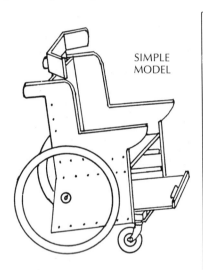

SIMPLE MODEL

HOW TO MAKE YOUR CHAIR

1. Review drawings of chair and adaptive equipment.
2. Cut out the two side pieces to the same shape; sand with sandpaper.
3. Cut out back support, seat, and bottom piece of chair; sand with sandpaper.
4. Screw or nail seat and bottom piece to back piece.
5. Screw or nail side pieces to seat, bottom, and back.
6. Check that all pieces are lined up straight. Then add glue and more screws or nails for strength.
7. Cut out footrest and guide brackets for footrest.
8. Screw or nail guide brackets to side pieces under seat.
9. Bolt front casters to chair and assemble rear axle tube.
10. Drill holes in side pieces for axle tube; mount tube and rear wheel.
11. Let glue dry 1 to 2 days; check for strength of all wood joints.

These measurements are for a 4 to 8-year-old child.

MATERIALS NEEDED

• 3/8" plywood (1 sheet)
• 20" bicycle wheels (2)
• small caster wheels (2)
• 1/2 steel tube (66 cm. long)
• wood glue
• sandpaper
• screws
• nails
• 1/2" by 1/4" wood strips (6 x 46 cm. long)

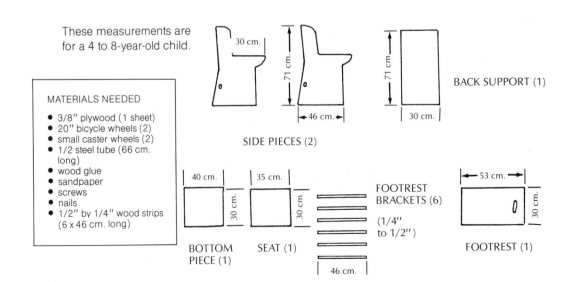

30 cm.

71 cm.

71 cm.

← 46 cm. →

30 cm.

SIDE PIECES (2)

BACK SUPPORT (1)

40 cm.

35 cm.

30 cm.

30 cm.

BOTTOM PIECE (1)

SEAT (1)

46 cm.

FOOTREST BRACKETS (6)

(1/4" to 1/2")

← 53 cm. →

30 cm.

FOOTREST (1)

A plywood wheelchair with many adaptations

This wheelchair has a variety of additions sometimes needed for a small child who has poor body control, head control, and urine or bowel control. The head support and armrests fit into wooden holders and can be easily removed. A lap table can be easily added. Holes can be cut out for chest and hip straps for extra support.

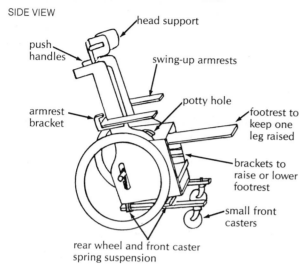

SIDE VIEW

head support

push handles

swing-up armrests

potty hole

armrest bracket

footrest to keep one leg raised

brackets to raise or lower footrest

small front casters

rear wheel and front caster spring suspension

BACK VIEW

removable head support

wood brackets for removable head support

20″ bicycle wheel

holes for chest support strap

holes for hip support strap

cut strips of used inner tube for springy ride

rear axle

head positioner

Wedge adjusts angle of head piece.

Important: Pad it well.

Bottom slides into slot on rear of chair.

swing-up armrests

brackets to hold armrests

padded hip and shoulder positioners

Tabs fit into slots in the wheelchair back and seat.

INSIDE

potty bowl holder with leg separator

Pull out to empty potty.

potty bowl

Tree branch holds stiff legs apart.

lap table

The lap table should be cut to fit closely around the wheelchair sides. The same wooden brackets for the armrests keep this table in place. If the table wobbles, you can use small slats to strengthen the table. If the knee separator is made a bit higher, the table can rest on top of it and prevent any dips.

Armrest brackets secure table here.

plywood (1/4″)

SPRINGS FOR ALL 4 WHEELS

This plywood wheelchair has a springy ride. Old inner tube rubber strips connect the rear wheel axle to the wood strips holding the front caster wheels. These wooden strips should be strong enough to withstand the springy motion of the front casters.

Special cut-away slots allow the rear axle to move up and down freely. Other cut-away slots in the bottom of the wheelchair allow for the inner tube strips to be wrapped around the wooden caster strips. The tighter the inner tube strips are wrapped, the less bouncy the ride becomes.

To build your own strong rear hub and axle, see p. 623. If you want to use hubs from bicycle wheels, see p. 597.

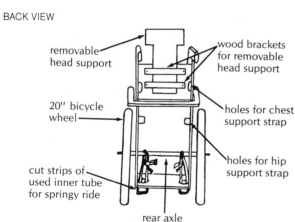

Strips of inner tube connect rear axle to front-caster arms.

A long hole here allows back axle to spring up and down.

2 loose-fitting bolts keep caster arms from moving sideways.

Wood strip separates caster arm from the bottom.

Rubber or wooden caster wheel bolts to wooden arm.

inner tube strips

Notches keep rubber strips from slipping.

Loose-fitting bolt acts as pivot.

WHIRLWIND STEEL TUBE WHEELCHAIR

The whirlwind (ATI-Hotchkiss) wheelchair is a very strong lightweight folding chair. On rough ground it rides more easily and lasts longer than more costly factory-made chairs. If it breaks, it can be fixed by the neighborhood metalworker. It is narrow and helps the rider to move about crowded rooms.

The frame of this chair is made of thin-wall steel tubing that is easy to shape by someone with basic mechanical and welding skills. It can be built in about 4 days in a small metalworking shop. More than 10 groups of disabled mechanics throughout Latin America are building this wheelchair—often at less than a quarter the cost of imported wheelchairs.

Most materials for this chair can be obtained locally. It uses standard 24" (or 26") bicycle wheels. The extra strong hubs (see p. 623) use standard small machinery bearings (which can often be obtained used for free or at low cost from electric machinery repair shops). The axles are 5/8" (1.6 cm.) steel bolts. Seating is canvas (heavy cloth). If the small front wheels are not available, you can make them out of wood (see p. 597 and 616).

The curved fender bar that follows the shape of the tire makes transfers easier. The lightweight folding footrests are narrow at the front, for moving more easily in crowded spaces.

Plans for making hubs, casters, and brakes are on the next page. Complete plans for making this wheelchair are in the book *Independence Through Mobility* (see p. 604). The book is essential for anyone planning to build this chair.

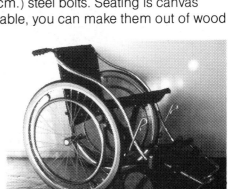

Model with wooden front wheels

MATERIALS NEEDED

- thin-wall tubing (from 1/2" to 1 1/4")
- thick-wall tubing (5/8" inside diameter)
- thick canvas or nylon cloth (2 meters)
- square tubing (thin-wall)
- bicycle rims and spokes (24" or 26" diameter)
- caster wheels (2)
- used sealed bearings (8)
- re-bar steel (3/8" round)

- flat bar steel (1/16" x 3/8")
- axle bolts (4) (5/8" x 5")
- washers (4) (1" diameter, 16 upholstery)
- screws (8 upholstery)
- machine screws (8) (1/4" x 1 1/2")
- paint or chroming chemicals
- bronze welding rod, flux
- bicycle tires and inner tubes (24")

FOLDING FOOTREST

TOP VIEW

Swing up when not in use.

footrest stop bar

bolt for length adjustment

X-BRACE

Seat hooks slide on frame to fold chair.

weld

axle socket of thick-wall steel tube

X-brace

bolt for attaching brake

Round tube turns on thinner tube inside it— allowing chair to fold.

seat tube

square tubing

Weld steel washers around center hole to add strength.

round tube

For a photo of this chair, see p. 536.

DETAILS OF HOW TO MAKE WHEELCHAIR PARTS
(can be used with many wheelchair designs)

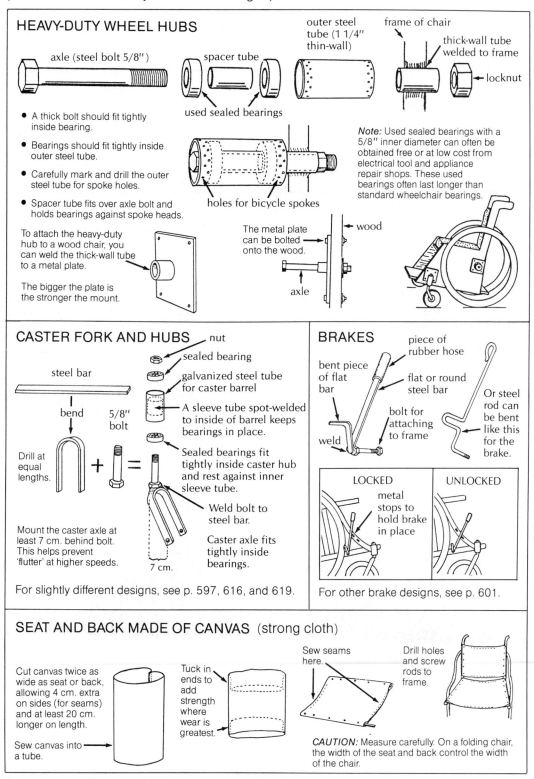

HEAVY-DUTY WHEEL HUBS

axle (steel bolt 5/8")

spacer tube

outer steel tube (1 1/4" thin-wall)

frame of chair

thick-wall tube welded to frame

locknut

used sealed bearings

- A thick bolt should fit tightly inside bearing.
- Bearings should fit tightly inside outer steel tube.
- Carefully mark and drill the outer steel tube for spoke holes.
- Spacer tube fits over axle bolt and holds bearings against spoke heads.

holes for bicycle spokes

Note: Used sealed bearings with a 5/8" inner diameter can often be obtained free or at low cost from electrical tool and appliance repair shops. These used bearings often last longer than standard wheelchair bearings.

To attach the heavy-duty hub to a wood chair, you can weld the thick-wall tube to a metal plate.

The bigger the plate is the stronger the mount.

The metal plate can be bolted onto the wood.

wood

axle

CASTER FORK AND HUBS

steel bar

bend   5/8" bolt

Drill at equal lengths.

Mount the caster axle at least 7 cm. behind bolt. This helps prevent 'flutter' at higher speeds.

7 cm.

nut

sealed bearing

galvanized steel tube for caster barrel

A sleeve tube spot-welded to inside of barrel keeps bearings in place.

Sealed bearings fit tightly inside caster hub and rest against inner sleeve tube.

Weld bolt to steel bar.

Caster axle fits tightly inside bearings.

For slightly different designs, see p. 597, 616, and 619.

BRAKES

piece of rubber hose

bent piece of flat bar

flat or round steel bar

bolt for attaching to frame

weld

Or steel rod can be bent like this for the brake.

LOCKED	UNLOCKED
metal stops to hold brake in place	

For other brake designs, see p. 601.

SEAT AND BACK MADE OF CANVAS (strong cloth)

Cut canvas twice as wide as seat or back, allowing 4 cm. extra on sides (for seams) and at least 20 cm. longer on length.

Sew canvas into a tube.

Tuck in ends to add strength where wear is greatest.

Sew seams here.

Drill holes and screw rods to frame.

CAUTION: Measure carefully. On a folding chair, the width of the seat and back control the width of the chair.

For designs of other wheelchair parts, see the following pages:

wheels: 594, 596, 597, 616, 619
seats and backs: 595, 615, 616, 617, 619, 620
tires: 596
armrests: 599, 621

footrests: 600, 616, 619, 621, 622
axle mounts: 597, 598, 615
handrims: 601
cushions: 200, 609

Examples of locally made wheelchairs

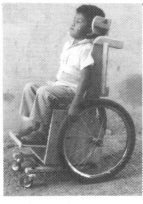
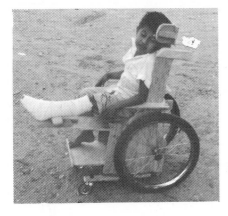
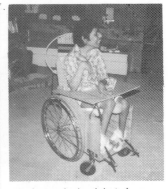

The plywood wheelchair on p. 620, with the armrest in place (left) and swung back (right).

A plywood wheelchair for a child with cerebral palsy with inner tube stretching aids to gently pull his feet and straighten his severe knee contractures.

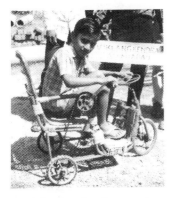
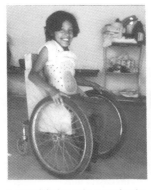
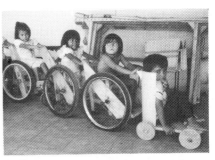

A bamboo hand-powered tricycle made at Viklang Kendra (People's Village), Allahabad, India.

A wheelchair made completely of paper, including the wheels. Paper is glued together using rice flour in water (Zimbabwe).

A wood design of the wheelchair on p. 617, two AHRTAG wheelchairs, and a 'trolley' made from half of a plastic bucket and wood wheels.

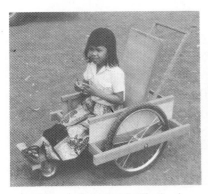
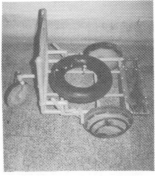
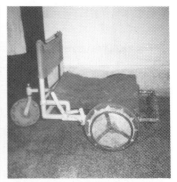

A wood wheelchair in Thailand. The bicycle wheel axles are supported on both sides to keep them from bending.

A metal frame, wood wheel 'trolley' in Bangladesh (see p. 572). The rubber tube serves as a cushion and also as a toilet seat.

This trolley, also from Bangladesh, uses a cushion made of coconut fiber covered with rubber (see p. 199).

For more examples of wheelchair designs, see p. 65, 86, 98, 189, 190, 229, 288, 343, 430, 441, and 526.

Artificial Legs

Artificial legs can be (and often are) made at home or in village shops. How well they work and how natural they look depend on many things, including costs, skills, and materials available.

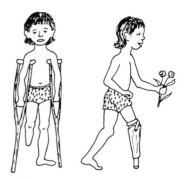

BELOW THE KNEE

The most common leg amputation is below the knee. A leg that has been amputated **halfway between the knee and ankle** works best for walking with an artificial *limb*. Here are some examples of artificial limbs, from simple to more complex.

Even a simple artificial limb can make a big difference.

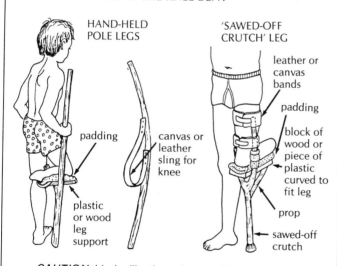

WITH THE KNEE BENT

HAND-HELD POLE LEGS

padding

canvas or leather sling for knee

plastic or wood leg support

'SAWED-OFF CRUTCH' LEG

leather or canvas bands

padding

block of wood or piece of plastic curved to fit leg

prop

sawed-off crutch

CAUTION: Limbs like these 3 are quick and easy to make, but **they cause knee contractures. As a result, the knee cannot be easily straightened** to fit a better, more useful limb. **Bent-knee limbs should only be for temporary or emergency use. Do exercises every day** to keep the knee straight and strong. (See p. 229 and 230.)

WITH THE KNEE STRAIGHT

BAMBOO AND PLASTER LEG (See p. 628.)

PLASTIC PIPE LEG WITH FOOT (See p. 632.)

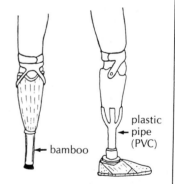

bamboo

plastic pipe (PVC)

These limbs are better because the knee has full range of motion. Walking is easier and more natural. However, **the person's weight must be supported evenly over the entire stump, not only at the end of the stump.** (See p. 631.)

Positions for
FITTING A LIMB

BAD

will only work with a bent-knee limb

DIFFICULT

knee does not straighten fully

GOOD

knee straightens completely

Exercises to strengthen and straighten the leg

From the time a leg has been amputated until
a limb is fitted, daily exercises are needed to
keep the hip and knee *muscles* strong and to avoid
contractures. If weakness and contractures
already exist, these should be corrected as much
as possible before a limb is fitted. Exercises
are discussed on p. 229 and 230.

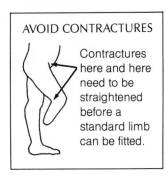

AVOID CONTRACTURES

Contractures here and here need to be straightened before a standard limb can be fitted.

How soon can an artificial limb be fitted?

**Children born without a foot or part of a
leg (or legs)** can be fitted with an artificial
limb as early as 10 or 12 months of age.

A child whose foot has been cut off can
and should be fitted with a temporary limb **as
soon as the wound has healed.** However, **be
very careful not to injure or put any
pressure on the new scars or end of the stump.**

Note: On a very young
or fat child, it may be
difficult to fasten the
limb firmly to the knee
(the bones may not
stick out enough).
Straps to a waistband
and even over the
shoulder may be needed.

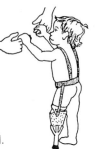

Temporary limbs—when to use them and why

Because a stump usually shrinks and changes shape in the first weeks after a limb
is fitted, it is often wise **first to fit a low-cost, temporary limb.** This is especially true
if the amputation is new or the stump is swollen. A better-looking, more permanent
limb can be made after 4 to 6 weeks, or when swelling is gone.

Preparing the stump

In the first weeks or months after an amputation, the stump tends to swell up. The
swelling may in time lead to a club-shaped, deformed stump, which is difficult to fit
with an artificial limb. For this reason, **it is important to wrap the stump with elastic
bandage from the time the leg is cut off until a limb is fitted,** or at least until there
is no more sign of swelling. Instructions for wrapping the stump are on page 228.

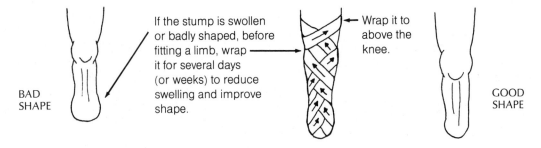

BAD SHAPE

If the stump is swollen
or badly shaped, before
fitting a limb, wrap
it for several days
(or weeks) to reduce
swelling and improve
shape.

Wrap it to
above the
knee.

GOOD SHAPE

NOTE: When the person is not wearing the artificial leg, he
should also wear an elastic bandage to control the stump shape.

The art of limb making

Making artificial limbs that fit and work well is both a science and an art. If possible,
try to learn from a skilled limb maker. 'On-the-job' training for even a few days can
make a big difference.

Before starting to make an artificial limb, STUDY THE PERSON'S LEG.

A good fit of the socket on the stump and at the knee is one of the most important—and difficult—parts of limb making. It helps to have an understanding of the bones and muscles in the leg.

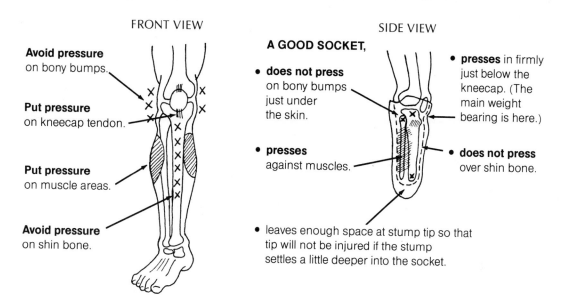

FRONT VIEW

Avoid pressure on bony bumps.

Put pressure on kneecap tendon.

Put pressure on muscle areas.

Avoid pressure on shin bone.

SIDE VIEW

A GOOD SOCKET,

- **does not press** on bony bumps just under the skin.

- **presses** against muscles.

- **presses** in firmly just below the kneecap. (The main weight bearing is here.)

- **does not press** over shin bone.

- leaves enough space at stump tip so that tip will not be injured if the stump settles a little deeper into the socket.

Before beginning, study the person's knee and stump carefully. Note the positions of the kneecap, the bony bumps on the sides of the knee, and the shin bone.

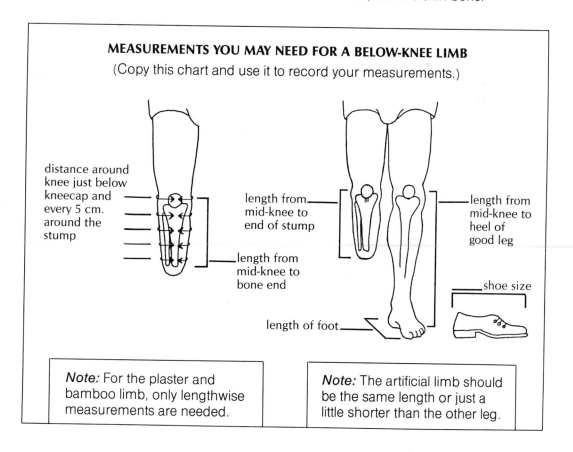

MEASUREMENTS YOU MAY NEED FOR A BELOW-KNEE LIMB
(Copy this chart and use it to record your measurements.)

distance around knee just below kneecap and every 5 cm. around the stump

length from mid-knee to end of stump

length from mid-knee to bone end

length from mid-knee to heel of good leg

shoe size

length of foot

Note: For the plaster and bamboo limb, only lengthwise measurements are needed.

Note: The artificial limb should be the same length or just a little shorter than the other leg.

PLASTER AND BAMBOO BELOW-KNEE ARTIFICIAL LEG

This simple, low-cost leg was developed for refugee amputees in Thailand by Operation Handicap Internationale. It is most useful as a temporary limb for learning to walk. However, if the inner (plaster) part of the socket is made with waterproof glue, or is protected from getting wet, the leg can last for a long time.

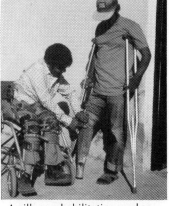

A village rehabilitation worker fits a young man with a bamboo limb. (PROJIMO)

Steps for making the plaster socket

1. Make a thick 'cup' or 'cap' of sponge or folded cloth and tape it over the end of the stump (to give it a little extra length).

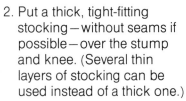

2. Put a thick, tight-fitting stocking—without seams if possible—over the stump and knee. (Several thin layers of stocking can be used instead of a thick one.)

Pull tight to avoid wrinkles.

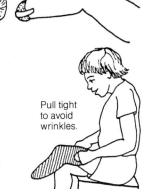

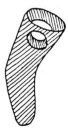

Putting holes near the top of the stocking makes it easy for the child to pull it up tight against the skin while the cast is put on.

3. Put a thin plastic bag over the stocking.

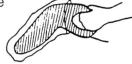

4. Put a thin cotton stocking or stockinette over the plastic bag and also pull tight to avoid wrinkles.

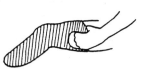

PALM OIL

Note: If you do not have a stocking, you can mold the socket directly on the stump. Shave any hair off the stump and cover it with vegetable oil (for example, coconut or palm oil).

5. With the stocking stretched tight, mark the important places with a 'grease pencil'. The pencil marks will 'print' onto the inside of the plaster cast when it is removed.

Mark all these places:

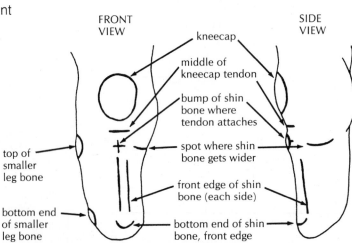

FRONT VIEW

SIDE VIEW

kneecap

middle of kneecap tendon

bump of shin bone where tendon attaches

spot where shin bone gets wider

front edge of shin bone (each side)

bottom end of shin bone, front edge

top of smaller leg bone

bottom end of smaller leg bone

6. Wrap the stump and knee with plaster bandage. **Be very careful to put the bandage on evenly and smoothly.** (Elastic plaster bandage works best, but is very costly. To reduce costs you can make your own plaster bandages for casting. See p. 569).

See p. 569

Cast the knee with the stump slightly bent.

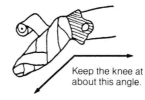

Keep the knee at about this angle.

MAKING THE PLASTER WATER-RESISTANT

The plaster cast of the stump will become the inner layer of the socket of the bamboo limb. So it should be strong and waterproof. To make the cast stronger and water-resistant, wet the plaster bandage with glue instead of water.

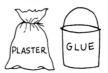

Use a water-base glue that is water-resistant when it dries.

Note: If the plaster cast is to be used only as a mold for making a leather or resin socket, use water, not glue.

---

7. As the plaster dries, hold the stump firmly below the knee.

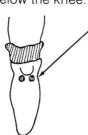

Press your thumbs on each side of the tendon just below the knee cap.

FRONT VIEW

BACK VIEW

With the 2 middle fingers of each hand, press into the hollow behind the knee.

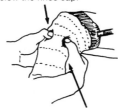

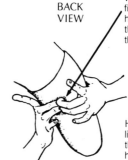

With the ball of the hand, press gently on the muscles on both sides of the leg.

Hold the stump like this until the plaster is hard enough to hold its shape.

---

8. When the cast becomes hard, mark where to cut the top edge (see below).

SIDE VIEW

BACK VIEW

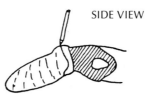

---

9. To remove the cast, roll the stocking over it. Put your hands over the pressure points (as shown above). Have the child wiggle the stump as you gently pull off the cast.

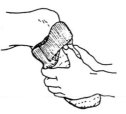

It may be necessary to cut the cast behind the knee, like this, to get it off.

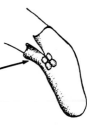

---

10. Cut the cast along the line you drew.

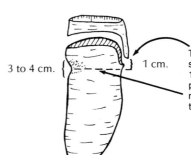

3 to 4 cm.

1 cm.

The dip behind the knee should reach at most 1/2 cm. above a line passing through the mid-point of the kneecap tendon.

Preparing the bamboo post

1. Select a piece of strong, green bamboo a little longer than the good leg from the knee to heel.

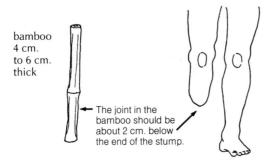

bamboo 4 cm. to 6 cm. thick

← The joint in the bamboo should be about 2 cm. below the end of the stump.

2. Split the bamboo to a little below the level of the stump end. Split into thin strips— each about 3/4 cm. wide.

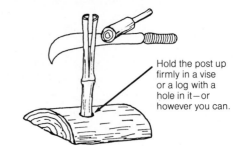

Hold the post up firmly in a vise or a log with a hole in it—or however you can.

3. Remove the softer inner layer from each of the thin strips.

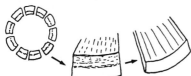

4. Spread the bamboo strips around the plaster socket.

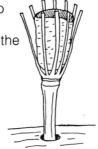

5. Position the socket as correctly as you can. Then, with a thin wire, wrap the bamboo tightly against the socket.

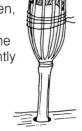

6. Put the limb on the stump and have the child stand on it. Check the length. If necessary, cut some off the post.

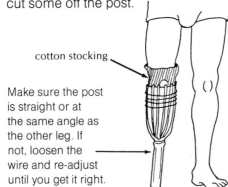

cotton stocking

Make sure the post is straight or at the same angle as the other leg. If not, loosen the wire and re-adjust until you get it right.

Note: If child uses a shoe or sandal, be sure to have her wear it when measuring the height of the limb.

7. After trimming the tops of the bamboo strips, cover the outside of the socket with several layers of glue, sawdust, and gauze bandage:

- Brush on one layer of glue.

- Press sawdust on the glue (with gloves).

- Wrap tightly with gauze bandage. Let it dry.

- Repeat 5 or 6 times.

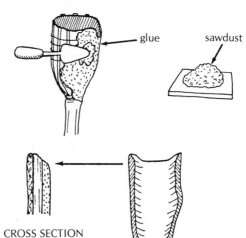

glue   sawdust

8. Smooth the outside of the socket with sandpaper. Also smooth and round the inner edges at the top.

CROSS SECTION

9. Make a 'cuff' to hold the limb on. (If attached correctly, it should also help keep the knee from over-straightening.)

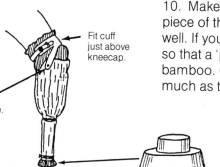

Fit cuff just above kneecap.

Rivet cuff to socket slightly behind mid-line. (Mark rivet points with tabs pulled tight when knee is a little bent.)

10. Make a rubber 'heel'—a piece of thick truck tire works well. If you can, cut the tire so that a 'plug' fits inside the bamboo. Cut off bamboo as much as the heel is thick.

(Be sure to allow for height of sandal or shoe on other foot.)

Design for the knee cuff

Use strong leather and line it on inside with soft smooth leather. It should be a few cm. longer than the distance around the knee.

Glue layers of leather and webbing together with rubber cement and sew at edges.

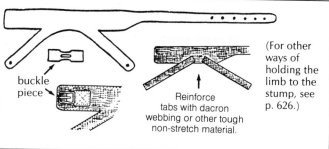

buckle piece

Reinforce tabs with dacron webbing or other tough non-stretch material.

(For other ways of holding the limb to the stump, see p. 626.)

---

11. Have the child stand and walk on the limb for several minutes. Then remove it and look for sore spots on the child's skin, or signs of too much pressure. Check especially over bony spots. An area that looks pale when the limb is removed and then turns red or dark, is a sign of too much pressure.

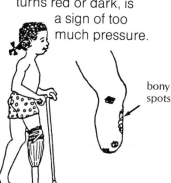

bony spots

12. Scrape shallow pits into the socket from the inside, at the points where it presses over bones. You may also need to build up around the area where pressure occurs.

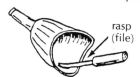

rasp (file)

(To help you find the right points, it helps to have marked 'bony spots' before casting. They will then be 'printed' inside the socket—see p. 628.)

If stump presses on bottom of socket, you may need to build up

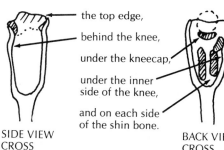

the top edge,

behind the knee,

under the kneecap,

under the inner side of the knee,

and on each side of the shin bone.

SIDE VIEW CROSS SECTION

BACK VIEW CROSS SECTION

To build up these spots, dig a few pits into the socket surface so new material will grip better. Fill with a paste of fresh plaster mixed with glue.

If socket presses on the end of the bone, scrape out a hollow here.

During the first few weeks of using an artificial limb, the stump becomes smaller, and several changes in limb size may be needed. To save time, use a shorter bamboo post so that the plaster socket can be replaced several times with new, smaller ones.

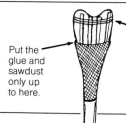

Put the glue and sawdust only up to here.

Hold the bamboo strips to the cast with wire. Cut the wire to change the plaster socket.

Artificial leg using PVC plastic pipe instead of bamboo

Where plastic PVC water pipe is available, it can be used instead of bamboo. Use a 3 cm. (1¼ inch) thick-walled PVC.

1. Measure the tube the same as bamboo, and cut it to form 4 strips.

2. Heat the PVC in an oven until it gets a little soft.

3. Fit the hot PCV around the socket piece and wrap it tightly with a long strip of cloth or rubber until it cools.

4. Fasten PVC firmly to socket with wire or rivets (or both). It is best to attach it temporarily with wire and to have the child try it before you fix it permanently.

5. Cover with sawdust and glue, or with resin-base casting bandage (very expensive) or with fiberglass and resin (also expensive).

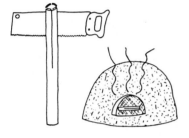 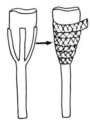 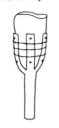 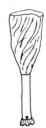

Note: For a stronger, water-resistant limb, the socket can also be made with resin-based casting bandage. But this is also expensive.

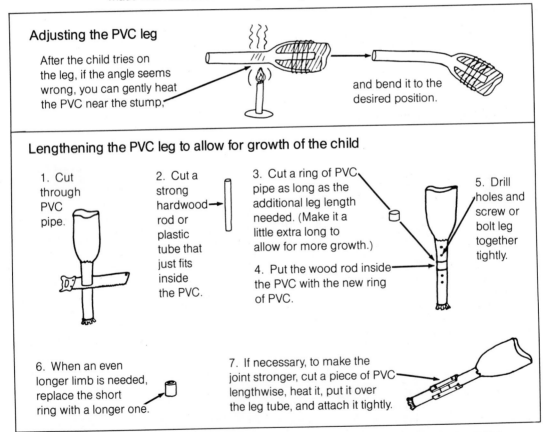

Adjusting the PVC leg

After the child tries on the leg, if the angle seems wrong, you can gently heat the PVC near the stump, and bend it to the desired position.

Lengthening the PVC leg to allow for growth of the child

1. Cut through PVC pipe.

2. Cut a strong hardwood rod or plastic tube that just fits inside the PVC.

3. Cut a ring of PVC pipe as long as the additional leg length needed. (Make it a little extra long to allow for more growth.)

4. Put the wood rod inside the PVC with the new ring of PVC.

5. Drill holes and screw or bolt leg together tightly.

6. When an even longer limb is needed, replace the short ring with a longer one.

7. If necessary, to make the joint stronger, cut a piece of PVC lengthwise, heat it, put it over the leg tube, and attach it tightly.

IMPORTANT: For both below-knee and above-knee limbs, try to **line up the limb** as well as possible so that its angle is similar to the other leg and 'feels right' when the child stands and steps. Often this requires repeated tries and adjustments. **Getting the limb to line up right is the key to successful limb fitting.** It helps to learn this from someone skilled at fitting limbs.

ABOVE-KNEE ARTIFICIAL LIMBS

Children who are growing quickly need a low-cost limb that can be easily replaced or lengthened. Small children usually learn to walk well with a straight leg limb that does not have a knee joint.

1. **A bamboo or PVC plastic tube above-knee limb** can be made in much the same way as for the below-knee limb.

The top edge of the socket should be rounded to form a wide lip on the back, where the butt can sit. Weight bearing should be on the butt bone and over the entire stump—and not just on the end of the stump.

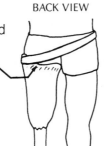

BACK VIEW   FRONT VIEW

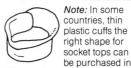

Note: In some countries, thin plastic cuffs the right shape for socket tops can be purchased in different sizes from *orthopedic* suppliers. They can be placed around the leg before casting and can be re-used. Ask for 'prefabricated ishial weight-bearing cuffs'.

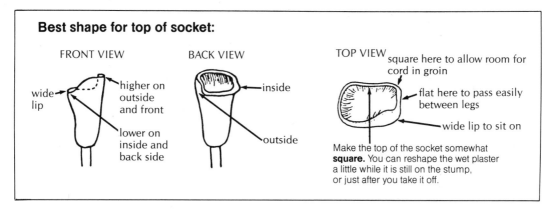

Best shape for top of socket:

FRONT VIEW

wide lip

higher on outside and front

lower on inside and back side

BACK VIEW

inside

outside

TOP VIEW square here to allow room for cord in groin

flat here to pass easily between legs

wide lip to sit on

Make the top of the socket somewhat **square.** You can reshape the wet plaster a little while it is still on the stump, or just after you take it off.

2. **A leather and metal rod limb** (adapted from *Simple Orthopaedic Aids,* see p. 642).

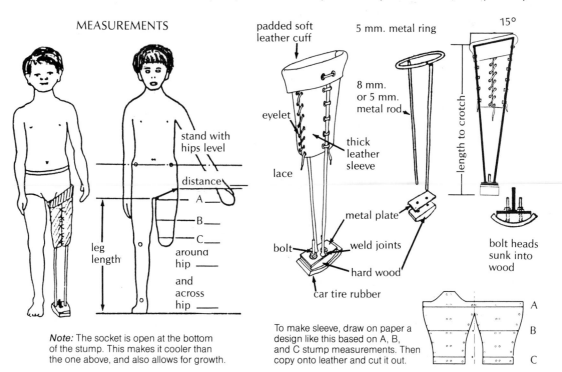

MEASUREMENTS

stand with hips level

distance

A ___
B ___
C ___

leg length

around hip ___

and across hip ___

Note: The socket is open at the bottom of the stump. This makes it cooler than the one above, and also allows for growth.

padded soft leather cuff

5 mm. metal ring

15°

eyelet

8 mm. or 5 mm. metal rod

thick leather sleeve

lace

metal plate

bolt   weld joints

hard wood

length to crotch

bolt heads sunk into wood

car tire rubber

To make sleeve, draw on paper a design like this based on A, B, and C stump measurements. Then copy onto leather and cut it out.

A
B
C

Above-knee limb with knee joint (for older children and adults)

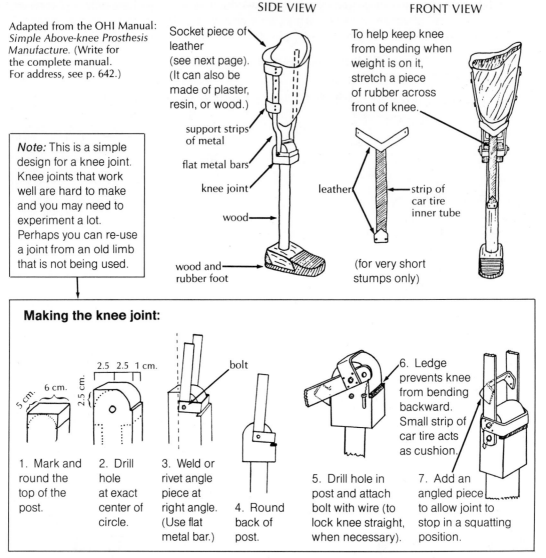

Adapted from the OHI Manual: *Simple Above-knee Prosthesis Manufacture.* (Write for the complete manual. For address, see p. 642.)

SIDE VIEW

FRONT VIEW

Socket piece of leather (see next page). (It can also be made of plaster, resin, or wood.)

To help keep knee from bending when weight is on it, stretch a piece of rubber across front of knee.

support strips of metal

flat metal bars

knee joint

wood

leather

strip of car tire inner tube

wood and rubber foot

(for very short stumps only)

Note: This is a simple design for a knee joint. Knee joints that work well are hard to make and you may need to experiment a lot. Perhaps you can re-use a joint from an old limb that is not being used.

Making the knee joint:

5 cm.   6 cm.   2.5 cm.   2.5 2.5 1 cm.

bolt

6. Ledge prevents knee from bending backward. Small strip of car tire acts as cushion.

1. Mark and round the top of the post.

2. Drill hole at exact center of circle.

3. Weld or rivet angle piece at right angle. (Use flat metal bar.)

4. Round back of post.

5. Drill hole in post and attach bolt with wire (to lock knee straight, when necessary).

7. Add an angled piece to allow joint to stop in a squatting position.

FEET

Putting feet on artificial legs makes them look better (with shoes, sandals, or boots). Also, the wide base helps prevent the leg from sinking into mud or sand. A well-made, flexible foot can make walking easier. Here are 2 possibilities.

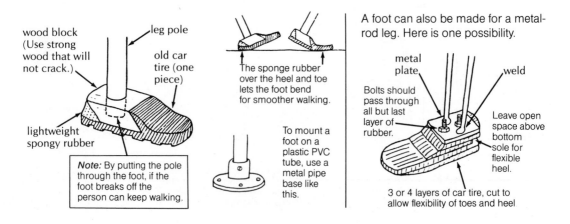

wood block (Use strong wood that will not crack.)

leg pole

old car tire (one piece)

lightweight spongy rubber

Note: By putting the pole through the foot, if the foot breaks off the person can keep walking.

The sponge rubber over the heel and toe lets the foot bend for smoother walking.

To mount a foot on a plastic PVC tube, use a metal pipe base like this.

A foot can also be made for a metal-rod leg. Here is one possibility.

metal plate

weld

Bolts should pass through all but last layer of rubber.

Leave open space above bottom sole for flexible heel.

3 or 4 layers of car tire, cut to allow flexibility of toes and heel

OTHER WAYS OF MAKING ARTIFICIAL LIMBS

Wooden legs

The oldest, traditional way of making artificial limbs is to make the socket out of wood.

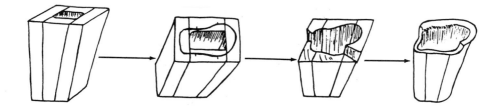

This is best learned from a skilled craftsperson. Unfortunately, this is a skill that is difficult to learn from a book. A book that describes the method step-by-step is *Manual of Above-Knee Wood Socket Prosthetics* by Miles Anderson, John Bray, and Charles Hennesey. It has gone out of print, but you may still be able to find it. Unfortunately, the methods described are complex and require a lot of special equipment. However, perhaps they could be simplified. (We have not tried this method.)

Leather socket: Self-adjusting prosthesis

This method uses flat metal bars, a wood post, and a thick, firm leather socket. To form the socket, wet leather is stretched over a plaster mold of the stump. Methods are clearly and simply described in *Simple Below-knee Prosthesis Manufacture*. (See reference, p. 642.)

A leather socket has several advantages. Leather is available almost everywhere, is more comfortable in hot weather, and can easily be adjusted to the stump as it becomes smaller. Also, leather is soft and easily takes the shape of the stump, and therefore self-corrects molding mistakes.

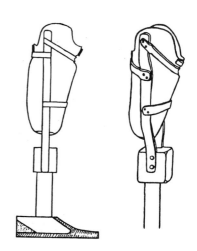

Stump protectors from old tires

For a child with both legs amputated above the knee, short artificial limbs or even simple 'stump protectors' may allow her to move about easier than long leg limbs.

thick stocking

adjustable straps

Cut an old tire like this.

Cut part way through rubber to bend.

Jaipur limb

The 'Jaipur limb' was developed in Jaipur, India to meet the need for a limb that would (1) allow working 'barefoot' in rice paddies, (2) look like a real bare foot, (3) bend at the foot in all directions enough so the person can squat easily and walk firmly on uneven ground, and (4) be low cost and quick to make.

The foot is made of wood and sponge rubber and then 'vulcanized' (heat molded) with rubber, using a metal mold. The rubber gives the foot its life-like form and color and makes it strong and waterproof.

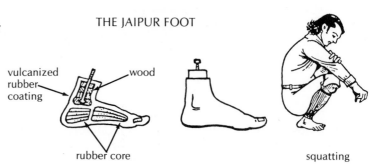

THE JAIPUR FOOT

vulcanized rubber coating — wood — rubber core

squatting

The limb is made of SHEET ALUMINUM.

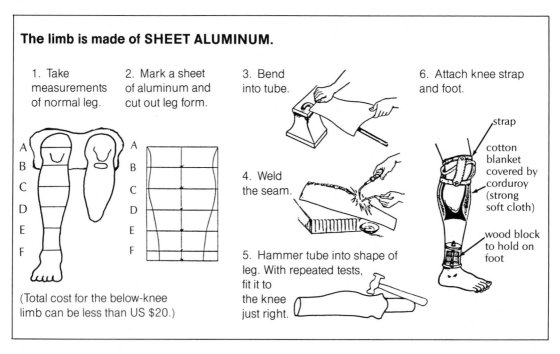

1. Take measurements of normal leg.

2. Mark a sheet of aluminum and cut out leg form.

3. Bend into tube.

4. Weld the seam.

5. Hammer tube into shape of leg. With repeated tests, fit it to the knee just right.

6. Attach knee strap and foot.

strap — cotton blanket covered by corduroy (strong soft cloth) — wood block to hold on foot

(Total cost for the below-knee limb can be less than US $20.)

To make the Jaipur limb requires a lot of skill as well as special equipment. But once a shop is set up and persons trained, the limb can be made at very low cost, and fitted very quickly (one hour from the first measurements until the person walks away on his new limb). For instructions, contact Rehab Centre, SMS Medical College, Jaipur 302004, India.

Ideas for a limb-making shop. On p. 521 there is a description of the OHI prosthetics shop in Thailand, where amputee workers make the bamboo and above-knee adjustable limbs shown in this chapter.

JAIPUR ABOVE-KNEE DESIGN

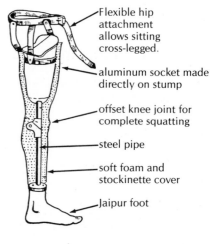

Flexible hip attachment allows sitting cross-legged.

aluminum socket made directly on stump

offset knee joint for complete squatting

steel pipe

soft foam and stockinette cover

Jaipur foot

REFERENCES
(Where to Get More Information)

In the first edition of this book we included a list of references. In that list we gave the names of publications from which we borrowed information to use in this book. We also included books and materials which we did not use, but that we felt could be useful to other people.

It has been many years since *Disabled Village Children* was written. Since then, many of the books that we recommended have gone out of print. This means that they are not published anymore. For this reason, the list of references in this edition is somewhat different from the original. We still give credit to books and authors whose materials we used. Whenever possible, we still include the name and address of the organization or publisher who distributes the materials, so anybody who wishes to can write directly to them.

In some cases, we were not able to find the producers or distributors of some books and we decided to take them out of the list to save you time and effort.

In this new list, we also include organizations and associations that offer information and materials on different disabilities. The services and materials they offer vary from one to the other. Some of them send free materials but most charge some money for them. Write to them directly to get information on the type of books they sell and their prices. Be as precise as you can in explaining what you need so they can do a good job helping you.

You will notice that most of the organizations that we list here are in the United States but there are others in many different countries. Find out what kind of organizations or associations of disabled people exist where you are. It may be easier to get appropriate information and materials locally.

DISABILITY AND REHABILITATION—GENERAL

Disability Dialogue. Healthlink Worldwide, Cityside, 40 Adler Street, London E1 1EE, UNITED KINGDOM. http://www.healthlink.org.uk/

Supports disabled people, service providers and policy makers with practical information. It promotes the social inclusion of disabled people through community-based rehabilitation and other social action. Issues are produced by regional partners of Healthlink Worldwide. Available in English (including Braille and audiocassette editions), Hindi, Tamil, Bengali, Gujarati, and Nepali.

Training in Community for People with Disability. World Health Organization, Distribution and Sales, Avenue Appia 20, 1211 Geneva 27, SWITZERLAND.

Very basic information—sometimes too basic. This latest edition has been improved, but it takes a rather top-down, authoritarian approach. Very simple language. Many pictures. Part of a total plan for a 'community-based', government-directed program.

Rehabilitation International. 25 East 21st Street, New York, NY 10010, USA. Tel: (212) 420-1500 www.rehab-international.org

A worldwide federation of organizations of disabled people. Publications about social issues and the politics of disability and rehabilitation. They also publish the newsletter *One in Ten*, a report on what is happening around the world that may be of interest to disabled persons and their advocates.

Special Needs Project. 324 State Street, Suite H, Santa Barbara, CA 93101 USA. Tel: (800) 333-6867, Fax: (805) 962-5087, books@specialneeds.com

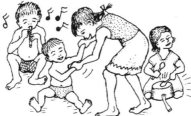

A bookstore that sells by mail. It offers a great selection of books on many different disabilities and rehabilitation.

Werner, David. *Project PROJIMO*. The Hesperian Foundation, 1919 Addison Street #304 Berkeley, CA 94704 USA. 65 pages. Tel: (510) 845-4507, Fax: (510) 845-0539, www.hesperian.org

A photographic report on the villager-run rehabilitation program in Mexico.

PRIMARY HEALTH CARE

Werner, David. *Where There Is No Doctor*. The Hesperian Foundation (see address above), 506 pages.

Widely used handbook for village health workers and families on basic curative and preventive health care. Second edition, revised and expanded.

Werner, David and Bower, Bill. *Helping Health Workers Learn*. The Hesperian Foundation (see address above). 632 pages.

A 'people-centered' educational approach to health care.

Dickson, Murray. *Where There Is No Dentist*. The Hesperian Foundation (see address above), 208 pages.

Basic information on care of teeth and gums.

King, Maurice and Felicity. *Primary Child Care: Book One*. Teaching Aids at Low Cost (TALC). PO Box 49, St. Albans, Herts, AL1 4AX, UNITED KINGDOM.

Excellent guide for health care of children.

POLIO

Huckstep, R.L. *Poliomyelitis: A Guide for Developing Countries—Including Appliances and Rehabilitation for the Disabled*. Churchill Livingstone, Robert Stevenson House, 1-3 Baxter's Place, Leith Walk, Edinburgh EH1 3AF, UNITED KINGDOM.

This is an excellent book that went out of print. Very complete. Includes braces, assistive equipment, rehabilitation, and information for hospital care and surgery. Well adapted for poor countries and community programs. You may still be able to locate a copy.

Post-Polio Health (formerly *Polio Network News*). Post-Polio Health International, 4207 Lindell Blvd #110, St. Louis, MO 63108-2915, USA. www.post-polio.org

Quarterly report with international circulation. Focuses on long-term effects of polio. It promotes scientific research on polio and proposes the creation of a worldwide network of people with polio.

CEREBRAL PALSY

Finnic, Nancy. *Handling the Young Cerebral Palsied Child at Home*. Penguin USA, PO Box 999, Dept. 17109, Bergenfield, NJ 07621 USA. 1975, 337 pages.

Excellent, complete and detailed information for home care. May be too much detail for some families—but a highly-recommended resource for a community program.

Levitt, Sophie. *Treatment of Cerebral Palsy and Motor Delay*. Blackwell Scientific Publications, PO Box 20, Williston, VT 05495-9957 USA. Third edition, 1995.

An advanced book, mostly on physiotherapy. Excellent information but difficult language and presentation. Many good pictures.

MUSCULAR DYSTROPHY

Muscular Dystrophy Association, Inc. 3300 E. Sunrise Drive, Tucson, AZ 85718-3208, USA. Tel: (800) 572-1717, www.mdausa.org, mda@mdausa.org

Lots of pamphlets on all the different types of muscular dystrophy. This association can be very helpful for children who live in the United States because they provide, and can help find, many services. (Their main focus is finding a cure.)

ARTHRITIS

Arthritis Foundation. PO Box 7669, Atlanta, GA 30357-0669, USA. Tel: (800) 283-7800, www.arthritis.org

A great variety of written materials on the different aspects of several types of arthritis, including juvenile arthritis. Updated information on current research and medical treatment to function with and manage arthritis.

SPINA BIFIDA

McLone, David. *Introduction to Spina Bifida*. Spina Bifida Association of America (SBAA), 4590 MacArthur Boulevard NW Suite 250, Washington DC 20007, USA. Tel: (800) 621-3141, Fax: (202) 944-3295, sbaa@sbaa.org

Basic information, especially useful for those who live in the USA and can access the care and services available.

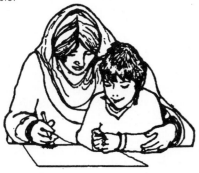

Sexuality and the Person with Spina Bifida. Available from SBAA (see address above).

An important topic explained in easy terms. Different aspects of sexuality—development, activity, society—relevant to persons with spina bifida.

Also from SBAA, *Bowel Continence and Spina Bifida*, and other publications; write for a list of their materials.

Welch, Collette. *Spina Bifida and You: A Guide for Young People*. Association for Spina Bifida and Hydrocephalus (ASBAH), 42 Park Road, Peterborough, PE1 2UQ, UNITED KINGDOM. Tel: (44-173) 355-5988, Fax: (44-173) 355-5985

This and many other publications on spina bifida are available from ASBAH. Some of their materials are excellent.

SPINAL CORD INJURY

Bromley, Ida. *Tetraplegia and Paraplegia: A Guide for Physiotherapists*. Churchill Livingston Sales, Elsevier Science, Footscray High Street, Sidcup, Kent DA4 5HP, UNITED KINGDOM. 1991, 219 pages.

Useful information on exercises, transferring, and how to shift weight to prevent pressure sores. Some good illustrations. Very technical.

Spinal Cord Injury— A Manual for Healthy Living. RRTC, Baylor College of Medicine, 1333 Moursund B-107, Houston, Texas 77030-3405 USA. Also available in Spanish.

Excellent (but expensive), accessibly written guide for people with spinal cord injuries and their families and caregivers. Many good illustrations. Has 29 sections, including bowel and urine management, skin care, sexual adjustment, medications, and others.

EPILEPSY

Vinig, Eileen P.G. and Pillas, Diana J. *Seizures and Epilepsy in Childhood—A Guide for Parents*. Johns Hopkins University Press, 2715 North Charles Street, Baltimore, MD 21218-4319, USA 1990, 87 pages.

Clearly explains many aspects of epilepsy in children. A good resource for a child with epilepsy and his family. It can also be bought from the Epilepsy Foundation.

Epilepsy Foundation of America. 4351 Garden City Drive, Landover, MD 20785, USA. Tel: (800) 332-1000 www.epilepsyfoundation.org

An organization that offers a great collection of publications and videos on all the different aspects of epilepsy. These are educational materials, designed for individuals with epilepsy, their families, teachers, and society in general.

LEPROSY

The resources listed under this category are available from ILEP at the following address: The Teaching and Learning Materials Co-ordinator, ILEP, 234 Blythe Road, LONDON W14 0HJ, UNITED KINGDOM, Tel: (44-20) 7602-6925, Fax: (44-20) 7371-1621, books@ilep.org.uk www.ilep.org.uk

Brand, P. *Insensitive Feet*. 1966, reprinted many times.

A good background to the problems of insensitive feet and the prevention of disability. Suitable for doctors and health workers.

ILEP Learning Guide No 1. *How to diagnose and treat leprosy*. 2001.

A new, well-illustrated publication suitable for the wide range of health professionals who need to recognize and treat leprosy.

ILEP Learning Guide No 2. *How to recognize and manage leprosy reactions*. 2002.

A comprehensive guide to identifying and managing leprosy reactions; includes details of how to safely prescribe corticosteroids.

Neville, P. Jane, editor. *A footwear manual for leprosy control programs*. Volumes I and II.

Two books about special footwear for persons with leprosy. The first book is a guide for setting up a footwear making shop. The second book deals with technical aspects of making footwear and has clear, easy to follow instructions for production of shoes, boots and sandals. Free for programs serving people with leprosy.

BLINDNESS

Blind Children Center. 4120 Marathon Street, Los Angeles, CA 90029, USA. www.blindcntr.org/

This is an organization dedicated to serving blind children 5 years of age and younger. They produce a lot of written materials for families with blind children.

Niemann, Sandy and Jacob, Namita, *Helping Children Who Are Blind: Family and community support for children with vision problems*. Hesperian Foundation (see address on p. 637). 2000, 192 pages.

The simple activities in this book can help parents, caregivers, teachers, health workers, rehabilitation workers and others help a child with vision problems develop all his or her capabilities. It also has sections containing innovative charts on child development and easy-to-make, low-cost learning toys.

Sandford-Smith, John. *Eye Diseases in Hot Climates*. Available from International Resource Centre, ICEH, London School of Hygiene & Tropical Medicine, Keppel St, London WC1E 7HT, UNITED KINGDOM. Tel: (44-20) 7612-7973, sue.stevens@lshtm.ac.uk www.jceh.co.uk 164 pages.

A valuable resource for health programs. It teaches how to identify, prevent, and provide basic care for the most common eye diseases found in the tropics.

World Blind Union. CBC-ONCE, C/ La Coruna 18, Madrid 28020, SPAIN. umc@once.es http://umc.once.es/

ONCE (National Spanish Association of the Blind) is also the home base of the World Blind Union. They have an international directory of organizations and programs for the blind. Write to them to get the names and addresses of programs in your region.

DEAFNESS

We have listed some producers of materials for deaf people. Remember that sign language differs from place to place. Investigate and observe what works well in your region and what materials are offered there.

Helping Children Who Are Deaf: A guide for family and community support. The Hesperian Foundation (see address on p. 637). 2003, 250 pages.

This book has activities for helping deaf children communicate to the fullest of their ability, including learning a language. It helps parents make good decisions about the development of a child who is deaf.

Wirz, Sheila W. and Winyard, Sally W. *Hearing and Communication Disorders*. Published by MacMillan but costs less from TALC (see address on p. 637).

A manual for rehabilitation programs that include or want to include services for deaf children or those with other communication problems. It simplifies a lot of techniques used by deafness professionals.

Gallaudet University Bookstore, 800 Florida Avenue NE, Washington, DC 20002-3695, USA. Tel: (202) 651-6876, http://bookstore.gaulladet.edu/ bookstore.mailorder@gaulladet.edu

This store specializes in all kinds of publications that deal with deafness—history, theory, education, etc. Popular children's books in sign language. Aids and equipment for deaf persons.

Medwid, Daria and Weston, Denise C. *Kid Friendly Parenting with Deaf and Hard of Hearing Children*. Gallaudet University Bookstore (see address above).

A good book on parenting deaf children. It teaches a fun, flexible method for building good relationships between parents and children.

The Dictionary. Signing Exact English. Box 1181, Los Alamitos, CA 90720, USA. 1993, 479 pages.

A very complete dictionary of sign language in English, very useful to anyone who wants to learn the North American system. Signing Exact English also offers many other publications and visual aids for teaching and learning sign language.

THERAPY, EXERCISES, AND POSITIONING

Hardinge, Elizabeth A., and Wilson, Patricia M.P. *A Manual of Basic Phyisiotherapy for the Use of Nurses in Rural Hospitals*. Tear Fund, 100 Church Road, Teddington, Middlesex, TW11 8QE, UNITED KINGDOM. 1981, 162 pages.

Basic, clearly presented, very useful for training rehabilitation workers.

Bergen, Adrienne Falk and Colangelo, Cheryl. *Positioning the Client With Central Nervous System Deficits: The wheelchair and other adapted equipment*. Valhalla Rehabilitation Publications, PO Box 195, Valhalla, NY 10595 USA. 1985 (second edition), 237 pages.

Detailed, in-depth discussion of adaptive seating to meet the needs of individual children with cerebral palsy. Excellent illustrations. Language is fairly complex.

Jaeger, D. LaVonne. *Home Program Instruction Sheets for Infants and Young Children*. The Psychology Corporation, Order Service Centre, PO Box 708906, San Antonio, TX, USA.

Excellent, well-illustrated book of instruction sheets for many exercises. It includes range of motion exercises. (Revised version of the first edition by Jaeger and Hewitt.)

Stern, Linda and Steidle, Kathryn. *Paediatric Strengthening Program*. Therapy Skill Builders, 555 Academic Court, San Antonio, TX 78204 USA.

Many playful activities to increase the strength of children with disabilities or those who are recovering from surgery. Pages can be copied and given to families so they will remember how to do the exercises with their children.

Physical Therapy Assistant's Manual. Operation Handicap International, Sectur Ventes, 14 Av. Berthelot, 69361 Lyon, Cedex 07, FRANCE.

Three volumes of 170 pages each. Simple manuals that teach how to provide physical therapy. The first book covers theory and basic anatomy. The second book shows therapy techniques. And the third one helps you choose an exercise program according to the particular disability. Good illustrations and clearly written.

CHILD DEVELOPMENT AND DEVELOPMENTAL DELAY

Miles, Christine. *Special Education for Mentally Handicapped Children—A Teaching Manual*. Mental Health Centre, Dabgari Gardens, Peshawar Cantt., North West Frontier Province, PAKISTAN. Revised edition, 1990, 277 pages. Email inquiries to: Humphrey Peters: humphrey@brain.net.pk

Excellent adaptation of special education to a developing community. Clearly written. A few good illustrations. Perhaps the best special education text for community programs.

Teaching Skills. Cheshire Homes, 515 Q Jalan Hashim, Tanjong Bungah, Penang, MALAYSIA.

A package of 6 video programs that describe teaching techniques to use with children and adults who are slow to learn. Well done and at prices that community programs can afford.

Sheda, Constance and Small, Christine. *Developmental Motor Activities for Therapy—Instruction sheets for children*. Therapy Skill Builders (see address above).

Well illustrated and organized activities to promote physical development and motor skills in children. Sheets can be reproduced and given to families.

National Down Syndrome Congress, 1370 Centre Drive Suite 102, Atlanta, GA 30338, USA.

An organization that provides many small pamphlets on different issues concerning Down syndrome. They also offer a reading list for families.

BEHAVIOR TRAINING AND TOILET TRAINING

Wipfler, Patty. *Listening to Children*. Parents Leadership Institute, PO Box 50492, Palo Alto, CA 94303, USA.

A series of 6 booklets that cover crying, fear, anger, special time, tantrums, and listening. A very new and revolutionary approach for dealing with feelings and behavior. Not written specifically for disabled children but the basic ideas work for everyone.

Azrin, Nathan and Foxx, Richard. *Toilet Training in Less Than a Day*. Simon & Schuster Mail Order, 100 Front Street, Riverside, NJ, USA. 1974, 189 pages.

Good instructions for 'the fast method'; oriented towards the USA and Europe.

TOYS AND GAMES

Ludins-Katz, Florence and Katz, Elias. *Arts and Disabilities*. Institute of Art and Disabilities, 551 23rd Street, Richmond, CA 94804, USA. 1983, 235 pages.

Ideas for starting an art center for disabled people. Materials, equipment, aids, and instruction needed for many crafts and art forms.

Sher, Barbara. *Extraordinary Play with Ordinary Things*. Therapy Skill Builders (see address above).

Play activities and games for children with varied levels of disability. Designed to encourage thinking, movement, coordination and balance. It uses materials and objects available in most homes.

Rogow, Sally M. *Shared Moments: Learning Games for Disabled Children*. The Disability Bookshop, PO Box 129, Vancouver, WA 98666, USA.

Learning games and activities designed to stimulate and encourage babies and children with physical, visual and developmental disabilities.

Hale, Karen. *Some Crafty Things to Do*. OXFAM Publishing, 274 Banbury Road, Oxford 0X2 7DZ, UNITED KINGDOM. 1992, 32 pages.

A manual for making toys from many different countries. Written for children, with good illustrations.

MIKKY: Visual Aids and Toys. Life Help Centre for the Handicapped, East Coast Road, Palavakkam, Madras 600-041, INDIA.

A manual on the therapeutic uses of crafts-making. Many different crafts and a list of suppliers. Very useful if you can find or afford the materials.

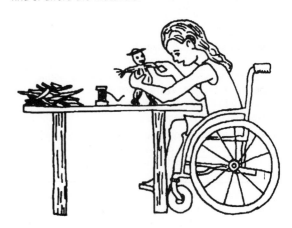

AWARENESS RAISING; POLITICS OF DISABILITY, REHABILITATION, AND MEDICINE

Jones, Ron. *The Acorn People*. Bantam Books, 2451 S. Wolf Road, Des Plaines, IL 60018, USA. 1976, 80 pages.

A good, very human story about disabled children and their need for freedom, adventure, and understanding.

Davidson, Margaret. *Louis Braille: The Boy Who Invented Books for the Blind*. Scholastic Book Services, PO Box 120, Bergenfield, NJ 07621 USA.

Excellent story for children about the accomplishments of a disabled child. Good reading for CHILD-to child activities.

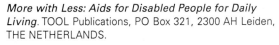

Melrose, Dianna. *Bitter Pills— Medicines and the Third World Poor*. OXFAM (see address on p. 640). 277 pages.

Excellent discussion of how drug companies often exploit people and endanger their health.

The Ragged Edge (formerly *The Disability Rag & Resource*), PO Box 145, Louisville, KY 40201, USA. www.raggededgemagazine.com editor@raggededgemagazine.com

A bi-monthly magazine by disabled people. A constant critic of disinformation and false ideas about people with disabilities. Good articles and analysis.

Disability Awareness in Action. 11 Belgrave Road, London SW1V 1RB, UNITED KINGDOM. Tel: (44-71) 834-0477, DAA_ORG@compuserve.com

An organization dedicated to fostering the integration of disabled people and advocating respect for their rights. Excellent materials on how to organize and maintain an organization of disabled people.

AIDS, APPLIANCES, AND SPECIAL EQUIPMENT, INCLUDING WHEELCHAIRS

How to Make Basic Hospital Equipment, compiled by Roger England. Intermediate Technology Publications, Sales Office, 103-105 Southampton Row, London WC1B 4HH, UNITED KINGDOM. 1979, 86 pages.

Simple tube metal wheelchairs and other designs from Africa. Well illustrated and with useful comments. Fairly simple language.

A Plastic Caliper for Children. Operation Handicap International (see address on p. 640).

A manual with all the instructions to make a plastic caliper (brace) similar to the ones we describe in Chapter 58. It includes information about choosing the correct caliper.

UPKARAN: A Manual of Aids For the Multiply Handicapped. Spastics Society of India, Upper Colaba Road, Opposite Afghan Church, Colaba, Bombay 400-005, INDIA. 106 pages.

Many excellent and mostly simple aids, well illustrated. Written in English and Hindi.

More with Less: Aids for Disabled People for Daily Living. TOOL Publications, PO Box 321, 2300 AH Leiden, THE NETHERLANDS.

Simply written in English, French, and Spanish, with illustrations on every page. Very good ideas.

Personal Transport for Disabled People. Available from Healthlink Worldwide (see address on p. 637). http://www.healthlink.org.uk/

For a description of this book see p. 604

How to Make Simple Disability Aids. Available from Healthlink Worldwide (see address on p. 637).

Many illustrations. Easy to make aids that are very useful. Many things that children can make themselves.

Hotchkiss, Ralf. *Independence Through Mobility: A Guide to the Manufacture of the ATI-Hotchkiss Wheelchair*. Wheeled Mobility Center, Dept. of Engineering, San Francisco State University, San Francisco, CA 94132, USA.

Complete instructions to make the 'Whirlwind', a high-quality, low-cost steel wheelchair. For a list of books about various types of personal transport for disabled people see pages 604 to 606.

ARTIFICIAL LIMBS

Pluyter, B. *Alternative Limb Making*. Available from Healthlink Worldwide (see address above).

Teaches how to manufacture and fit low-cost, below-knee prostheses. Detail on innovative products. Provides theory and technical information.

Simple Below-knee Prosthesis Manufacture and Simple Above-knee Prosthesis Manufacture. Operation Handicap International (see address on p. 640).

Excellent. Fairly simple method for making prostheses. See page 634 for a brief overview.

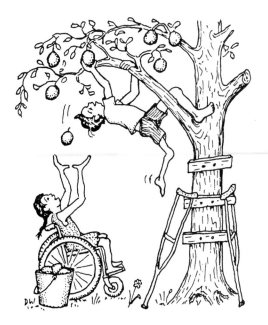

Other books from the Hesperian Foundation

Helping Children Who Are Blind, by Sandy Niemann and Namita Jacob, aids parents and other caregivers in helping blind children from birth through age 5 develop all their capabilities. Topics include: assessing how much a child can see, preventing blindness, moving around safely, teaching common activities, and many others. 192 pages.

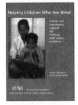

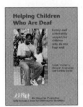

Helping Children Who Are Deaf, by Darlena David, Devorah Greenstein and Sandy Niemann, aids parents, teachers, and other caregivers in helping deaf children learn basic communication skills and a full language. It also gives simple methods to assess hearing loss and develop listening skills, explores how communities working together can help deaf children, and offers ways parents and caregivers can support each other. 250 pages.

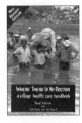

Where There Is No Doctor, by David Werner with Carol Thuman and Jane Maxwell, is perhaps the most widely used health care manual in the world. The book provides vital, easily understood information on how to diagnose, treat and prevent common diseases. Special importance is placed on ways to prevent health problems, including cleanliness, a healthy diet and vaccinations. The authors also emphasize the active role villagers must take in their own health care. 512 pages.

Where There Is No Dentist, by Murray Dickson, shows people how to care for their own teeth and gums, and how to prevent tooth and gum problems. Emphasis is placed on sharing this knowledge in the home, community, and school. The author also gives detailed and well-illustrated information on using dental equipment, placing fillings, taking out teeth, and more, and suggests ways to teach dental hygiene and nutrition. A new chapter includes material on HIV/AIDS and oral health. 208 pages.

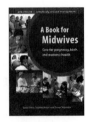

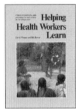

Helping Health Workers Learn, by David Werner and Bill Bower, is an indispensable resource for anyone involved in teaching about health. This heavily illustrated book shows how to make health education fun and effective. Includes activities for mothers and children; pointers for using theater, flannel-boards, and other techniques; and many ideas for producing low-cost teaching aids. Emphasizing a people-centered approach to health care, it presents strategies for effective community involvement through participatory education. 640 pages.

A Book for Midwives, by Susan Klein, Suellen Miller, and Fiona Thomson. This completely revised edition is for midwives, community health workers, and anyone concerned about the health of women and babies in pregnancy, birth and beyond. An invaluable tool for training as well as a practical reference, it covers helping pregnant women stay healthy, care during and after birth, handling obstetric complications, breastfeeding, and includes expanded information for women's reproductive health care. 544 pages.

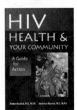

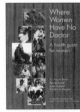

Where Women Have No Doctor, by A. August Burns, Ronnie Lovich, Jane Maxwell, and Katherine Shapiro, combines self-help medical information with an understanding of the ways poverty, discrimination, and cultural beliefs limit women's health and access to care. Clearly written and with over 1000 drawings, this book is an essential resource for any woman who wants to improve her health, and for health workers who want more information about the problems that affect only women, or that affect women differently from men. 584 pages.

HIV, Health, and Your Community, by Reuben Granich and Jonathan Mermin, is an essential resource for community health workers and others confronting the growing HIV/AIDS epidemic. This clearly written guide emphasizes prevention and also covers virus biology, epidemiology, and ideas for designing HIV prevention and treatment programs. Contains an appendix of common health problems and treatments for people with HIV/AIDS, along with other practical tools for health workers. Now updated to include antiretroviral treatments and new advances in therapy. 245 pages.

All titles are available from Hesperian in both English and Spanish. For information regarding other language editions, prices and ordering information, or a description of Hesperian's work, please visit our website or write to us.

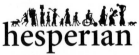

hesperian

Publishing for community health and empowerment

the Hesperian Foundation
1919 Addison St., #304
Berkeley, California 94704 USA
tel: (510) 845-4507, fax: (510) 845-0539
email: bookorders@hesperian.org
Visit our website: www.hesperian.org

LIST OF SPECIAL OR DIFFICULT WORDS

This is a list in alphabetical order of words used in this book that you may not understand. The first time one of these words is used in the book, or in a chapter, it is written in *italics* so that you know you can look it up here, where we explain each word. Sometimes, we also refer you to a page of the book that explains the word more completely. If this list does not have a word you want explained, look in the INDEX. The word may be explained on a page that the INDEX refers you to. For example, 'arthrogryposis' is explained on p. 122.

A

Action nerves (motor nerves) Nerves that carry messages from the brain to parts of the body, telling muscles to move.

Acute Sudden and short-lived. An acute illness is one that starts suddenly and lasts a short time. It is the opposite of 'chronic'.

Adaptation Change or changes to better fit a specific child or local area. A seat may be adapted by the addition of straps and pads to better support the body.

Antibiotic A medicine that fights infections caused by bacteria. Penicillin and tetracycline are antiobiotics. For discussion of antibiotics and their use, see *Where There Is No Doctor*, p. 55-58.

Arthritis Pain and inflammation in one or several joints of the body such as the knees, elbows, or hips.

Ataxia Difficulty with balance and with coordination. (See p. 90.)

Atrophy A progressive wasting or weakening of the muscles that comes from a problem in the nerves. (Compare with 'dystrophy'.)

B

Behavior A person's way of doing things; pattern of actions. The way a child acts, or relates to others. (See Chapter 40.)

Bladder A muscular bag in the belly in which urine collects before it leaves the body.

Bowel The part of the gut or intestine where solid waste (stool, shit) collects before it leaves the body.

Bowel movement Emptying of the bowel; shitting.

Butt Buttocks; backside; rear end; the part of the body on which a person sits.

C

Caliper British word for "brace." An aid which gives support to a weak or injured leg. (See Chapter 58.)

Caster A wheel that is mounted so that it turns from side to side to go around corners. The small wheels of a wheelchair are usually made with casters.

Chronic Long-term or frequently returning. A chronic disease is one that lasts a long time. Compare with 'acute'.

Circulation The flow of blood through the blood vessels (veins and arteries). Good circulation is necessary for healthy body parts.

Clog A wooden sandal or shoe, often used with a brace.

Contracture Reduced range of motion in a joint, often due to muscle shortening. (See Chapter 8.)

Cord A simple name for 'tendon', a part of the body that connects muscle to bone. For example, the 'heel cord' or 'Achilles Tendon' joins the calf muscle to the heel. (*Note:* The 'spinal cord' is not a tendon. It is made of nerves. See p. 35.)

D

Diaper (nappy) A cloth to soak up urine, usually worn by a child.

Diplegia Paraplegia in which the upper part of the body is also slightly affected. (See p. 90.)

Disability A long-lasting or permanent defect or problem that in some way makes it more difficult for a person to do certain things than for a 'non-disabled' person. A disability can be:

mild: Causes some inconvenience but the person can learn to do everything he or she needs to.

moderate: Person needs to make adaptations to be independent in self-care and other activities.

severe: Person will always need help for some or all self-care and other activities.

Dislocation Damage to a joint; the bone ends have slipped out of their normal position. Dislocation can be from birth, from an accident, or from weakness and 'muscle imbalance'.

Dystrophy A progressive muscle weakness that comes from a problem in the muscles themselves. Compare with 'atrophy'.

E

Evaluation Observations and study to find out how well something is working and where the problems are.

F

Functional Useful; serving some purpose for day-to-day life. Exercise or therapy is functional when it is done as part of some useful activity.

Flacid Lacking firmness; soft.

Functional Useful; serving some purpose for day-to-day life. Exercise or therapy is functional when it is done as part of some useful activity.

G

Gene A hereditary unit; something that controls or acts in the passing down of features from parent to child.

H

Hemiplegia Paralysis or loss of movement in the muscles of the arm and leg on one side of the body only.

Hereditary Familial; a feature that passses from parent to child when the baby is first made (conceived). If a disease is hereditary, there is a factor or characteristic in the father and/or mother which is passed on to their children, and then to their children's children. Inherited.

Hygiene Actions or practices of personal cleanliness that protect health.

I

Infantile Of infants (babies) or young children.

Infection A sickness caused by germs (bacteria, virus, worms, or other small living things). Some infections affect part of the body only, others affect all of it.

Inherited Familial; a feature that passes from parent to child when the baby is first made (conceived). If a disease is inherited, there is a factor or characteristic in the father and/or mother which is passed on to their children, and then to their children's children. Inherited.

J

Joint capsule The tough covering around a joint.

Juvenile Of children.

L

Ligament Tough strips or bands inside the body that hold joints and bones together. Ligaments join bones with other bones, while tendons or cords' join bones with muscles.

Limb An arm or leg.

M

Mental Having to do with the mind or intelligence. A child who is mentally handicapped or retarded does not learn as quickly as other children.

Multiple disability Several disabilities, often both physical and mental, in the same child. (See page 283.)

Muscles Meaty parts of the body that pull or 'contract' to make the body and limbs move.

N

Nappy (diaper) A cloth to soak up urine, worn by a child who does not have bladder control.

Nerve A thin line along which messages travel in the body. Nerves are the 'messengers' of the body. Some nerves let us feel things, and tell us when something hurts. Other nerves let us move parts of the body when we want to. (See p. 35.)

O

Occupational Having to do with work or function. An occupational therapist is a person who helps figure out how a disabled person can do things better.

Orthopedic Aids, procedures, or surgery to help correct a physical deformity or disability.

Orthotist A brace maker.

P

Paralysis Muscle weakness; decrease or loss of ability to move part or all of the body.

Paraplegia Paralysis or loss of movement in the muscles of both legs (sometimes with slight involvement elsewhere) caused by disease or injury to the spinal cord.

Physical Having to do with the body and how it works, as distinct from 'mental', which has to do with the mind.

Physical therapist, physiotherapist A person who designs and teaches exercises and activities for physically disabled persons.

Positioning Helping a person's body stay in healthy or helpful positions—through special seating, padding, supports, or in other ways.

Procedure Some kind of medical, surgical, or technical action. For example, casting, strapping, and surgery are 3 procedures for correcting a club foot.

Progressive A progressive illness or disability is one that steadily gets worse and worse. For example, muscular dystrophy.

Prosthesis An artificial limb or other part of the body—for example, a wooden leg. 'Prosthetics' is the art of making prostheses.

Q

Quadriplegia (tetraplegia) Paralysis or loss of movement in the muscles of both arms and legs caused by disease or injury to the spinal cord, in the neck.

R

Rehabilitation The art of helping a person learn to live as best she can and do as much as possible for herself, given her limitations or disability.

Retarded Slow to develop. A mentally retarded child does not learn as quickly or remember as well as other children.

S

Sensory nerves Nerves that bring messages from parts of the body to the brain about what the body sees, hears, smells, and feels.

Social Having to do with the actions, values, decisions, and relationships within groups of people.

Spasticity Uncontrolled tightening or pulling of muscles that make it difficult for a person to control her movements. A muscle or a child with spasticity is said to be 'spastic'. Spasticity often occurs with brain damage, cerebral palsy, and spinal cord injury.

Spinal Having to do with the spine or backbone.

Spinal cord The main 'trunk line' of nerves running down the backbone. It provides communication (for movement and feeling) between the brain and all parts of the body. (See p. 175.)

Spine Backbone; spinal column; the chain of bones, called vertebrae, that runs down the back.

Stimulation Sounds, sights, activities, toys, smells, touch, and anything else that makes a child take interest in things and develop the use of his body and senses. 'Early stimulation' refers to activities that help a baby develop his first responses and skills. (See p. 301.)

Stool Shit; body waste that is usually solid; also known as bowel movement or feces.

T

Tendon A strong rope-like structure in the body that connects muscles to bones. In this book we mostly call tendons 'cords'.

Tetraplegia (see quadriplegia).

Therapy Treatment; planned exercise and activity for a person's rehabilitation. See 'physical therapy' and 'occupational therapy'.

Toxic Poisonous.

Transfer Moving from (or to) a wheelchair to a bed, chair, cot, car seat, toilet, or floor.

Trunk The body, not including the head, neck, arms, and legs.

U

Urine Liquid body waste, also known as "pee," or "piss."

V

Vaccination Immunization; to give certain medicines (vaccines) by injection or mouth to protect against infectious diseases such as polio and measles.

Velcro A strong, fuzzy plastic tape that sticks to itself. (The surface of one piece of the tape has little plastic hooks that catch onto the curly hairs on the other piece of the tape.) Useful to use instead of buttons, buckles, or laces on clothes, braces and shoes—especially for children with poor hand control. (See p. 335.)

Virus Germs smaller than bacteria, that cause some infectious (easily spread) diseases. Most viruses are not killed by antibiotics.

W

Weight-bearing Supporting the weight of the body on a particular joint or limb. For example, weight-bearing on the knee is possible if the strength of the thigh muscle is good, but not if it is poor.

INDEX